# CARDIAC ANESTHESIA *for* INFANTS *and* CHILDREN

*Jay Kambam,* M.D., F.A.C.A.

Professor and Vice-Chairman,
Director of Cardiothoracic Anesthesia,
Department of Anesthesiology,
Vanderbilt University Hospital,
Nashville, Tennessee

*with* 205 *illustrations*

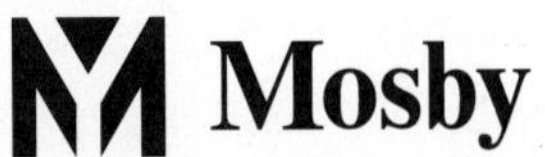

St. Louis Baltimore Boston Chicago London Madrid Philadelphia Sydney Toronto

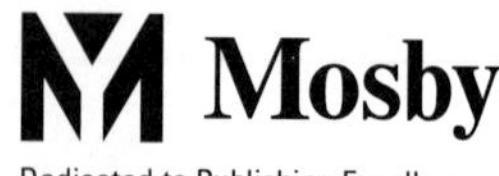

Dedicated to Publishing Excellence

*Executive Editor:* Susan M. Gay
*Developmental Editor:* Sandra E. Clark
*Project Manager:* Peggy Fagen
*Cover Design:* Elizabeth Rohne Rudder
*Cover Illustration:* Don O'Connor
*Editing and Production:* Graphic World Publishing Services
*Manufacturing Supervisor:* John Babrick



Printed in the United States of America
Composition by Graphic World, Inc.
Printing/binding by Maple-Vail Book Mfg. Group

Mosby–Year Book, Inc.
11830 Westline Industrial Drive
St. Louis, MO 63146

**Library of Congress Cataloging in Publication Data**

Kambam, Jay.
Cardiac anesthesia for infants and children / Jay Kambam.
p. cm.
Includes bibliographical references and index.
ISBN 0-8016-7289-9
1. Congenital heart disease in children—Surgery. 2. Anesthesia in cardiology. 3. Pediatric anesthesia. I. Title.
[DNLM: 1. Heart Surgery—in infancy & childhood. 2. Anesthesia——in infancy & childhood. WO 440 K15c 1993]
RD87.3.H43K35 1993
617.4'12'0083—dc20
DNLM/DLC
for Library of Congress 93-41430
CIP

95 96 97 98 GW/MY 9 8 7 6 5 4 3 2 1

# Contributors

*Kumar G. Belani,* M.B.B.S., M.S.
Associate Professor,
Director of Pediatric Anesthesia and Anesthesia for Liver Transplantation,
Department of Anesthesiology,
University of Minnesota,
Minneapolis, Minnesota;
Associate Clinical Professor,
Department of Anesthesiology,
University of California,
San Francisco, California

*Scott H. Buck,* M.D.
Assistant Professor of Pediatrics,
Division of Pediatric Cardiology,
University of Wisconsin Medical School,
University of Wisconsin Children's Hospital,
Madison, Wisconsin

*Jayant K. Deshpande,* M.D.
Associate Professor of Pediatrics and Anesthesiology,
Director, Division of Pediatric Critical Care and Anesthesia,
Vanderbilt University School of Medicine,
Nashville, Tennessee

*Frank A. Fish,* M.D.
Assistant Professor of Pediatrics and Medicine,
Vanderbilt University School of Medicine,
Nashville, Tennessee

*William H. Frist,* M.D.
Associate Professor of Surgery,
Surgical Director, The Vanderbilt Transplant Center,
Vanderbilt University Medical Center,
Nashville, Tennessee

*Thomas P. Graham,* M.D.
Professor of Pediatrics,
Director of Pediatric Cardiology,
Vanderbilt Medical Center,
Nashville, Tennessee

*Steven J. Hoff,* M.D.
Resident,
Department of Cardiac and Thoracic Surgery,
Vanderbilt University School of Medicine,
Nashville, Tennessee

*James A. Johns,* M.D.
Assistant Professor of Pediatrics,
Division of Pediatric Cardiology,
Vanderbilt University School of Medicine,
Nashville, Tennessee

*Jay Kambam,* M.D., F.A.C.A.
Professor and Vice-Chairman,
Director of Cardiothoracic Anesthesia,
Department of Anesthesiology,
Vanderbilt University Hospital,
Nashville, Tennessee

*Wesley W. Kinney,* M.D.
Clinical Assistant Professor of Anesthesiology,
Vanderbilt University Hospital,
Nashville, Tennessee

*Sandra Lowe,* M.D.
Assistant Professor of Pediatric Anesthesia,
Department of Anesthesiology,
Vanderbilt University,
Nashville, Tennessee

*Walter H. Merrill,* M.D.
Professor of Surgery,
Department of Cardiac and Thoracic Surgery,
Vanderbilt University School of Medicine,
Nashville, Tennessee

*James Phythyon,* M.D.
Associate Clinical Professor,
Department of Anesthesiology,
Vanderbilt University School of Medicine,
Nashville, Tennessee

*P. Syamasundar Rao,* M.D.

Professor of Pediatrics,
Head, Division of Pediatric Cardiology,
University of Wisconsin Medical School,
University of Wisconsin Children's Hospital,
Madison, Wisconsin

*James R. Stewart,* M.D.

Assistant Professor of Surgery,
Department of Cardiac and Thoracic Surgery,
Vanderbilt University School of Medicine,
Nashville, Tennessee

*Volker Striepe,* M.B.B.C.h., D.A., F.F.A. (S.A.)

Assistant Professor of Anesthesiology,
Vanderbilt University Medical Center,
Assistant Chief of Anesthesia,
VA Medical Center,
Nashville, Tennessee

*Mike Sweeney,* M.D.

Assistant Professor of Anesthesiology and Pediatrics,
Associate Medical Director of Pediatric Critical Care,
University of Minnesota School of Medicine,
Minneapolis, Minnesota

*Joseph D. Tobias,* M.D.

Associate Professor of Anesthesiology and Pediatrics,
Assistant Director, Division of Pediatric Critical Care and Anesthesia,
Vanderbilt University School of Medicine,
Nashville, Tennessee

*Michael S. Vinas,* B.A., R.R.T., C.C.P.

Perfusion Program Director,
Cardiovascular Perfusion Technology,
Programs in Allied Health,
Vanderbilt University Medical Center,
Nashville, Tennessee

*Allen D. Wilson,* M.D.

Professor of Pediatrics,
Division of Pediatric Cardiology,
University of Wisconsin Medical School,
University of Wisconsin Children's Hospital,
Madison, Wisconsin

*Margaret Wood,* M.D.

Professor of Anesthesiology,
Department of Anesthesiology,
Vanderbilt University School of Medicine,
Nashville, Tennessee

*Dedicated to my wife, Veni, and sons, Shravan and Praveen.*

# Foreword

The surgical management of patients with congenital cardiac malformations had its infancy in the 1940s with the development of operative techniques to manage patent ductus arteriosus, coarctation of the aorta, and the creation of systemic pulmonary arterial shunts. From that time there has been rapid development of the specialty, particularly following the advent of successful extracorporeal circulation and the understanding of the benefits derived from hypothermic diminution in oxygen requirement during periods of circulatory arrest.

It has been my good fortune to be involved in the surgical management of patients with congenital cardiac malformation since the 1950s. The advances that have been made in the management of these desperately ill infants and children has been phenomenal, with tremendous improvement in survival figures for even the most complex intracardiac malformations. When one looks back at the evolution in surgical procedures and the management of patients in the perioperative period, it is difficult to single out specific changes that were instrumental in the resultant improvement in survival. Obviously important among those improvements were the better understanding of the pathologic anatomy of the various malformations and the ability to perform precise reparative procedures even in the smallest neonate. In addition to the obvious operative advances, the understanding and the ability to measure arterial blood gases, cardiac output, and electrolyte changes rapidly had a significant role in the perioperative management of these patients.

Commensurate with the development of children's cardiac surgery as a specialty has been the development of pediatric cardiac anesthesiology. The pediatric cardiac anesthesiologist's understanding of the pathophysiologic changes in infants with congenital cardiac malformations has been extremely important. The role of ventilation in the management of oxygen and $CO_2$ concentrations with respect to pulmonary vascular resistance is but one example. The drugs that are now available for the conduct of anesthesia and the management of patients in the postoperative period has had enormous impact on the survival of infants with complex cardiac malformations.

This textbook was written with the idea that it would be useful to students and house officers in anesthesiology. It was thought that it would provide a broad picture of the population of patients with congenital cardiac disease and the pathophysiologic changes related to the various specific abnormalities. As the book has evolved, it has become directed to a broader audience. The authors have managed to address each of the major groups of malformations with respect to the changes in pulmonary blood flow, changes in pulmonary vascular resistance, the degree or absence of cyanosis, and the degree or absence of congestive cardiac failure that may be present. In each chapter the authors have outlined the embryology, the pathologic anatomy and the changes in physiology that will have direct impact on the administration of anesthetic agents. As a result, this book will be of considerable interest to surgeons and surgical students as they approach patients with congenital heart disease.

I am confident that this book will be well received by pediatricians, surgeons, and anesthesiologists, and I am honored to be asked to write this foreword.

*Harvey W. Bender, Jr.,* M.D.
Professor of Surgery
Chairman, Thoracic and Cardiac Surgery
Vanderbilt University Medical Center
Nashville, Tennessee

# Foreword

***—Ah, what would the world be to us***
***If the children were no more?***
***We should dread the desert behind us***
***Worse than the dark before.—***
**H.W. Longfellow: *"Children"***

It has been said that as many as 1% of all infants are born with some degree of congenital heart anomaly, and that, uncorrected, these would result in approximately 40% mortality before the fifth year of life.[6] Yet surgical correction of these anomalies was not attempted until the 1939 report by Gross and Hubbard of the surgical ligation of a patent ductus arteriosus,[5] and even palliative surgery awaited the 1945 description by Blalock and Taussig of their shunting procedure.[3]

The application to children of extracorporeal techniques approximately similar to current practice was not reported in a significant series until 1955 by Kirklin et al.[9] However, by 1966 surgical mortality was still as great as 30% for relatively conservative repairs of major cardiac anomalies even at leading centers.[15] The refinement process continued from approximately 1972 to the present until pediatric cardiac surgery reached a point where such ominous lesions as transposition of the great vessels have now been repaired in significant numbers of patients with a mortality rate less than 6%.[1]

Today techniques as formidable as intentional deep hypothermic cardiac arrest have become so routine in children as to allow a series of nearly 160 cases to be collected within 26 months in the editor's hospital.[12]

Although they have been the leaders and the risk takers in achieving this progress, cardiac surgeons have been enthusiastic in enrolling help from a field of specialists ranging from physicians to engineers. Thus the flowering of congenital cardiac surgery has been a remarkable team effort. Anesthesiologists have contributed much to this progress, not only in the operating room, but also by their participation in the development of postoperative mechanical ventilation[8] and other critical care support methods.[4] However, specific advances in diagnosis such as enhanced radiographic and radionuclide procedures[13] and expanded uses of echocardiography[10]; new pharmacology for preoperative, intraoperative, and postoperative medications such as prostaglandin[11] and indomethacin infusions[7]; the appearance of a variety of useful new catecholamines, positive inotropes, and receptor blockers and agonists; and a variety of advances in laboratory medicine, materials, engineering, extracorporeal life support disciplines[14], and many other sources, have each made critical contributions.

More prominently than in many other areas of medicine, many of these advances have been made by the astute observations and expressed opinions of busy experienced clinicians in all of these fields, because of the relatively small numbers of patients and the intrinsic difficulty of controlled systematic research concerning alternative therapies. Perhaps fewer than 15,000 total surgical invasions for congenital heart problems requiring extracorporeal life support are required annually in the United States even now, and certainly far fewer were attempted per annum in the recent past.[16] Furthermore, objective research in the presence of a seriously ill child is frequently not technically difficult, but often is not ethically supportable.

Because of these limitations, the format chosen by the editor, Professor J.R. Kambam, is particularly appropriate and effective in delineating the problems of anesthesia in cardiac surgical patients. He brings to the task extensive practical personal experience in anesthesia for the surgery of congenital heart lesions gained in one of the busiest and most successful centers. In addition, he has chosen co-authors who, although many are internationally recognized authorities in their own field, are also busy clinicians, and most of whom are members of the same team in the same center. Thus the descriptions of the basic background, as well as the narration of diagnosis, therapy, and surgical procedures, are all formulated and influenced by the experience of a team of busy and practical clinician academics who have familiarity with the literature and with the actual practices of their co-authors in the care of these patients.

Professor Kambam has successfully coordinated the literary efforts of this authoritative group of friends into an enjoyable and concise, yet thorough, treatise. Enormous credit should also be acknowledged to the surgeon who has coordinated the efforts of this team through the past two decades, whose surgical achievements are enviable, and who has immeasurably influenced the philosophies expressed in this book, Professor H.W. Bender.[2] This book will be valuable not only to the anesthesiologist, but to surgeons, specialists, generalists, and nursing professionals who wish to become familiar with the many ways in which the anesthesiologist's involvement impacts the total care of patients with congenital heart defects. The editor, his co-authors, and colleagues are to be congratulated!

*Bradley E. Smith, M.D.*
Professor of Anesthesiology
Vanderbilt University Medical Center
Nashville, Tennessee

## REFERENCES

1. Bender HW Jr, Stewart JR, Merrill WH: Ten years' experience with the senning operation for transposition of the great arteries: physiological results and late follow-up, *Ann Thorac Surg* 47:218, 1989.
2. Bender HW Jr: Preparation, trust, and responsibility, *Ann Thorac Surg* 51:351, 1991.
3. Blalock A, Taussig HB: The surgical treatment of malformations of the heart in which there is pulmonary stenosis or pulmonary atresia, *JAMA* 112:189, 1945.
4. Gregory GA, Edmunds LH, Kellerman JA et al: Continuous positive pressure and pulmonary and circulatory function after cardiac surgery in infants less than three months of age, *Anesthesiology* 43:426, 1975.
5. Gross RE, Hubbard JP: Surgical ligation of a patent ductus arteriosus: report of first successful case, *JAMA* 112:729, 1939.
6. Hamilton DI: The surgery of congenital heart defects. In Lester J, Irving IM, editors: *Neonatal surgery,* London, 1990, Butterworths.
7. Heymann MA, Rudolph AM, Silverman NH: Closure of the ductus arteriosus in premature infants by inhibition of prostaglandin synthesis, *N Eng J Med* 295:530, 1976.
8. Kirby RR, Robinson EJ, Shultz J et al: A new pediatric volume ventilator, *Anesth Analg* 50:533, 1971.
9. Kirklin JW et al: Intracardiac surgery with the aid of a mechanical pump-oxygenator system (Gibbon type): report of eight cases, *Mayo Clin Proc* 30:201, 1955.
10. Muhiudeen IA, Roberson DA, Silverman NH et al: Intraoperative echocardiography for evaluation of congenital heart defects in infants and children, *Anesthesiology* 76:165, 1992.
11. Olley PM, Coceani F, Bodach E: E type prostaglandins: a new emergency therapy for certain cyanotic heart malformations, *Circulation* 53:728, 1976.
12. Phythyon JP: Deep hypothermia and circulatory arrest. In Kambam J, editor: *Cardiac anesthesia for infants and children,* St Louis, 1994, Mosby.
13. Rao PS, Wilson AD, Sideris EB: Transcatheter closure of patent ductus arteriosus with "buttoned" device: first successful clinical application in a child, *Am Heart J* 121:1799, 1991.
14. Roberts CP, McCarthy P, Wildman D et al: Left ventricular assist with the biomedicus pump on a 4-month-old infant with anomalous left coronary artery, *J Ext Corp Tech* 21:73, 1989.
15. Strong MJ, Keats AS, Cooley DA: Anesthesia for cardiovascular surgery in infancy, *Anesthesiology* 27:257, 1966.
16. Vinas MS: Extracorporeal circulation. In Kambam J, editor: *Cardiac anesthesia for infants and children,* St Louis, 1994, Mosby.

# Preface

Anesthesia for surgery involving congenital heart defects has experienced tremendous breakthroughs over the past 15 years. The creation of *Cardiac Anesthesia for Infants and Children* has been based on several personal communications with friends in the field of anesthesiology, particularly cardiac anesthesiology. The purpose of this book is to provide a single source of the information necessary for optimal perioperative care of an infant or a child with congenital heart disease. As a cardiac anesthesiologist for more than 15 years, I have long felt the need for such a book.

*Cardiac Anesthesia for Infants and Children* was written by groups of pediatric cardiologists, cardiac surgeons, and pediatric anesthesiologists. It provides basic knowledge of the subject, as well as guidelines for perioperative management of a child with congenital heart disease undergoing cardiac or noncardiac surgery. The latest advances in pediatric cardiac surgery and anesthesia are described from several vital perspectives, including embryology, pathologic anatomy and physiology, medical and surgical management, and anesthesia management. Figures and drawings were designed for easy understanding of pathologic anatomy and physiology of complex congenital heart lesions.

Most chapters involving particular malformations were written by groups of pediatric cardiologists, surgeons, and anesthesiologists. Thus each chapter provides a balanced analysis of its subject, and each is presented in a coherent manner by experts familiar with the latest research. These chapters were deliberately designed to be read separately rather than in a generalized fashion (for example, L-to-R shunt lesions). Though this book was primarily written for anesthesiologists at all levels, I believe pediatricians and pediatric surgeons will also find it very useful.

We have written this book in a period of one year, and I wish to thank all of the contributors who have worked so hard to finish their chapters in such a short time. I also would like to thank Kathleen Finn and Steven Wasserman for their editorial advice, Paul Gross for the outstanding drawings he produced for this book, Susan Britt for her secretarial assistance, and all the publishers and their authors who gave us permission to reproduce figures and tables. A special thank you goes to Susan Gay and Sandy Clark of Mosby–Year Book publishers for their help and support in creating this book.

Finally, I must express my deep appreciation to my wife, Veni, for her patience and support during the hectic period of preparation of the book.

*Jay Kambam*

# Contents

*PART ONE*
**General Principles**

*PART TWO*
## Particular Malformations
### SECTION A. LEFT-TO-RIGHT SHUNTS



### SECTION B. RIGHT-TO-LEFT SHUNTS



### SECTION C. OBSTRUCTIVE LESIONS

## SECTION D. MISCELLANEOUS DEFORMITIES

# CARDIAC ANESTHESIA

## *for* INFANTS *and* CHILDREN

# *PART ONE*

# General Principles

# 1 Embryology

*Allen D. Wilson and P. Syamasundar Rao*



Knowledge of the steps in development of the heart and great vessels is useful for understanding and anticipating many of the variations and combinations of congenital heart defects. Knowledge of great artery and vein anomalies is especially important for the pediatric cardiac anesthesiologist who places various intravascular lines for perioperative monitoring. In addition, development of fetal echocardiography has recently allowed prenatal diagnosis of many congenital heart defects and raised the possibility of fetal cardiac surgery, especially for defects with known poor prognosis.

The goals of this chapter are to provide an overview of cardiac and vascular development, emphasizing points in cardiogenesis where defects may occur, defects for which mechanisms are known or suspected, and abnormalities of development not covered elsewhere in this book.

## EARLY DEVELOPMENT OF THE CARDIOVASCULAR SYSTEM

During the first 2 weeks of development, when the embryo has only two cell layers, there is no cardiovascular system.[10,11] Shortly after development of the splanchnic mesoderm, however, cells from this layer rapidly proliferate into angiogenic cell clusters, which then form luminae connected in the form of capillary plexi.[5,6] These plexi enlarge, grow, and remodel into a paired, connected system of larger longitudinal vessels. Two medial dorsal aortae travel down the back of the embryo, and they are connected anteriorly to the first aortic arch, which bends around to the paired primordial heart tubes in the ventral aspect of the embryo.[2] The paired heart tubes grow together and fuse into a straight heart tube by approximately 20 days of age, and shortly thereafter the heart begins to beat.[10] The straight heart tube develops a series of dilations along its length (Fig. 1–1). The most caudal dilation is the sinus venosus, which receives the two sinus horns, each of which receives a vitelline, umbilical, and cardinal vein. The other four dilations in order, moving forward along the primary heart tube, are the primitive atrium, primitive ventricle, bulbus cordis, and truncus arteriosus.

### Looping of the heart tube

Until the embryo is 3 weeks of age (length 2.2 mm), the heart is a straight tube inside the pericardial cavity. The bulboventricular portion of the heart tube grows more rapidly than the pericardial cavity. During the process of growth, the cephalic portion of the straight tube bends in a ventral and caudal direction and slightly to the right (D-loop). The cardiac tube folds up with the atria slightly to the left with the primitive ventricle and the bulbus cordis anteriorly and to the right.[5] The mechanism for this is probably a combination of differential tissue pressure of matrix around the cardiac tube and differential cell growth in the myocardial mantle.[3,4] The bulbus cordis becomes the morphologic right ventricle. If the heart tube loops to the left (L-loop), then the morphologic right ventricle is on the left side and ventricular inversion results and is associated with L-transposition, or corrected transposition.

Next, both the atria and ventricles rapidly expand. The proximal part of the bulbus cordis grows

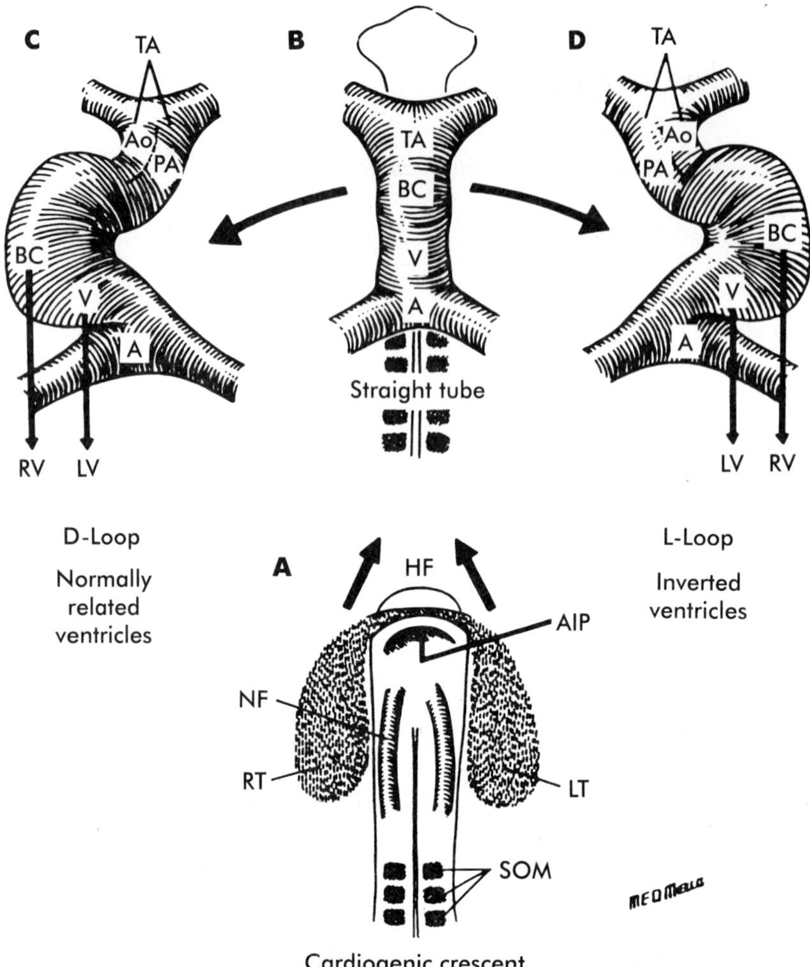


**Figure 1–1** Cardiac loop formation. **A,** Cardiogenic crescent of precardiac mesoderm. **B,** Straight heart tube or preloop stage. **C,** D-loop, with solitus (noninverted) ventricles. **D,** L-loop with inverted (mirror-image) ventricles. *A,* atrium; *AIP,* anterior intestinal portal; *Ao,* aorta; *BC,* bulbus cordis; *HF,* head fold; *LT,* left; *LV,* morphologically left ventricle; *NF,* neural fold; *PA,* (main) pulmonary artery; *RT,* right; *RV,* morphologically right ventricle; *SOM,* somites; *TA,* truncus arteriosus. (From Van Praagh R, Weinberg PM, Matsuoka R et al: Malpositions of the heart. In Adams FH, Emmanouilides GC, editors: *Heart disease in infants, children and adolescents,* ed 3, Baltimore, 1983, Williams & Wilkins.)

caudally to become the morphologic right ventricle, and the primitive proximal ventricle grows caudally to become the morphologic left ventricle.

Besides the looping of the tube, at this point there is an important shift of the bulbus cordis to the center of the heart tube on top of the atria, which allows the right side of the atrium to establish communication with the bulbus cordis. If this does not occur or if the bend goes too far, then later both atrioventricular valves enter the same ventricle and the condition of single (double-inlet) ventricle can occur and be associated with varying outflow anatomy.[1]

### Atrial septation

Atrial septum formation begins in the fourth week of life, concurrently with separation of right and left sides of the atrioventricular canal by the anterior and posterior endocardial cushions (Fig. 1–2).[10] The septum primum grows down from the superior wall of the primitive atrium to meet fusing cushion tissue, and this closes the ostium primum. While the ostium primum is being obliterated, some resorption of tissue at the mid and upper portion of the septum primum takes place, resulting in ostium secundum. Presence of a defect in the atrial septum is vital for the fetus. A second atrial

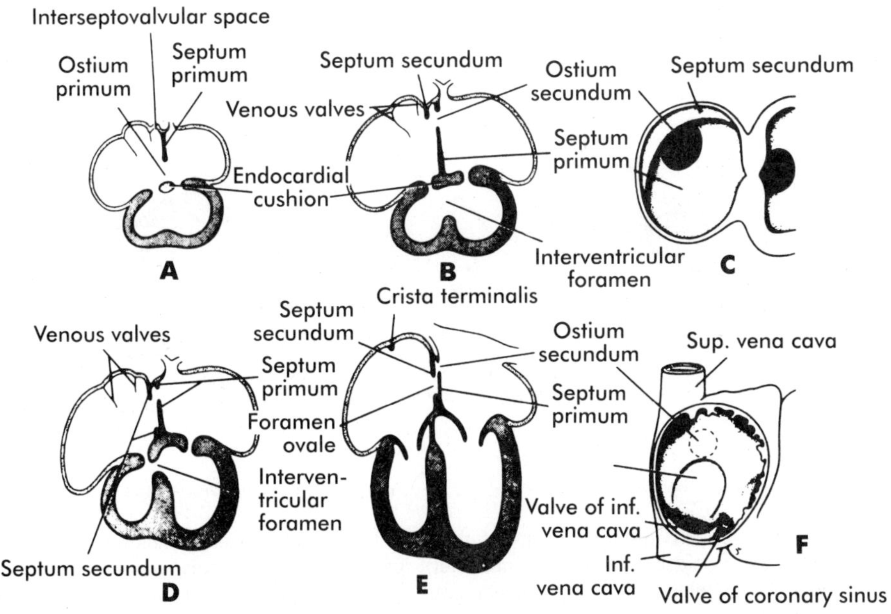


**Figure 1–2** Schematic representation of the atrial septa at successive stages of development. **A,** At 6 mm (approximately 30 days). **B,** 9 mm (approximately 33 days). **C,** Same stage as in *B*, but seen from the right. **D,** 14 mm (approximately 37 days). **E,** Newborn. **F,** View of the atrial septum seen from the right, same stage as in *E*. Note the interseptovalvular space to the right and the pulmonary vein to the left of the septum primum in *A*. (From Clark EB, Van Mierop LHS: Development of the cardiovascular system. In Adams FH, Emmanouilides GC, Riemenschneider TA, editors: *Moss' Heart disease in infants, children and adolescents,* ed 4, Baltimore, 1989, Williams & Wilkins.)

septum forms by an infolding flap of the superior wall of the atrium, the septum secundum.[5] This septum does not grow all the way down to separate the two atria completely but partially covers the ostium secundum, leaving an opening between it and the flap of the septum primum; this allows shunting of blood from the right atrium to the left atrium, vital for adequate development of the left heart chambers and aorta in the fetus.

If the septum primum cannot fuse with the endocardial cushions, then an ostium primum atrial defect occurs. If the midportion of the atrial septum remains patent, a secundum atrial septal defect occurs. A defect in the superior (anterior or posterior) atrial septum, called a sinus venosus atrial defect, is often associated with partial anomalous pulmonary venous return of the right pulmonary veins to the right superior vena cava–right atrial junction.

### Ventricular and great artery septation

Septation of the ventricles and great arteries occurs between days 27 and 37,[5] and while this very complicated process goes on rapidly, the developing heart must continue to support the embryo's circulatory requirements. Clinically, four regions of the ventricular septum during development correspond to the four different parts of the ventricular septum where defects may occur: inlet (posterior), muscular (trabecular), conotruncal (infundibular), and membranous septum (Fig. 1–3).[1]

The inlet septum forms when fusion of the anterior and posterior endocardial cushions divides the atrioventricular canal into left- and right-sided rings (Fig. 1–4). Abnormal development at this stage can lead to posterior (or inlet) ventricular septal defect or an inlet ventricular defect as part of a common atrioventricular canal defect (as is common in Down syndrome). Lesser abnormality in the septal cushion development may lead to anterior medial leaflet or septal tricuspid leaflet abnormalities, such as a cleft mitral valve. It is also important at this stage of septation that tissue separating the right side of the atrioventricular canal from the bulbus cordis regress so that the newly formed right atrioventricular ring empties into the right ventricle.

The largest part of the ventricular septum is the muscular septum, and this is formed as a by-product of the rapid growth of the ventricles and fusion of their medial common walls during this rapid growth.[5] During this stage the ventricles become trabeculated, possibly as a mechanism to improve blood flow to the heart muscle before the coronary circulation is completely established or possibly to

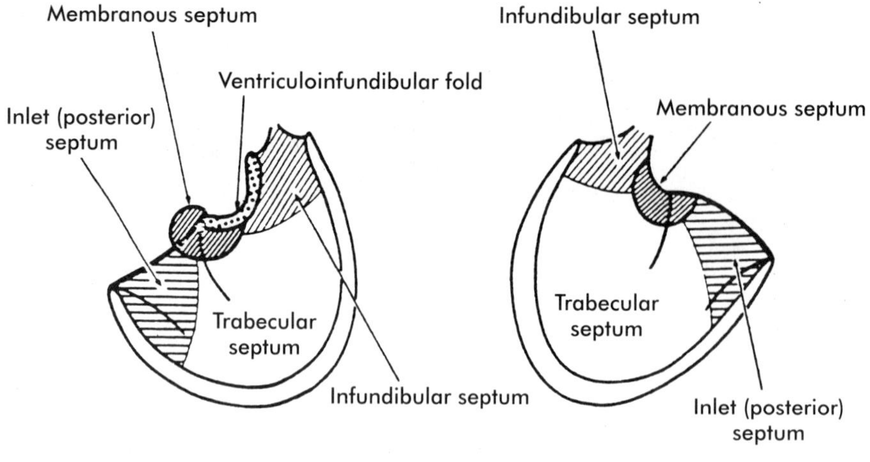


**Figure 1–3** Diagram of the components of the ventricular septum (in the definitive heart the margins between muscular segments are indistinct). There are three muscular portions: inlet, trabecular, and infundibular. The fibrous membranous portion completes the septum. Note the ventriculoinfundibular fold in the right ventricle between the atrioventricular and arterial valves. (From Anderson RH: Another look at cardiac embryology, *Progress in Cardiology,* Philadelphia, 1978, Lea & Febiger.)

help distribute stresses of ventricular wall contraction. Defects in the muscular septum are thought most likely to be due to areas of cell death[4] or excessive resorption. Muscular defects may be very difficult for the surgeon to visualize because of the large amount of trabeculation on the right side of the ventricular septum.

The conotruncal septum is normally a spiral structure that is formed by two sets of opposing ridges. One pair of ridges at the caudal end of the truncus arteriosus grows rapidly downward and together and then fuses. The other pair arises in the outflow part of the bulbus cordis, grows together, then fuses with tissue growing up from the inlet septum (Fig. 1–4).[5] The mechanism for the spiral course of the septum is unclear, though it is known that neural crest cells are very important in outflow tract development. Failure of spiraling may place the aorta anteriorly and pulmonary artery posteriorly, that is, transposing the great arteries. Failure of fusion of the ridges may easily cause ventricular septal defect in the outflow septum (supracristal ventricular septal defect). If in addition the spiral septation is asymmetrical, tetralogy (ventricular septal defect and small right ventricular outflow tract and pulmonary artery) can occur.

The last part of the septum to close is the membranous septum, which lies along the inner curvature between the tricuspid valve and pulmonary valve (Fig. 1–3). Closure of this part of the septum seems to depend on both timing and position of the three septa noted above.[4] Clinically, the membranous septum is the site of most septal defects, and in this position the defects are not usually difficult for the surgeon to reach. Many small or moderate-sized ventricular defects will narrow or close spontaneously.

## Valves

The cardiac valves are formed after the cardiac septa are complete, and all four valves are found at sites of cushion tissue.[5] The atrioventricular valves develop from loose folds in the endocardial cushions, which then erode in a selective fashion, leaving the atrioventricular valves connected by chordae tendineae to papillary muscles deeper in the ventricle.[4] An alternative hypothesis is that portions of atrioventricular valves develop from the ventricular muscle. The atrioventricular valves develop by undermining of a skirt of ventricular muscle tissue (with mesenchymal tissue on the atrial side).[7,8,12] The process of undermining extends until the atrioventricular junction is reached. Subsequent resorption of the muscle results in normal-appearing valve leaflets and chordae tendineae. Should the process of undermining of the tissue stop short of atrioventricular annulus, various degrees of Ebstein's malformation will result.[7,8,12] The semilunar valves develop from three pyramid-shaped cushions inside the pulmonary artery and aorta.[4] After outgrowth the cushions are remodeled with help of flow stresses and become thinner and smoother.[4]

If the developing cushion leaflets fuse during development, stenosis of the valve occurs. If the

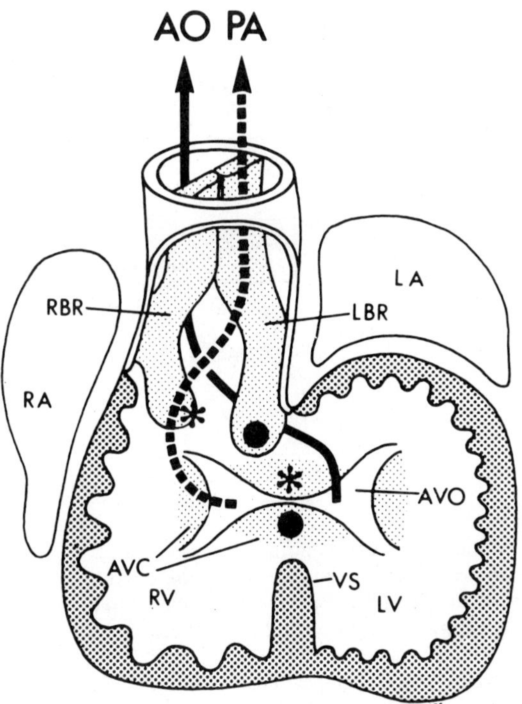


**Figure 1–4** Conal (infundibular) septation. The lower margin of the right bulbar ridge grows spirally downward and backward and joins the posterior atrioventricular cushion *(asterisks)*. The left bulbar ridge grows downward and forward to join the anterior atrioventricular cushion, thus separating the systemic pathway *(solid dark line)* from the pulmonary pathway *(dotted line)*. *AO*, Aorta; *AVC*, atrioventricular cushions; *AVO*, atrioventricular orifice; *LA*, left atrium; *LBR*, left bulbar ridge; *LV*, left ventricle; *PA*, pulmonary artery; *RA*, right atrium; *RBR*, right bulbar ridge; *RV*, right ventricle; *VS*, ventricular septum. (From Reller MD, McDonald RW, Gerlis LM et al: *J Am Soc Echocardiogr* 4(5):519, 1991.)

obstruction is severe enough, then fetal flow patterns are altered and the opposite side of the heart carrying more flow increases in size, the obstructed side of the ventricular cavity becomes hypoplastic, and the muscle thickens. If the obstruction is mild, no abnormality is evident until later in life. Valvar insufficiency is less common but in utero is more likely to be tricuspid than mitral and may be poorly tolerated by the fetus (for example, tricuspid insufficiency in Ebstein's anomaly).

### The venous system

The systemic venous system, by the time the embryo is 4 mm in length, has three pairs of veins entering the sinus venosus.[5] The three pairs are the vitelline veins from the yolk sac and later from the foregut, the umbilical veins from the placenta, and the cardinal veins from the head and body of the embryo.[1,2] The vitelline system contributes part of later hepatic, splenic, and superior messenteric as well as portal veins. The umbilical vein carries the flow from the chorionic villi to the sinus venosus, then involutes after birth.[9] The cardinal system grows and develops as the embryo enlarges in all directions. The superior vena cava is normally formed by the right common cardinal vein and proximal part of the right anterior cardinal veins (Fig. 1–5). The inferior vena cava is a more complicated fusion of several embryonic veins, especially the right sacrocardinal (lower extremities), the right subcardinal (renal), and the right hepatocardiac channel. The superior parts of the supercardinal (embryo body wall) system form the azygos and hemiazygos veins. Usually the azygos and hemiazygos veins are smaller than the vena cava, but if the intrahepatic part of the inferior vena cava fails to develop, then they are larger, and one or the other carries the bulk of the inferior vena cava flow back to the heart.[9] Normally the left common cardinal vein partially regresses and persists as ligament of Marshal on the back of the heart and the coronary sinus. But if the left common cardinal vein does not regress, a left superior vena cava persists and drains some of the upper body blood into the coronary sinus.

The pulmonary veins form initially as outpouching of venous channels from the lung bud mesenchymal tissue at approximately 8 weeks of age. These channels join and form a common pulmonary vein, which then grows toward and fuses with the primitive left atrium, responding to some signal from the left atrium itself. The fusion of the common vein into the left atrium enlarges the left atrium. Incomplete fusion of the common pulmonary vein with the left atrium causes cor triatriatum, which has several forms. Before establishing connection with the left atrium, the pulmonary venous system is connected with and drains into the systemic veins. These veins are connected to the left innominate vein, superior vena cava, portal venous system, and others. These connecting veins involute once the common pulmonary vein establishes connection with the left atrium. If the fusion between left atrium and common pulmonary vein does not take place, one of these connecting veins persists. The type of total anomalous pulmonary venous connection therefore depends on the vein that persists. The most common type is supracardiac drainage into the left innominate vein via the vertical vein. The most common type in the neonate, however, is infradiaphragmatic type, draining into the portal venous system. This usually results in pulmonary venous obstruction, causing severe problems in the neonatal period. In patients with

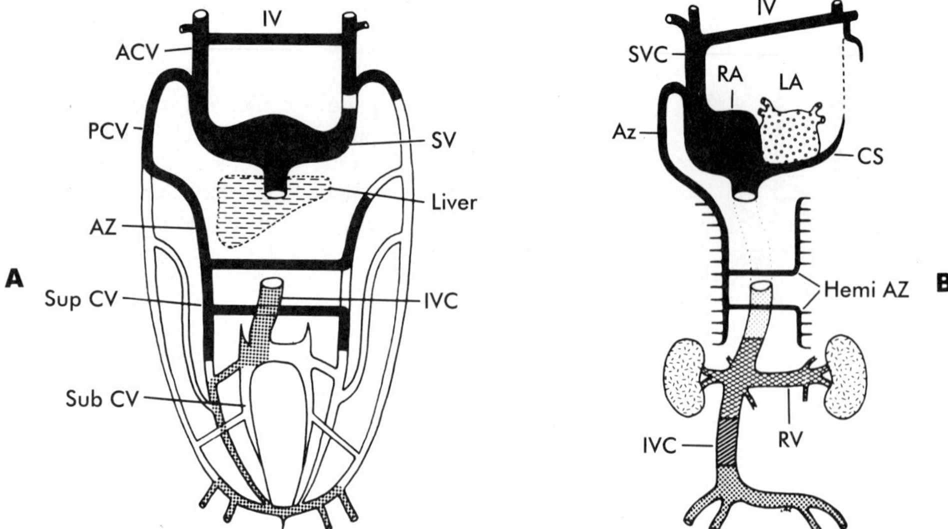


**Figure 1–5** Development of the systemic veins. **A,** The constituent embryonic components. Vessels that persist and drain into the superior vena cava are shown in black. Those that form the inferior vena cava are shaded. **B,** The mature systemic venous pattern. The constituent portions of the inferior vena cava are indicated. *ACV,* anterior cardinal vein; *AZ,* azygos vein; *CS,* coronary sinus; *Hemi* AZ, hemiazygos vein; *IV,* innominate vein; *IVC,* inferior vena cava; *LA,* left atrium; *PCV,* posterior cardinal vein; *RA,* right atrium; *RV,* renal vein; *Sub CV,* subcardinal vein; *Sup CV,* supracardinal vein; *SVC,* superior vena cava. (From Reller MD, McDonald RW, Gerlis LM et al: *J Am Soc Echocardiogr* 4(5):519, 1991.)

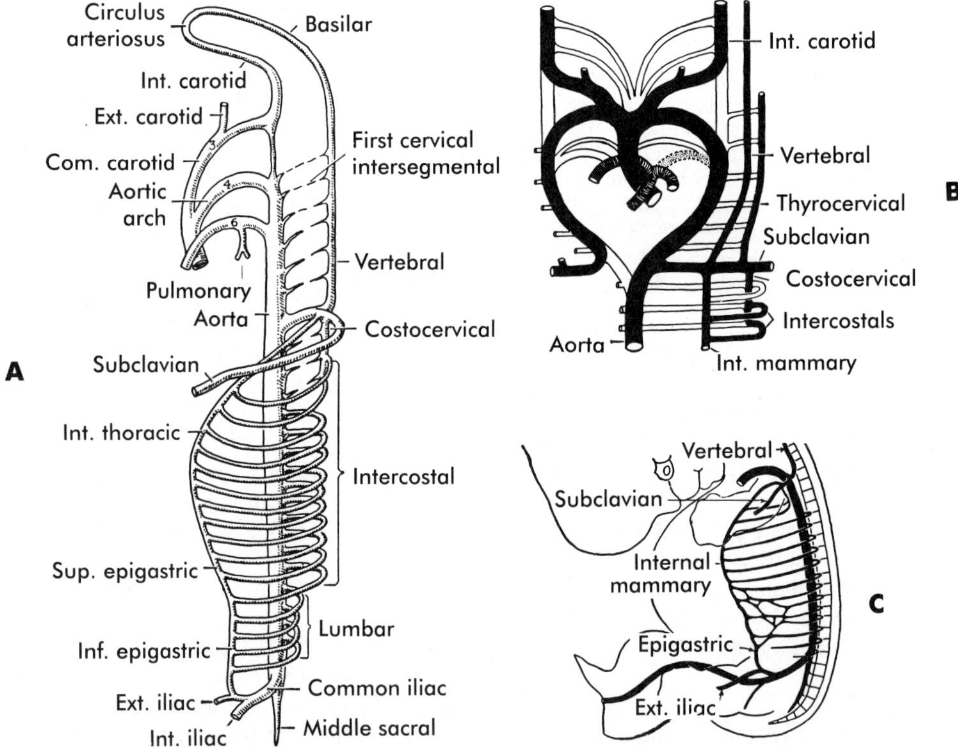


**Figure 1–6** Derivatives of the dorsal branches (intersegmental arteries) of the human aorta. **A,** Diagram, viewed from the left side. **B,** Scheme in ventral view showing origins in the vicinity of the subclavian artery. **C,** Relations of the internal thoracic (or mammary) and epigastric arteries at 16 mm, viewed from the left side (after Mall). (From Arey LB: *Developmental anatomy: a textbook and laboratory manual of embryology,* ed 7, Philadelphia, 1965, Saunders.)

visceral and cardiac heterotaxy (in other words, bilateral left- or right-sidedness) anomalous pulmonary venous return occurs more frequently than in those with normal visceroatrial situs (solitus). In bilateral left-sidedness the pulmonary veins attach to both sides of the atrium. In bilateral right-sidedness the pulmonary veins do not attach to the atrium at all. Instead, the common pulmonary vein persists and connects to more primitive venous channels of the cardinal system, as detailed earlier.[4]

### The arterial system

As the embryo forms successive branchial arches, successive paired aortic arches develop and connect the heart tube ventrally with the paired dorsal aortae in the back. Much of this early arch system regresses and disappears.[4] By 14 mm of embryo length, the aortic arch system is no longer symmetric. The third aortic arch with help from the first and the second arches forms the common carotid artery and the first part of the internal carotid artery (Fig. 1–6). The fourth aortic arch on the left forms part of the transverse aorta. On the right the fourth arch contributes the proximal right subclavian artery. The sixth arch gives bilateral branches that grow toward the lung buds. The proximal sixth arch becomes the proximal part of the right and left pulmonary arteries.[5] If the right fourth arch and a right dorsal aorta persist, then right aortic arch occurs. If both the right and left fourth arch persist, then double aortic aortic arch occurs and has a strong potential for vascular ring formation and airway compression.

Fig. 1–6 shows the main aortic branches, which persist during development, along with the collateral connections from the upper body arteries to the lower body arteries, which can persist in some cardiac defects such as coarctation and interrupted aortic arch.

### Cardiac control systems

Tissue level mechanisms seem to control the embryonic circulation during most of the period of morphogenesis. The Frank-Starling mechanism does operate even early on, and adrenergic receptors are present and operating with great sensitivity.[4] Later on, during the growth phase of development, first the parasympathetic and then the sympathetic nervous system develop connections in the heart in close association with the developing coronary artery system, which is relatively late in formation.[4]

The main steps in cardiac development have been traced, and points where defects are likely to occur have been discussed. A great deal of research is now under way regarding the actual mechanisms operating in normal and abnormal development.[4] These studies, along with continued developments in fetal echocardiography and fetal surgery, will hopefully allow better definition of natural history of cardiac defects and earlier medical and surgical intervention in cases of known poor prognosis.

## REFERENCES


1. Anderson RH: Another look at cardiac embryology, *Progress in cardiology #7,* Philadelphia, 1978, Lea and Febiger.
2. Arey LB: *The vascular system and developmental anatomy,* ed 7, Philadelphia, 1965, Saunders.
3. Clark EB: Cardiac embryology: its relevance to congenital heart disease, *Am J Dis Child* 140:41, 1986.
4. Clark EB: Growth, morphogenesis, and function: the dynamics of cardiac development. In Moller JH, Neal WA, editors: *Fetal, neonatal, and infant cardiac disease,* Norwalk, Connecticut, 1990, Appleton-Lange.
5. Clark EB, VanMierop LHS: Development of the cardiovascular system. In Adams FH, Emmanouilides GC, Riemenschneider TA, editors: *Moss' heart disease in infants, children, and adolescents,* ed 4, Baltimore, 1989, Williams & Wilkins.
6. Langman J: *Medical embryology,* ed 4, Baltimore, 1981, Williams & Wilkins.
7. Patten BM: *Human embryology,* ed 3, New York, 1968, McGraw Hill.
8. Rao PS, Jue KL, Isabel-Jones J, et al: Ebstein's malformation of the tricuspid valve with atresia, *Am J Cardiol* 32:1004, 1973.
9. Reller MV, McDonald RW, Gerlis LM, et al: Cardiac embryology: basic review and clinical correlations, *J Am Soc Echocardiogr* 4 (5):519, 1991.
10. VanPraagh R: Embryology. In Fyler DC, editor: *Nadas pediatric cardiology,* Philadelphia, 1992, Hanley and Belfus.
11. VanPraagh R, Takao A, editors: Etiology and morphogenesis of congenital heart disease, Mt. Kisco, NY, 1980, Futura.
12. VanMierop LHS, Gessner IH: Pathogenetic mechanisms in congenital cardiovascular malformations, *Prog Cardiovasc Dis* 15:67, 1972.

# 2 Fetal and Neonatal Circulations

*P. Syamasundar Rao*



The fetal circulation is designed to use the placenta for gas exchange, but the postnatal circulation must rely on the lungs for gas exchange. The circulatory systems must therefore adapt to these changing requirements. The placenta also serves as a site for exchange of metabolic end products with fresh sources of energy and metabolism such as glucose, amino acids, fatty acids, and electrolytes, as well as the transfer of hormones.[6] Knowledge of the fetal circulation and the normal changes it undergoes at birth is essential for a better understanding of the postnatal adaptation of the circulation of the various types of congenital cardiac defects.

For characteristic features of adult and fetal circulation, see the box on p. 11. The objectives of this chapter are (1) to present an outline of the fetal circulation; (2) to describe postnatal changes; and (3) to discuss circulatory adaptation to certain important congenital cardiac defects.

## FETAL CIRCULATION

Although some data from human fetuses are available, most of the information with regard to the fetal circulation is derived from the experimental observations of the animal models,[2-4,14,34,35,42,48,49,50,51] particularly the lamb. It is generally believed that the lamb model offers the closest approximation to human physiology.[47] Quantitative measurements of blood flow have been derived from oxygen saturation differences (Fick principle), from electromagnetic flow transducers, and by radionuclide-labeled microspheres. In the postnatal circulatory states the cardiac output is expressed as the volume ejected by each ventricle, but in the fetal circulatory states the cardiac output is conventionally represented as the combined output of both the ventricles.

### Course of the fetal circulation

The fetal circulatory pathways are depicted in Fig. 2-1. The oxygenated blood from the placenta is returned by way of the umbilical vein, which enters the inferior vena cava via the ductus venosus. Approximately one half of the umbilical venous blood goes through the liver and is returned to the inferior vena cava via the hepatic veins. A significant proportion of the inferior vena caval blood streams preferentially into the left atrium. This preferential shunting of the arterialized blood into the left atrium occurs mainly because the free margin of the septum secundum, the crista dividens (forming

## CHARACTERISTICS OF CIRCULATION

**Adult**

No communication between systemic and pulmonary circuits exists.

Resistances are in series.

The systemic circuit is a high-pressure circuit, and the pulmonary circuit is a low-resistance, low-pressure circuit.

Pulmonary arterioles are widely dilated and thin walled as compared with muscular systemic arterioles.

**Fetal**

Intercirculatory communication exists.

Resistances are parallel.

Pulmonary circuit has high resistance; low-resistance systemic circuit (secondary to low-resistance placental circuit) has equal pressures in the ventricles and great arteries.

The pulmonary vascular bed has thick-walled muscular arterioles.

From Rao PS: *Indian J Pediatr* 58:441, 1991.

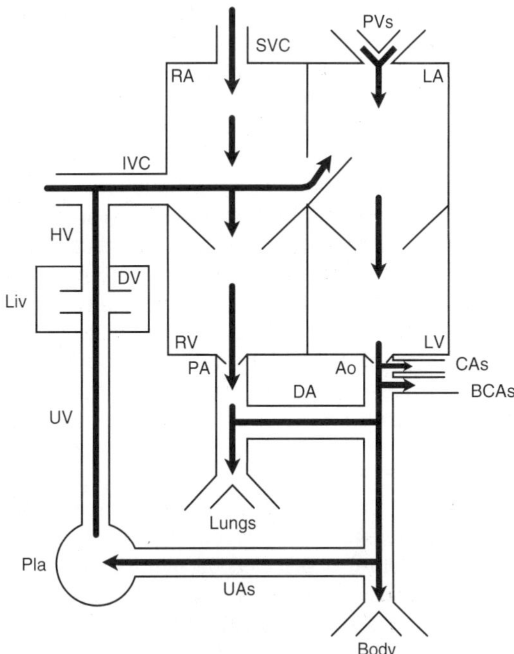


**Figure 2–1** Diagrammatic depiction of fetal circulatory pathways. *Ao,* aorta. *BCAs,* Brachiocephalic arteries. *CAs,* Coronary arteries. *DA,* Ductus arteriosus. *DV,* Ductus venosus. *HV,* Hepatic vein. *IVC,* Inferior vena cava. *LA,* Left atrium. *Liv,* Liver. *LV,* Left ventricle. *PA,* Pulmonary artery. *Pla,* Placenta. *PVs,* Pulmonary veins. *RA,* Right atrium. *RV,* Right ventricle. *SVC,* Superior vena cava. *UAs,* Umbilical arteries. *UV,* Umbilical vein. *CS, Coronary sinus.* (From Rao PS: *Indian J Pediatr* 58:441, 1991.)

the upper margin of the foramen ovale), overrides the inferior vena cava.[3] The septum primum, forming the lower margin of the foramen ovale, has its free edge on the left side of atrial septum, and the foramen ovale is kept open by the inferior vena caval stream. In addition, the eustachian valve (a prominent shelflike structure at the opening of the inferior vena cava) diverts the inferior vena caval blood stream toward the atrial septum.[26] Thus, the oxygenated blood mixes with the pulmonary venous blood and enters the left ventricle and then the ascending aorta. The heart (via the coronary arteries) and the upper part of the body, including the brain (via the brachiocephalic vessels), receive oxygenated blood. The superior vena caval and coronary venous returns, along with a portion of the inferior vena caval blood that did not stream into the left atrium, enter the right ventricle via the tricuspid valve. This desaturated blood is ejected by the right ventricle into the main pulmonary artery, from which a small quantity enters the lungs. The rest enters the descending aorta via the ductus arteriosus. In this manner the deoxygenated blood makes its way into the placenta via the umbilical arteries.

### Mechanisms for maintaining fetal circulatory pathways

***The foramen ovale.*** This is kept patent in the fetus, it is believed, because of the mechanical effect of streaming of the inferior vena caval blood into the left atrium. The same thing may be held true for the ductus venosus and umbilical vessels.

***The ductus arteriosus.*** Because of its muscular content the ductus arteriosus may have to be kept actively dilated. Recent studies suggest that prostaglandins ($E_2$ and possibly $I_2$) actively keep the ductus open. Both the locally produced and circulating prostaglandins may be responsible for this phenomenon. In postnatal life the prostaglandins are rapidly cleared by passage through the lungs, but in the fetus the pulmonary blood flow is very low (7% of combined ventricular output) and there is therefore a higher concentration of circulating prostaglandins. Furthermore, the placenta produces large quantities of prostaglandins. It is generally believed that these prostaglandins keep the ductus widely patent. Ductal patency may also be related to circulating concentration of adenosine.[37]

***Pulmonary vascular resistance.*** Because of the large size of the ductus arteriosus, the pressures in the main pulmonary artery and descending aorta are equal. Therefore the relative amounts of flow to the placenta and lungs depend upon their relative resistances. The placental circulation is a low-resistance circuit, and therefore a large proportion of the blood goes to the placenta. The pulmonary circulation is a high-resistance circuit, and therefore only a small proportion of the combined ventricular output is distributed to the lungs.

The cause of this high pulmonary vascular resistance is variously hypothesized. Tortuosity and kinking of the small pulmonary vessels has been proposed,[46] but this theory is not generally agreed upon. Several studies[8,13] have shown that the pulmonary arterioles, which have a thick smooth muscle layer, are responsible for the high resistance. The pulmonary arterioles are regulated by partial pressure of oxygen to which they are subjected. Changes in the pH, carbon dioxide pressure,[8,13] and autonomic nervous system may also influence the pulmonary vascular resistance. The fetal pulmonary vasculature is affected by many endogenous and exogenous vasoactive materials. Several recent studies have shown dramatic effects of pharmacologic doses of prostaglandins on the fetal pulmonary circulation.[8,28] The prostaglandins $E_1$, $E_2$, and $I_2$ produce pulmonary vasodilatation, and prostaglandin $F_2\alpha$ and leukotrienes ($LTD_4$) produce pulmonary vasoconstriction.[9] However, their role in maintaining a normally high pulmonary vascular resistance is not clearly defined; perhaps the hypoxic stimulus may be mediated by prostaglandins.

## Distribution of the cardiac output and oxygen saturation in the fetus

As mentioned above, the cardiac output is expressed as combined output of both ventricles. Rudolph[47] estimates that the combined ventricular output (CVO) in the lamb is 200 ml/kg/min. Rudolph and his associates[22,48] determined the relative distribution of the CVO in chronically instrumented lambs, and these will be summarized here (Fig. 2–2). The inferior vena cava carries 69% of the CVO. Of this, 27% is diverted into the left atrium across the foramen ovale, where it is joined by venous return from the lungs (7% of CVO). Thus, one third of the CVO enters the left ventricle and aorta. The majority of this blood flow (24%) is distributed to the heart and upper part of the body via the coronary arteries and brachiocephalic vessels, and 10% traverses the isthmus of the aortic arch. The superior vena caval return (21% of CVO) joins with the remaining inferior vena caval return (42% of CVO) and coronary venous return (3% of CVO) and traverses the tricuspid valve. The right ventricle and pulmonary artery therefore carry two thirds of the CVO. Only 7% of CVO is distributed to the lungs, and the remaining (approximately

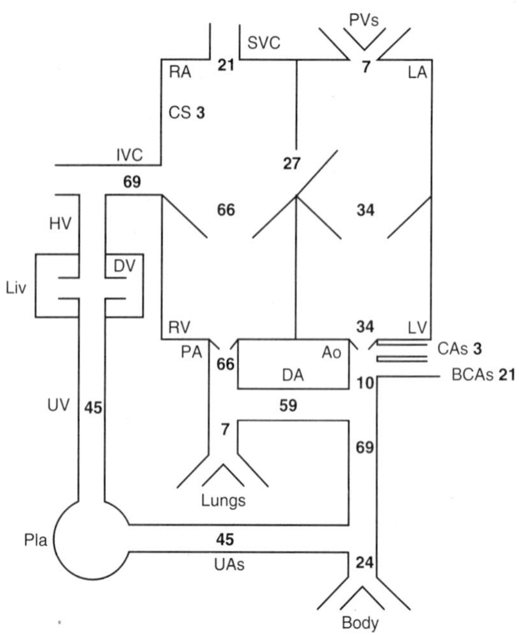


**Figure 2–2** Distribution of cardiac output.[23,47,48] The numbers indicate percent of combined ventricular output. *Ao,* aorta. *BCAs,* Brachiocephalic arteries. *CAs,* Coronary arteries. *DA,* Ductus arteriosus. *DV,* Ductus venosus. *HV,* Hepatic vein. *IVC,* Inferior vena cava. *LA,* Left atrium. *Liv,* Liver. *LV,* Left ventricle. *PA,* Pulmonary artery. *Pla,* Placenta. *PVs,* Pulmonary veins. *RA,* Right atrium. *RV,* Right ventricle. *SVC,* Superior vena cava. *UAs,* Umbilical arteries. *UV,* Umbilical vein. *CS, Coronary sinus.* (From Rao PS: *Indian J Pediatr* 58:441, 1991.)

59% of CVO) blood crosses the ductus arteriosus to enter the descending aorta. Thus, 69% of CVO reaches the descending aorta. A large proportion (45% of CVO) reaches the placenta for oxygenation. The remaining blood goes to the abdomen and lower extremities.

Oxygen saturations and partial pressures of oxygen and carbon dioxide in various vessels are shown in Table 2–1.[23,48] As can be seen from the table, these oxygen levels are much lower than those in neonates, infants, and children. This difference is probably related to the lower efficiency of the placenta as an organ of oxygen transport compared with the lungs. The fetus adapts to lower levels of oxygen saturation by virtue of high levels of fetal hemoglobin with low P50 of 18 to 19 torr, facilitating oxygen uptake from the placenta at relatively low levels of oxygen pressure. In addition, there is most advantageous distribution of the blood to the various organs and the placenta; the highly saturated blood to the heart and brain and less-saturated blood to placenta.

**Table 2–1** Blood gas and pH values in the fetus[23,48]

| Site | $O_2$ saturation (%) | $P_{O_2}$ (torr) | $P_{CO_2}$ (torr) | pH |
|---|---|---|---|---|
| Umbilical vein | 75-80 | 32-35 | 37-38 | 7.36-7.38 |
| Inferior vena cava | 70 | 28-30 | — | — |
| Left ventricle, aorta, carotid artery | 65 | 26-28 | 29-45 | 7.34-7.36 |
| Superior vena cava | 40 | 12-14 | — | — |
| Right ventricle, main pulmonary artery | 50-55 | 16-18 | — | — |
| Descending aorta | 55-60 | 20-22 | 42-45 | 7.32-7.34 |

From Rao PS: *Indian J Pediatr* 58:441, 1991.

## MYOCARDIAL FUNCTION IN THE FETUS

The structure of the fetal myocardium differs greatly from that of the adult. In the adults the myocardial cells are compact with small nuclei and with little connective tissue surrounding them, but in the fetus the myocardial cells are less well organized, have large nuclei, are sometimes even multinucleated, and have a smaller number of sarcomeres per unit of mass. In addition, the organization and function of the sarcoplasmic reticulum are incomplete and progressively increase with advancing fetal age, as does the development of the t-tubule system.[21] A large amount of areolar tissue lies between the fetal myocardial cells.[17] There is also evidence that the sympathetic innervation of the heart is not completely developed in most species studied.[17,48] Furthermore, there are differences between fetal, neonatal, and adult myocardium in regard to the type of substrates used, the type of contractile protein activated, production and delivery of high energy phosphate, the method of calcium delivery, and the response of contractible elements to calcium ions; Gingell[21] has reviewed and referenced these well.

The physiologic counterparts of the structural differences are greater resting tension at a given muscle length in the fetus than in the adult and a lesser tension developed at any resting length in the fetus than in the adult.[17]

It has been thought that the fetal cardiac output is mostly regulated by a change in the heart rate rather than by a change in the stroke volume, in contrast to the adult, who first changes the stroke volume, that is, uses the Frank-Starling mechanism.[22,48] More recent studies[30] suggested that the Frank-Starling mechanism is indeed operative in the fetus within the narrow physiologic ranges. The fetal heart is also sensitive to increase in afterload.[20]

## POSTNATAL CIRCULATORY CHANGES

The major changes at birth include elimination of the placenta, development of pulmonary circulation, and closure of fetal circulatory pathways. There is a dramatic, immediate change at birth followed by a gradual change until a mature cardiovascular system is achieved; the time sequence of the latter varies.

### Elimination of the placenta

At birth, with elimination of placental circulation, either by clamping the umbilical cord or by vasoconstriction in a natural birth, the systemic vascular resistance increases markedly because of exclusion of low-resistance placental circuit, and there is an acute need for the lungs to assume the gas exchange function.

### Development of pulmonary circulation

Within a few seconds following delivery, respiration begins, and almost complete expansion of the lungs occurs within a few minutes after birth. There is a marked decrease in the pulmonary vascular resistance and a marked increase in the pulmonary blood flow at birth. There is a concomitant decrease in pulmonary arterial pressures. Expulsion of the fluid from the alveoli and ventilation of the lungs are to some extent responsible for the fall in the pulmonary vascular resistance.[8,14,31,53] Decrease in partial pressure of carbon dioxide also decreases the pulmonary resistance,[13] although its effect may in part be related to changes in pH. However, a more important factor in producing reduction of pulmonary vascular resistance appears to be an increase in oxygen pressure in the alveoli and blood. It is the consensus that the alveolar gaseous oxygen diffuses in sufficient quantities into the region of precapillary vessels to cause them to dilate. The mechanism of action of oxygen in producing the pulmonary arteriolar dilation is not clearly understood. The oxygen may directly affect the smooth muscle cells of the pulmonary arterioles, or it may act through a chemical mediator. Some studies have indicated that oxygen may help activate kininogen to bradykinin in the lung[7,25,36]; bradykinin, a potent pulmonary vasodilator, produces the desired pulmonary vasodilation. The bradykinin effect may be mediated through prostacyclin.[40] Although there is a rapid increase in bradykinin levels in the left atrial blood following oxygen ventilation, these increased levels last for only a short period and therefore raise questions as to the validity of this hypothesis as the sole factor responsible for pulmonary vasodilation. Oxygen-induced pulmonary vasodilatation appears to have two phases. The first, the rapid phase, appears not to be dependent on prostacyclin mediation and cannot be inhibited by indomethacin. The prostaglandins may play a role in the second, the slow phase, of the oxygen-mediated pulmonary vasodilator effect,[32,33] but this has not yet been completely elucidated. With the fall in the pulmonary vascular resistance, the pulmonary blood flow increases markedly.

Subsequent fall in the pulmonary vascular resistance and regression of the medial musculature of the pulmonary arterioles are parallel and occur more gradually. By the age of 6 to 8 weeks the pulmonary vasculature looks very similar to that of the adult. Decreased inspired oxygen such as in high altitude and disease states causing alveolar hypoxia may prevent normal maturation of pulmonary vasculature. Congenital heart defects that cause elevation of pulmonary artery pressure also cause retardation of the normal involution of the pulmonary vasculature.

### Closure of the fetal circulatory pathways

***Patent foramen ovale.*** With the decrease in the pulmonary arteriolar resistance there is an increase in the pulmonary flow with resultant increase in the volume of blood in the left atrium. This will raise the left atrial pressure. Concomitantly, because of elimination of the placenta, the umbilical venous and consequently the inferior vena caval flow decrease markedly. This alteration will produce a slight decrease in the right atrial pressure. These two factors together will produce apposition of the septum primum and septum secundum, resulting in functional closure of the foramen ovale. The functional closure occurs within the first few hours after birth. The closure is incomplete in that any factor that causes an increase in the right atrial pressure (e.g., crying,[42] hypoxic pulmonary vasoconstriction,[35] severe right ventricular or atrial obstruction), and/or a decrease in the left atrial pressure will result in right-to-left interatrial shunting. Marked enlargement of the left atrium secondary to a large pulmonary blood flow (due to a patent ductus arteriosus or ventricular septal defect) will stretch the patent foramen ovale and may cause left-to-right shunting.[27,52]

Anatomic closure of the foramen ovale usually occurs within about 2 to 3 months of life.[10,45] However, approximately 20% of older infants, children, adolescents, and adults may have a patent foramen ovale.[43]

***Ductus venosus.*** The ductus venosus also closes soon after birth. The mechanism of closure is less well delineated and may be similar to the closure of ductus arteriosus.

***Ductus arteriosus.*** Closure of ductus arteriosus at birth occurs in two stages,[19] functional closure by constriction of ductal muscle within 10 to 15 hours of age,[10,14,29,39,47] and anatomic closure by endothelial destruction, subintimal layer proliferation, and connective tissue formation within 2 to 3 weeks of age. Increase of oxygen pressure following birth is associated with ductal closure.[29] Several studies have shown that an increase in oxygen tension causes muscular constriction of ductal muscle, causing ductal closure.[2,5,24,29] On the contrary, the ductal closure is delayed at high altitudes or when the infant is exposed to low oxygen concentration.[1,38,41] The mechanism of action of oxygen is not clearly understood but appears to be direct stimulation of constriction of the smooth muscle cells of the ductal tissue, although mediation through cytochrome[11,15,16] and thromboxane[18] systems has been postulated. Hemodynamic changes, release of vasoactive substances such as histamine, 5-hydroxytryptamine, acetylcholine, bradykinin, and catecholamine may contribute to the ductal closure but are thought not to be essential.

Recent research has raised questions with regard to the role of prostaglandins in either initiating ductal constriction or mediating ductal constrictive effect of oxygen. However, the current evidence supports oxygen as a primary factor. The prostaglandin-mediated ductal relaxing mechanism develops in early fetal life[12]; this prostaglandin function is more active at about 0.7 gestation than at term. Although the ductal muscle is becoming less responsive to prostaglandins with increasing gestational age, it acquires increasing sensitivity to oxygen. Thus, prostaglandins indirectly contribute to ductal closure by becoming less effective after birth, and they potentiate constrictor action of oxygen.[12]

## POSTNATAL CHANGES AND CONGENITAL HEART DEFECTS

Congenital heart disease is usually well tolerated during fetal life. However, postnatal circulatory changes have marked effects on the clinical presentation and on the course of the heart disease in the early newborn period. The influence of these postnatal changes on congenital heart defects will be summarized in the ensuing paragraphs.

**Ductus arteriosus**

***Hypoplastic left heart syndrome.*** In this defect complex, the mitral valve, left ventricle and/or the ascending aorta are markedly stenotic or atretic, and the entire systemic circulation depends on the flow through the patent ductus arteriosus. As the oxygen pressure increases, the ductus tends to constrict and thus compromises the systemic blood flow (Fig. 2–3). This, along with the decrease in the pulmonary vascular resistance, will produce a markedly increased pulmonary blood flow. This combination of events causes severe acidemia (reflecting decreased systemic perfusion) and a rise in arterial oxygen pressure, reflecting an increase in pulmonary-to-systemic flow ratio. In this condition it seems logical to avoid increasing oxygen pressure by not increasing ambient oxygen concentration so as not to hasten the ductal closure. As a matter of fact, some workers advocate lower fractional inspired oxygen concentration than in room air so as to increase pulmonary vasoconstriction and thus facilitate systemic perfusion through the ductus arteriosus. Also, administration of prostaglandin $E_1$ will keep the ductus patent, thus maintaining systemic perfusion.

***Pulmonary atresia.*** In this condition with com-

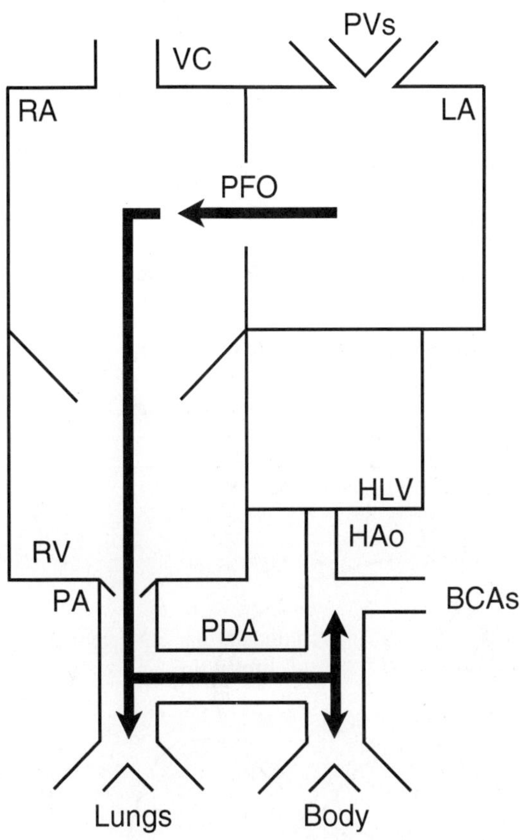


**Figure 2–3** Box diagram of hypoplastic left heart syndrome. In hypoplastic left heart syndrome (or mitral atresia) pulmonary venous return cannot exit into the left ventricle *(HLV)*, and its egress has to be into the right atrium *(RA)* via the patent foramen ovale *(PFO)*. If the foramen ovale is obstructed, the infant will develop signs of pulmonary venous obstruction. Because there is no forward flow from the left ventricle into the hypoplastic aorta *(HAo)*, the systemic perfusion depends on the patency of the ductus arteriosus. *RA*, Right arium. *PVs*, Pulmonary veins. *LA*, Left atrium. *RV*, Right ventricle. *PA*, Pulmonary artery. *BCAs*, Brachiocephalic arteries. *PFO*, Patent foramen ovale. *HLV*, Left ventricle. (From Rao PS: *Indian J Pediatr* 58:441, 1991.)

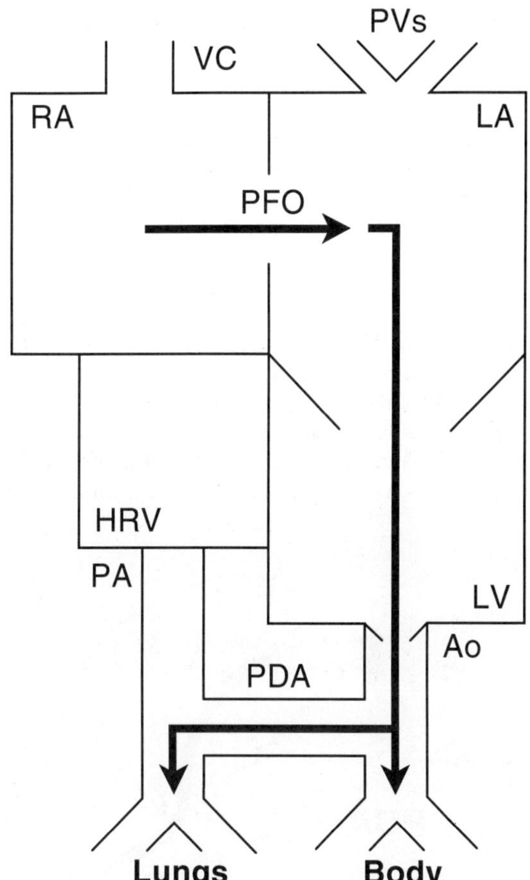


**Figure 2–4** Box diagram of hypoplastic right heart syndrome. In pulmonary atresia (or tricuspid atresia) the right atrial blood has to egress into the left atrium *(LA)* via the patent foramen ovale *(PFO)*. If the PFO is obstructive, signs of systemic venous obstruction will develop. Since there is no forward flow into the pulmonary artery *(PA)* from the right ventricle *(HRV)*, the pulmonary flow is dependent upon the patency of the ductus arteriosus. *RA*, Right atrium. *PVs*, Pulmonary veins. *LA*, Left atrium. *PA*, Pulmonary artery. *VC*, Venae cavae. *PDA*, Patent ductus arteriosus. *Ao*, Aorta. (From Rao PS: *Indian J Pediatr* 58:441, 1991.)

plete blockage of the pulmonary valve, pulmonary blood flow is entirely dependent on the patency of the ductus (Fig. 2–4). While the ductus is widely patent the pulmonary blood flow is adequate, and arterial oxygen pressure is maintained. However, as the ductus begins to constrict during the natural process of closure, marked hypoxemia and metabolic acidosis will result. Prostaglandin $E_1$ infusion will help keep the ductus open. Many other cardiac defects (see the box at right) involving severe stenosis or atresia of the pulmonary outflow tract are similarly ductus-dependent and will benefit from prostaglandin $E_1$ infusion.

***Total anomalous pulmonary venous connection.*** In this congenital cardiac anomaly the pulmonary veins drain into the systemic veins. Frequently in the neonate pulmonary venous obstruction is present (particularly common with infradiaphragmatic type). This phenomenon will result in pulmonary edema and marked elevation of pulmonary arteriolar resistance and pressures. If the ductus is open, decompression of the pulmonary arterial tree may occur with some relief of suprasystemic pulmonary pressures.

***Transposition of the great arteries.*** An open ductus may enhance intercirculatory mixing in transposition of the great arteries (see section on the patent foramen ovale earlier in this chapter), thus improving arterial oxygen pressure.

***Coarctation of the aorta.*** Postnatal development of coarctation is in part related to a shelflike structure with infolding of medial and intimal tissue of the aortic wall and in part the result of constriction of the ductus arteriosus. Blood flow from the isthmus of the aorta into the descending aorta around the posterolateral shelf of coarctation is facilitated by an open ductus (Fig. 2–5, *A*). When the ductus arteriosus closes (Fig. 2–5, *B*), this bypass mechanism is no longer available, and acute aortic obstruction follows quickly with consequent development of symptoms.[45] Temporary relief can be obtained by prostaglandin $E_1$ infusion.

**DUCTUS-DEPENDENT CARDIAC DEFECTS**

**Ductus-dependent pulmonary blood flow**

Pulmonary atresia with intact ventricular septum
Pulmonary atresia with ventricular septal defect
Severe tetralogy of Fallot
Complex cyanotic heart disease with pulmonary atresia or severe stenosis
Tricuspid atresia
Critical pulmonary stenosis
Ebstein's anomaly of the tricuspid valve
Hypoplastic right ventricle

**Ductus-dependent systemic blood flow**

Interruption of the aortic arch
Severe coarctation of the aorta syndrome
Hypoplastic left heart syndrome

From Rao PS: *Indian J Pediatr* 58:441, 1991.

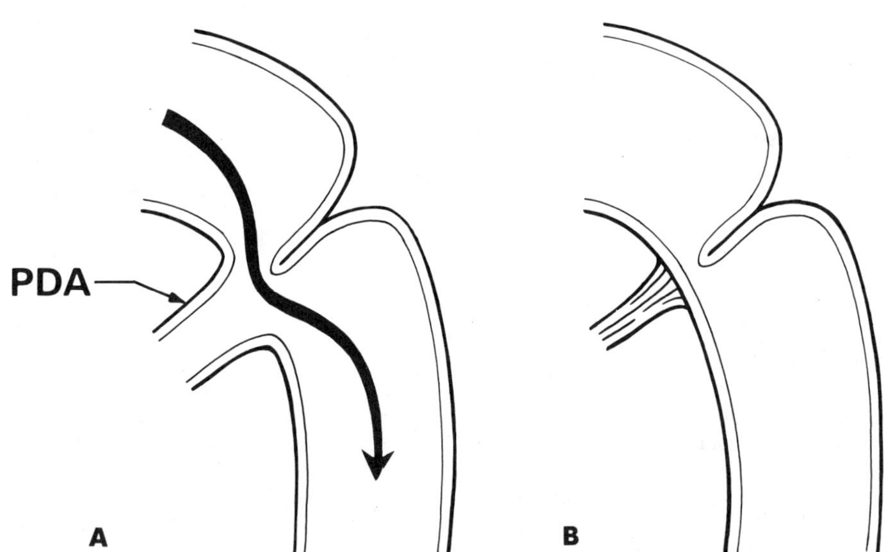


**Figure 2–5** Diagrammatic portrayal of the flow from the aortic isthmus to the descending aorta in coarctation of the aorta. **A,** With open ductus. **B,** With closed ductus. (From Rao PS, Solymar L: *Am Heart J* 116:1558, 1988.)

### Ductus venosus

In **total anomalous pulmonary venous connection** to the portal vein,[44] or ductus venosus, the clinical picture depends on the patency of the ductus venosus. If the ductus is open, the pulmonary venous flow is unobstructed and the infant may be asymptomatic. If the ductus venosus closes, signs of pulmonary venosus obstruction, namely, tachypnea, cyanosis, and pulmonary edema, will develop rapidly because of the necessity of the blood passage through the liver and because of high impedance to the passage of blood through the liver.

### Patent foramen ovale

***Right-sided obstructive lesions.*** In lesions such as **tricuspid** or **pulmonary** atresia, the pressure in the right atrium is higher and will keep the foramen ovale open; indeed this right-to-left shunting at the atrial level (Fig. 2–4) is essential for survival of the patient.

***Total anomalous pulmonary venous connection.*** The systemic blood flow depends upon the adequacy of patent foramen ovale because all the pulmonary venous blood returns to systemic veins and all the systemic output must pass through the patent foramen ovale.

***Left-side obstruction lesions.*** In **mitral** or **aortic atresia,** the foramen ovale has to remain open to direct the pulmonary venous return to the right side (Fig. 2–3). Should the foramen ovale close in any of the above conditions, surgical or balloon atrial septostomy can relieve the interatrial obstruction.

***Transposition of the great arteries.*** In this cardiac anomaly with the aorta arising from the right ventricle and the pulmonary artery from the left ventricle, the pulmonary and systemic circulations are in parallel arrangement (Fig. 2–6) rather than in the normal series arrangement. In the absence of intercirculatory mixing across a patent foramen ovale, patent ductus arteriosus, or a ventricular septal defect, the infant does not survive. If the fetal circulatory pathways close, as they usually do, creation or enlargement of atrial septal defect by surgery or balloon atrial septostomy is mandatory. Such an atrial communication may be necessary even in a patient with patent ductus arteriosus.

***Left-to-right shunt lesions.*** In lesions such as large **patent ductus arteriosus** and **ventricular septal defect,** the pulmonary blood flow is markedly increased and so consequently is the left atrial size. This left atrial enlargement will cause stretching of the patent foramen ovale, resulting in an additional left-to-right atrial shunting. However, such shunting maintains low pulmonary venosus pressure and may even prevent pulmonary edema.

### Pulmonary vascular bed

If a large systemic-to-pulmonary communication such as ventricular septal defect is present, the pressures in both ventricles are nearly equal. Therefore the degree of left-to-right shunt is largely dependent on the level of pulmonary vascular resistance. If the pulmonary vascular resistance decreases in a normal fashion, the neonate has a large left-to-right shunt and congestive heart failure during the first few days to weeks of life. Usually this does not happen until the age of 4 to 12 weeks, and it occurs because of delayed regression of the pulmonary vascular resistance. Increased pressure to which the pulmonary arterioles are exposed is thought to be responsible for this delayed regression, but the exact mechanism through which the high pressure acts is not known.

Any cardiac defect with large intercirculatory

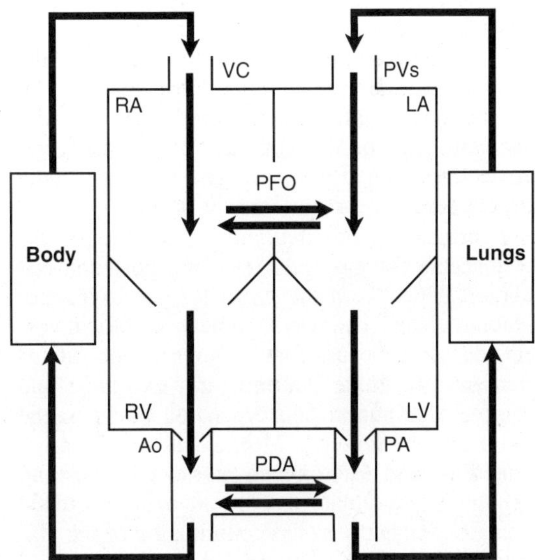


**Figure 2–6** Box diagram of the heart showing parallel circulations in transposition of the great arteries. Note that right ventricle *(RV)* pumps into the aorta *(Ao)* because of transposition, which goes to the body and returns to the right atrium *(RA)* and body. Similarly, left ventricular output goes to the pulmonary artery *(PA)* and lungs and returns to the left atrium *(LA)* and left ventricle *(LV)* to be pumped back into the lungs. Unless there are intercirculatory communications via either a patent foramen ovale *(PFO)* or patent ductus arteriosus *(PDA)*, the infant cannot survive. Mixing across a ventricular septal defect *(VSD)* if such is present (not shown) would also prevent progressive hypoxemia and death. *VC,* Venae cavae. *PVs,* Pulmonary veins. *RV,* right ventricle. (From Rao PS: *Indian J Pediatr* 58:441, 1991.)

connection, such as large patent ductus arteriosus, double outlet right ventricle, truncus arteriosus, single ventricle, and others, affects the pulmonary vascular bed in a manner similar to that described for ventricular septal defect.

Chronic hypoxia also delays regression of pulmonary vasculature. Pulmonary disease or decreased ambient oxygen at high altitude may delay the development of large left-to-right shunt and congestive heart failure.

As mentioned above, the development of fetal pulmonary vasculature is dependent upon the oxygen pressure to which it is exposed, and therefore, if the oxygen pressure of pulmonary blood is increased because of cardiac defect, pulmonary vasculature (arterioles) remain underdeveloped and less muscular. Hence the pulmonary vasculature can regress rapidly, producing a decrease in the pulmonary vascular resistance and a large left-to-right shunt much earlier than expected.

In premature infants, because of lack of complete development of the media of the pulmonary arterioles, there is less pulmonary arterial smooth muscle to regress; therefore, the infants with large systemic-pulmonary communications develop heart failure much earlier than expected. If they have pulmonary disease producing hypoxia, this event may be delayed, but as the infant improves from lung disease, a large left-to-right shunt and congestive heart failure will develop.

In summary, fetal circulation is designed to use the placenta for gas exchange, and postnatal circulation depends on the lungs for gas exchange. Fetal circulatory pathways, namely, umbilical vessels, ductus venosus, foramen ovale, and ductus arteriosus, facilitate placental gas exchange and promote distribution of oxygenated blood to the vital organs of the fetus. Mechanical factors, prostaglandins, and low oxygen pressure in the lung keep the fetal circulatory pathways open. Postnatal circulatory changes include elimination of the placenta, development of pulmonary circulation, and closure of fetal circulatory pathways. Postnatal circulatory changes markedly influence the clinical presentation and clinical course of the neonate with congenital heart defects.

## REFERENCES


1. Alzamora-Castro V, Baltilana G, Abrugattas R et al: Patent ductus arteriosus and high altitude, *Am J Cardiol* 5:761, 1960.
2. Assali NS, Morris JA: Maternal and fetal circulations and their interrelationships, *Obstet Gynecol Surg* 19:923, 1964.
3. Barclay AE, Franklin KJ, Prichard MML: *The foetal circulation and cardiovascular system and the change that they undergo at birth,* Oxford, 1944, Blackwell Scientific.
4. Bancroft J: *Researches on prenatal life,* Oxford, 1946, Blackwell Scientific.
5. Born GVR, Dawes GS, Mott JC et al: The constriction of the ductus arteriosus caused by oxygen and by asphyxia in the newborn lambs, *J Physiol (Lond)* 132:304, 1956.
6. Boyd JD, Hamilton WI: The human placenta. Cambridge, 1970, Heffer.
7. Campbell AGM, Dawes GS, Fishman AP et al: The release of bradykinin-like pulmonary vasodilator substance in foetal and newborn lambs, *J Physiol (Lond)* 195:83, 1968.
8. Cassin S, Dawes GS, Mott JC et al: The vascular resistance of the fetal newly ventilated lung of the lamb, *J Physiol (Lond)* 171:61, 1964.
9. Cassin S, Tyler T, Leffler C et al: Role of prostaglandins in control of fetal and neonatal pulmonary circulation. In Lango L, Reneau DD, editors: *Fetal and newborn cardiovascular physiology,* New York, 1978, Garland STPM Press.
10. Christie A: Normal closing time of the foramen ovale and the ductus arteriosus: an anatomic and statistical study, *Am J Dis Child* 40:323, 1930.
11. Coceani F, Hamilton NC, Labue J et al: Cytochrome P 450–linked mono-oxygenase: involvement in the lamb ductus arteriosus, *Am J Physiol* 246:H640, 1984.
12. Coceani F, Olley PM: Prostaglandins and the ductus arteriosus, *Pediatr Cardiol 4* (suppl 2):33, 1983.
13. Cook CD, Drinker PA, Jacobsen HN et al: Control of pulmonary blood flow in the fetal and newly born lamb, *J Physiol (Lond)* 169:10, 1963.
14. Dawes GS: *Foetal and neonatal physiology,* Chicago, 1968, Mosby.
15. Fay FS: Guinea pig ductus arteriosus I: cellular and metabolic basis for oxygen sensitivity, *Am J Physiol* 221:470, 1971.
16. Fay FS, Cooke PH: Guinea pig ductus arteriosus II: irreversible closure after birth, *Am J Physiol* 222:841, 1972.
17. Friedman WF: The intrinsic physiologic properties of the developing heart, *Prog Cardiovasc Dis* 15:87, 1972.
18. Friedman WF, Printz MP, Kirkpatrick SE et al: The vasoactivity of the fetal lamb ductus arteriosus studied in utero, *Pediatr Res* 17:331, 1983.
19. Gérard G: De l'oblitération du canal artérial, les théories et les faits, *Journal d'Anatomie (Paris)* 36:323, 1900.
20. Gilbert RD: Effect of afterload and baroreceptors on the cardiac function in fetal sheep, *J Dev Physiol* 4:299, 1982.
21. Gingell RL: Developmental biology of mammalian myocardium. In Freedom RM, Benson LN, Smallhorn JF, editors: *Neonatal heart disease,* London. 1992, Springer-Verlag.
22. Heymann MA, Creasy RR, Rudolph AM: Quantitation of blood flow patterns in the foetal lamb in utero. In *Foetal and neonatal physiology:* proceedings of Sir Joseph Barcroft centenary symposium, Cambridge University Press, 1973, Cambridge, England.
23. Heymann MA, Rudolph AM: Effects of congenital heart disease on fetal and neonatal circulations, *Prog Cardiovasc Dis* 15:115, 1972.
24. Heymann MA, Rudolph AM: Control of ductus arteriosus, *Physiol Rev* 55:62, 1975.
25. Heymann MA, Rudolph AM, Niles AS et al: Bradykinin production associated with oxygenation of the fetal lamb, *Circ Res* 25:521, 1969.
26. Ho SY, Angelini A, Moscoso G: Developmental cardiac anatomy. In Long WA, editor: *Fetal and neonatal cardiology,* Philadelphia, 1990, Saunders.
27. James LS, Burnard ED, Rowe RD: Abnormal shunting through the foramen ovale after birth, *Am J Dis Child* 102:550, 1961 (abstract).
28. Kadowitz PJ, Joiner PD, Hyman AIL et al: Influence of $PGE_1$ and $F_2\alpha$ on pulmonary vascular resistance, isolated

lobar vessels, and cyclic nucleotide levels, *J Pharmacol Exp Ther* 192:677, 1975.
29. Kennedy JA, Clark SL: Observations on the physiologic reactions of the ductus arteriosus, *Am J Physiol* 136:140, 1942.
30. Kirkpatrick SE, Pitlick PT, Naliboff J et al: Frank-Starling relationship as an important determinant of fetal cardiac output, *Am J Physiol* 231:495, 1976.
31. Lauer RM, Evans JA, Acki H et al: Factors controlling pulmonary vascular resistance in fetal lamb, *J Pediatr* 67:568, 1965.
32. Leffler CW, Hassler JR, Terrango NA: Ventilation-induced release of prostaglandin-like material from fetal lungs, *Am J Physiol* 238:H282, 1980.
33. Leffler CW, Tyler TL, Cassin S: Effect of indomethacin on pulmonary vascular response to ventilation in fetal goats, *Am J Physiol* 234:H346, 1978.
34. Lind J, Stern L, Wegelius C: *Human foetal and neonatal circulation,* Springfield, Ill, 1964, Charles C Thomas.
35. Lind J, Wegelius C: Changes in circulation at birth, *Acta Paediatr Scand* 41:495, 1952.
36. Lloyd TC Jr: Hypoxic pulmonary vasoconstriction: role of perivascular tissue, *J Appl Physiol* 25:560, 1988.
37. Mentzer RM, Ely SW, Lasley RD, et al: Hormonal role of adenosine in maintaining patency of the ductus arteriosus in the fetal lambs, *Ann Surg* 202:223, 1985.
38. Moss AJ, Emmanouilides GC, Adams FH et al: Response of ductus arteriosus and pulmonary and systemic arterial pressure to changes in oxygen environment in newborn infants, *Pediatrics* 33:937, 1964.
39. Moss AJ, Emmanouilides GC, Duffie ER Jr: Closure of ductus arteriosus, *Lancet* 1:703, 1963.
40. Nasjletti A, Malik KU: Relationship between the Kalli-Krein-Kinen and prostaglandin systems, *Life Sci* 25:99, 1979.
41. Penaloza D, Arias-Stella J, Sime F, et al: The heart and pulmonary circulation in children at high altitudes, *Pediatrics* 34:568, 1964.
42. Prec KJ, Cassels PE: Oxymeter studies in the newborn infants during crying, *Pediatrics* 9:756, 1952.
43. Rao PS: the femoral route for cardiac catheterization of infants and children, *Chest* 63:239, 1973.
44. Rao PS: Perinatal circulatory physiology, *Indian J Pediatr* 58:441, 1991.
45. Rao PS, Solymar L: Transductal balloon angioplasty of coarctation of the aorta in the neonate: preliminary observations, *Am Heart J* 116:1558, 1988.
46. Reynolds SRM: Fetal and neonatal pulmonary vasculature in guinea pig in relation to hemodynamic changes at birth, *Am J Anat* 98:97, 1956.
47. Rudolph AM: The changes in circulation at birth: their importance in congenital heart disease, *Circulation* 41:343, 1970.
48. Rudolph AM: *Congenital diseases of the heart,* Chicago, 1974, Mosby.
49. Rudolph AM: Fetal and neonatal pulmonary circulation, *Annu Rev Physiol* 41:383, 1979.
50. Rudolph AM, Heymann MA: The circulation of the fetus in utero: methods for studying distribution of blood flow, cardiac output, and organ blood flow, *Circ Res* 21:163, 1967.
51. Rudolph AM, Heymann MA: Circulatory changes during growth in the fetal lamb, *Circ Res* 26:289, 1970.
52. Rudolph AM, Scarpalli EM, Golinko RJ et al: Hemodynamic basis for clinical manifestation of patent ductus arteriosus, *Am Heart J* 68:477, 1964.
53. Teitel DF, Iwamoto HS, Rudolph AM: Effect of birth related events on the central flow patterns, *Pediatr Res* 22:557, 1987.

# 3 Extracorporeal Circulation

*Michael S. Vinas*



The application of extracorporeal circulation (ECC) was pioneered by the experiments of Gibbon in 1934. However, it was not until 1953 that the first successful human open-heart procedure, closure of an atrial septal defect, was performed by this surgeon on a young female patient.[4]

It is estimated that there are 250,000 cardiopulmonary bypass (CPB) procedures performed annually in the United States and 400,000 worldwide. Of the number performed in the United States approximately 6% are infant or pediatric interventions.[21]

The conduct of ECC mandates that the cardiovascular perfusionist be experienced with the anatomy and pathophysiology of premature, neonate, infant, and pediatric patients. It is also important to know the corresponding cardiac defect and the corrective or palliative surgical procedure.

A 1990 pediatric perfusion survey cited 127 responses from community, government, and university medical centers performing infant and pediatric open-heart surgery (OHS). The centers reported performing 14,473 OHS procedures requiring ECC.[21] This averages to 114 OHS surgical cases per institute. Stammers and Riley[35] compiled data on over 1016 infant and pediatric patients treated with CPB at University of Michigan Hospitals between 1986 and 1990. They were able to categorize 869 of these into the procedures listed in Table 3–1.

The cardiac surgical procedures and their percentiles will vary from institution to institution. Many community and some university programs do not perform infant and pediatric OHS procedures.

## HEMATOCRIT AND HEMOGLOBIN

The hemoglobin in infants and children ranges between 12.5 and 22 gm/dl.[18] Laboratory values should be assessed serially, since samples obtained

**Table 3–1** Infant and pediatric surgical procedures

| Procedure | Percentage |
|---|---|
| Atrial septal defect | 9.3 |
| Atrial or ventricular septal defect | 2.1 |
| Atrioventricular canal | 8.2 |
| Conduction disturbances | 5.2 |
| Double outlet of the right ventricle | 3.1 |
| Left ventricular outflow tract abnormalities | 9.0 |
| Heart transplantation | 2.1 |
| Hypoplastic left heart syndrome | 6.6 |
| Mitral valve lesions | 2.9 |
| Partial anomalous pulmonary venous return | 1.8 |
| Pulmonary atresia | 3.5 |
| Pulmonary stenosis | 7.9 |
| Tetralogy of Fallot | 12.9 |
| Transposition of the great arteries | 12.5 |
| Truncus arteriosus | 2.3 |
| Ventricular septal defect | 10.7 |

from a fasting patient may vary dramatically from the status in the surgical suite following the fluid reconstitution of the patient by intravenous infusion of crystalloid and/or blood products.

Our 1992 institutional survey depicted an average preoperative hematocrit of 38% plus or minus 3% from patients 1 day to 5 years of age. Patients with compensatory polycythemia were not included. Patients with cyanotic heart disease, for example tetralogy of Fallot, may have nonhemodilutional hematocrit values between 50% and 75%. A nonhemic or asanguinous prime of the heart-lung console circuit may dilute a standard hematocrit to a calculated value of less than 15%, an individual with polycythemia less critical. It is the cardiovascular perfusionist's responsibility to estimate via calculations the degree of hemodilution and any blood product requirements needed to adjust the hematocrit to a value of 20% to 30% or greater during ECC.

Nonhemic primes with circulating hematocrits of 13% to 18% have been reported.[10,18,24,36] Our hemodilutional protocol requires a 30% packed cell volume (PCV) or Hematocrit during ECC for infants, 25% PCV for pediatric patients.

To augment the hematocrit during ECC, an online hemoconcentrator (ultrafilter) should be integrated into the circuit.[17,34,38] Ultrafiltration promotes the elimination of excessive extracellular solutions between 17,000 and 20,000 daltons at a maximum rate of 10 to 30 ml/min. The hematocrit

**Table 3–2** Blood volume in neonate, infant, child, and adult patients

| Patient's age | Blood volume (ml/kg) |
|---|---|
| 0-3 months | 90 |
| 3-6 months | 85 |
| 6-12 months | 80 |
| > 12 months | 70 |

at the termination of ECC should average 25% to 30% or greater to enhance oxygen-carrying capacity and prevent hemodilutional acidosis caused by inadequate oxygen delivery.

## PLASMA VOLUME

Plasma volume contains critical clotting factors, fibrinogen, and platelets. Plasma includes antithrombin III, which is essential for binding to heparin to induce anticoagulation.[43] Plasma volume normally makes up 55% to 65% of estimated blood volume. A 3-kg infant, for example, may have a plasma volume of 180 ml. A 700-ml nonplasma prime would dilute the respective clotting factors, fibrinogen, and platelets below 20%, which is virtually inadequate for proper hemostasis. The plasma volume should be calculated to determine the degree of hemodilution of these factors with the possibility of adding fresh frozen plasma to the extracorporeal circuit.

## HEMODILUTION AND TARGET HEMATOCRIT

Infant and pediatric patients have a higher blood volume factor than adults. This value decreases with human development (Table 3–2). At our institution we have adopted the blood volume factors described in the following table.

Several calculations are required to assess hemodilution and blood product requirements. Assume a patient with a weight of 10 kg, a hematocrit of 40% ($HCT_1$) and an ECC priming volume of 700 ml. The following calculations will derive the patient's predicted blood volume (PBV), red cell mass ($RCM_1$), total system volume (TSV) or ECC circulating volume, hemodilutional hematocrit ($HCT_2$), and hemodilutional or ECC circulating red call mass ($RCM_2$) required.[41]

### Calculations for hemodilution

For a 10-kg patient the predicted blood volume (PBV) is 850 ml (85 ml/kg).

$$\begin{aligned}\text{Patient's red call mass } (RCM_1) &= PBV \times HCT1\\ &= 850 \times 0.40\\ &= 340 \text{ ml}\end{aligned}$$

Hemodilutional hematocrit ($HCT_2$) =
$RCM_1 \div TSV \times 100$
$340 \div 1550 \times 100 = 22\%$

RCM at target or minimally accepted hemodilutional hematocrit at 30% ($RCM_2$) = TSV × HCT
= 1550 × 0.3
= 465 ml

RCM difference ($RCM_1 - RCM_2$) =
340 ($RCM_1$) − 465 ($RCM_2$) = − 125 ml

To achieve a circulating hematocrit of 30%, add 125 ml RCM to the ECC prime.

Due to relative body size, considering the perfusate required to prime the extracorporeal circuit, a neonate or infant will be more adversely affected by hemodilution than a child. Comparing an infant with a pediatric patient with similar hematocrit levels reveals the potential impact of this hemodilution (Table 3–3).

**Table 3–3** Effect of pump prime on hemodilutional HCT in infant and pediatric patients

| | Infant | Pediatric |
|---|---|---|
| Body weight (kg) | 5 | 25 |
| Blood volume factor (ml/kg) | 85 | 70 |
| Estimated blood volume (ml) | 425 | 1750 |
| Hematocrit (%) | 40 | 40 |
| Estimated red cell mass (ml) | 170 | 700 |
| Estimated plasma volume (ml) | 255 | 1050 |
| Prime-extracorporeal circuit (ml) | 700 | 1000 |
| Calculated hemodilutional HCT (%) | 15 | 25 |

## Adenine saline versus citrate phosphate dextrose adenine

As a rule, a unit of packed red blood cells with CPD-A preservation solution contains a volume of 250 ml and hematocrit of 76%. This provides 190 ml (250 × 0.76) of red cell mass or volume. An average unit of adenine saline (ADSOL) preservative solution contains 310 ml with a hematocrit of 59%, or approximately 183 ml of red cell mass (310 × 0.59). The deficit red cell mass divided by these standard figures equals the number of packed red blood cell units to administer. Therefore, a deficit of 125 ml divided by 190 equals 0.65 units of a CPD-A preserved unit of packed red blood cells, 0.68 units if the unit has been preserved with adenine saline. There is not a significant difference in the red cell mass of either unit.

Adenine saline is becoming more prevalent as a blood bank preservative solution for packed red blood cells. This is due to the extended storage period (Table 3–4).

If the patient is under 4 months of age, the CPDA-1 or adenine saline preservative solution is removed and the unit is reconstituted with fresh frozen plasma.

## Fibrinogen dilution

A critical consideration is that of plasma fibrinogen dilution. Normal fibrinogen levels are 150 to 400 mg/dl.[13] Because of the infant or pediatric patient's relatively low blood volume compared with the priming requirements of the ECC circuit, the fibrinogen concentration may be adversely affected. During CPB it is desirable to maintain the plasma fibrinogen concentration above 100 mg/dl to prevent impairment of post-ECC hemostasis.[13]

For example, for a 10-kg patient with a prebypass fibrinogen level of 250 mg/dl, a 40% HCT, and a 700-ml ECC prime volume, additional fi-

**Table 3–4** Characteristics of ADSOL and CPDA-1

| | ADSOL solution AS-1 RBCs | CPDA-1 RBCs | CPDA-1 Whole blood |
|---|---|---|---|
| Storage period (days) | 42 | 35 | 35 |
| In vivo recovery (%) | 82 | 78 | 78 |
| Volume (ml) | 310 | 250 | 513 |
| Hematocrit (%) | 59 | 76 | 37 |
| Red cell mass (ml/unit) | 181 | 190 | 190 |
| pH | 6.65 | 6.6 | 6.7 |
| Potassium (mEq/pack) | 6.2 | 5.2 | 9.0 |
| Sodium (mEq/pack) | 15 | 6 | 50 |
| Glucose (mg/pack) | 717 | 58 | 830 |

brinogen via fresh frozen plasma is calculated as follows:

Patient's blood volume (PBV) = 10 × 85 = 850 ml
Plasma volume = (PBV × 0.60) [1 − (HCT/100)]
= 850 × 0.60 = 510 ml
250 mg/dl or 2.5 mg/ml = patient's fibrinogen level
Total plasma fibrinogen = 510 × 2.5 = 1275 mg
Total system volume = PBV + pump volume
= 510 + 700 = 1210 ml
Fibrinogen level in the total system volume =
1275/1210 = 1.05 mg/ml or 105 mg/100 ml

Therefore, no additional 140 ml of fresh frozen plasma should be administered to raise the ECC fibrinogen level to 100 mg/dl.

### Platelet dilution

Platelet concentration values range from 200,000 to 400,000/mm$^3$. Blood exposure to the foreign components of the extracorporeal circuit, in conjunction with the effects of hemodilution, may further decrease the platelet concentration. This phenomenon may be observed in electron photomicrographs of the arterial filter and blood reservoirs. Albumin added to the ECC circuit reduces platelet aggregation on these foreign surfaces, thus minimizing platelet loss to the ECC circuit.[16] Platelet reconstitution, if indicated, should be reserved until after the bypass to optimize the effects of platelet administration and their contribution to hemostasis.

### Colloidal osmotic pressure and oncotic dilution

The loss or hemodilution of plasma may lead to protein deficiency. Third spacing, the migration of intravascular fluid into the interstitium, which causes edema, should be realized as a possibility during ECC, especially in infants and children. This phenomenon may be deterred by the use of an isooncotic (protein) priming solution. Reductions of the colloidal osmotic pressure (COP) by 30% to 60% during ECC have been reported without chronic complications in the adult patient.[3] However, the literature does not address the same for infant and pediatric patients. The balance of infant priming solution, after the addition of packed red blood cells, whole blood, and/or fresh frozen plasma, should approach isooncotic concentrations.

Assuming a 10-kg patient with a 40% HCT requiring 125 ml of packed red blood cells (PRBCs) and 140 ml of fresh frozen plasma (FFP) with a prime requirement of 700 ml, the estimated hemodilutional COP may be derived by the following:

850 ml = PBV × 0.60 [1 − [HCT/100)] =
510 ml = plasma blood volume

510 ml plasma blood volume + 140 ml
FFP = 650 ml total plasma volume

$$\frac{650 \text{ ml total plasma volume}}{1350 \text{ ml (patient pump noncellular volume)}} \times 25 = 12 \text{ mm Hg}$$

In the example, the COP has been diluted to 12 mm Hg compared with 20 to 25 mm Hg for normal COP if a nononcotic solution is used. Therefore, the remainder of the prime should consist of 5% albumin derived from plasma unless contraindicated.

Pediatric patients not requiring packed red blood cells or fibrinogen via fresh frozen plasma may be administered an isotonic physiologic solution such as Plasmalyte-A, Normosol, or lactated Ringer's. However, the dilution of protein should be considered. Each milliliter of 12.5 gm, 25% albumin is oncotically equivalent to five times its volume of normal human plasma (American Red Cross). Therefore 50 ml may be included to reconstitute 250 ml of crystalloid perfusate to an isooncotic solution.

## COMPOSITION OF THE CIRCULATING FLUID

### Hespan

Hespan (hetastarch 6%) is synthesized by the hydroxyethylation of polysaccharides and approximates the behavior of albumin. It has been used successfully for nonprotein primes of the ECC circuit[28] and as an agent to increase the COP in patients exhibiting hypovolemia circulatory shock.[19] However, being a nonprotein agent, the plasma protein, albumin, and/or COP levels should be monitored along with ionized calcium when employing this agent.

### Crystalloid solutions

In the event that crystalloid priming solutions are administered, they should be pH balanced and isotonic. The electrolyte composition should approach the values of normal blood chemistry to ensure normal electrolyte levels. The clinician should be cognizant of the potential dilution of critical serum electrolytes and pH, as well as osmolarity and the successful resuscitation to normal values. The composition of standard isotonic solutions is compared with that of normal human blood chemistry in Table 3–5.

Calcium may be added to solutions that do not contain it to a value of 100 mg/l. Blood chemicals such as sodium, potassium, magnesium, chloride,

**Table 3–5** Composition of isotonic solutions versus plasma

| | Normosol R | Plasmalyte | Lactated Ringer's | 0.9% NaCL | Human plasma |
|---|---|---|---|---|---|
| **Each 100 ml contains** | | | | | |
| Calcium chloride (mg) | | | 20 | | |
| pH | 7.4 | 7.4 | 6.5 | 5.0 | 7.4 |
| Potassium chloride (mg) | 37 | 30 | 20 | | |
| Sodium acetate (mg) | 222 | 368 | | | |
| Sodium chloride (mg) | 526 | 526 | 600 | 900 | |
| Sodium lactate | | | 310 | | |
| Sodium gluconate (mg) | 502 | 502 | | | |
| Trihydrate USP (mg) | | 37 | | | |
| Acetate (mEq/L) | 27 | 27 | | | |
| Calcium (mEq/L) | | | 3 | | 4.9 |
| Chloride (mEq/L) | 98 | 98 | 109 | 154 | 100 |
| Gluconate (mEq/L) | 23 | 23 | | | |
| Lactate | | | 28 | | |
| Magnesium (mEq/L) | | 3 | 4 | | 1.7 |
| Osmolality (mOsm/L) | 295 | 294 | 273 | 308 | 285 |
| Potassium (mEq/L) | 5 | 5 | 4 | | 4.5 |
| Sodium (mEq/L) | 140 | 140 | 130 | 154 | 140 |

glucose, total protein, and total and ionized calcium should be monitored.[9,14] Typically, some if not all of these components are monitored every 20 to 30 minutes during cardiopulmonary bypass.

Patients with relatively high potassium levels, in renal failure for example, should not be administered solutions containing potassium, or at least caution is advised. Sodium chloride at 0.9%, buffered to a pH of 7.4, may be substituted. Lactated Ringer's solution should not be administered to patients exhibiting clinical signs of lactic acidosis.

### Cardiopulmonary priming compositions

The compositions of priming volumes are as varied as the institutions performing OHS procedures. Some institutions may use lactated Ringer's, Normosol-R or Plasmalyte-A. To this they may add mannitol or furosemide (Lasix), 5% dextrose, 6% hetastarch, albumin, sodium bicarbonate, and sodium heparin.[18,28,37] During neonatal and infant ECC our average prime may be composed of the following:

750 ml *reconstituted red blood cells
1500 units heparin–beef lung
200 mg calcium chloride
15 mEq 8.5% sodium bicarbonate

A nonhemic or asanguinous prime for a pediatric patient not adversely affected by hemodilution may consist of the following:

950 ml Plasmalyte-A (pH 7.4)
2000 units heparin–beef lung
100 mg calcium chloride
50 ml 12.5 gm albumin

## BODY SURFACE AREA

The DuBois and DuBois chart is used to calculate body surface area according to height and weight. The chart is not sex specific. The infant and pediatric version, as well as the adult, is based on the following equation:

$$BSA\ M^2 = [kg^{0.425} \times cm^{0.725}] \times 0.007184$$

The BSA value is used in calculating ECC blood flow rates, basal and hypothermic oxygen requirements, and conversions of pharmacologic doses for infants and children.

## METABOLIC REQUIREMENTS

### Basal oxygen consumption

The basal oxygen consumption in the neonate and infant is higher than in the adult. The respiratory quotient ($Vco_2/Vo_2$) may be reduced by 15%–20% by anesthesia, skeletal muscle paralysis, and mechanical ventilation.[26,31] Hypothermia during ECC further reduces this value.

The basal oxygen consumption of a neonate may vary according to a variety of factors. Extracorporeal flow rate requirements are predicated on the predicted basal and hypothermic oxygen requirements, level of anesthesia, degree of hemodilution, oxygen-carrying capacity, degree of hypothermia, and so on.

Pediatric perfusion groups have reported the application of extracorporeal perfusion flow rate

*Adenine saline or CPD-A removed, 240 ml fresh frozen plasma added to PRBC.

**Table 3–6** Extracorporeal circulation flow rate based on $L/M^2$ and ml/kg

| $L/M^2$ | ml/kg |
|---|---|
| Newborns to 2 yrs = 2.6 × BSA | 2-5 kg, 150 ml/kg |
| 2-4 yrs, 2.5 × BSA | 6-10 kg, 125 ml/kg |
| 4-6 yrs, 2.4 × BSA | 11-15 kg, 100 ml/kg |
| 6-9 yrs, 2.3 × BSA | 16-25 kg, 95 ml/kg |
| >9 yrs, 2.2 × BSA | 26-35 kg, 80 ml/kg |
| | >35 kg, 70 ml/kg |

ranges between 2.2 and 3.21 l/min/$M^2$. Others use 70 to 150 ml/kg/min.[2,18,26,32]

In the flow rate guidelines in Table 3–6 the higher of the two calculations is considered the optimal, and the lower value is considered the minimum flow rate.

Extracorporeal perfusion flow rates are adjusted during hypothermia to ensure adequate arterial and venous oxygen transferability. Oxygen consumption in humans normally decreases at a rate of 7% per degree Celsius. Therefore, decreasing the temperature from 37° C to 30° C reduces oxygen requirements to 50%; the requirement is 25% at 23° C. A pediatric patient with a calculated basal $VO_2$ of 84 ml/min at 37° C may experience a reduction to 42 ml/min at 30° C or 21 ml/min at 23° C via hemodilution and hypothermia. Greeley[15] has reported a 50% to 60% reduction in total body oxygen consumption at 28° C and an 85% to 90% reduction at 18° C.

The following is an estimation of basal perfusion flow rate using a variant of the Fick equation[2]:

$$\frac{\text{Oxygen requirement in ml/min}}{(\text{A} - \text{VO}_2 \text{ saturation}) \times 1.34 \text{ Hgb}} = \text{Perfusion flow rate}$$

Given: Hgb of 10 gm/dl, an arterial saturation of 100%, and a desired venous oxygen saturation of 65%.

$$\frac{42 \text{ ml/min}}{(1 - 0.65) \times 1.34 \times 10 \text{ gm}/100 \text{ ml}} = 896 \text{ ml/min}$$

Satisfactory ECC flow rates should result in acid-base homeostasis without lactic acid production. Such a scenario may be difficult to obtain. Reversal of metabolic acidosis with an 8.4% sodium bicarbonate or tromethamine (THAM) solution is almost always required.

Formulas are subject to estimations and do not allow for alterations in cardiopulmonary and hemodynamic pathophysiology. Adequacy of extracorporeal perfusion flow rates and accommodation of oxygen metabolic requirements necessitate frequent reliable arterial and venous blood gas analysis in conjunction with hematology and chemistry values. The assessment of oxygen delivery versus oxygen consumption via continuous or serial arterial and venous blood gas analysis is advisable to determine the adequacy of perfusion flow rates.

### Pulsatile versus nonpulsatile perfusion

Pulsatile versus nonpulsatile perfusion has been debated for several years. The pulse is generated by a specially designed DeBakey roller pump that can be programmed to deliver an intermittent flow and amplitude that emulates an arterial pressure tracing. Proponents cite improved perfusion to the vital organs, enhanced oxygen use, and decreased systemic vascular resistance.[8]

### Cerebral blood flow

Cerebral activity is dependent on the level of anesthesia and its management as well as the degree of hypothermia. Electroencephalographic monitoring should be considered an adjunct to such management.[22,23]

Recently investigators have been able to measure cerebral metabolic rate for oxygen ($CMRO_2$) and cerebral blood flow (CBF) by direct measurement in neonate, infant, and pediatric patients before, during, and after hypothermic cardiopulmonary bypass with and without deep hypothermic circulatory arrest (DHCA). Brain ischemic tolerance during hypothermia, or hypothermic metabolic index (HMI), has been reported by the same scientists. Based on this index they have reported a predictable "safe" cerebral ischemic time of 11 to 19 minutes at 28° C and 39 to 65 minutes at 18° C.[15]

## EQUIPMENT

### Extracorporeal circuitry

The components for the extracorporeal circuit tubing are selected so as to minimize hemodilution while accommodating blood flow rate requirements without excessive resistance to perfusion flow rates. The tubing of the extracorporeal circuit is clear polyvinyl chloride. The cannula, catheter, and tubing connectors, as well as the casings of the oxygenators, arterial filters, and hemoconcentrators usually are polycarbonate.

The ECC circuit usually comprises the arterial line, arterial pump boot (unless a centrifugal pump is used), venous line, suction lines, and a bubbler or membrane oxygenator. A cardiotomy reservoir with oxygenators such as bubblers and nonintegrated cardiotomy membrane oxygenators is required. Arterial filters should be incorporated to filter particulate matter between 20 and 40 μm as well as gaseous microemboli during ECC.[6,12,21,23,37] The caridiotomy allows for recycling and filtration of blood suctioned from the surgical field. Table 3–7 shows recommended arterial and venous line diameters predicated on the average flow rate requirements of infant and pediatric patients based on weight.[11]

### Arterial cannula and venous catheter sizes

Arterial cannulas are normally inserted into the ascending aorta or femoral artery. The recommended flow rate varies according to length and internal diameter (ID) (Table 3–8). A cannula is selected to provide the recommended ECC perfusion flow rate without excessive resistance that may lead to increased shear stress with resulting hemolysis.[39]

Venous catheters inserted into the right atrium or inferior and superior vena cava must be able to provide total right heart drainage. The average height difference between the tip of the venous cannula and the venous drainage port of the oxygenator is approximately 18 to 20 inches. This differential will produce an average negative hydrostatic pressure of 34 to 37 mm Hg or 46 to 51 cm of water pressure (CWP). This differential may be altered by augmenting the height of the column.

### Venous cannulas

Venous cannulas are manufactured in a variety of diameters (Table 3–9). They may be right-angled or straight and wire-wound or not.

Single venous cannulation of the right atrium is applicable if the patient is subjected to profound hypothermia, decannulation, and circulatory arrest (Table 3–10).

Proper arterial and venous circuitry ensures adequate arterial perfusion without excessive resistance and venous drainage with minimal priming volumes to minimize or prevent blood product usage.

Accidental reversal of arterial and venous lines to the arterial cannula and venous catheters with

**Table 3–7** Recommended arterial and venous line cannulas

| Patient's weight (kg) | Arterial line (ID) | Venous line (ID) |
|---|---|---|
| Up to 6 kg | 3/16″ | 1/4″ |
| 6-12 | 1/4″ | 1/4″ |
| 13-17 | 1/4″ | 5/16″ |
| 18-22 | 1/4″ | 3/8″ |
| 23-32 | 5/16″ | 3/8″ |
| 33-43 | 3/8″ | 3/8″ |
| >43 | 3/8″ | 1/2″ |

**Table 3–8** The flow rates for different sizes of aortic cannulas

| Maximum flow rates (ml/min) | mm | French |
|---|---|---|
| Up to 500 | 2.7 | 8 |
| 500-800 | 3.3 | 10 |
| 700-1600 | 4.0 | 12 |
| 1400-3500 | 5.3 | 16 |
| 3500-5500 | 6.7 | 20 |

**Table 3–9** The flow rates for different sizes of venous cannulas

| DLP—right-angled metal tip, wire wound | | |
|---|---|---|
| Maximum venous flows (ml/min) | SVC F size | IVC F size |
| 700 | 12 | 16 |
| 1400 | 16 | 16 |
| 2000 | 16 | 20 |
| 2700 | 20 | 20 |

**Table 3–10** The flow rates of single venous cannula

| Maximum venous flows (ml/min) | French |
|---|---|
| up to 600 | 18 |
| 600-800 | 20 |
| 800-1200 | 22 |
| 1200-1800 | 24 |
| 1800-2400 | 26 |
| 2400-3000 | 28 |

**Table 3–11** The recommended tubing boot sizes

| Tubing boot size (inches) | Maximum blood flow rate (ml/min) |
|---|---|
| 3/16 × 3/32 | Up to 600 |
| 1/4 × 3/32 | 1,500 |
| 5/16 × 3/32 | 2,200 |
| 3/8 × 3/32 | 3,500 |
| 1/2 × 3/32 | >3,500 |

tubing of the same caliber has been reported. The practice of selecting identical arterial and venous tubing calibers is discouraged to avoid this hazard.

The tubing boot is the portion of the ECC circuit that comes in contact with the DeBakey roller pump head to provide negative flow at the inlet and positive flow on the outlet ports of the tubing raceway (Table 3–11). Some tubing boots consist of silicon rubber (Silastic), others of polyvinyl chloride.

Circuits bonded or coated with heparin are available from several manufacturers. These circuits present evidence of increased biocompatibility with a corresponding decreased heparin requirement as well as complement activation.[1,42]

### Bubbler versus membrane oxygenator

The debate continues concerning the use of bubbler versus membrane oxygenators. Many authors have reported that there is virtually no difference in the two systems for procedures lasting less than 3 hours. However, bubbler oxygenators have a direct blood to gas (100% oxygen) interface that is not conducive to extended cardiopulmonary bypass. The fractional inspired oxygen concentration is not adjustable in bubbler oxygenators, which is a concern during ECC of the premature infant. Retrolental fibroplasia is caused by hyperoxia-induced vasoconstriction of the retinal arteries. Permanent retinal damage has been reported when arterial oxygen pressure is greater than 110 for longer than 1 to 2 hours.

Semipermeable polypropylene membrane oxygenators, on the other hand, do not have a direct blood to gas interface. These oxygenators may be used for more than 3 hours of ECC, with recommendations up to 6 hours. The exception is with extracorporeal membrane oxygenator (ECMO) applications. The SciMed or Kolobow Lung, which is composed of a silicone rubber membrane oxygenator, is the only alternative for extracorporeal circulation lasting several days.

Listed are the more common polypropylene infant and pediatric membrane oxygenators (Table 3–12). Note that the Cobe VPCML is a two-compartment folded-sheet polypropylene membrane. The first compartment may accommodate infant, and the second pediatric, perfusion flow rates. The two compartments combined may accommodate large pediatric or small adult ECC flow rates.

Several refinements in recent years, including increased affordability, have made the membrane oxygenator increasingly popular with the cardiovascular perfusion community. The membrane oxygenator has proved to be a safe, reliable product with predictable performance and improved arterial and venous blood sampling capabilities.

### ECC priming volumes

The amount of priming volume for infant and pediatric circuits is dependent on the size of arterial and venous lines, static prime of the oxygenator, and any accessories incorporated, such as prebypass and arterial filters, hemoconcentrators, ECC arterial line pressure monitoring devices, and so on. The following are standard priming volumes for average infant and pediatric extracorporeal circuits.

***Infant ECC circuit.*** Volume, 700 ml; 3⁄16-inch arterial line; 1⁄4-inch arterial boot, 1⁄4-inch venous line with an integrated membrane oxygenator.

***Pediatric ECC circuit.*** Volume, 1000 ml; 1⁄4-inch arterial line, 1⁄4-inch arterial boot, 3⁄8-inch venous line with an integrated membrane oxygenator. Extracorporeal circuit priming volumes vary according to the components and accessories used. The values presented are an average depiction of typical infant and pediatric ECC circuits providing

**Table 3–12** Various types of membrane oxygenators

| | | Membrane surface | Static maximum | |
|---|---|---|---|---|
| **Manufacturer** | **Model** | **Area-M²** | **Prime (ml)** | **Flow rate (L/min)** |
| Cobe | VPCML Plus | 0.40 | 142 | 1.3 |
| Cobe | VPCML Plus | 0.85 | 283 | 2.7 |
| Cobe | VPCML Plus | 1.25 | 425 | 4.0 |
| Medtronic | Minimax | 0.60 | 140 | 1.5 |
| SARNS | SMO/INF | 0.70 | 170 | 2.5 |
| SciMed | 0.60 | 0.60 | 90 | 1.0 |
| SciMed | 0.80 | 0.80 | 100 | 1.2 |
| Shiley | Plexus 2.0 | 0.42 | 135 | 2.0 |
| Shiley | Plexus 3.5 | 0.62 | 160 | 3.5 |
| Terumo | 308 | 0.80 | 80 | 0.8 |

200 to 300 ml residual volume in the perfusate reservoir.

### Central and online pressure monitoring

An ECC arterial line pressure transducer or manometer with a fluid-blood barrier should be integrated to monitor the ECC arterial line pressure. During ECC the delivery pressure should not exceed 300 mm Hg. Occasionally the arterial cannula may be displaced. Excessive line pressures may indicate the problem. Also, during and post CPB, a peripheral arterial line pressure may be dampened via vasoconstriction. The ECC arterial line pressure may be used to determine whether there is a pressure differential, thus avoiding the treatment of a pseudohypotensive event. Pressure monitoring devices may also be used to monitor the pressure drop across a membrane oxygenator. The pressure drop should not exceed 100 mm Hg at full flow rates.

## BLOOD PRODUCT REQUIREMENTS

Fresh heparinized, recalcified whole blood drawn less than 24 hours prior to ECC is the preferred perfusate for the prime of neonatal and infant extracorporeal circuits requiring blood products. Fresh whole blood contains viable elements in the plasma for post-ECC hemostasis. These factors deteriorate precipitously after 24 hours and are in effect nonfunctional after 48 to 72 hours. If citrated fresh whole blood is not available, packed red blood cells may be reconstituted with fresh frozen plasma. However, reconstituted blood lacks platelets and may have to be replaced after the bypass, depending on blood platelet concentration.

Most packed red blood cells are preserved in CPD-A or adenine saline preservative solution. The blood bank preservation solution should be removed and replaced with either saline or fresh frozen plasma if the infant is less than 4 months of age. Irradiated blood poses a special problem. Irradiation destroys leukocytes and lymphocytes. Blood units that have been irradiated and stored longer than 24-48 hours will contain excessive levels of potassium that may be sufficient to induce cardiac arrest during the initiation of ECC. As a precaution the plasma or preservative solution should be removed from these units to eliminate the possibility of hyperkalemia.

## PRIMING CONSIDERATIONS

Once the required perfusion flow rate, blood volume, and hemodilutional data have been obtained, the extracorporeal circuit is designed. An updated hematocrit should be obtained in the surgical suite to determine whether hemodilution from intravenous fluids has changed the predicted hemodilutional and target hematocrit. On occasion the reported hematocrit before fasting may vary 10% to 15% from the updated hematocrit prior to bypass. In this event all calculations must be refigured and additional blood products may be needed.

### Hypothermia

Bigelow in 1949 suggested the use of hypothermia in conjunction with intracardiac surgery requiring circulatory arrest.[26] Today most cardiac surgical cases are performed during hypothermia between 18° and 22° C. The lower temperatures decrease the basal metabolic rate and provide myocardial protection. Cooling and rewarming the patient are accomplished by subjecting the perfusate in the oxygenator to an integrated heating and cooling coil. The regulated water temperature circulates countercurrent to the perfusate for maximum efficiency.

Hypothermia, among other factors, causes the oxyhemoglobin dissociation curve to shift to the left. This readily binds the hemoglobin to the oxygen. This leftward shift is observed while monitoring venous blood oxygen saturation levels during normothermia versus hypothermia. A shift of the oxyhemoglobin dissociation curve to the right presents the opposite effect.[26,37]

### Deep hypothermic circulatory arrest and profound hypothermia

Infants under 12 months or 10 kg body weight who undergo profound hypothermia and circulatory arrest may be precooled with a Subramanian Cooling Chamber. Another possibility is systemic hypothermia via ECC. The patient's head should be packed in ice. The Subramanian device externally cools the patient to 30° C. All patients scheduled for circulatory arrest are administered dextran 40 at 10 ml/kg to prevent aggregation of blood elements at the hypothermic ranges encountered, usually 18° to 20° C.

## PREBYPASS RECIRCULATION OF THE PERFUSATE

Infant circuits will most certainly require blood products. An asanguinous extracorporeal circuit prime would hemodilute the patient to hematocrit levels approaching 15% or less. The addition of banked blood products will yield an extremely acidotic prime. Once the prime is circulated and vented, the pH of the perfusate will approach 7 or below, depending on the carbon dioxide pressure value. The base excess is approximately minus 20. However, the base excess value should be used to calculate the amount of sodium bicarbonate required to adjust the pH to 7.4. The following is a calculation for the amount of bicarbonate required to buffer an acidotic prime:

$HCO_3$ (mEq) =
amount of perfusate (L) × base excess (ABS)

The $H^+$ ions in the acidotic prime will combine with $H_2CO_3^-$ to form $H_2CO_3^-$ carbonic acid. This further dissociates into carbon dioxide and water. Immediate dissociation may produce carbon dioxide pressure values in excess of 70 to 80 mm Hg. Therefore the prime should be ventilated for several minutes to reduce the associated hypercapnia of the perfusate.

## HEPARINIZATION

Beef lung sodium heparin is the anticoagulant of choice during ECC. It inhibits thrombin formation and blood coagulation factors Xa, IXa, and XIa. An average dose is 300 IU/kg to obtain an activated clotting time over 400 seconds.[37] It is preferable to perform a heparin titration analysis or the Bull protocol to determine heparin resistance or sensitivity. During ECC an activated clotting time should be performed every 30 minutes to determine that anticoagulation exceeds 400 seconds. Bull concluded that the response to heparin administration is linear. Therefore, once a dose-response curve is established, addition of heparin or reversal with protamine is a matter of plotting the heparin dose-response graph.[5]

## PHARMACOLOGIC CONSIDERATIONS

As a rule, dividing the pediatric patient's BSA ($M^2$) by 1.7 $M^2$ will derive the pediatric equivalent (Orlando). Thus, a pediatric patient with a BSA of 0.56 $M^2$ would require 33% (0.56/1.7) of an adult drug dose. However, the circuit should be considered as an adjunct to the patient during ECC. Therefore, an infant with a blood volume of 700 ml and a circulating prime of 700 ml should be considered as having a blood volume of 1400 ml, since a pharmacologic agent will be diluted to 50% of its strength predicated on hemodilution. An isooncotic perfusate will have a weight approximating 1 mg/ml. Therefore, a 700-ml prime will weigh 700 gm. This is the equivalent blood volume of an 8.2 kg patient (700 ml/85 ml/kg blood volume factor).

## INITIATION OF EXTRACORPOREAL CIRCULATION

After the administration of sodium heparin, the heart-lung machine arterial pumphead should be increased to the patient's maximum blood flow rate, and the lines should be tapped to dislodge residual air bubbles. The surgical assistant at the operative field should do likewise. The ECC should be slowly terminated and the arterial and venous lines clamped. Three to 5 minutes after heparin administration, the heart-lung machine pump sucker may be activated to recover mediastinal shed blood. Once aortic and vena cava cannulation has been achieved and the arterial and venous lines connected, the patient is prepared for ECC.

Upon initiation of ECC the patient's arterial blood pressure will generally be between 30 and 40 mm Hg with full flow rates. The perfusion pressure should be kept between 50 and 70 mm Hg to maintain adequate cerebral perfusion at normocapnia levels.[25]

Many surgeons prefer to cool the patient immediately to the target temperature, thus decreasing metabolic rate. If circulatory arrest is the goal, an arteriovenous (AV) blood gas sample is obtained after 5 minutes of cardiopulmonary bypass to assess oxygenation and acid-base status. Any acidotic pH, carbon dioxide pressure, and base excess levels are adjusted immediately, prior to circulatory arrest. If the patient is not to be subjected to circulatory arrest, it is advisable to obtain a routine blood gas profile after 5 minutes of ECC or upon obtaining the target temperature.

Hypothermia increases the solubility and affinity of oxygen and carbon dioxide. The pK and thus the pH are also affected, causing the oxyhemoglobin dissociation curve to shift to the left. Hyperthermia has the opposite effect.[31]

The correction of membrane oxygen pressures may be accomplished by the reduction of the fractional inspired oxygen concentration (percent of oxygen divided by 100). A bubbler oxygenator does not allow this feature, and oxygen pressure in excess of 300 to 400 mm Hg may be experienced. Carbon dioxide pressures may be adjusted with this formula[7]:

Adjusted gas flow =
(Measured $P_{CO_2}$ ÷ target $P_{CO_2}$) × gas flow

## ANALYSIS OF BLOOD GAS SAMPLES

There are two methods for analyzing blood gas samples during ECC: alpha-stat and pH-stat. Alpha-stat measures the blood gas sample at 37° C regardless of the patient. pH-stat measures the blood gas sample at 37° C, then adjusts for the temperature change of the patient (Tables 3–13 and 3–14). Some authors cite that the increased carbon dioxide pressure levels caused by the pH-stat method are responsible for increased cerebral blood flow during ECC. Others dispute this theory and advocate the alpha-stat method as safer for reporting ECC AV blood gases.[20,27,31]

A 1990 pediatric perfusion survey documented that approximately 80% of the reported surgical centers used alpha-stat. The remaining 20% used the pH-stat method. Some centers reported blood

**Table 3–13** pH and $Pco_2$ values of alpha-stat method

| | 37°C | Actual results (temp. corrected to 25°C) |
|---|---|---|
| Normothermia | pH, 7.4 | pH, 7.4 |
| | $Pco_2$, 40 | $Pco_2$, 40 |
| Hypothermia | pH, 7.4 | pH, 7.57 |
| | $Pco_2$, 40 | $Pco_2$, 23 |

Alpha-stat perfusion goal is constant blood $CO_2$ content

A. Hypothermia will increase $CO_2$ plasma solubility.
B. To maintain constant $CO_2$ content during cooling, more carbon dioxide must be removed than with pH-stat.
C. To maintain constant $CO_2$ content, the gas ventilation rate will be higher than with pH-stat.

**Table 3–14** pH and $Pco_2$ values of pH-stat method

| | 37°C | Actual results (temp. corrected to 25°C) |
|---|---|---|
| Normothermia | pH, 7.4 | pH, 7.4 |
| | $Pco_2$, 40 | $Pco_2$, 40 |
| Hypothermia | pH, 7.22 | pH, 7.4 |
| | $Pco_2$, 67 | $Pco_2$, 40 |

pH stat perfusion goal is constant pH/increasing $CO_2$ content

A. pH stat corrects all blood gases to the patient's temperature (hypothermia samples not at 37°C)
B. Goal: maintain $Pco_2$ at 40 mm Hg (pt. temp. corr.)
   Maintain pH at 7.4 (pt. temp. corr.)
C. Increasing levels of hypothermia and corresponding $CO_2$ plasma solubility will increase total $CO_2$ content to maintain temperature-corrected Pco of 40 mm/Hg

gas values using both methods. Ironically, the AV content difference does not change, possibly as a result of the shift of the oxyhemoglobin dissociation curve.

On-line or continuous AV oxygen blood gas monitoring has been available clinically for the past several years. These devices allow for continuous display of pH, oxygen and carbon dioxide pressures, base excess and hematocrit.[29,31] Some online monitors analyze electrolytes.[29] A survey reported that 62% of the infant and pediatric cardiac surgical centers used on-line AV blood gas monitoring.[21]

Correction of metabolic acidosis via sodium bicarbonate is obtained by application of the American Heart Association standard for sodium bicarbonate administration:

$$[\text{Body weight (kg)} \times 0.3] \times \text{base excess} \div 2$$

One vital factor that is often ignored is the addition of the ECC circuit volume to the calculation. This is critical in the neonate. For example a 3-kg patient attached to a 700-ml ECC circuit presents the following, given a base excess of minus 6 during ECC:

$$(3 \text{ kg} \times 0.30) \times 6 \div 2 = 2.7 \text{ mEq of } NaHCO_3$$

The addition of a 700-ml prime to obtain the total system volume alters this figure:

$$[(3 \text{ kg} \times 0.3) + 0.7] \times 6 \div 2 = 4.8 \text{ mEq of } NaHCO_3$$

Nearly 78% of additional sodium bicarbonate is required in comparison with the dose from the previous calculation. Therefore it is imperative that ECC prime be considered as an adjunct to the neonate, infant, and pediatric total body water for correct reversal of acidosis.

## REWARMING DURING EXTRACORPOREAL CIRCULATION

When the surgical procedure is complete or near completion, the surgeon will give the command to rewarm the patient. The heating blanket and the heater-cooler are activated. The temperature of the water in the heat exchanger should not exceed 42° C and a gradient versus the patient's blood temperature should be 12° C in an adult, 8° C in the pediatric patient.

As the patient is rewarmed, the solubility of oxygen decreases and the metabolic oxygen demands of the patient increase. Therefore, during rewarming the patient's blood flow rates and fractional inspired oxygen concentration are increased at incremental rates. Carbon dioxide production is less prevalent during rewarming than during normothermia and cooling. Therefore caution must be used not to hyperventilate the patient and induce hypocapnia. This is especially likely when the anesthesiologist is ventilating the patient while the patient is on partial bypass. Partial bypass occurs when some of the venous return is diverted to the right ventricle and ejected into the pulmonary system. Rewarming times vary with the size of the patient and the level of hypothermia, and 25 to 45 minutes may be necessary to obtain a 37° C core temperature. Warming the room to 70° to 75° F enhances rewarming and reduces the possibility of post-bypass hypothermia.

**Table 3–15** Infant and pediatric intraaortic balloon catheters

| Balloon/prefill volume (cc) | Catheter size (French) | Approximate age range | Approximate weight range |
|---|---|---|---|
| 2.5/6 | 4.5 | <1 yr | 3–8 kg |
| 5.0/10 | 5.5 | 1–2.5 yrs | 8–13 kg |
| 7.0/12 | 5.5 | 2.5–5 yrs | 13–18 kg |
| 12.0/17 | 7.0 | 5–12 yrs | 18–40 kg |
| 20.0/26 | 7.0 | >12 yrs | >40 kg |

## BALANCE VOLUME

The balance volume should be estimated following cardiopulmonary bypass. The balance volume is the input volume minus the output volume. The amount of perfusate required to prime the extracorporeal circuit delivers a circulating volume at the required maximum perfusion flow rate, usually 200 to 300 ml in the AV reservoir. At static, or resting, volume the amount may be 50 to 100 ml higher because of the compliance of the circuit during circulation. The balance volume is computed by adding the difference between the input volume and the output volume to the static or resting volume. For example, given a 5-kg patient with a perfusate prime of 700 ml and a resting volume of 300 ml, calculate the input versus output as follows:

| | | |
|---|---|---|
| Static volume | 300 ml | |
| Input volume | | |
| Cardioplegia | 50 ml | |
| Added volume | 100 ml | |
| | = 150 ml | |
| Output volume | | |
| Floor suction | 150 ml | (floor suction minus irrigation) |
| Urine output | + 10 ml | |
| Residual volume | + 75 ml | (equals the volume required to wet the surface of the ECC circuitry) |
| | = 235 ml | |
| Input − output | 150 ml | input volume |
| | = 235 ml | output volume |
| Balance | − 85 ml | |

## DEPRIMING THE PERFUSATE OF THE ECC CIRCUIT

If ECC is terminated with minimal blood loss, the ECC perfusate may be salvaged. This is performed by circulating the remaining volume into a sterile transfusion transfer pack at the surgical field or using a stopcock adaptor for attaching a transfer pack onto the AV manifold of a membrane oxygenator. Either way the volume in the venous and arterial lines may be emptied into the blood reservoir. The perfusate is then slowly circulated into the transfer pack until reaching the zero level in the reservoir. Attach a 1-liter bag of Plasmalyte-A or similar physiologic solution, then chase the perfusate through the system. An infant circuit should recover an additional 500 ml, a pediatric, 750 ml, via chasing a physiologic solution through the system.

## INTRAAORTIC BALLOON COUNTERPULSATION

Intraaortic balloon counterpulsation is used to increase oxygen delivery to the heart via increased coronary perfusion while decreasing oxygen demands through mechanical afterload reduction. This is accomplished by augmenting the tension time index (TTI) and diastolic pressure index (DPI) ratio[3,37]:

$$\frac{\text{DPI}}{\text{TTI}} = \frac{\text{Supply}}{\text{Demand}}$$

If properly timed, the diastolic augmentation increases myocardial oxygen supply via increased perfusion to the coronaries while decreasing the myocardial oxygen demand by reducing the resistance caused by afterload by deflating the balloon just prior to isovolumetric contraction.

Intraaortic balloon catheters are available in infant and pediatric sizes (Table 3–15).[30,32,40] The reported use of intraaortic balloon counterpulsation in infant and pediatric patients is not nearly so frequent as with adults.

The application of extracorporeal circulation or cardiopulmonary bypass is complex. Infant and pediatric patients present many variables not readily addressed during ECC for adults. The clinician must be cognizant of the pathophysiology of the defect, the cardiac catheterization values, and cardiopulmonary, hemodynamic, hematologic, and chemistry data.

Much preparation is required to assess the influence of hemodilution and to accommodate the basal metabolic rate of the mechanically ventilated anesthetized patient during normothermia and hypothermia. Oxygen consumption, perfusion flow rates, ECC circuitry, effects of hemodilution, the reconstitution of hemodiluted blood, hematocrit, and coagulation factors are all critical. All computational data must be checked and rechecked to prevent an error that may result in ECC mismanagement with catastrophic results.

## REFERENCES


1. Bennett J, Hill J, Long W et al: Biocompatible circuits: an adjunct to noncardiac extracorporeal cardiopulmonary support, *J Extr Corp Circ* 24:6, 1992.
2. Berryessa R, Hydrick D, McCormick J et al: Refinements in pediatric perfusion, *J Extr Corp Circ* 18:140, 1986.
3. Beshere GA, Camerlengo LJ, Dearing JP: Estimation of colloid osmotic pressure during hemodilutional cardiopulmonary bypass, *J Extr Corp Tech* 14:381, 1982.
4. Bone DK, William WH, Hatcher CR: Techniques of cardiopulmonary bypass and its complications. In Hurst JW, editor: *The heart,* New York, 1982, McGraw-Hill.
5. Bull B, Huse W, Brauer FS: Heparin therapy during extracorporeal circulation II: the use of a dose curve to individualize heparin and protamine dosage, *J Thorac Cardiovasc Surg* 69:685, 1975.
6. Butler BD: Gaseous micro emboli: concepts and considerations, *J Extr Corp Circ* 15:148, 1983.
7. Cameriengo LJ, Dearing JP: Precise control of $Pco_2$ during cardiopulmonary bypass, *J Extr Corp Tech* 13:183, 1981.
8. Casper M: Pulsatile flow during cardiopulmonary bypass: is it beneficial? *J Extr Corp Circ* 20:25, 1988.
9. Chernow B, Smith J, Rainey T et al: Hypomagnesemia: implications for the critical care specialist, *Crit Care Med* 10:193, 1982.
10. Conley JC, Zografos CA: Bloodless prime in pediatric cardiopulmonary bypass circuits, *J Extr Corp Tech* 23:80, 1991.
11. Courtney PH, Wansley DE, Heath BJ: Three-sixteenth inch perfusion tubing: a new concept for the pediatric patient, *J Extr Corp Tech* 191:100, 1987.
12. Demierre D, Maass D, Turina M: ECC sources of gaseous microemboli, *J Extr Corp Tech* 17:20, 1985.
13. Ecklund JM, Riley JB, Sutton RG et al: Estimation of fibrinogen concentration during extracorporeal circulation in pediatric cardiac surgery, *J Extr Corp Tech* 23:72, 1992.
14. Graziano CC, Howland WS, Kahn RC et al: Calcium chloride administration in normocalcemic critically ill patients, *Crit Care Med* 8:209, 1980.
15. Greeley WJ, Kern FH, Ungerleider RM et al: The effect of hypothermic cardiopulmonary bypass and total circulatory arrest on cerebral metabolism in neonates, infants, and children, *J Thorac Cardiovasc Surg* 101:783, 1991.
16. Gurjar U, Bowman JM: Prevention of platelet adhesion to extracorporeal surfaces, *J Extr Corp Circ* 16:104, 1984.
17. Han YQ, Zhu DM, Su ZK: Ultrafiltration in pediatric cardiac surgical procedures, *J Extr Corp Tech* 23:63, 1992.
18. Hartley-Winkler M, Lamberti JJ, Rohrer C: Perfusion considerations for infants weighing 10 kg or less, *J Extr Corp Tech* 17:31, 1985.
19. Haupt MT, Rackow EC: Colloid osmotic pressure and fluid resuscitation with hetastarch, albumin and saline solutions, *Crit Care Med* 10:159, 1982.
20. Hering JP, Schroder T, Singer D et al: Influence of pH management on hemodynamics and metabolism in moderate hypothermia, *J Thorac Cardiovasc Surg* 104:1388, 1992.
21. Hill AG, Groom RC, Bechara F et al: 1990 Pediatric perfusion survey II: expanded multivariate data analysis, *Proceedings of the American Academy of Cardiovascular Perfusion* 12:96, 1991.
22. Kern FH, Jonas RA: Temperature monitoring during CPB in infants: does it predict efficient brain cooling? *Ann Thorac Surg* 54:749, 1992.
23. Massimino RJ, Gough JD, Stearns GT et al: Gaseous emboli removal efficiency in arterial screen filters: a comparative study, *J Extr Corp Tech* 15:25, 1983.
24. McCormick JS, Berryessa RG, Clark DR et al: Lactic acid generation during pediatric cardiopulmonary bypass: a comparison of blood and crystalloid primes, *J Extr Corp Tech* 26:84, 1988.
25. Miller MF, Luckenbach J, Chen C: Clinical evaluation of a new saturation/hematocrit monitor, *J Extr Corp Tech* 24:55, 1992.
26. Mitchell BA: Optimal perfusion flow rates for cardiopulmonary bypass, *J Extr Corp Tech* 22:165, 1990.
27. Murkin JM: Alpha-stat versus pH-stat: implications for the brain during cardiopulmonary bypass, *J Extr Corp Tech* 22:137, 1990.
28. Palanzo DA, Martin GT, Gough JD et al: Hetastarch as a clear prime for cardiopulmonary bypass, *J Extr Corp Tech* 16:55, 1984.
29. Parault BG, Conrad SA: The effect of extracorporeal circulation time and patient age on platelet retention during cardiopulmonary bypass: a comparison of roller and centrifugal pumps, *J Extr Corp Tech* 2:34, 1991.
30. Pennington DG, Swartz MT: Circulatory support in infants and children, *Ann Thorac Surg* 55:233, 1993.
31. Riley JB, Justison GA: Alpha-stat and pH-stat management techniques in artificial blood oxygenators, *J Extr Corp Tech* 16:77, 1984.
32. Roberts CP, McCarthy P, Wildman D et al: Left ventricular assist with the Bio-Medicus pump on a 4-month-old infant with anomalous left coronary artery, *J Extr Corp Tech* 21:73, 1989.
33. Rung GW: Thiopental as an adjunct to hypothermia for EEG suppression in infants prior to circulatory arrest, *J Cardiothorac Vasc Anesth* 5:337, 1992.
34. Shannon T, Truog R, Harmon W et al: A prospective analysis of creatinine clearance during ECMO and ultrafiltration, *J Extr Corp Tech* 23:90, 1992.
35. Stammers AH, Riley JB: Does cardioplegia protection of the pediatric heart vary according to the cardiac defect? *J Extr Corp Tech* 23:8, 1992.
36. Stammers AH, Bove EL: The Neonatal Heart: Developmental Differences to Ischemia, and Protection during Cardiopulmonary Bypass. *J Extr Corp Tech* 18:210, 1986.
37. Taylor KM: Cardiopulmonary bypass, Principles and Management. Williams and Wilkins, Baltimore, MD, 1990.
38. Traynor L, Sutton R, Riley J et al: Comparing Ultrafiltration and Centrifugation During and After Pediatric Cardiopulmonary Bypass. *J Extr Corp Tech* 23:140, 1992.
39. Van Meurs KP, Mikesell GT, Seale WR et al: Maximum Blood Flow Rates for Arterial Cannulae Used in Neonatal ECMO, *ASAIO Trans* 36:679, 1990.
40. Veasy GL, Blalock BA, Orth JL et al: Intra-Aortic Balloon Pumping in Infants and Children, *Circulation* 68:1095, 1983.
41. Vinas MS: The Volume Allowance Formula as a Guide to Non-Haemic Solution Administration, *J Extr Corp Tech* 22:70, 1990.
42. von Segesser LK, Turina M: Cardiopulmonary Bypass without Systemic Heparinization, *J Cardiovasc Surg* 98:386, 1989.
43. Zimmerman J, Baugh R: Heparinsase in Hemostasis Management, *Perfusion Review* 1:8, 1992.

# 4 Deep Hypothermia and Circulatory Arrest

*James Phythyon*



Profound hypothermia for circulatory arrest is a technique that has achieved considerable popularity over the past 2 decades. It is designed for the operative management of small children undergoing surgical procedures for the correction of complex congenital cardiac defects. The technique allows nearly ideal conditions for the operating surgeon—a still, bloodless heart wherein no cannulae obstruct either the view of or the access to the heart.

## HISTORY

The first use of induced hypothermia for the problems of cardiac surgery was by McQuiston[7] in 1949. Severely cyanotic children undergoing heart surgery were made hypothermic on the assumption that hypothermia would decrease metabolic rate and hence oxygen consumption to a par with available oxygen supply. This would increase the duration of hypoxia that the children could tolerate without causing irreversible tissue or organ damage.

In 1950 Bigelow and his associates[3] published a series of investigations on experimental animals. They showed that a period of cessation of the circulation could be lengthened according to the degree to which hypothermia had depressed the metabolism. Dogs that had been cooled to 30° C were able to survive 8 to 10 minutes of circulatory arrest in contrast to the allowable 3 to 4 minutes at normothermia. By 1959 Drew and his associates[4] had shown that the period of circulatory arrest could be extended to 60 minutes at nasopharyngeal (presumably brain) temperatures of 10° C. These results are in keeping with the general trend reported by virtually all investigators in the field. They follow the general tenet of van't Hoff's law, which states that chemical reaction rates double for each 10° C increase in temperature and halve for each corresponding decrease.

More recently, Hickey and Anderson[5] have argued that the decreases in cerebral metabolic rates and oxygen consumption induced by hypothermia are insufficient to explain cerebral tolerance to ischemia. Decreased flow rates at hypothermic levels induce an increased level of oxygen extraction by the brain at the expense of other areas of the body. If intracellular pH is allowed to rise in the cold (see section on gas transport later in this chapter) in keeping with fundamental theory as proposed by Rahn, Reeves, and Howell[11] in 1975, high-energy phosphate levels are maintained within the cell, and this preservation is an important mechanism in hypothermic protection.

These initial applications of hypothermia achieved by surface cooling were combined with circulatory arrest in the early 1950s. The advent of extracorporeal circulation in the 1960s all but led to the abandonment of surface cooling. Repairs could be accomplished by cardiopulmonary bypass combined with moderate core cooling. However, in the late 1960s Hikasa and associates[6] reintroduced surface cooling. They followed surface cooling by core cooling using cardiopulmonary bypass and a heat exchanger to produce profound hypothermia. They were seeking to enlarge the numbers and variety of congenital lesions amenable to operative repair. It is now generally agreed that initial surface cooling followed by core cooling produces more even total body cooling than core cooling alone, which may allow some peripheral areas isolated by reflex vasoconstriction to remain uncooled. Modifications quickly followed and the modern technique was enunciated by Barratt-Boyes and colleagues[1] in 1971.

## DEFINITIONS

The defined levels of hypothermia were proposed by Okamura[10] in 1969. They are shown in Table 4–1.

The transition of an unanesthetized infant at normothermia to a state of circulatory arrest at 18° C can be divided into two stages. The first of these stages, surface cooling under general anesthesia and muscle paralysis, is less easily controlled and thus more dangerous than the second stage, that of core cooling with a pump oxygenator and a heat exchanger. The danger of sudden ventricular fibrillation and consequent failure of the circulation no longer pertains. The physiologic changes brought about as hypothermia deepens admit no such clear-cut dichotomy.

## PHYSIOLOGIC CONSIDERATIONS

### The antimetabolic effect of hypothermia

Many estimates of the antimetabolic effect of hypothermia have been made. All of them vary slightly according to conditions, but all are in substantial agreement that within limits cold suppresses oxygen consumption. Metabolic energy is ultimately derived from the oxidation of substrates to carbon dioxide and water. Investigators have generally chosen to measure oxygen consumption rather than carbon dioxide production because of the hideous complexity of dealing with its changing solubility in the cold and the shifting characteristics of various buffer systems in the cold. This choice allows the possibility of error in that lactate metabolism may supervene, but estimates of this anaerobic effect can be computed from the changes in base deficit.

These estimates of the antimetabolic effect of hypothermia achieve a general agreement that oxygen consumption falls approximately 7% for each 1° C drop in core temperature. The data provided by Benazon[2] and Nagashima[9] vary slightly but achieve considerable agreement at 18° C (Fig. 4–1).

Not surprisingly, survival times in humans have never been accurately determined. Allowable durations of circulatory arrest have been guided by evidence derived from experimental animals. Most investigators are of the opinion that the younger the subject, the higher the degree of tolerance to circulatory arrest. The data provided by Swan[12] and Benazon[2] again achieve considerable agreement (Table 4–2).

### Effects on the central nervous system

Cooling slows all nervous system activity, including conduction velocity in peripheral nerves. Thus, central function slows and narcosis supervenes in the range of 25° C to 28° C. Anesthetic requirements thus become negligible. Electroencephalo-

**Table 4–1** Levels of hypothermia

| Level | Temperature (°C) |
|---|---|
| Mild hypothermia | 30–37 |
| Moderate hypothermia | 25–30 |
| Deep hypothermia | 20–25 |
| Profound hypothermia | 10–20 |
| Severe hypothermia | Less than 10 |

**Table 4–2** Survival times in relation to body temperature

| | Survival time, minutes | |
|---|---|---|
| Body temp (°C) | Swan | Benazon |
| >32 | | 3–9 |
| 30 | 4–5 | |
| 29 | 8–10 | 9–15 |
| 22 | 16–20 | 15–45 |
| <18 | 32–80 | 45–60 |

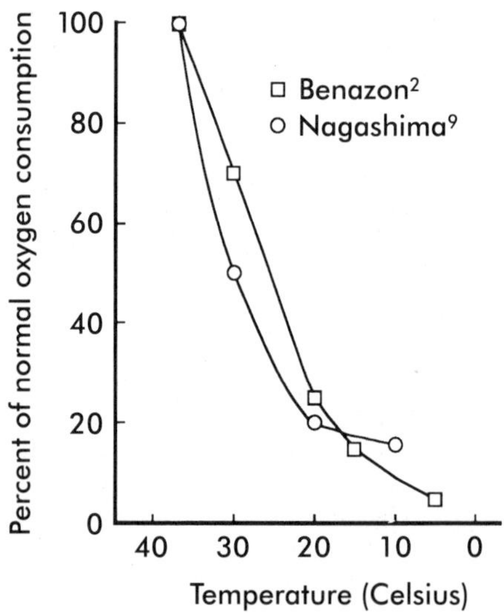


**Figure 4–1** Effect of hypothermia on oxygen consumption.

graphic activity disappears in the range of 15° C to 20° C whether or not circulatory arrest ensues. Cerebrospinal fluid pressure and brain size both decrease.

### Respiratory function

Should ventilation not be controlled, respiratory depression ensues and is enhanced by most anesthetic agents. Spontaneous ventilation ceases or becomes negligible at about 20° C. Dead space increases because of bronchial dilatation, and there may be a mismatch between ventilation and perfusion.

### Blood and gas transport

Cold increases the solubility of both oxygen and carbon dioxide in the blood. The ionization constant of water increases as temperature falls so that the maintenance of electroneutral concentrations of hydrogen and hydroxyl ions requires a gradually increasing pH. This is necessary to maintain protein structure and function (read enzyme structure and function) and to maintain ionization of many different intermediate metabolites, preventing them from diffusing out of the cell as uncharged lipophilic molecules. The retention of these intermediary compounds within the cell is necessary to maintain and to regenerate high-energy phosphate compounds after a period of nonsupply of oxygen.

The oxyhemoglobin dissociation curve shifts to the left, making oxygen release more difficult. In the past, many workers added carbon dioxide to the pump gases. This was designed to reverse this left shift of the dissociation curve, to improve cerebral circulation (except for the period of circulatory arrest), and to correct the pH of the blood gases in the cold. Murkin and co-workers[8] have shown that this pH-stat strategy, which adds carbon dioxide or allows it to be retained, actually induces excess cerebral blood flow and may contribute to increased intracranial pressure.

Viscosity of the circulating blood increases, both directly as the result of the lower temperature and indirectly from hemoconcentration, thought to be due to fluid shifts to the tissues. Accordingly, most workers have attempted to compensate for it. The addition of low–molecular weight dextran decreases viscosity, and most workers have attempted to adjust the hematocrit of the pump prime to achieve a mixed pump and patient hematocrit of approximately 30% during bypass.

Above 30° C vasoconstriction in the cold tends to impede the circulation, but at some lower point, thought to be about 25° C, generalized vasodilatation ensues.

## DESCRIPTION OF THE TECHNIQUE AND ITS EVOLUTION

The technique was first established by Barratt-Boyes and co-workers.[1] It is described here, more or less completely as it was originally enunciated. The careful reader will easily spot the changes that have subsequently been made.

The infant is placed supine on a cooling blanket. Anesthesia is induced with nitrous oxide, oxygen, and halothane in concentrations of 0.5% to 1%. Muscle relaxation is obtained using 1 mg/kg curare. Surface cooling is obtained by packing the infant in ice-filled plastic bags placed over the trunk, upper portions of the limbs, and the crown of the head. This cooling is continued until core temperature reaches 26° C, at which time the ice bags are removed and the operation is begun, using a median sternotomy incision. Following heparinization the atrium and the aorta are cannulated, and cooling bypass takes the temperature to 22° C. At this point the arterial line is clamped, venous blood is drained, and the repair is undertaken, allowing some 60 to 70 minutes of arrest time.

Following the repair, air is evacuated from all chambers and warming bypass is used to bring the temperature up to 32° C. At this point bypass is discontinued, the chest is closed, and surface rewarming supervenes.

Barratt-Boyes has published time figures for the various portions of the procedures (Table 4–3).

I have restricted this technique to children who weigh 10 kg or less. Analysis of approximately 160 consecutive cases between January 1990 and May 1992 showed an average weight of 4.8 kg and a median weight of 4.4 kg. The range was 2.2 to 10.9 kg (Fig. 4–2).

Ages of the children have ranged from newborn to 2.5 years (Fig. 4–3). Of the 43 children aged 1 month or less, 28 were in the first week of life. It is worthwhile to point out that of the 9 infants operated on in the first 2 days of life, 8 had a diagnosis of total anomalous pulmonary venous

**Table 4–3** Time pattern for the various portions of the operative procedure under deep hypothermia and circulatory arrest

| | Average (min) | Range (min) |
|---|---|---|
| Surface cooling | 153 | 98–217 |
| Bypass cooling | 9 | 2–18 |
| Circulatory arrest | 48 | 30–69 |
| Bypass rewarming | 21 | 11–34 |
| Total operative time | 320 | 240–420 |

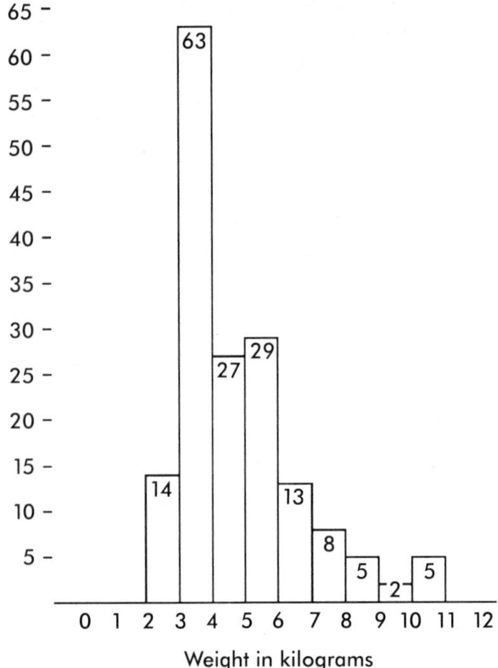


**Figure 4–2** Cases divided according to body weights of the children in kilograms, between January 1991 and May 1992 at Vanderbilt University Medical Center.

drainage. These infants contribute significantly to the overall mortality rate.

Diagnoses have ranged widely but are not entirely characteristic of congenital cardiac lesions in that these children are selected for a reparative rather than a palliative operation.

Five diagnoses comprise nearly three quarters of this recent series:

| | |
|---|---|
| Ventricular septal defect | 22% |
| Teratology of Fallot | 17% |
| Atrioventricular canal | 15% |
| Transposition of great vessels | 13% |
| Total anomalous pulmonary venous drainage | 8% |

The remaining diagnoses include the following:

Aortic stenosis
Hypoplastic left heart syndrome (for transplant)
Pulmonary atresia
Pulmonary valvular stenosis
Truncus arteriosus
Pulmonary venous stenosis
Aortic-pulmonary window
Tricuspid atresia
Sinus of valsalva fistula
Common atrium
Interrupted aortic arch

The basic monitoring that I have applied are electrocardiogram, central venous pressure, arterial cannula (generally radial artery, sometimes umbilical artery), esophageal and nasopharyngeal temperature probes, pulse oximetry, and urinary catheter.

Induction of anesthesia has varied according to the circumstances of the child. The average child who is stable generally arrives in the operating room without an intravenous line and without supplemental oxygen. My practice has been to measure oxygen saturation in room air, and if it is higher than 80%, to induce anesthesia by mask inhalation of halothane. A few of the staff have chosen to induce anesthesia by intramuscular ketamine. Children with shunts may require prolonged mask inductions, but I have found that it is rarely necessary to go above 1% halothane. This prolonged induction by mask may be safely accomplished provided the pulse rate is maintained.

It has been my experience that children who are quite sick and unstable will generally arrive in the operating room with an intravenous line in place. Induction may then be accomplished by a variety of combinations of intravenous ketamine or fentanyl and muscle relaxants.

Children who arrive desaturated without an intravenous line generally receive intramuscular ketamine. On a few occasions intravenous lines have been established before the induction, but I have not attempted mask induction in badly desaturated children.

Maintenance of anesthesia has generally been by continuation of halothane or by switching to intravenous fentanyl. Relative overdoses of long-acting muscle relaxants have been applied, and no attempt has been made to reverse them at the end of the case. These children have been routinely ventilated for some time in the immediate postoperative period.

When anesthesia is adequate and the appropriate monitors have been placed, 10 ml of dextran per kilogram of body weight is given. The child is then placed in the cooling chamber and the esophageal temperature is lowered to 30° C. This period is the most dangerous from an anesthetic standpoint, as there is an increasing probability of sudden ventricular fibrillation as the temperature drops. I carefully monitor the pulse rate as it falls and often discontinue the cooling above 30° C if the pulse rate drops too precipitously. The few instances of ventricular fibrillation that have occurred during this period have been in relatively sick children who were previously digitalized and/or treated with diuretics to control congestive failure. The risk of obstructive lesions of the aortic valve or of the aortic arch is particularly high during this period of surface cooling. Ventricular fibrillation may be very difficult to reverse, and restoration of the circulation may not be possible. In any event, the core

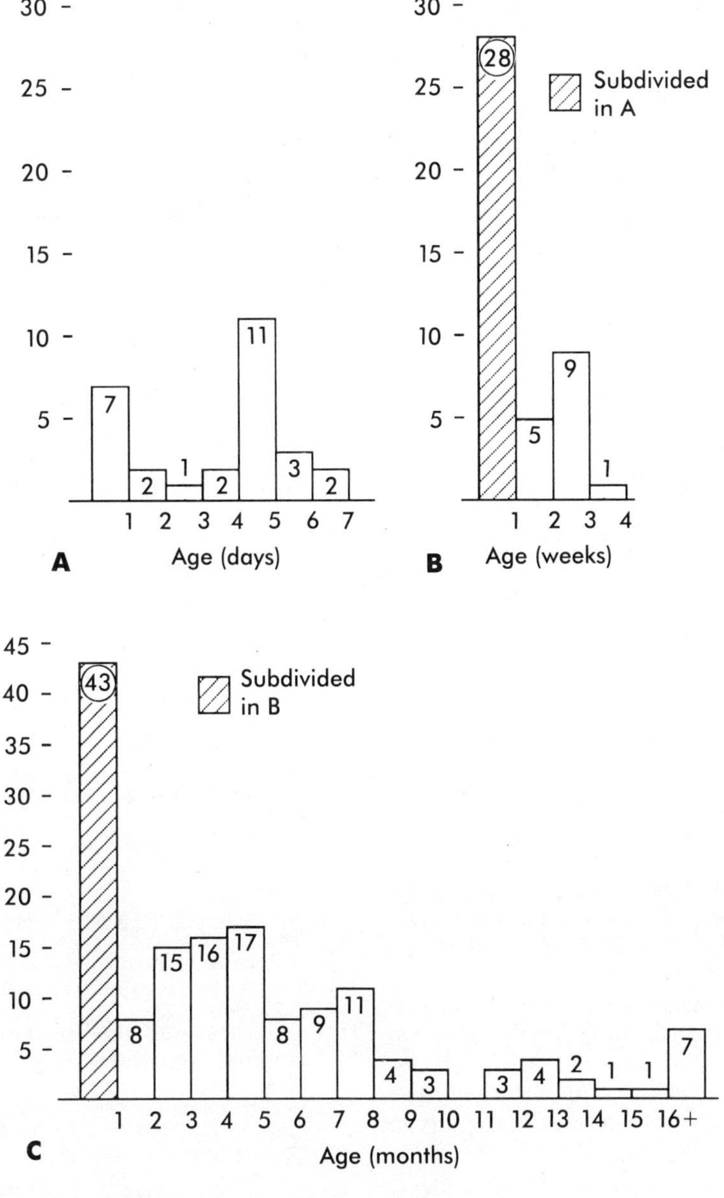


**Figure 4–3** Cases divided according to ages of the children in days, weeks, and months between January 1991 and May 1992 at Vanderbilt University Medical Center.

temperature almost always continues to fall a few degrees after the child has been removed from the chamber.

At 30° C or when appropriate (see earlier section on technique) the child is placed supine on the table, prepped, and draped, and the operation is begun with a median sternotomy. Venous and arterial cannulas are placed, the pump prime is buffered and adjusted to achieve a packed cell volume of 30, and bypass is started. Cardioplegia is instituted through the aortic root. Cooling is continued to achieve a core temperature of 18° C. Blood gases are tested at this point, and any base deficit is corrected prior to circulatory arrest.

The pump is stopped and the blood volume is drained into the pump canister. When drainage is complete, the venous cannulas are removed from the atrium. The arterial cannula is doubly clamped and disconnected from the arterial limb. The two limbs, venous and arterial, are connected to each other, and the blood volume is gently circulated through the pump during the course of the operative circulatory arrest.

When the repair is complete, the venous cannulas are reintroduced into the right atrium, and the arterial and venous limbs are reconnected. Air is evacuated from the chambers, and bypass is gently resumed with the perfusate no more than 10° C higher than the core temperature. The core temperature is then gently raised to 36° or 37° C. Often sinus rhythm spontaneously resumes during the rewarming. Occasionally electric defibrillation is necessary.

When temperature has been achieved, separation from bypass is accomplished by adjusting blood volume to adequate preload. I have often used a dilute isoproterenol infusion to enhance contractibility and to maintain an adequate pulse rate. The cannulas are removed, protamine is given to counteract the heparin, bleeding is controlled, ventricular pacing wires are applied, pericardial and mediastinal tubes are placed, the sternotomy is closed, and the infant is returned to the recovery room.

## OUTCOMES AND CONCLUSIONS

Nearly 2 decades of using this technique have convinced me of its utility and have allowed a steady improvement in outcome.

Many questions remain about the present and the future of this technique. One question seems to have been answered. Lowering the temperature below 16° to 18° C produces only an unacceptable level of bleeding, pulmonary edema, and neurologic complications. The future seems best served by taking the knowledge, now rapidly accumulating, about the nature of ischemic and reperfusion injury and applying it in an antecedent and protective manner to this process.

The crux of the matter lies in brain cell preservation. There does not seem to be any long-term damage to any organ system other than the brain. Two avenues of approach seem to be apparent. The first is the maintenance of intracellular integrity in the cold by the maintenance of proper pH and high-energy phosphate compounds that will preserve enzyme (protein) function. The second is the prevention of cellular lipid membrane destruction brought about by lipid peroxidation, the production of superoxide free radicals, and the failure of calcium channel integrity as adenosine triphosphate levels fall. The interested reader is referred to the seminal article by Hickey and Anderson.[5]

## REFERENCES


1. Barratt-Boyes B, Simpson M, Neatze J: Intracardiac surgery in neonates and infants using deep hypothermia with surface cooling and limited cardio pulmonary bypass, *Circulation* 53:25, 1971.
2. Benazon D: *Hypothermia in Scientific Foundations of Anesthesia,* ed 2, Chicago, 1974, Year Book Medical Publishers.
3. Bigelow WG, Lindsay WK, Harrison RC et al: Oxygen transport and utilization in dogs at low body temperature, *Am J Physiol* 160:125, 1950.
4. Drew CE, Keen CT, Benazon DB: Profound hypothermia, *Lancet* 1:745, 1959.
5. Hickey PR, Anderson NP: Deep hypothermic circulatory arrest, *J Cardiovasc Anesth* 1:137, 1987.
6. Hikasa Y, Shiratami H, Satumarak K et al: Open heart surgery in infants with an aid of hypothermic anesthesia II. *Nippon Geka Hokan-Archivfur Japanishe Chirurgie* 37:399, 1968.
7. McQuiston WO: Anesthetic problems in cardiac surgery in children, *Anesthesiology* 10:590, 1949.
8. Murkin JM, Farrar JK, Tweed WA et al: Relationship between cerebral blood flow and $O_2$ consumption during high-dose narcotic anesthesia for cardiac surgery, *Anesthesiology* 63:44, 1985.
9. Nagashima H: Hypothermia, *Int Anesthesiol Clin* 18:133, 1980.
10. Okamura H: Inhalational anesthesia for simple deep hypothermia induced by surface cooling, *Med J Osaka Univ* 20:29, 1969.
11. Rahn H, Reeves RB, Howell BJ: Hydrogen ion regulation, temperature and evolution, *Am Rev Respir Dis* 112:165, 1975.
12. Swan H, Zeavin I, Blount GS Jr et al: Surgery by direct vision in the open heart during hypothermia, *JAMA* 153:1081, 1953.

# 5 Myocardial Protection for Corrective Congenital Heart Surgery

*James R. Stewart*

Special concerns for infants and children
Coronary physiology during cardiopulmonary bypass
Strategies to limit intraoperative injury
Reperfusion
Operative techniques
Cardiopulmonary bypass
Assessment of myocardial protection of patients
Future research

Early in the era of open cardiac surgery there was little mention of the possible role of intraoperative myocardial ischemia as an important cause of postoperative low cardiac output. As long as the ischemic interval was relatively short, to accomplish valvotomies and close simple septal defects, few sequelae were noted. As longer ischemic times were required to accomplish complex intracardiac repairs or myocardial revascularization, it became apparent that different operative strategies would be required to ensure successful outcome. Taber[31] and Najafi[23] noted areas of myocardial necrosis after successful cardiac surgery and postulated alterations in the myocardial supply demand ratio as well as inadequate perfusion of the subendocardium as problems during cardiopulmonary bypass. As surgical myocardial revascularization began in the early 1970s, it soon became clear that transmural perioperative myocardial infarction was an important complication of all corrective cardiac surgery.[6,13] Since then intraoperative myocardial protection has been a concern of all heart surgeons and anesthesiologists.

## SPECIAL CONCERNS FOR INFANTS AND CHILDREN

While the hearts of infants and children are unique in several physiologic and metabolic respects, there is no compelling evidence that a fundamentally different form of intraoperative myocardial protection is required for them than for older patients. In general the normal neonatal and infant heart is believed to be more resistant to ischemia-reperfusion injury than the adult heart.[3,10]

There is experimental evidence that recovery of systolic and diastolic postischemic function is better in the immature mammalian heart. Postischemic dysfunction is probably related to changes in calcium-mediated excitation-contraction coupling. My colleagues and I have demonstrated that alterations in the calcium uptake velocity of the sarcoplasmic reticulum and ventricular dysfunction after global ischemia appear to be related to the generation of oxygen-free radicals during reperfusion.[27] In the immature myocardium a higher extracellular calcium is required to achieve maximal contractile force. The newborn mammalian heart experiences a net efflux of calcium, probably the result of sodium influx, during ischemia,[16] and that may account for the newborn heart's greater ability to recover function after ischemia. A number of experimental and clinical investigations have extolled the excellent protective virtues of systemic hypothermia and cold potassium cardioplegia solution. Below 15° C the addition of potassium to the cardioplegia solution appears to add little to the protective effects of hypothermia alone. It appears that hypothermia is responsible for the greatest reduction of myocardial oxygen consumption in the neonatal heart and that potassium-induced arrest at this temperature adds little to reduction in oxygen consumption.[15]

While most experimental studies support the contention that the mature myocardium is less tolerant of ischemia and reperfusion than the immature heart, the notable exceptions to this are the hearts of patients with cyanosis, uncompensated heart failure, and ventricular hypertrophy. It has been shown that immature hearts in the setting of hypoxia or acute cardiac failure develop profound functional depression when subjected to ischemia that is well tolerated by the normal immature heart.[14,17] As most neonates and infants coming to operation do not have normal hearts, they are probably not resilient to the effects of global ischemia and reperfusion.

Among patients with long-standing experimental cyanosis, recovery of postischemic function is impaired compared with that of acyanotic controls.[8,21,32] Mechanisms are unclear, but there may be down-regulation of intracellular antioxidant defenses.[7] With the institution of cardiopulmonary bypass, with high arterial oxygen pressure followed by global ischemia, oxidant stress may be amplified. Long-term cyanosis may lead to abnormal ventricular function and hypertrophy. Many operations for congenital heart disease involve incisions in the heart and great vessels. The transection of nutrient coronary arteries with resultant regional ischemia and possible introduction of air into the coronary circulation may account for the observed dysfunction. Some patients with cyanotic heart disease, especially pulmonary atresia with ventricular septal defect, have large aortopulmonary collaterals. A surgical connection between the systemic and pulmonary circulation may exist. During the operation these connections flood the operative field with blood, reducing the perfusion pressure on cardiopulmonary bypass and warming the ischemic myocardium.

Ventricular hypertrophy is an important aspect of many congenital heart defects. Hypertrophied ventricles have long been known to be particularly susceptible to ischemic injury.[24] The hypertrophied myocardium presents increased resistance to coronary blood flow, and reperfusion of the subendocardium is more difficult than in the normal heart. Uniform cooling of the myocardium may be incomplete, having important hypertrophy that requires larger volumes of cardioplegia solution than the usual case. Xanthine oxidase levels have been found to be increased, with a reduction in superoxide dismutase levels, when experimental hypertrophy reduces natural defenses against postischemic free radical injury.[2] During cardiopulmonary bypass, perfusion pressure may be low, leading to subendocardial ischemia in the setting of significant hypertrophy.

The fundamental principles of rapid induction of myocardial hypothermia and electromechanical arrest as well as use of hypothermic cardiopulmonary bypass apply in all patients. In this chapter I shall review some of the special circumstances associated with congenital cardiac surgery and suggest one intraoperative strategy that has proven successful over 20 years of experience.

## CORONARY PHYSIOLOGY DURING CARDIOPULMONARY BYPASS

While coronary blood flow is autoregulated continuously with intact circulation, blood flow may be very abnormal during cardiopulmonary bypass. Mean arterial pressure may be low (50 to 70 mm Hg). The heart is empty, minimizing intracavitary pressure, but because it is small, intramyocardial tension is increased.[26] Ventricular fibrillation further increases intramyocardial tension, decreasing subendocardial perfusion. Coronary arterial anatomy and myocardial blood supply are rarely normal in patients requiring heart surgery.

The probability of a precise and complete operation is greatest in the arrested, bloodless heart. This requires global myocardial ischemia and appropriate intraoperative management to limit the injury that would otherwise result. Injury may be irreversible (infarction) or temporary (stunning).

Temporary myocardial dysfunction after cardiac surgery in the absence of myocardial necrosis, which has been recognized for many years, may be of variable duration. It is thought that this injury is in part mediated by the release of oxygen-derived free radicals, presumably from activated neutrophils.[12,19,20,27,29,30]

Many components of a systemic inflammatory response are responsible for dysfunction after heart surgery: complement activation, platelet and leukocyte activation, prostaglandin synthesis, expression of adherence molecules in the endothelium, increase in capillary permeability. Many of these factors are at least minimized by the routine use of heparin anticoagulation, systemic hypothermia, and hemodilution during cardiopulmonary bypass.

## STRATEGIES TO LIMIT INTRAOPERATIVE INJURY

Alterations of the circumstances of ischemia were the first steps taken to prevent ischemic injury. It was apparent for many years that hypothermia is protective. To increase the length of the safe ischemic interval, topical hypothermia was advocated,[25] and it improved early results. Systemic hypothermia allowed for safe reduction in total flow rates during cardiopulmonary bypass, therefore the amount of noncoronary collateral flow returning to and rewarming the ischemic heart. The importance of avoiding distention (increasing wall tension and oxygen consumption) with left ventricular venting was established. To minimize energy requirements rapidly, immediate cessation of electromechanical activity was recognized as important. Since the early 1970s the most widely accepted technique of myocardial protection has been systemic hypothermic cardiopulmonary bypass with a cold antegrade cardioplegia solution to assure rapid myocardial cooling and cessation of electrical activity.[9] A vast body of experimental work has studied the "best" protection solution for a particular circumstance, the majority associated with adult ischemic heart disease.

Substrate enhancement has been investigated in the laboratory and appears advantageous but has not been evaluated carefully in clinical trials. The infusion of warm substrate-enriched blood before and/or after the onset of global myocardial ischemia (myocardial resuscitation) has been shown to be advantageous in hearts that have become acutely ischemic preoperatively.[1]

## REPERFUSION

It has recently been determined that the circumstances surrounding the reintroduction of blood and oxygen into the ischemic myocardium may play an important role in myocardial injury: ischemia-reperfusion injury.[12,19,20,27,29,30] This injury is thought to be related in part to the generation of oxygen-derived free radicals and intracellular calcium overload. Certain other factors have been proposed to be important to minimize reperfusion injury and postischemic myocardial dysfunction:

1. Reduction in the amount of ionized calcium in the reperfusate to minimize intracellular calcium accumulation
2. Avoidance of arterial hypertension in the first few minutes of coronary reperfusion to minimize injury and edema in the endothelium
3. Minimizing production of oxygen-free radicals
4. Adjusting the pH of the initial reperfusate to ameliorate accumulated myocardial acidosis and to allow for more rapid recovery of function
5. Increasing the availability of substrate for myocardial energy production

## OPERATIVE TECHNIQUES

The surgeon has available a number of strategies and techniques to accomplish operative repair:

1. Continuous coronary artery perfusion
2. Hypothermic fibrillating heart
3. Intermittent aortic cross-clamp with moderate hypothermia
4. Profound hypothermia and global ischemia
5. Cold cardioplegia
   a. Single dose
   b. Multidose
   c. Blood versus crystalloid
   d. Antegrade versus retrograde
6. Warm blood cardioplegia
   a. Intermittent
   b. Continuous retrograde

All these techniques have a role in the management of certain patients requiring cardiac surgery, with the particular patient's condition determining the best operative approach. The most common method of myocardial protection during heart surgery for neonates, infants, and children is the administration of cold blood or crystalloid cardioplegia solution, 10 to 20 ml/kg, usually in an antegrade fashion, in combination with moderate systemic (25° C) hypothermic bypass or profoundly hypothermic (18° C) circulatory arrest.

## CARDIOPULMONARY BYPASS

The conduct of cardiopulmonary bypass has a great influence on myocardial protection. Profound hypothermia with circulatory arrest has some distinct advantages with respect to operative exposure and myocardial protection. During circulatory arrest the heart is cold and flaccid, and a precise operative repair can be accomplished in a very small heart. The body is maintained near the temperature of the heart (18° C), minimizing myocardial rewarming by contact with the lungs and diaphragm. Bronchial and aortopulmonary collateral blood flow, with attendant myocardial rewarming, is avoided. At Vanderbilt University Medical Center we have reserved this method for patients less than 1 year of age and less than 10 kg in weight. Circulatory arrest time is usually limited to about 60 minutes to minimize multiorgan (brain, kidney, liver) dysfunction.

With improvements in arterial and venous cannulas, cardiopulmonary bypass has become more popular for congenital heart operations in all but the smallest neonates and infants. Pediatric oxygenators with small priming volumes are commonly used. Moderate hypothermia (25° to 22° C) allows reduction of arterial blood flow to approximately half the calculated flow (2.2 l/min/$M^2$) for the patient's surface area. Low flow perfusion has the advantage of limiting organ damage, but it makes myocardial protection more difficult. Relatively warm blood returning to the heart from bronchial or aortopulmonary collaterals may make intracardiac repair more difficult and necessitate multiple infusions of cardioplegia solution or additional topical hypothermic techniques. It is essential in this setting to maintain optimal left ventricular venting to prevent distention and rewarming. Because most surgery for congenital heart defects is performed with the heart open, a topical cold solution or iced saline slush may be applied to the endocardial as well as epicardial surfaces to achieve optimal cooling. It is generally desirable to maintain myocardial temperature at 15° C or less during global ischemia.

To administer cardioplegia solution in infants and small children, an 18-gauge catheter is introduced into the aortic root and connected to the cardioplegia perfusion device. At our institution we have used a crystalloid cardioplegia solution in a 500-ml bag placed in an inflatable cuff, pressurized to 150 mm Hg. The solution is maintained in ice at 4° C until used. Standard intravenous tubing containing a bubble trap is used as the infusion line. A stopcock with 50-ml syringe is connected in line and used to administer the cardioplegia solution. Immediately after the aorta is cross-clamped, 10 ml/kg of cold hyperkalemic cardioplegia solution is infused into the aortic root at physiologic pressure. In our experience this volume is satisfactory to achieve uniform cooling with mechanical arrest and a motionless, flaccid heart. As most operations can be completed expeditiously, a single dose is satisfactory in most patients. For more complex operations requiring cross-clamp times in excess of 60 minutes (arterial switch, aortic valve autograft) a different approach is often used. In this case multidose cold blood cardioplegia is often employed with initial administration through the aortic root and subsequent doses retrograde through the coronary sinus. In patients with severe preoperative dysfunction or heart failure, terminal warm blood reperfusion with substrate enhancement may be used.

To administer retrograde cardioplegia solution in the small heart a purse-string suture is made in the right atrium adjacent to the orifice of the coronary sinus. Through a stab wound in the middle of the purse-string a pediatric retrograde infusion catheter (9 or 10 French) is introduced into the right atrium and with digital control into the orifice of the coronary sinus. Care must be taken to advance the catheter until the balloon is completely within the coronary sinus. The stylet is then removed and the catheter drained of air and connected to the cardioplegia perfusion device. Pressure in the coronary sinus is measured continuously during retrograde cardioplegia infusion and should not exceed approximately 30 mm Hg. Operations performed through the right atrium conveniently lend themselves to repeated administration of cardioplegia solution through the coronary sinus by direct ostial cannulation. When repeated intermittent infusions are performed, it is important to flush out the warm solution remaining in the tubing before beginning the infusion to avoid myocardial rewarming during the initial reinfusion.

Special circumstances surround the operations performed for aortic valve disease with concomitant left ventricular hypertrophy. Unless the aortic valve is completely competent, the induction of hypothermic arrest is best performed with direct coronary ostial infusion. If subsequent cardioplegia infusions are required, these may be administered by the same route or retrograde through the coronary sinus. Special attention is given to the use of topical cold saline or iced saline slush to maintain myocardial hypothermia. Because the aortic root is open, topical endocardial cooling can also be accomplished.

## ASSESSMENT OF MYOCARDIAL PROTECTION OF PATIENTS

Because of the many different types of congenital heart defects and the subtle differences among patients, meaningful clinical investigation of specific operative techniques and methods of myocardial protection has been difficult. The best measurements would involve following serum enzymatic assays for myocardial oxidant stress and injury (malonaldehyde, glutathione, creatine kinase, and isoenzymes) and bedside monitoring of load-independent left ventricular function. While I have recently made inroads into the feasibility of measuring preload recruitable stroke work at the bedside in an on-line fashion using a nonimaging gamma detector, these techniques have not been used in children and are not readily available.[5,28] Transesophageal and surface two-dimensional echocardiography have been used to determine left ventricular (LV) wall stress in children. With the introduction of smaller and multiplane probes, estimation of LV volume for pressure-volume determinations may be possible.

The metabolic aspects of myocardial protection have been extensively investigated clinically using intraoperative myocardial biopsies and assays for adenine nucleotides. These appear to have some correlation with measurement of ventricular function in experimental investigations. Measurements of cardiac output and other simple hemodynamic descriptors of cardiac performance have not been helpful to evaluate myocardial protection.

The easiest, albeit not independent, variable to measure is perioperative mortality. Kirklin and associates[18] demonstrated a decline in hospital mortality in their institution with the advent of cold cardioplegia arrest to facilitate corrective surgery for congenital heart disease. Bull and associates[4] in London used measurements of myocardial high-energy phosphates and showed their hospital mortality to be directly related to the duration of ischemic arrest and preoperative clinical status of the patient. In our institution a series of patients with congenital heart disease was evaluated with LV biopsies at the end of the ischemic arrest period. LV function was evaluated using radionuclide ventriculography during the first postoperative week. Postoperative ventricular ejection fraction appeared to be related to the level of high-energy phosphates at the end of operation. High-energy phosphates did decrease during the ischemic interval. When comparing moderate hypothermia and cardioplegia arrest with profound hypothermia, myocardial high-energy phosphates were better preserved in the latter group.[11]

## FUTURE RESEARCH

It will be important to determine the best preoperative and early intraoperative management of patients with congenital heart disease to evaluate the autoregulation of endogenous antioxidant defense systems in experimental models of different forms of congenital heart disease. Just as it is important to avoid high oxygen tensions in patients with hypoplastic left heart syndrome to maintain systemic perfusion, it may be important for myocardial protection to avoid hyperoxia in cyanotic patients, especially if antioxidant defenses are down-regulated. The potential effects of certain cytokines (TNF$\alpha$, interleukins) on the regulation of protective enzyme systems and potential preconditioning have not been systematically studied among congenital heart models.

While a number of well-planned laboratory investigations will lead to improved management in patients, there is a paucity of clinical investigation of myocardial protective strategies in patients with congenital heart disease. For continued progress, prospective trials of different protective regimens and additives to the cardioplegia solution should be carried out.

### REFERENCES


1. Allen BS, Buckberg GD, Schwaiger M et al: Studies of controlled reperfusion after ischemia XVI: early recovery of regional wall motion in patients following surgical revascularization after 8 hours of acute coronary occlusion, *J Thorac Cardiovasc Surg* 92:605, 1986.
2. Batist G, Mersereau W, Malashenko B-A et al: Response to ischemia-reperfusion injury in hypertrophied heart: role of free-radical metabolic pathways, *Circulation* 80(suppl 2):III-10, 1987.
3. Bove EL, Gallagher KP, Drake DH et al: The effect of hypothermic ischemia on recovery of left ventricular function and preload reserve in the neonatal heart, *J Thorac Cardiovasc Surg* 95:814, 1988.
4. Bull C, Cooper J, Stark J: Cardioplegia protection of the child's heart, *J Thorac Cardiovasc Surg* 88:287, 1984.
5. Carey JA, Stewart JR, Merrill WH et al: Continuous radionuclide monitoring: a valuable adjunct to evaluate myocardial preservation into the 21st century, *J Mol Cell Cardiol* 22(suppl 5):S30, 1990.
6. Cooley DA, Reul GJ, Wukasch DC: Ischemic contracture of the heart: "stone heart," *Am J Cardiol* 29:575, 1972.
7. Del Nido PJ, Mickle DAG, Williams WG et al: Evidence of myocardial free radical injury during elective repair of tetralogy of Fallot, *Circulation* 74(suppl 2):II-77, 1986.
8. Fujiwara T, Kurtts T, Anderson W et al: Myocardial protection in cyanotic neonatal lambs, *J Thorac Cardiovasc Surg* 96:700, 1988.
9. Gay WA, Ebert PA: Functional, metabolic, and morphologic effects of potassium-induced cardioplegia, *Surgery* 74:284, 1973.
10. Grice WN, Konishi T, Apstein CS: Resistance of neonatal myocardium to injury during normothermic and hypothermic ischemic arrest and reperfusion, *Circulation* 76(part 2):V-150, 1987.
11. Hammon JW Jr, Boucek RJ Jr: The techniques of myocardial protection in infants and children. In Roberts AJ, editor: *Myocardial protection in cardiac surgery,* New York, 1987, Marcel Dekker.
12. Hammond B, Hess ML: The oxygen free radical system: potential mediator of myocardial injury, *J Am Coll Cardiol* 6:215, 1985.
13. Hultgren HN, Miyagawa M, Buch W et al: Ischemic myocardial injury during cardiopulmonary bypass surgery, *Am Heart J* 85:167, 1973.
14. Jarmakani JM, Nagamoto T, Nakazawa M et al: Effect of hypoxia on myocardial high-energy phosphates in the neonatal mammalian heart, *Am J Physiol* 235:H475, 1978.
15. Jessen ME, Hanan SA, Abd-Elfattah AS et al: Oxygen consumption in the empty beating, fibrillating, and potassium chloride-arrested neonatal heart, *Surg Forum* 39:233, 1988.
16. Jimenez E, del Nido P, Feinberg H et al: Immature myocardium effluxes calcium during reversible ischemia, *Surg Forum* 41:206-207, 1990.
17. Julia P, Kofsky ER, Buckberg GD et al: Studies of myocardial protection in the immature heart III: models of ischemic and hypoxic injury in the immature puppy heart, *J Thorac Cardiovasc Surg* 101:14, 1991.
18. Kirklin JK, Blackstone EH, Kirklin JW et al: Intracardiac surgery in infants under age 3 months: incremental risk factors for hospital mortality, *Am J Cardiol* 48:500, 1981.
19. Lee RB, Stewart JR, Merrill WH et al: Pharmacokinetics of superoxide dismutase during hypothermic cardiopulmonary bypass, *Circulation* 80(suppl 3)3:25, 1989.
20. Lee RB, Stewart JR, Morley SA et al: Optimal dose of superoxide dismutase in hypothermic global myocardial ischemia, *Surg Forum* 39:216-218, 1988.
21. Lupinetti FM, Wareing TH, Huddleston CB et al: Pathophysiology of chronic cyanosis in a canine model, *J Thorac Cardiovasc Surg* 90:291, 1985.
22. McCord JM: Superoxide radical: a likely link between reperfusion injury and inflammation, *Adv Free Radical Biol Med* 2:325, 1986.
23. Najafi H, Henson D, Dye WS et al: Left ventricular hemorrhagic necrosis, *Ann Thorac Surg* 7:550, 1969.
24. Schaper J, Scheld HH, Schmidt U et al: Ultrastructural study comparing the efficacy of five different methods of intraoperative myocardial protection in the human heart, *J Thorac Cardiovasc Surg* 92:47, 1986.
25. Shumway NE, Lower RE: Topical cardiac hypothermia for extended periods of anoxic arrest, *Surg Forum* 10:563, 1960.

26. Steed D, Follette D, Foglia R et al: Unavoidable subendocardial underperfusion during bypass, especially in infants, *Circulation* 55,56(suppl 3):3-248, 1977.
27. Stewart JR, Blackwell WH, Crute SL et al: Inhibition of surgically induced ischemia-reperfusion injury by oxygen free radical scavengers, *J Thorac Cardiovasc Surg* 86:262, 1983.
28. Stewart JR, Carey JA, Merrill WH et al: Continuous radionuclide monitoring of left ventricular systolic performance in postoperative cardiac surgery patients: validation of the Capintec vest, *J Am Coll Cardiol* 15:130A, 1990.
29. Stewart JR, Crute SL, Loughlin V et al: Prevention of free radical induced myocardial reperfusion injury with allopurinol, *J Thorac Cardiovasc Surg* 90:68, 1985.
30. Stewart JR, Gerhardt EB, Wehr CJ et al: Free radical scavengers and myocardial preservation during transplantation, *Ann Thorac Surg* 42:390, 1986.
31. Taber RF, Morales AR, Fine G: Myocardial necrosis and the postoperative low-cardiac-output syndrome, *Ann Thorac Surg* 4:12, 1967.
32. Visner MS, Arentzen CE, Ring WS et al: Left ventricular dynamic geometry and diastolic mechanisms in a model of chronic cyanosis and right ventricular pressure overload, *J Thorac Cardiovasc Surg* 81:347, 1981.

**Table 6–4** Comparison of half-lives in newborns and adults of drugs with low or high hepatic extraction

| Drug | T½ in newborn (hours) | T½ in adults (hours) |
|---|---|---|
| **Drugs with low hepatic clearance** | | |
| Aminophylline | 24-36 | 3-9 |
| Amylobarbitone | 17-60 | 12-27 |
| Caffeine | 103 | 6 |
| Carbamazepine | 8-28 | 21-36 |
| Diazepam | 25-100 | 15-25 |
| Mepivacaine | 8.7 | 3.2 |
| Phenobarbitone | 21-100 | 52-120 |
| Phenytoin | 21 | 11-29 |
| Tolbutamide | 10-40 | 4.4-9 |
| **Drugs with intermediate or high hepatic clearance** | | |
| Bromosulfophthalein | 0.16 | |
| Meperine | 22 | 3-4 |
| Nortriptyline | 56 | 18-20 |
| Morphine | 2.7 | 0.9-4.3 |
| Lidocaine | 2.9-3.3 | 1.0-2.2 |
| Propoxyphene | 1.7-7.7 | 1.9-4.3 |

From Rane A: Drug disposition and action in infants and children. In Yaffe SJ, Aranda JV editors: *Pediatric pharmacology,* Philadelphia, 1992, Saunders.

**Table 6–5** Pathways in drug metabolism

| Reactions | Examples |
|---|---|
| Phase I | |
| Oxidation reactions | Narcotics, halogenated anesthetics |
| Phase II | |
| Conjugation reactions | Lorazepam, morphine, fentanyl, naloxone, procainamide |
| Hydrolysis reactions | |
| Ester hydrolysis | Ester and amide local anesthetics, succinylcholine, acetylsalicyclic acid |

From Tucker GT: Pathways in drug metabolism, *Br J Anaesth* 51:603, 1979.

infant because the hepatic enzymes systems—cytochrome P-450 system, NADPH (reduced nicotinamide-adenine dinucleotide phosphate), and molecular oxygen—are incompletely developed in the neonate (Table 6–5). Postnatal age determines the maturity of the hepatic systems. Therefore premature and term birth infants develop the ability to metabolize drugs at the same rate. The most affected parts of hepatic metabolism are phase I reactions, which require oxidation of the drug because the oxidative and reductive enzymes are not well developed until a few days of life. Phase II reactions, which are the conjugation reactions, including sulfate, acetate, glucuronide, or amino acids, are absent at birth. The ability to conjugate pharmacologic agents matures with age: postnatal conjugation with acetate occurs by 1 month of age; with glucuronide by 2 months of age; and with amino acids by 3 months of age. After conjugation most of these metabolites are excreted in the urine, and some metabolites or unmetabolized drugs can be excreted in bile. The activity of the cytochrome P-450 enzyme is system stimulated by repeated administration of various drugs that require these systems for metabolism. In infants phenobarbital is a particularly good induction agent for enhancing the hepatic cytochrome P-450 system.

Simple renal excretion is the most common route of elimination of drugs or their metabolites. The neonate's glomerular filtration rate (GFR) is approximately 30% of that of the adult. It approaches adult values by about 3 months of age when compared on the basis of body surface area. Proximal tubular secretion of drugs and their metabolites is significantly decreased at birth but assumes adult values by the fourth to sixth month of life. Therefore, renal clearance of drugs and their metabolites should not be a major influence in pediatric pharmacology beyond the sixth month of life unless renal function is compromised because of low renal perfusion or renal failure.

## EFFECT OF INTRACARDIAC SHUNTS ON UPTAKE AND DISTRIBUTION

Newborn infants and children with congenital heart disease may have intracardiac shunts that permit admixture of venous and arterial blood. The presence of intracardiac shunts can significantly alter the uptake and distribution of inhalation and intravenous anesthetics. Uptake of inhalation agents that are relatively insoluble such as nitrous oxide is more markedly influenced (see section on Inhalation Anesthetics). A right to left shunt will divert blood away from the pulmonary circulation and therefore slow the uptake of anesthetic. In turn, the anesthetic concentration (Fa) rises more slowly in the arterial blood than normal. In such children the induction of anesthesia is prolonged. The use of overpressure techniques will increase the rate of induction. However, the cardiovascular depressant effect of such overpressure techniques may prove hazardous to the patient.

Conversely, a left to right shunt will direct more blood through the pulmonary circulation and increase the uptake through the lungs. Distribution of anesthetic to the tissue beds may be decreased in these patients because of the decrease in systemic circulation. The presence of a right to left shunt also will influence the distribution of drugs administered intravenously. An agent injected into a peripheral vein will reach the systemic circulation more quickly and in a higher dose because it bypasses the pulmonary vascular bed. Therefore, a dose of an intravenous induction agent may have a more rapid onset than in a normal patient. The presence of a left to right shunt, on the other hand, will have minimal effect on the rate of induction and distribution of an intravenous drug.

## SPECIFIC AGENTS

### Narcotics and opiates

Narcotics act as agonists at opioid receptors in the brain and other tissues (Table 6–6). The intravenous anesthetics, in particular the narcotics and opiates, have emerged as pharmacologic mainstays of cardiac anesthesia. Since the first report in 1963 on the use of high-dose morphine for cardiac anesthesia,[62] high-dose narcotics have become the agents of choice for open heart procedures and cardiac operations in general. The scope of this chapter does not permit an extensive discussion of the pharmacology of narcotics. We will highlight the cardiovascular effects of the narcotics and their usage in and specific concerns for pediatric patients. Table 6–6 shows the relative potency of various narcotic and opiate agents.

Narcotics depress the newborn's respiration to a greater degree than the adult's on a dose per weight basis. High-dose narcotics have been demonstrated to have greater central nervous system (CNS) toxicity in newborn animals than in older ones. As discussed earlier, the infant blood-brain barrier is immature and therefore quite permeable to many agents. Morphine and the opiates can traverse the infant's blood-brain barrier more easily and manifest higher CNS levels than the adult's. In rodent studies the brain concentration of morphine several hours after injection was 2 to 4 times greater than in adult rats despite equal blood concentrations.[54] One might expect similar results with fentanyl and its analogues, which have a relatively high lipid solubility. The age-dependent changes in blood-brain barrier permeability do not affect a more lipid-soluble drug such as meperidine to the same degree.

Morphine is metabolized through N-demethylation and conjugation with glucuronide, and the inactive forms are excreted in the urine. The elimination half-life of morphine in the newborn is longer than in the older infant or child.[63,77] Meperidine also is demethylated and conjugated with glucuronide. Therefore, the metabolism of meperidine is also lower in newborns than in adults. There seems to be no significant difference in volume of distri-

**Table 6–6** Classification of opioid receptors

| | Effect | Agonist | Antagonist |
|---|---|---|---|
| Mu-1 | Supraspinal analgesia | β-endorphin<br>Meptazinol*<br>Morphine | Naloxone<br>Pentazocine<br>Nalbuphine |
| Mu-2 | Hypoventilation<br>Bradycardia<br>Physical dependence<br>Euphoria<br>Ileus | Meperidine<br>Fentanyl<br>Sufentanil<br>Alfentanil | |
| Delta | Modulate mu receptor activity | Leuenkephalin | Naloxone<br>Metenkephalin |
| Kappa | Analgesia<br>Sedation<br>Hypoventilation(?)<br>Miosis | Dynorphin<br>Pentazocin<br>Butorphanol<br>Nalbuphine<br>Buprenorphine<br>Nalorphine | Naloxone |
| Sigma | Dysphoria<br>Hypertonia<br>Tachycardia<br>Tachypnea<br>Mydriasis | Pentazocine(?)<br>Ketamine(?) | Naloxone |

*Relatively selective for mu-1 receptors.

From Stoelting RK: *Pharmacology and physiology in anesthetic practice,* ed 2, Philadelphia, 1991, Lippincott.

bution of either drug from that of adults. Fentanyl is a synthetic opiate with relatively few hemodynamic consequences. The primary problems associated with rapid administration of fentanyl include bradycardia and chest wall rigidity. The chest wall rigidity may be avoided by infusing fentanyl slowly. When used with an anticholinergic agent such as atropine, the bradycardia associated with the fentanyl can be averted. At doses used for cardiovascular surgery (50 to 100 μg/kg), the hemodynamic effect of the agent is minimum. A modest decrease in mean arterial pressure may occur, particularly if the patient has a high sympathetic tone. Other indicators of cardiac function usually remain unchanged.

It is unclear what dose of fentanyl will result in satisfactory anesthesia in infants. Yaster (1987) has noted that in neonates anesthetized with fentanyl, metocurine, and oxygen and undergoing a variety of medical procedures, fentanyl provided hemodynamic stability for up to 75 minutes. Neonatal clearance of fentanyl is comparable with that in the older child and adult. The premature infant, however, has a markedly decreased clearance of fentanyl.[13] Plasma concentrations in infants and children are less than those achieved in adults with the same dosage (μg/kg).[91] These differences may be attributed to the larger volume of distribution and the lower renal clearance in infants.

Sufentanil has claimed a significant role in cardiac anesthesia for adults and children.[12] A derivative of fentanyl, sufentanil is a highly lipophilic compound that is rapidly distributed and taken up in all tissues. Sufentanil is 10 times more potent than fentanyl and has a higher margin of safety. Metabolism of sufentanil occurs by o-demethylation and dealkylation. Sufentanil demonstrates higher protein binding than fentanyl and has a higher clearance rate.[69] This results in a shorter elimination half-life and shorter duration of action. Serum pH will also affect protein binding of sufentanil: a pH of 7 increases protein binding by 28% over the normal of 7.4; alkalosis to a pH of 7.8 will decrease protein binding by 28%.[73] The hemodynamics of fentanyl and sufentanil appear to be similar. Sufentanil provides a comparable level of hemodynamic stability with respect to mean arterial pressure, systemic vascular resistance, and other measured variables. Alfentanil is a fentanyl analogue of lesser potency (20% to 33%) and shorter duration of action than fentanyl. The drug is metabolized by N-dealkylation and glucuronidation. Like fentanyl and sufentanil, alfentanil is associated with hemodynamic stability.[105] At high doses the drug is associated with a decrease in heart rate and mild decrease in mean arterial pressure and systemic vascular resistance. However, the clinical effects of these changes are negligible.

All of the narcotic and opiate drugs affect the respiratory system similarly; that is, the ventilatory response to carbon dioxide is shifted to the right and manifested as an elevated resting $PaO_2$. The degree of shift is dose dependent, with respiratory depression occurring at subanalgesic doses. With the fentanyl analogues the respiratory depressant effect of intravenous agents is dissipated by 30 to 60 minutes after injection. At the doses used for cardiothoracic surgery, the respiratory depression may last up to 24 hours.

### Ketamine

Ketamine is a frequently used induction agent for children undergoing cardiothoracic surgery. The drug is a cyclohexamine derivative that produces a dissociative state. Ketamine blocks afferent impulses in the diencephalon and the associated cortical pathways. It also may exert its effect on the brain stem.[61] Seizurelike activity, particularly from cortical and limbic areas, may be observed on the electroencephalogram (EEG). The clinical effects of ketamine include analgesia at lower doses (0.5 to 1mg/kg) of skin, muscle, and bone but not of the viscera. Higher doses are associated with general anesthesia (1 to 2 mg/kg). The respiratory effects of the drug are minimal and the gag reflex is preserved. Laryngeal irritability also is preserved to slightly increased and muscle tone is unaffected. Significant bronchorrhea may occur. The clinically effective doses of ketamine are high in young patients, particularly those under 6 months of age. This is probably due to the immaturity of the N-methyl-D-asparate (NMDA) receptor to which ketamine binds. NMDA is an excitatory amine that may act on or modulate sigma opiate receptors. Ketamine may act as an antagonist at these NMDA sites.[111]

The anesthetic state produced by higher doses of ketamine is associated with minimal effects on respiration and blood pressure. In infants the doses required for lack of movement may produce respiratory depression and apnea. However, with doses commonly used for induction of anesthesia (1 to 2 mg/kg) or sedation the hemodynamic and respiratory effects are minimal. Acute increases in pulmonary artery pressure have been seen in infants with congenital heart disease undergoing cardiac catheterization.[30] However, the increase in pulmonary artery pressure is proportionate to that seen in systemic vascular resistance and mean arterial pressure. Therefore, an intracardiac shunt is usually minimally affected by ketamine.[43,75] The changes in pulmonary vascular resistance are further minimized with appropriate support of the airway and ventilation.

The etiology of the cardiorespiratory stimulation is not clear. Administration of ketamine is associated with a release of systemic catecholamines. The pressor effect of increased circulating epinephrine and norepinephrine may account for maintained or increased blood pressure, heart rate, and cardiac output.

Undesirable effects of ketamine include increased laryngeal irritability and bronchorrhea in children. Intracranial cerebrospinal fluid (CSF) pressure may be significantly increased following ketamine administration. Therefore, the use of ketamine in children at risk for intracranial hypertension should be avoided. There are no documented reports of toxic effects of ketamine on liver, kidneys, or other organ systems in older children and adults. The agent is associated with dysphoric reactions and hallucinations that can persist for several hours. The incidence of hallucinations is as high as 50% in adults but significantly less in the younger age group. The psychotomimetic effects of ketamine can be reduced by pretreatment with benzodiazepines.

### Barbiturates

Short-acting barbiturates are commonly used to induce the anesthetic state. In most patients with cardiovascular disease these agents can be used safely for induction. However, the drugs do exert significant idiosyncratic and dose-dependent effects on hemodynamics. In particular, the short-acting barbiturates can act as direct myocardial depressants. The negative inotropic effect is exerted on left ventricular function and results in prolonged left ventricular ejection time, prolonged ejection, and decreased stroke work index.[26] Increased venous capacitance leads to a decrease in venous return and decreased filling volume. The heart rate may increase following administration of barbiturates because of baroreceptor stimulation. In addition, injection of barbiturate is commonly associated with histamine release leading to peripheral vasodilatation and associated hypotension. Anaphylactoid reactions may also occur. Furthermore, barbiturates decrease sympathetic response to hypotension, further exacerbating the hypotensive effect. Because of their hemodynamic side effects these agents should be used with caution in patients with depressed myocardial function, systemic hypotension, or hypovolemia.

Of particular interest in patients undergoing cardiothoracic surgery is the role of thiopental and other barbiturates in neurologic and myocardial protection during hypoxia and severe hypotension. In animals pretreatment with barbiturates reduces the loss of neurons following ischemia.[99] A similar protective effect is seen in the myocardium, where large doses of thiopental may reduce the loss of myocardial enzymes after ischemia. However, the high doses of the drug may exacerbate hypotension and hemodynamic compromise.

### Etomidate

Etomidate, an imidazole compound, is a potent short-acting sedative hypnotic that possesses no analgesic properties. It is almost completely metabolized through ester hydrolysis. The onset of action of etomidate is similar to that of short-acting barbiturates. Etomidate produces less hemodynamic depression than do other barbiturates. With induction doses of 0.3 to 0.6 mg/kg, minimal depression of myocardial function is seen and the heart rate does not change. This is true for normal as well as hemodynamically compromised patients.[36,37] Therefore, the use of etomidate for induction of anesthesia seems desirable in the child undergoing cardiac surgery. However, the drug produces a significant amount of pain and burning on injection and is associated with myoclonic movements.[31] The pain of injection can be minimized by pretreatment with intravenous lidocaine. Myoclonic movements may be minimized by treatment with benzodiazepines, barbiturates, or narcotics. Etomidate has one significant side effect that can produce significant morbidity and mortality—the suppression of adrenal steroidogenesis.[28] Although this effect can be seen after a single dose, it is more likely to occur with higher doses and sustained administration. Therefore, the routine use of etomidate for induction of anesthesia has not been popularized.

### Propofol

Propofol, an isopropylphenol derivative, is a short-acting rapid-onset hypnotic agent with no analgesic properties. The drug is rapidly redistributed and metabolized, accounting for its short duration of action. It is suspended in oil (10% soybean oil; 2.25% glycerol, and 1.2% egg phosphatide) because of its lack of water solubility. The drug undergoes nearly complete metabolism via conjugation with glucuronide and sulfate. In doses used for induction of anesthesia (2 to 2.5 mg/kg) it has minimum excitatory and other side effects. Because of its extremely short duration of action and rapid metabolism, repeated doses can be given, or continuous infusions (100 to 200 μg/kg/min) can be used to administer the drug without major side effects. The hemodynamic consequences of induction doses, mild tachycardia and mild hypotension, are minimal. Therefore, propofol may be a good agent for induction in children undergoing cardiac surgery or in maintaining the sedative state in children in the cardiac catheterization lab.

**Benzodiazepines**

The three most commonly used intravenous benzodiazepines in the United States are diazepam, midazolam, and lorazepam (Table 6–7). Of these, midazolam has become the most frequently used because of its water solubility and short duration of action. All of these agents produce a pleasant sedation and hypnosis with few respiratory or hemodynamic side effects in children. Acting through the GABA (γ-aminobutyric acid) receptors in the amygdala of the limbic system and spinal neurons, the agents produce hypnosis, sedation, and amnesia (Fig. 6–1).[65] They are commonly used as premedications and postoperative sedatives in children with cardiovascular disease. All of them are associated with cardiovascular stability with minimum effect on blood pressure, cardiac output, and heart rate at doses that produce sedation. Respiratory depression may occur following bolus doses or high doses of the agents. Metabolism of the three agents occurs primarily in the liver. Diazepam undergoes N-demethylation, producing two active metabolites. Urinary excretion of the metabolites is in oxidized and glucuronidated forms. Midazolam undergoes extensive hydroxylation and glucuronidation prior to excretion in the urine. Lorazepam also undergoes glucuronidation and urinary excretion. These agents are most commonly used for premedication, postoperative sedation, and adjuncts for sedation during cardiac catheterization procedures.

**Narcotic antagonists**

Narcotic antagonists are used to counteract the side effects or undesirable effects of the narcotics and

**Table 6–7** Comparative pharmacology of benzodiazepines

| | Equivalent dose (mg/kg$^{-1}$) | Volume of distribution (l/kg$^{-1}$) | Protein binding (percent) | Clearance (ml/kg$^{-1}$ × min$^{-1}$) | Elimination half-life (h) |
|---|---|---|---|---|---|
| Diazepam | 0.3-0.5 | 1-1.5 | 96-98 | 0.2-0.5 | 21-37 |
| Midazolam | 0.15-0.3 | 1-1.5 | 96-98 | 6-8 | 1-4 |
| Lorazepam | 0.05 | 0.8-1.3 | 96-98 | 0.7-1 | 10-20 |

From Stoelting RK: *Pharmacology and physiology in anesthetic practice,* ed 2, Philadelphia, 1991, Lippincott.

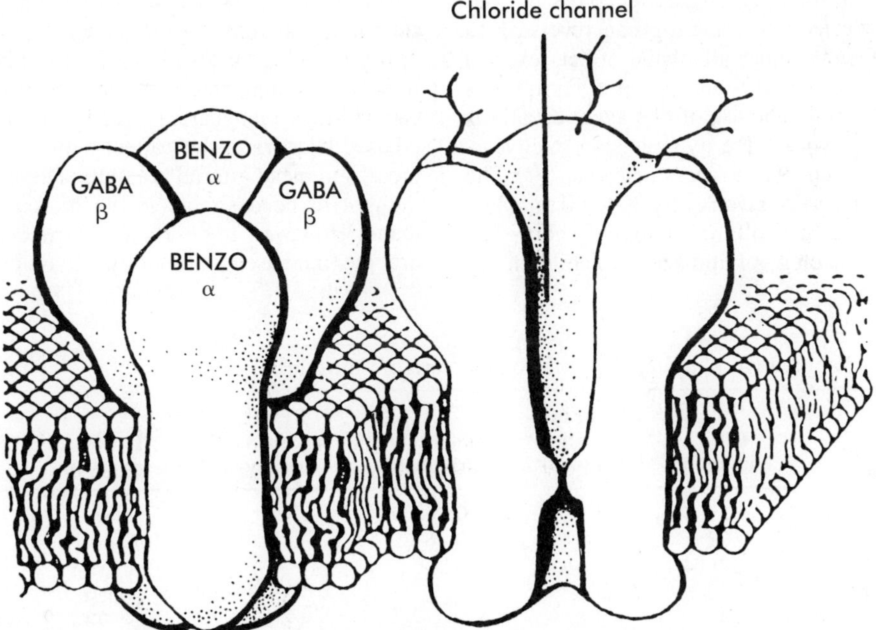


**Figure 6–1** Model of γ-aminobutyric acid (GABA) receptor forming a chloride channel. (From Richards JG, Mohler H: *Eur J Anaesth* 2:15, 1988.)

opiates. The only pure antagonist available is naloxone. This agent is a competitive antagonist at all of the four opiate receptors and is usually given intravenously (IV) in doses of 1 to 4 μg/kg. The peak effect of intravenously administered naloxone occurs at 30 to 60 minutes, with total duration of action of approximately 4 hours. In patients who have been given narcotics, reversal of the analgesic effects may result in significant adverse cardiovascular and neurologic effects. In particular, the reversal of high-dose narcotic anesthesia such as that used in cardiothoracic surgery can produce a massive release of catecholamines resulting in ventricular irritability, increased mean arterial pressure, and increases in various cardiovascular parameters. If administered in the absence of anesthesia, naloxone has few hemodynamic consequences. In patients who have undergone cardiothoracic surgery or those with compromised cardiovascular function who have received narcotics for analgesia, naloxone should be used with extreme caution if at all. If used to counteract significant respiratory depression associated with high-dose narcotics or opiates, naloxone can be titrated in small incremental doses. Most commonly it is better to support the child's respiratory system until the effects of the narcotic have subsided.

### Benzodiazepine antagonist

Flumazenil, a competitive antagonist of benzodiazepines at the GABA receptor, has recently been released for use in the United States. The agent has a very high affinity for GABA receptors but has few agonist effects.[40] The drug can reverse in a dose-dependent manner all of the effects exerted by benzodiazepines. It is administered IV in doses of 8 to 15 μg/kg. The use of this agent usually is not associated with acute hypertension, tachycardia, or a neuroendocrine stress response.[52,106] The agent may have to be given every 30 to 60 minutes, as the half-life in adults is relatively short. The precise pharmacology of flumazenil in children has not been defined. However, with children experiencing hypoventilation or oversedation because of benzodiazepine use in clinical situations such as cardiac catheterization, use of flumazenil may be appropriate.

## NEUROMUSCULAR BLOCKING AGENTS

Neuromuscular blocking agents are most frequently used in association with high-dose narcotics in the practice of cardiothoracic anesthesia (Table 6–8).

### Succinylcholine

Succinylcholine is a depolarizing neuromuscular blocker with a rapid onset and a short duration of action. As a cholinergic agonist, the agent can produce transient bradycardia. It also may have negative inotropic effects, particularly in low doses.[33] Occasionally bradyarrhythmias, nodal rhythms, and premature ventricular contractions (PVC) may follow succinylcholine administration. The use of succinylcholine in cardiothoracic surgery is limited by the agent's short duration of action.

### Pancuronium

Pancuronium has been a mainstay of neuromuscular blockade in children undergoing surgery in general and in cardiothoracic surgery in particular. Pancuronium is a steroidal noncompetitive neuromuscular blocker that produces a dose-dependent increase in blockade. There is evidence for a β-adrenergic–mediated positive inotropic effect of pancuronium.[47] Associated with increased isometric force and maximum velocity of force development, the agent also has anticholinergic effects mediated through cardiac muscarinic receptors that can produce tachycardia.[87] In addition to the increased heart rate, the patient may experience increases in mean arterial pressure. These effects are thought to be desirable in the presence of halothane. However, in children with myocardial failure the increased chronotropy may prove detri-

**Table 6–8** Comparative pharmacology of nondepolarizing muscle relaxants

| | $ED_{95}$ (mg/kg$^{-1}$) | Onset to max twitch supp (min) | Volume of distribution | Renal excretion (% unchanged) | Hepatic degradation | Intubating (mg/kg$^{-1}$) |
|---|---|---|---|---|---|---|
| d-Tubocurarine | 0.51 | 3-5 | 0.30 | 45 | NS | 0.6 |
| Pancuronium | 0.07 | 3-5 | 0.26 | 80 | 10%-40% | 0.1 |
| Doxacurium | 0.03-0.04 | 4-6 | | 70 | Unknown | 0.5-0.8 |
| Atracurium | 0.20 | 3-5 | | NS | Modest | 0.4-0.5 |
| Vecuronium | 0.05 | 3-5 | | 15-25 | 20%-30% | 0.08-0.1 |
| Mivacurium | 0.08 | 2-3 | | NS | NS | 0.16 |

From Stoelting RK: In *Pharmacology and physiology in anesthetic practice,* ed 2, Philadelphia, 1991, Lippincott.

mental. The drug is primarily excreted unchanged in the kidney. In patients undergoing hypothermia during surgery, neuromuscular blockade seems to be unaffected.[18,45]

### d-Tubocurarine

d-Tubocurarine, a curare derivative, is a competitive neuromuscular blocker. Although the clinical impression is that newborns may be sensitive to the effects of d-tubocurarine, electromyogram (EMG) studies show no increase in sensitivity in infants. d-Tubocurarine can produce a dose-dependent decrease in isometric force and maximum velocity of force development but in the heart does not seem to have a clinically relevant effect. The agent can also decrease the cardiac output to various organs, including spleen, small intestine, and adrenals while increasing the blood flow to the stomach and possibly the brain. Blood flow to the mesentery and the heart remains relatively unchanged. The most profound effect on hemodynamics is a decrease in vascular resistance of the vessels in the stomach, brain, and large intestine as a result of a large histamine release.[76,89] In turn, the mean arterial blood pressure is reduced and the heart rate increases. In patients undergoing cardiac surgery or those with hemodynamic compromise, the hypotensive effects of d-tubocurarine may prove quite detrimental. These effects can be attenuated by administration of intravenous fluids. Curare undergoes extensive hepatic metabolism and subsequently hepatic and renal excretion.

### Vecuronium

Vecuronium is a relatively new steroidal muscle relaxant similar to pancuronium. The agent is metabolized by the liver and excreted in the hepatobiliary system (up to 50%) and through the kidneys (up to 15%). A few active metabolites are present, including 3-hydroxy, 17-hydroxy, and 3,17-dihydroxy metabolites. The dihydroxy compound is a weak neuromuscular blocker. With the commonly used clinical doses vecuronium has few cardiovascular effects. With high doses cardiac output to the brain may increase,[89] although, generally regional blood flows are unchanged. Vascular resistance is also minimally affected by clinically relevant doses of vecuronium but may be decreased with higher doses. In clinical use the heart rate, mean arterial pressure, and cardiac output do not change after a dose of vecuronium. However, there is an associated decrease in systemic vascular resistance and an increase in cardiac output when the drug is used with halothane.[76] The heart rate and blood pressure are not affected. With concurrent fentanyl anesthesia, patients with coronary disease or myocardiopathy may show slight decrease in heart rate and cardiac index in response to a vecuronium bolus.

### Atracurium

Atracurium is an intermediate-acting neuromuscular blocker metabolized by plasma (nonspecific) esterases. It undergoes spontaneous decomposition by Hofmann degradation. Both of these reactions are pH and temperature sensitive. Under usual clinical circumstances, it is the ester hydrolysis that is responsible for most of the breakdown of atracurium. The absence of pseudocholinesterase has no effect on atracurium metabolism.[93] In normal patients an intubating dose of atracurium (0.6 mg/kg) has minimal effects on heart rate and blood pressure.[3] However, patients with hypovolemia or myocardial dysfunction may experience decreases in mean arterial pressure, heart rate, systemic vascular resistance, cardiac output, left ventricular filling pressure, and central venous pressure (CVP). The clinical consequences of these changes usually are limited.[82] Because the metabolism of atracurium is temperature and pH dependent, there is an increase in the neuromuscular blockade that is potentiated with hypothermia, which is frequently used in cardiothoracic surgery for children. Though statistically significant, the prolongation has been demonstrated to have little clinical relevance. In the presence of halothane and nitrous oxide anesthesia children given atracurium or vecuronium had no changes in blood pressure or heart rate.[9,27]

### Doxacurium

Doxacurium is a new nondepolarizing muscle relaxant that has recently been introduced into clinical use. The duration of action of doxacurium is similar to that of pancuronium. Unlike pancuronium, doxacurium has few cardiovascular effects.[88] The effective dose of doxacurium in children is similar to that in adults; however, the duration of action in children may be shorter.

The neuromuscular blocking agents with few hemodynamic effects usually are desirable in patients undergoing anesthesia. In children, however, the presence of relatively high parasympathetic tone may lead to profound bradycardia with the use of volatile anesthetics such as halothane. In this setting pancuronium may provide an advantage because its vagolytic effect produces tachycardia.

### Mivacurium

Mivacurium is a new short-acting nondepolarizing neuromuscular blocker. The unique feature of this agent is its metabolism by plasma cholinesterases. The drug has a recovery rate of 5 to 7 minutes

(25% to 75% recovery).[4] In children the effective dose ($ED_{95}$) is 115 μg/kg.[108] When titrated to 95% blockade by monitor, children recovered spontaneously within 10 minutes after discontinuation of the drug.[7] The hemodynamic side effects are limited.[82] Because of its short duration, predictable offset of action, and lack of hemodynamic effects, mivacurium may be a useful drug for short procedures. Its use in surgery for cardiothoracic procedures probably is limited.

## INHALATION ANESTHETICS

The pharmacology of inhalation anesthetics in adults and children is fairly well described in standard anesthesia textbooks. The most commonly used agents in pediatrics are halothane and isoflurane; enflurane is rarely used. Sevoflurane and desflurane are new volatile agents that have been suggested to be useful in children as well.[102] The uptake and distribution of volatile anesthetics in children is greatly affected by the physiology of the maturing child. Children have different respiratory and pulmonary variables from those of adults (Table 6–9). The relatively high respiratory rate, low functional residual capacity, and higher cardiac output in infants produce a more rapid uptake of volatile anesthetics. Because of differences in body composition (greater vessel-rich group than vessel-poor group in infants) the amount of anesthetic reaching the brain is greater during induction in infants (Fig. 6–2). Thus, the concentration of halothane in the brain and other vessel-rich tissues will increase more rapidly in infants at the same inspired halothane concentration.[7,14]

The presence of intracardiac shunts in children with congenital heart disease can affect the uptake of volatile anesthetics. The rate of induction of anesthesia will be slower than with no shunt. The influence of the shunt on uptake and distribution depends on the degree of an intracardiac shunt (Fig. 6–3). In particular, anesthetic agents that have low solubility are affected more than those that have a higher solubility.[96] Inhalation anesthesia is associated with a higher incidence of bradycardia, hypotension, and significant cardiac depression during induction of anesthesia in infants than in adults.[29,53,58,79]

The volatile agents depress the force of contraction in neonatal arterial tissue to a greater extent than they do in adult tissue. Furthermore, the higher parasympathetic tone in children exacerbates the bradycardia seen with volatile agents, especially halothane. Because of higher respiratory rates, the uptake of inspired volatile agents is more rapid in infants and small children than in adults. The use of overpressure techniques may lead to

**Table 6–9** Comparison of lung function in newborn infants and adults

| Respiratory variable | Newborn | Adult |
|---|---|---|
| VT (ml) | 17 | 500 |
| f (breaths/min) | 34 | 12 |
| V̇A (ml/min) | 385 | 4140 |
| FRC (ml) | 75 | 3030 |
| VC (ml) | 100 | 4620 |

VT, Tidal volume; f, breathing frequency; V̇A, alveolar ventilation; FRC, functional residual capacity; VC, vital capacity.
From Cook RD, Marcy JH: Pediatric anesthetic pharmacology. In Cook RD, Marcy JH, editors: *Neonatal anesthesia,* Pasadena, 1988, Appleton and Davies.

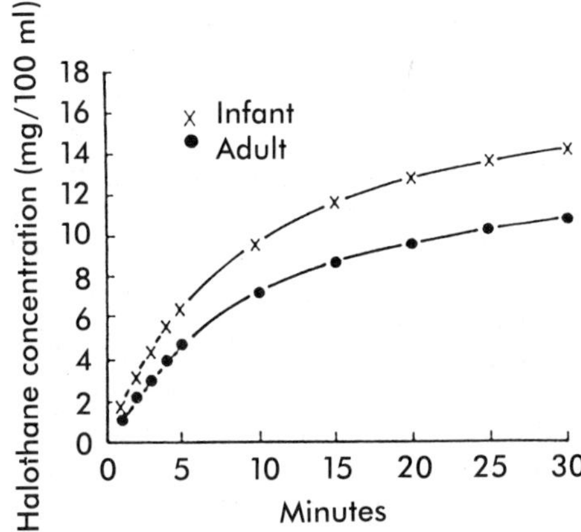


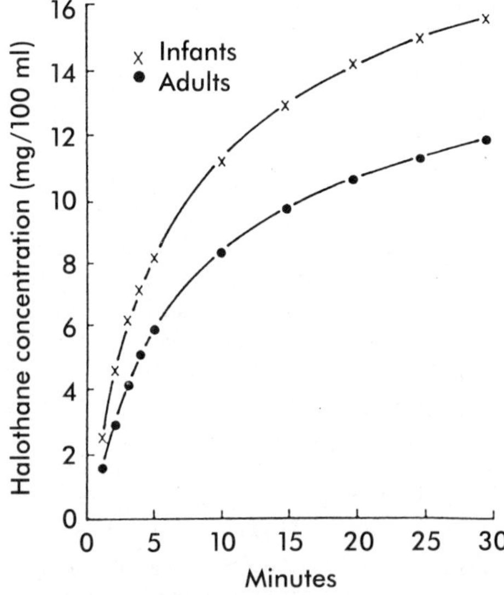


**Figure 6–2** Predicted concentration of halothane in the brain. (From Brandom BW, Cook DR, Brandom RB: *Anesth Analg* 62:404, 1983.)

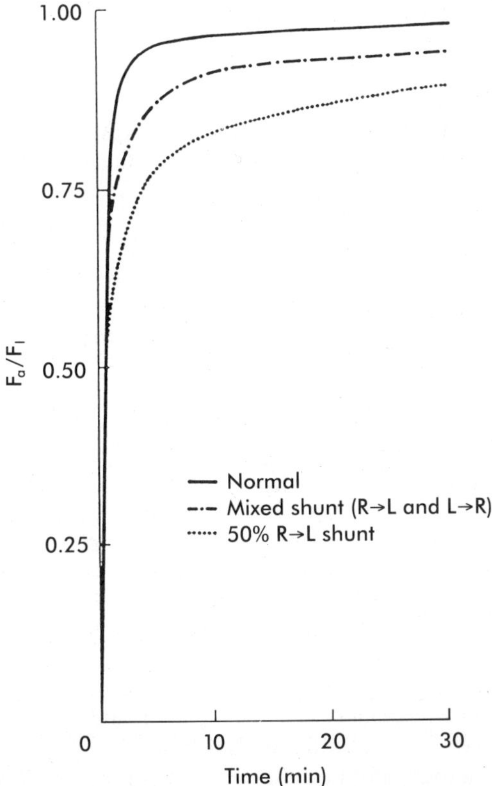


**Figure 6–3** Effect of left to right, mixed left to right, and right to left shunts on inhalation anesthetic induction in children: a computer model. (From Tanner G, Angus D, Barash P et al: *Anesth Analg* 64:101, 1985.)

higher than necessary inspired concentrations during induction. The net result may be significantly elevated concentrations of volatile anesthetics in the brain and heart, producing profound CNS depression and hemodynamic compromise.

The MAC (minimum alveolar concentration) of inhaled anesthetics is different in infants than in adults. As shown in Table 6–10, the MAC of halothane is higher in newborns than in the older age group. This most probably is related to the higher metabolic rate and increased oxygen consumption in infants. Subsequent to the newborn period, the MAC of inhaled anesthetics decreases progressively toward the adult range. Although the precise mechanism for the age-related differences is still unclear, the difference in the coefficient of blood gas solubility likely is the determining factor for the differences in MAC. In infants the blood gas coefficient for halothane decreases with age.

Volatile anesthetics can have significant hemodynamic consequences (box on p. 56). Halothane can cause bradycardia, hypotension, and subsequently cardiac arrest in high doses. As discussed earlier, the untoward effects may result from higher parasympathetic tone in association with higher brain and myocardial concentrations achieved in the infant. The volatile anesthetics have a profound effect on protective baroreceptor reflexes. In particular, halothane can produce direct myocardial depression, bradycardia, and decreased peripheral vascular resistance.[23,24,34] If atropine is administered prior to induction, the cardiovascular effects may be attenuated.[86,94] In animal studies Boudreaux and associates[5] found that cardiac indices, including cardiac output, mean arterial pressure, heart rate, and contracile indices, decreased in piglets

**Table 6–10** Characteristics of four potent inhalation anesthetic agents

| | **Sevoflurane** | **Halothane (Fluothane)** | **Isoflurane (Forane)** | **Desflurane** |
|---|---|---|---|---|
| Boiling point (°C) | 58 | 50.2 | 48.5 | 23.5 |
| Molecular weight (daltons) | 200.1 | 197.4 | 184.5 | 168 |
| Vapor pressure at 20° (mm Hg) | 160 | 243 | 250 | 664 |
| *Solubility or partition coefficients* | | | | |
| Oil/gas | 47.2 | 236 | 99.0 | 19 |
| Blood/gas | 0.59 | 2.3 | 1.4 | 0.4 |
| Odor | Mild | Mild | Pungent | Pungent |
| *MAC (%)* | | | | |
| Infant, 0-3 yrs | — | 1.08 | 1.7 | 8-10a |
| Child, 3-10 yrs | — | 0.9 | 1.4 | |
| Adult | 1.71 | 0.76 | 1.15 | 6.0 |
| Induction speed | Very rapid | Rapid | Less rapid | Very rapid |
| Metabolism | 2.9% | 10%-20% | Nil or minimal | |

From Cook DR, Davis PJ: Pharmacology of pediatric anesthesia. In Motoyama ED, Davis PJ, editors: *Smith's anesthesia for infants and children,* St. Louis, 1990, Mosby, and Taylor RH, Lerman J: Minimum alveolar concentration of desflurane and hemodynamic responses in neonates, infants and children, *Anesthesiology* 75:975, 1991.

**CARDIOVASCULAR EFFECTS OF INHALATION ANESTHETICS**

- Hypoxic pulmonary vasoconstriction *attenuated*
- Systemic blood pressure, myocardial contractility, vascular resistance *decreased*
- Cerebral blood flow autoregulation *attenuated* (blood flow *increases*/becomes dependent on mean arterial pressure, least with isoflurane)
- Renal blood flow, glomerular filtration rate, urine output *decreased* (potential for toxicity halothane>ENF>isoflurane)
- Liver blood flow *decreased* (possible hepatotoxicity halothane>ENF>isoflurane)

following exposure to halothane. When the heart was electrically paced at a more rapid rate, only the rate of change in pressure (dP/dT), cardiac index, and mean arterial pressure decreased. The other cardiac indices improved. Therefore, halothane predominantly seemed to exert a negative inotropic action. The degree of cardiovascular depression did not seem to vary with age.[5,72] The major age-related difference seems to be that of a lower heart rate in the piglet. Similarly, isoflurane exerts a negative inotropic effect and decreases peripheral vascular resistance. However, there ensues a reflex tachycardia that may account for preservation of cardiac output under isoflurane anesthesia.[90]

Volatile anesthetics significantly affect the function of baroreceptor reflexes. These reflexes are responsible for modulating the hemodynamic changes in blood pressure by influencing heart rate, myocardial contractility, and systemic vascular resistance. Baroreceptor function may not be fully developed in the neonate.[38] In a study by Gregory in 1982, premature infants undergoing PDA ligation were anesthetized with halothane.[25] After ductus ligation the systemic blood flow and the arterial pressure increased without a change in heart rate, indicating possible absence of baroreceptor activity in the anesthetized infant. Studies in adult and infant rabbits demonstrated the differences in baroreceptor response in immature and mature animals.[20,104] The baroreceptor reflex was less sensitive in the awake immature animal than in the awake mature animal. Moreover, at equal MAC doses of halothane, reflexes were affected more in the infants than in the adults. The attenuation or elimination of baroreceptor reflexes by a volatile agent can put the immature patient at risk for adverse events during anesthesia. In particular, premature or term infants undergoing cardiovascular or noncardiac surgery may be at significant risk for hemodynamic compromise if inhalation agents are used.

## CARDIOTONIC AGENTS

The pharmacologic support of cardiovascular function (Table 6–11) requires basic understanding of the functioning of the circulatory system. Lack of adequate cardiac output and systemic perfusion can lead to profound and irreversible damage to brain, kidney, and other tissues that cannot tolerate long periods of hypoperfusion. Appropriate pharmacologic support may be necessary in the perioperative state for children with cardiac dysfunction.

Perfusion inadequate to meet the needs of the tissue bed involved defines the shock state. Low cardiac output for any of a variety of reasons is the principal cardiac reason for the shock state. Myocardial (pump) failure may occur in high cardiac output states, such as arteriovenous malformations or other vascular shunts, thyrotoxicosis, or extreme increases in metabolism, or in low cardiac output states, such as primary myocardial failure. The purpose of this section is to discuss pharmacologic means available to support circulatory failure caused by myocardial dysfunction.

The scope of this chapter does not permit a full discussion on myocardial performance. Nevertheless, a brief review of the Frank Starling phenomenon will demonstrate the aims of pharmacologic intervention (Fig 6–4). The Frank Starling phenomenon is an oversimplified explanation of myocardial performance. It states that the "force of contraction of a muscle fiber is dependent on the initial fiber length." In the intact heart the fiber length is directly associated with the diastolic volume, which determines the length of the muscle fiber (sarcomere) and the eventual force of contraction. The tension against which the muscle works is termed the afterload. This is the tension in the ventricular wall during systole, and it is dependent on the diastolic radius of the ventricle, systemic vascular resistance, and ventricular wall thickness. In the intact animal, afterload may be considered directly proportional to systemic vascular resistance. As systemic vascular resistance increases, the afterload of the ventricle increases, and as it decreases, so does the afterload. The inotropic state of the heart is the ability of the ventricular musculature to develop the force of contraction independent of preload and afterload. Changes in the inotropic state can occur because of intrinsic weakness of the muscle, ischemic disease, myocardiopathy, age of the muscle, and other conditions. Assessment of the patient's inotropic state can be made by measuring the rate of pressure change (dP/dT) over various preloads while main-

**Table 6–11** Comparative pharmacology of sympathomimetics

| | Receptors stimulated | | | Mechanism of action | Cardiac effects | | | Peripheral vascular resistance | Renal blood flow | Mean arterial pressure | Airway resistance | Central nervous system stimulation | Single intravenous dose (70-kg adult) | Continuous infusion dose (70-kg adult) |
|---|---|---|---|---|---|---|---|---|---|---|---|---|---|---|
| | Alpha | Beta-1 | Beta-2 | | Cardiac output | Heart rate | Dysrhythmias | | | | | | | |
| **Natural catecholamines** | | | | | | | | | | | | | | |
| Epinephrine | + | ++ | ++ | Direct | ++ | ++ | +++ | ± | – – | + | – – | Yes | 2-8 μg | 1-20 μg/min$^{-1}$ |
| Norepinephrine | +++ | ++ | 0 | Direct | – | – | + | +++ | – – – | +++ | NC | No | Not used | 4-15 μg/min$^{-1}$ |
| Dopamine | ++ | ++ | + | Direct | +++ | + | + | + | +++ | + | NC | No | Not used | 2-20 μg/kg$^{-1}$ min$^{-1}$ |
| **Synthetic catecholamines** | | | | | | | | | | | | | | |
| Isoproterenol | 0 | +++ | +++ | | +++ | +++ | +++ | – – | – | ± | – – – | Yes | 1-4 μg | 1-5 μg/min$^{-1}$ |
| Dobutamine | 0 | +++ | 0 | | +++ | + | ± | NC | ++ | + | NC | | Not used | 2-10 μg/kg$^{-1}$ min$^{-1}$ |
| **Synthetic noncatecholamines** | | | | | | | | | | | | | | |
| ***Indirect-acting*** | | | | | | | | | | | | | | |
| Ephedrine | ++ | + | + | Indirect, some direct | ++ | ++ | ++ | + | – – | ++ | – – | Yes | 10-25 mg | Not used |
| Mephentermine | ++ | + | + | Indirect | ++ | ++ | ++ | + | – – | ++ | – | Yes | 10-25 mg | Not used |
| Amphetamines | ++ | + | + | Indirect | + | + | + | ++ | – – | + | NC | Yes | Not used | Not used |
| Metaraminol | ++ | + | + | Indirect, direct | – | – | + | +++ | – – – | +++ | NC | No | 1.5-5 mg | 40-500 μg/min |
| ***Direct-acting*** | | | | | | | | | | | | | | |
| Phenylephrine | +++ | 0 | 0 | Direct | – | – | NC | +++ | – – – | +++ | NC | No | 50-100 μg | 20-50 μg/min$^{-1}$ |
| Methoxamine | +++ | 0 | 0 | Direct | – | – | NC | +++ | – – – | +++ | NC | No | 5-10 mg | |

0, none; +, minimal increase; ++, moderate increase; +++, marked increase; –, minimal decrease; – –, moderate decrease; – – –, marked decrease; NC, No change
From Stoelting RK: *Pharmacology and physiology in anesthetic practice,* ed 2, Philadelphia, 1991, Lippincott.

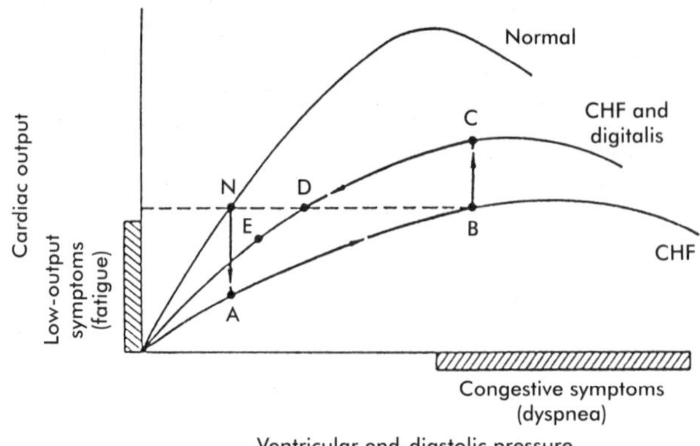


**Figure 6–4** Digitalis and allied cardiac glycosides. (From Hoffman BF, Bigger JT: Digitalis and allied cardiac glycosides. In Goodman LS and Gilman AG, editors: *The pharmacological basis of therapeutics,* ed 8, Pergamon Press, 1990, New York.)

taining constant afterload and heart rate. The final determinant of myocardial performance is heart rate. Increased heart rate may result in a slight increase in inotropic state. Unfortunately, increases in heart rate also are associated with significant increases in myocardial oxygen consumption. These usually are not compensated by concurrent increases in myocardial blood flow. Thus, the myocardium may be compromised because of a relative reduction in myocardial perfusion. Several sympathetic adrenergic agents are available clinically for hemodynamic support. The agents most commonly used in pediatric patients are isoproterenol, epinephrine, norepinephrine, and phenylephrine. Recently amrinone has gained popularity as postoperative inotropic agent for the child.

Epinephrine is a naturally occurring catecholamine with both α- and β- adrenergic effects. It is used to provide an increase both in inotropic state and in heart rate. Epinephrine infusion decreases peripheral vascular resistance at low doses but will increase it at higher doses. Coronary blood flow is increased, but renal blood flow is significantly decreased. With moderate to high dose infusions, myocardial oxygen demand is increased, producing a potentially detrimental state of lower coronary blood flow and increased myocardial oxygen demand. Furthermore, moderate to high doses and prolonged usage of epinephrine may increase the likelihood of ventricular ectopy.

Isoproterenol is a pure β (β-I and β-II) agonist and as such is a potent inotropic agent.[84] However, it significantly increases heart rate and myocardial oxygen demand simultaneously. Isoproterenol decreases peripheral vascular resistance because of its effect on β-II receptors. This action may have the beneficial effect of increasing cardiac output. The agent also decreases pulmonary vascular resistance, thus decreasing the afterload to both the right and left ventricle. However, because of the profound increase in myocardial oxygen demand associated with tachycardia and the risk of tachyarrhythmias, isoproterenol should be used with caution.

Dopamine is another naturally occurring catecholamine that affects both dopaminergic and adrenergic α- and β-receptors. Dopamine increases inotropy greater than chronotropy, thus producing a more advantageous hemodynamic state. In addition, ventricular ectopy is less likely than with epinephrine or isoproterenol. At higher doses, the α-adrenergic effects of dopamine are associated with increased systemic vascular resistance similar to the effects of epinephrine. In children dopamine exerts an inotropic effect in premature and term infants even at "lower" doses. In this age group dopaminergic receptors in the myocardium can lead to increased contractility without the concurrent increase in heart rate or systemic vascular resistance seen with higher doses. Dopamine has additional advantageous effects at lower doses (3 to 5 μg/kg/min) in decreasing renal vascular resistance and increasing renal blood flow. This renal protective dopaminergic effect is the reason dopamine is frequently used in the intensive care setting.

Dobutamine is a synthetic catecholamine derivative of isoproterenol. The agent is a strong β-I adrenergic agent with little β-II effect. As such, dobutamine is a potent inotropic agent without the significant increase in heart rate (chronotropy) that is seen with isoproterenol. The drug also has few of the undesirable side effects of the other inotropes—such as ventricular arrhythmias and effects on peripheral vascular activity and chronotropy. Dobutamine has no effect on dopaminergic receptors and therefore does not affect renal perfusion.

### Noncatecholamine, nonglyceride cardiac inotropes

Amrinone is a bipyridine derivative that has dose-dependent effects on cardiac inotropy and peripheral vasodilation. These actions lead to an increase in cardiac output, decrease in systemic vascular resistance, and therefore decrease in left ventricular end diastolic pressure (LVEDP).[59,110] With the infusion of amrinone the heart rate may increase, and because of the vasodilation the blood pressure may decrease. Amrinone seems to have no antidysrhythmic or arrhythmogenic properties.

Amrinone inhibits the phosphodiesterase enzyme and produces an increase in intracellular cyclic adenosine monophosphate. This leads to increased calcium in the myocardial contractile system.[35] The increased availability of calcium produces greater contractility, which is not altered by the presence of α- or β-adrenergic blockade or inhibition of the $Na^+ - K^+ -$ ATPase system. Amrinone has a half-life of approximately 6 hours and is excreted primarily through the kidneys. The drug can be given either orally or intravenously. In the perioperative state, it is usually given intravenously at 0.5 to 1.5 mg/kg, usually followed by an infusion of 2 to 10 μg/kg/min. A maximum recommended dose is 10 mg/kg/day. The most common undesirable effects of amrinone are hypotension due to vasodilation and thrombocytopenia, which is seen with chronic use of amrinone.

Milrinone is bipyridine derivative that has positive inotropic and vasodilating effects. It can be given orally or intravenously. Compared with amrinone it may produce a greater reduction in LVEDP and blood pressure.[39] However, the side effects of thrombocytopenia and possible hepatic dysfunction may be less with milrinone.[2]

## VASODILATORS

Vasodilators are frequently used in the postoperative period or in patients with pump failure to improve myocardial performance and systemic perfusion.[95] The use of vasodilators is aimed at decreasing left ventricular afterload and thus improving left ventricular dysfunction. The systemic vasodilators most commonly used in the perioperative period are those that can be titrated in an infusion: sodium nitroprusside, trinitroglycerin, and trimethaphan.

Sodium nitroprusside (SNP) is the most frequently used vasodilating agent. It is a direct-acting relaxer of arteriolar and venular smooth muscle that affects both preload and afterload. The agent decreases both systemic vascular resistance and mean arterial blood pressure. The infusion of SNP also is associated with slightly decreased systemic blood pressure and decreased pulmonary vascular resistance. Furthermore, patients with left ventricular dysfunction (who are on the right side of the Frank Starling curve) will exhibit an increase in cardiac output and systemic perfusion. The decreased resistances induce a reflex tachycardia associated with an increase in myocardial oxygen consumption. Thus, the beneficial effects of decreased systemic vascular resistance may be counteracted by the increase in $M\dot{V}O_2$. The effect on systemic perfusion including renal perfusion is dependent on the effect on cardiac output. In patients who have increased cardiac output, renal blood flow is increased. In patients whose systemic perfusion is decreased because of a significant reduction in mean arterial blood pressure, renal blood flow may actually decrease.

Nitroglycerin primarily affects venous capacitance and therefore the preload. It has little effect on afterload (or systemic vascular resistance). The drug also decreases pulmonary artery pressure. In patients with myocardial dysfunction, a decrease in preload may shift the cardiac function toward the left on the Frank-Starling curve, improving cardiac output for a given left ventricular end diastolic volume.

Trimethaphan is a short-acting ganglionic blocking agent that alters arterial and venous tone. The agent decreases both preload and afterload, although the effect on venous capacitance is greater than that on systemic vascular resistance. Because the drug blocks transmission in sympathetic ganglia, a reflex tachycardia does not occur with the use of trimethaphan. Trimethaphan is associated with a rapid onset of tachyphylaxis and a variable response to blood pressure. Therefore this agent has fallen into disfavor for routine use.

Recently, a tremendous amount of interest has been generated by the proposed multiple biological roles of endothelium derived relaxing factor (EDRF), which is thought to be nitric oxide (NO). NO is a potent vasodilator. The use of inhaled NO for selective pulmonary vasodilation suggests an exciting and innovative therapeutic use. In the new born lamb, NO has been shown to reverse pulmonary vasoconstriction caused by hypoxia and acidosis. Preliminary studies in lambs and in infants with congenital heart disease have demonstrated that NO at concentrations of 20-80 particles per min rapidly reverses hypoxic pulmonary vasoconstriction without producing systemic hypotension. Thus, if further clinical trials support these findings, NO may be extremely useful in the management of children with pulmonary hypertension.

## ANTIARRHYTHMICS

Antiarrhythmic drugs can be classified into several categories according to their mechanism of action (Table 6–12). These agents exert their effects by altering the myocardial action potential in various

**Table 6–12** Classification of antiarrhythmic agents by mechanism of action

| Class | Mechanism of action | Drug | Effect on ECG |
|---|---|---|---|
| I | Fast sodium channel blockade: depress phase 0 depolarization and prolong conduction | | |
| IA | Prolong repolarization and refractory period | Quinidine<br>Procainamide<br>Disopyramide | Prolong QRS and QTc |
| IB | Shorten repolarization | Lidocaine<br>Tocainide<br>Mexiletine<br>Phenytoin | Minimal effect on PR, QRS, and QTc |
| IC | Slow conduction; little effect on repolarization | Encainide<br>Flecainide<br>Lorcainide<br>Propafenone | Prolong PR, QRS, and QTc |
| Uncl | Combined effects of IA, IB, and/or IC | Ethmozine | May prolong PR and QRS |
| II | β-adrenergic blockade | Propranolol<br>Timolol<br>Metoprolol | Prolong PR |
| III | Prolong repolarization and refractory period | Amiodarone<br>Bretylium | Prolong PR and QTc |
| IV | Slow calcium channel blockade | Verapamil<br>Diltiazem<br>Nifedipine | Prolong PR |

Uncl, unclassified; QTc, QT interval corrected for heart rate.
From Gorodischer R, Koren G: Cardiac drugs. In Yaffe SF, Aranda JV, editors: *Pediatric pharmacology,* ed 2, New York, 1992, McGraw Hill.

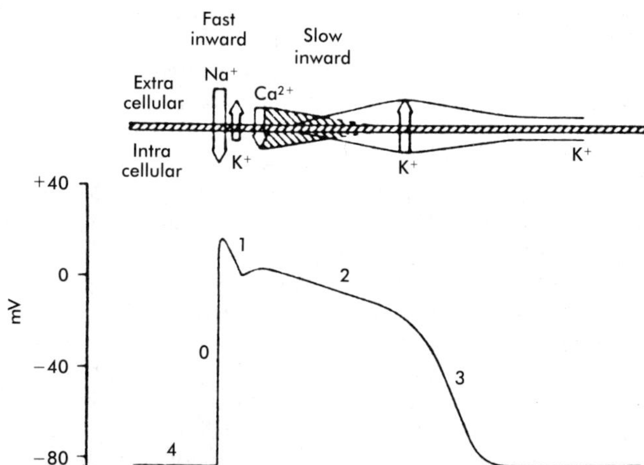


**Figure 6–5** Ventricular action potential and major associated ionic currents. Phase 0 is associated with rapid $Na^+$ influx, phase 1 with $K^+$ efflux. During early phase 2 there is a slow inward $Ca^{++}$ movement that gradually decreases while $K^+$ efflux slowly accelerates, eventually restoring the negative resting membrane potential. (From Radde IC, MacLeod SM: Cardiovascular pharmacology. In Radde IC, McLeod SM, editors: *Pediatric pharmacology and therapeutics,* ed 2, St Louis, 1993, Mosby.)

**Table 6–13** Pharmacokinetics of cardiac antidysrhythmic drugs

| | Principal clearance mechanism | Protein binding (%) | Elimination half-life (h) | Therapeutic plasma concentration |
|---|---|---|---|---|
| Quinidine | Hepatic | 80-90 | 5-12 | 2-8 μg/ml$^{-1}$ |
| Procainamide | Renal/hepatic | 15 | 2.5-5 | 4-10 μg/ml$^{-1}$ |
| Disopyramide | Renal/hepatic | 15 | 8-12 | 2-4 μg/ml$^{-1}$ |
| Lidocaine | Hepatic | 55 | 1.4-1.8 | 1-5 μg/ml$^{-1}$ |
| Tocainide | Hepatic/renal | 10-30 | 12-15 | 4-10 μg/ml$^{-1}$ |
| Mexiletine | Hepatic | 60-75 | 6-12 | 0.75-2 μg/ml$^{-1}$ |
| Phenytoin | Hepatic | 93 | 8-60 | 10-20 μg/ml$^{-1}$ |
| Flecainide | Hepatic | 35-45 | 13-30 | 0.3-1.5 μg/ml$^{-1}$ |
| Encainide | Hepatic/renal | 70 | 1-3 | 0.3-0.6 μg/ml$^{-1}$ |
| Propranolol | Hepatic | 90-95 | 2-4 | 10-30 ng/ml$^{-1}$ |
| Bretylium | Renal | <10 | 8-12 | 75-100 ng/ml$^{-1}$ |
| Amiodarone | Hepatic | 96 | 8-107 days | 1.5-2 μg/ml$^{-1}$ |
| Verapamil | Hepatic | 90 | 4.5-12 | 100-300 ng/ml$^{-1}$ |

From Stoelting RK: *Pharmacology and physiology in anesthetic practice,* ed 2, Philadelphia, 1991, Lippincott.

ways (Fig. 6–5). Class I contains local anesthetics or membrane stabilizers. Class II is composed of β-adrenergic blocking agents. Class III consists of bretylium, amiodarone, and other antiadrenergic agents. The calcium entry blocking agents comprise the class IV agents. The pharmacology of antiarrhythmics is summarized in Tables 6–13 through 6–15 and the box on p. 63.

### Class I agents

Lidocaine is a local anesthetic that depresses the automaticity of the Purkinje fibers and reduces the refractory period of the His-Purkinje fibers. Lidocaine may alter the intraventricular and AV nodal conduction in a variety of manners, including increasing, decreasing, or not affecting the time. Although lidocaine has no effect on the resting membrane potential of the muscle, it does suppress spontaneous diastolic depolarization and automatic impulse initiation or automaticity. Phase IV depolarization also is decreased because of a reduction in the potassium conduction (outward current). This effect is more pronounced in ventricular muscle and the conduction tissue of the atrium. In addition, lidocaine increases the depolarization threshold to ventricular stimulation, thus reducing the chance of PVCs. The drug has a negative inotropic effect on left ventricular contractility and is a potent peripheral vasodilator at higher doses. Usually the antiarrhythmic effects are exerted at lower doses, and cardiac contractility and cardiac output are not affected.

Lidocaine is used to treat arrhythmias caused by digitalis intoxication. Arrhythmias occurring during cardiac catheterization or postoperatively will also respond to lidocaine treatment. PVCs following myocardial infarction and recurrent severe ventricular tachycardia also will respond favorably to lidocaine therapy. Ventricular fibrillation may respond to a combination of IV lidocaine and cardioversion. The drug is usually administered as a loading dose (1 to 2 mg/kg) followed by repeat bolus dosing or continuous infusion (1 to 2 mg/min 20 to 50 μg/kg/min). The agent equilibrates rapidly in the perfused tissue beds and is taken up by fat tissues. At least 90% of lidocaine is metabolized in the liver and subsequently excreted in the urine. A bolus dose will last approximately 20 minutes. An IV infusion that follows bolus dosing can sustain therapeutic lidocaine levels (1 to 2 μg/ml, up to 5 μg/ml) for a prolonged period.

Lidocaine is contraindicated in patients with AV disassociation and idioventricular or slow nodal rhythms. On occasion complete heart block has occurred in patients who were given lidocaine. Lidocaine is not particularly effective in supraventricular arrhythmias and junctional tachycardias. The most common form of lidocaine toxicity occurs in the CNS. Patients become drowsy and may be euphoric or dysphoric. This is quickly followed by disorientation and seizures. Respiratory depression also may occur and lead to respiratory arrest.

Phenytoin depresses the sympathetic nervous system and efferent sympathetic activity. The drug shortens the duration of the action potential and decreases the amplitude and the maximum upstroke velocity of phase 0. Conduction in ventricular muscle or in Purkinje fibers is not affected at the usual drug concentrations and usual levels of potassium. Phenytoin is an effective agent in treating both atrial and ventricular arrhythmias. Adverse reactions that can occur with rapid intravenous infusion include hypotension, decreased myocardial con-

**Table 6–14** Therapeutic indications for antiarrhythmic drugs

| Drug | Therapeutic indications | Comments | Route | Dose |
|---|---|---|---|---|
| Quinidine | PVD, VT | Contraindicated in long QT syndrome | PO | 15-60 mg/kg/day (q6h) (Test dose 2 mg/kg) |
| Procainamide | PVD, VT | Contraindicated in myasthenia gravis and complete heart block | IV | Initial: 3-6 mg/kg over 5 min (max dose 500 mg); maintenance: 0.02-0.08 mg/kg/min (max 60 mg/kg/day) |
| Disopyramide | PVD, VT (non–life-threatening) | | PO | 15-50 mg/kg/day (q4-6h) (max 4 gm/day) |
| Lidocaine | VT | | PO | 3-6 mg/kg/day (q6h) adjusted for plasma conc >2 μg/ml |
| Phenytoin | Digoxin-induced tachyarrhythmias | Infuse slowly | IV | Initial: 1-5 mg/kg; maintenance: 0.01-0.05 mg/kg/min |
| Mexiletine | VA in CHD | May replace phenytoin in patients with phenytoin side effects | IV | 2-4 mg/kg over 5 min |
| Encainide | PJRT, SVT refractory to digoxin, propranolol, verapamil | Greater efficacy when combined with verapamil or propranolol | PO | 2-5 mg/kg/day (q12h) |
| Flecainide | Refractory and life-threatening arrhythmias | | PO | 60-120 mg/m²/day (q6-8h) |
| Propafenone | Life-threatening postoperative JET | Infuse colloid during loading to maintain BP | IV | 0.4-2 mg/kg over 5-10 min |
| Ethmozine | AET originating in right atrium | | PO | 3-6 mg/kg/day (q8-12h) increase if necessary to max 20 mg/kg |
| Propranolol | SVA, VA, digitalis-induced arrhythmias | Contraindicated in asthma and heart block | IV | Loading: boluses of 0.2 mg/kg q10min until ventricular rate <150/min or max 2 mg/kg<br>Maintenance: 0.004-0.0077 mg/kg/min |
| Amiodarone | Refractory and life-threatening arrhythmias in CHD, myocarditis, cardiomyopathies | Screen thyroid function, monitor HR in sick sinus syndrome, use with caution with other antiarrhythmics. Decrease digoxin dose to ½ (kinetic and dynamic interaction) | PO | 200 mg/m²/day (q8h) |
| Verapamil | Reentrant SVT | Contraindicated in severe low cardiac output, intracardiac right to left shunt, patient receiving beta blockers. Use with extreme caution in infants | IV | 0.01-0.02 mg/kg over 10 min (may repeat q6-8h) |
| | | | PO | 0.2-4 mg/kg/day (q6-8h) |
| | | | IV | 5-7 mg/kg over 30 min, followed by 1-2 mg/kg/h for 24-48 h |
| | | | PO | Loading: 10 mg/kg/day (q12h) for 7-10 days<br>Maintenance: 5 mg/kg/day for 1-2 mos; then decrease (to 2.5 mg/kg/day) or increase (to 10-15 mg/kg/day) according to response |
| | | | IV | 0.1 mg/kg over 30 s; may repeat ×2 after 15-min intervals |
| | | | PO | 0.01-0.3 mg/kg/day (q6-8h) |

From Gorodischer R, Koren G: Cardiac drugs. In Yaffe SJ, Aranda JV, editors: *Pediatric pharmacology,* ed 2, Philadelphia, 1992, Saunders.

**Table 6–15** Efficacy of antidysrhythmic drugs for treatment of specific cardiac dysrhythmias

| | Conversion of atrial fibrillation | Paroxysmal supraventricular tachycardia | Premature ventricular contractions | Ventricular tachycardia |
|---|---|---|---|---|
| Quinidine | + | + + | + + | + |
| Procainamide | + | + + | + + | + + |
| Disopyramide | + | + + | + + | + + |
| Lidocaine | 0 | 0 | + + | + + |
| Tocainide | 0 | 0 | + + | + + |
| Mexiletine | 0 | 0 | + + | + + |
| Phenytoin | 0 | 0 | + + | + + |
| Flecainide | 0 | + | + + | + + |
| Encainide | 0 | + | + + | + + |
| Propranolol | + | + + | + | + |
| Bretylium | 0 | 0 | + | + + |
| Amiodarone | + | + + | + + | + + |
| Verapamil | + | + + | 0 | 0 |

0, no effect; +, effective; + +, highly effective
From Stoelting RK: *Pharmacology and physiology in anesthetic practice,* ed 2, Philadelphia, 1991, Lippincott.

**UNTOWARD EFFECTS OF ANTIARRHYTHMIC DRUGS**

| Drug | Untoward effect |
|---|---|
| Quinidine | Cardiotoxicity (SA and AV blocks, VT, asystole), hypotension, cinchonism, nausea, vomiting, diarrhea, hypersensitivity reactions |
| Procainamide | Cardiotoxicity, hypotension, nausea, vomiting, psychosis, systemic lupus syndrome, hypersensitivity reactions |
| Disopyramide | Atropine-like symptoms (dry mouth, constipation, blurred vision, urinary retention), nausea, vomiting, cardiac depression |
| Lidocaine | Paresthesias, behavior changes, hypocusia, convulsions, respiratory arrest |
| Phenytoin | Nystagmus, ataxia, vertigo, nausea |
| Mexiletine | Headache, tremor, paresthesias, mood changes, nausea, rash |
| Encainide | Headache, fatigue, dizziness, proarrhythmic effects, heart failure, blurred vision, tremor |
| Flecainide | Proarrhythmic events, nausea |
| Propafenone | Hypotension, nausea, vomiting, congestive heart failure, proarrhythmic events, personality changes, sleep disturbances |
| Ethmozine | Headache, allergic reactions, neurologic, gastrointestinal, and proarrhythmic effects |
| Propranolol | Hypotension, heart failure, AV block, asystole |
| Amiodarone | Corneal microdeposits, gritty eyes, rash, headache, peripheral neuropathy, abnormal thyroid function, sleep disturbances, personality changes, photosensitivity, gray pigmentation of skin, abnormal liver function, liver failure, encephalopathy, cardiotoxicity (sinus bradycardia, AV block, deterioration of sinus or AV node function, VT, VF, Torsade de pointes with QTc prolongation.) Pulmonary fibrosis (in adults) |
| Verapamil | Cardiotoxicity (sinus node depression, bradycardia, AV block, asystole, heart failure), hypotension, shock, nausea, vomiting, constipation, hepatotoxicity |

From Gorodischer R, Koren G: Cardiac drugs. In Yaffe SJ, Aranda JV, editors: *Pediatric pharmacology: therapeutic principles in practice,* ed 2, Philadelphia, 1992, Saunders.

tractility, and bradycardia. The toxicity of the agent primarily is depression of the myocardium, associated with bradycardia, hypotension, and possibly asystole. The drug commonly is used in doses of 1 to 2 mg/kg administered over a 5-minute period. Repeat doses may be given in 5-minute intervals to treat persistent arrhythmias.

Quinidine, a highly lipid soluble agent, affects cation transfer in the cell membrane and depresses the membrane potential. Quinidine blocks sodium entry through the fast sodium channel and depresses diastolic depolarization in phase IV. The drug has numerous effects on the heart: increased threshold of ventricular tissue to electrical excitability, reduced myocardial contractility, direct dilatation of peripheral arteries, slower heart rate because of vagolytic actions in the S-A node, increased AV nodal conduction, and decreased depolarization in phase 0. The quinidine-induced decrease in conduction affects ectopic pacemaker tissue to a greater extent than normal tissue, accounting for its antiarrhythmic action. Quinidine is most commonly used to treat atrial fibrillation, atrial tachycardias, paroxysmal supraventricular tachycardia (PSVT), and ventricular tachycardia. Premature atrial contractions (PACs) and PVCs are suppressed because of the prolongation of the refractory period. The drug is contraindicated in complete AV block. In addition, an idiosyncratic effect also makes it contraindicated in thrombocytopenic purpura. Hypotension, myocardial depression, and exacerbation of conduction disorders may also occur with quinidine. Commonly, quinidine is administered IV in doses of 2.5 to 5 mg/kg/60 min. The drug is metabolized by the liver and excreted through the kidneys. Up to 50% may be excreted unchanged.

Procainamide depresses the excitability of both the atrium and the ventricle. The amplitude of the atrial, ventricular, and Purkinje action potentials are reduced following procainamide administration. Concurrently, the affected refractory period is prolonged. The threshold of ventricular and atrial fibrillation is increased, and phase IV depolarization and conduction velocity are both decreased. Hypotension may occur with intravenous administration of procainamide, particularly if administered rapidly. Procainamide can prolong the PR and Q-T intervals on the ECG, which may induce PVCs or PSVT. This agent is contraindicated in complete AV block. Normally procainamide is administered in a dose of 4 to 6 mg/kg given over 10 minutes. Toxic effects include conduction defects, arrhythmias, and hypotension. At least 60% of the drug is metabolized and is excreted in the urine. Idiosyncratic effects include agranulocytosis, rashes, psychosis, and convulsions.

### Class II β-adrenergic blocking agents

β-adrenergic antagonists bind selectively to the β-adrenergic receptors and interfere with the action of catecholamines and other sympathomimetic agents. Of particular clinical importance are the β-adrenergic effects on the heart, smooth muscles of the airways, and blood vessels. Adrenergic agents are commonly used in the treatment of arrhythmias and hypertension. Chronic administration of these agents is associated with upregulation or increased number of β-adrenergic receptors.

Most of the beta antagonists are derivatives of isoproterenol (Fig. 6–6). Because of the structural changes, these agents can attach to the β-receptors but not activate intracellular processes. The receptor binding is reversible and depends on the concentration of both the agonist and the antagonist at the receptor site. β-Adrenergic agents are classified as selective or nonselective for the subtypes β-I and β-II receptors. Even antagonists that selectively bind to β-I or β-II receptors exert cross-effects on the other receptor subtypes at higher doses (a loss of specificity). At high doses β-adrenergic agents can produce membrane stabilization in the myocardium because of the receptor blockade. Bradycardia and myocardial depression may ensue because of the lack of reflex action in the sympathetic nervous system. The pharmacologic characteristics of β-receptor antagonists are listed in Table 6–16.

***Nonselective antagonists.*** Propranolol is the classic nonselective β-adrenergic receptor antagonist. The drug, a pure antagonist, affects β-I and β-II receptors equally. The most important actions of propranolol are exerted on the heart. The drug decreases both heart rate and cardiac output. The bradycardia is more profound and longer lasting than the effect on myocardial contractility. Simultaneous β-II blockade can result in increased vascular resistance, including in coronary vessels. Conversely, the decrease in heart rate and in myocardial contractility result in decreased $M\dot{V}O_2$, improving the bioenergetics of the heart. Therefore, in conditions of myocardial ischemia the drug can actually improve the relationship between supply and demand.

Propranolol is rapidly absorbed and distributed through the gastrointestinal tract. With oral administration the drug is extensively metabolized (up to 70%) through first passed metabolism. Propranolol is highly protein bound (up to 95%), and this may reduce its overall clearance.[103] The primary mode of clearance of propranolol is through hepatic metabolism, with one active metabolite (4-hydroxypropranolol) being formed. The remaining metabolic by-products are not active and are excreted in the urine within 2 to 3 hours of admin-

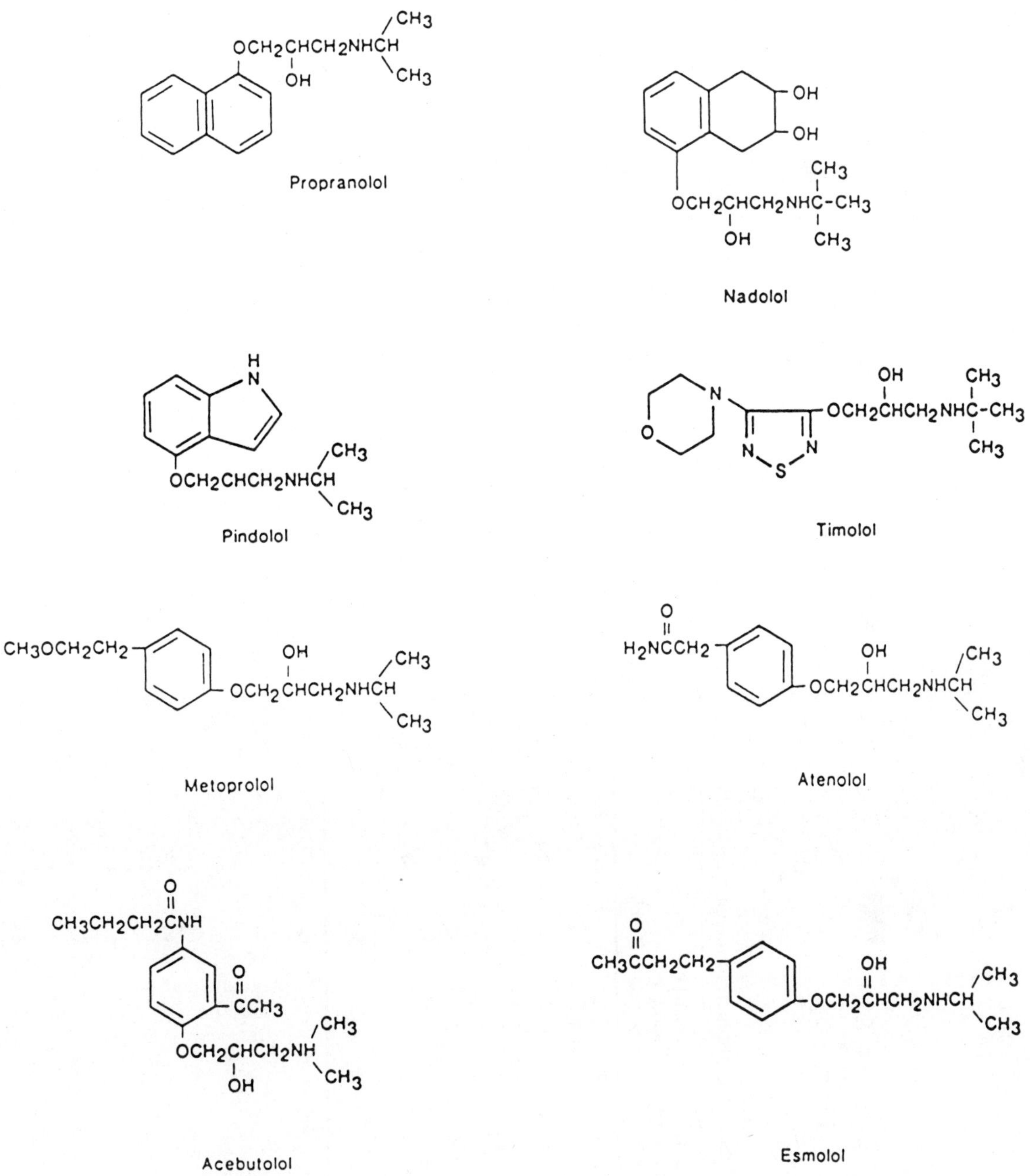

Propranolol

Nadolol

Pindolol

Timolol

Metoprolol

Atenolol

Acebutolol

Esmolol

**Figure 6–6** Structure of β-adrenergic antagonists. (From Stoelting RK: *Pharmacology & physiology in anesthetic practice,* Chapter 14, ed 2, Philadelphia, 1991, Lippincott.)

istration. In low perfusion states such as congestive heart failure and cardiopulmonary bypass, the elimination of propranolol is greatly reduced because of decreased hepatic blood flow, and the effects of propranolol may be prolonged.

In combination with local anesthetics, propranolol will reduce the clearance of amide anesthetics.[6] The reduction in clearance may reflect both reduced hepatic blood flow and metabolism of the anesthetics. The systemic toxicity of the local anesthetics, in particular bupivacaine, may be increased with the use of propranolol. This is of particular interest for children who undergo epidural anesthesia in the perioperative period.

Propranolol most frequently is used in the treatment of PATs, PATs secondary to digitalis toxicity, PVCs in the presence of myocardial ischemia or after surgery, and hypertrophic cardiomyopathy. In

**Table 6–16** Comparative characteristics of β-adrenergic receptor antagonists

| | Cardio-selective activity | Intrinsic sympathomimetic activity | Membrane stabilizing activity | Protein binding (%) | Clearance | Active metabolites | Elimination half-life (h) | Adult oral dose (mg) |
|---|---|---|---|---|---|---|---|---|
| Propranolol | No | 0 | + + | 90-95 | Hepatic | Yes | 2-3 | 40-1000 |
| Nadolol | No | 0 | 0 | 30 | Renal | No | 20-24 | 40-640 |
| Pindolol | No | + | +/− | 40-60 | Hepatic<br>Renal | No | 3-4 | 5-40 |
| Timolol | No | +/− | + | 10 | Hepatic | No | 3-4 | 5-45 |
| Metoprolol | Yes | 0 | +/− | 10 | Hepatic | No | 3-4 | 50-400 |
| Atenolol | Yes | 0 | 0 | 5 | Renal | No | 6-7 | 50-300 |
| Acebutolol | Yes | + | + | 25 | Hepatic<br>Renal | Yes | 3-4 | 200-800 |
| Esmolol | Yes | | | | Plasma hydrolysis | | 0.15 | 10-80 mg IV<br>100-300 $\mu \cdot kg^{-1} \cdot min^{-1}$ IV |

From Stoelting RK: *Pharmacology and physiology in anesthetic practice*, ed 2, Philadelphia, 1991, Lippincott.

addition, it is quite useful in the treatment of pheochromocytoma to reduce the systemic effects of circulating catecholamines. In children the doses recommended for supraventricular tachycardia (SVT) are 1 to 2 μg/kg. For treatment of infundibular spasm in tetralogy of Fallot, propranolol may be given orally 1 to 4 mg/kg or intravenously 1 mg at a time up to 3 mg. The hemodynamic effects of propranolol may be potentiated under anesthesia with volatile agents (halothane or enflurane). In particular, bradycardia and hypotension may be significantly exaggerated with concurrent use of inhalational anesthesia.

Treatment of side effects or toxicity is symptomatic. Atropine may be useful to counteract the bradycardia. If the response to atropine is inadequate or myocardial failure is present, isoproterenol may be indicated.

Because of its side effects propranolol is contraindicated in the presence of bradycardia, congestive heart failure, AV dissociation, significant reactive airways disease (asthma), and pulmonary hypertension. In addition, because propranolol can inhibit hepatic gluconeogenesis and glycogenolysis, it may be associated with profound hypoglycemia.

Nadolol is a nonselective β-adrenergic antagonist of long duration of action. It is incompletely absorbed from the gastrointestinal tract and not well metabolized. Approximately 75% of the drug is excreted in the urine. The elimination half-life of the agent is 20 to 40 hours, which permits its being administered once a day. Because of its long duration of action and lack of titratability its usefulness in the perioperative or perianesthetic time is limited. Pindolol is another nonselective antagonist with intrinsic sympathomimetic activity. The drug is well absorbed from the gastrointestinal tract and is highly protein bound (50% to 60%). The elimination half-life is 3 to 4 hours. Timolol is a nonselective β-adrenergic antagonist that is as effective as propranolol in the treatment of hypertension. Timolol also has been shown to be effective in the treatment of glaucoma because it reduces intraocular pressure when administered in eyedrop preparations. However, the drug can be systemically absorbed and can result in bradycardia and hypotension in children and adults.[74] Furthermore, in neonates timolol may impair respiratory drive and result in apnea.[1]

***Selective antagonists.*** Metoprolol is a selective β-I antagonist that has inotropic and chronotropic effects. The bronchodilator, vasodilator, and metabolic effects of β-II receptors are not affected by metoprolol as they are by propranolol. Therefore, patients with reactive airways disease, peripheral vascular disease, and hypoglycemia may not be adversely affected. As mentioned earlier, this selectivity is dose dependent and is lost at higher doses of metroprolol. The drug is quite easily absorbed from the GI tract but also undergoes substantial rate of first pass metabolism (up to 60%). It is not as highly protein bound as the other β-adrenergic antagonists and therefore may have a higher clearance rate. The half-life is approximately 3 to 4 hours. Atenolol is another selective β-I antagonist. Approximately 50% of the oral dose is absorbed from the GI tract and the agent undergoes very little hepatic metabolism. It is eliminated primarily by the kidneys and has a half-life of 6 to 7 hours. Because its antihypertensive effect may be prolonged, atenolol is commonly administered on a daily basis for the treatment of hypertension.

Esmolol is a new rapid-onset ultra-short-acting β-I antagonist. Esmolol has gained favor for the perioperative treatment of hypertension and tachycardia. Administered as an intravenous bolus (300 μg/kg) followed by intravenous infusion (100 to 200 μg/kg/min), esmolol will prevent tachycardia associated with noxious stimuli during surgery.[32] The drug also may be useful during treatment of pheochromocytoma in blocking the vascular effects of high circulating catecholamines without adversely affecting the systemic circulation.[78,81,83,98,113] Esmolol is rapidly metabolized in the blood by ester hydrolysis.[68] The short duration of action results in a return to baseline heart rates within 10 or 15 minutes of discontinuing the infusion. The elimination half-life is approximately 10 minutes.[17]

As mentioned earlier, the adrenergic antagonist agents have many side effects in common. These include bradycardia and hypotension, increased airway resistance, and hypoglycemia. In addition, extracellular potassium may increase because of the metabolic action. The synergistic or additive effects of general anesthesia and β-antagonists can result in profound bradycardia and hypotension. Conversely, unnecessary withdrawal of β-antagonist therapy in patients prior to surgery may result in rebound hypertension. In patients with excessive bradycardia or hypotension, the first line of therapy is IV atropine. The resulting tachycardia may improve cardiac output. If this proves ineffective, isoproterenol infusion should be used. The dose can be titrated to the desired increase in heart rate or blood pressure (starting dose 0.05 μg/kg/min). Dopamine is not recommended because of its α-adrenergic effects, which can result in profound unbalanced α-stimulation and significant increases in peripheral vascular resistance. Calcium chloride IV to treat hypotension or glucagon to treat hypoglycemia may also be useful.

### Combined α- and β-adrenergic receptor antagonists

Labetalol is a selective α-I and nonselective β-adrenergic antagonist.[64,101] Labetalol exerts its effect on postsynaptic α-I receptors, sparing the α-II receptors. It is metabolized in the liver by conjugation with glucuronic acid and has an elimination half-life of approximately 5 to 8 hours. Following intravenous administration of labetalol there is a decrease in systemic blood pressure because of a decrease in systemic vascular resistance. The expected reflex tachycardia is attenuated because of the β-blockade. Therefore the cardiac output may also decrease. A single IV bolus of labetalol (40 μg/kg) has a duration of action of approximately 5 to 10 minutes. Most commonly, labetalol is used to treat acute increases in blood pressures in the perioperative period.[60] The side effects and the toxic effects of labetalol, discussed previously, are related to the β-antagonists. In addition, labetalol may produce orthostatic hypotension because of its α-I blockade.

### Class III antiarrhythmic agents

***Bretylium.*** Bretylium tosylate, a bromobenzyl quaternary ammonium compound, is an antihypertensive and antiarrhythmic. The drug prolongs ventricular action potential and the refractory period. Therefore it is extremely effective in treating ventricular dysrhythmias. As an adrenergic agonist it initially causes the release of epinephrine from sympathetic nerve endings. Subsequently, bretylium prevents the additional release of epinephrine, which can produce orthostatic hypotension as well as bradycardia. The drug also increases the ventricular fibrillation threshold in animals. Therefore bretylium is quite useful in the treatment of life-threatening ventricular arrhythmias, including tachycardia and fibrillation. The elimination half-life of an intravenous dose of bretylium is 8 to 12 hours. The drug is cleared primarily through the kidneys (approximately 70% excreted in unchanged form). The initial loading dose is 5 to 10 mg/kg intravenously administered over 10 to 15 minutes. Repeated doses may be used to suppress ventricular arrhythmias. The primary side effects include an initial rise in blood pressure and heart rate. Subsequent hypotension may result because of the adrenergic blockade.

***Amiodarone.*** Amiodarone is a benzofurane derivative similar in structure to thyroxine. The agent prolongs the duration of action potential in both the atrium and the ventricle without altering the resting membrane potential delaying repolarization. In turn, the effective refractory period is increased. In addition, amiodarone decreases sinoatrial and AV nodal activity and slows conduction through the AV node. In Wolff-Parkinson-White syndrome, amiodarone is therapeutically effective because it increases the refractory period of the underlying accessory pathways. The drug produces a sodium channel blockade during phase II of the cardiac action potential, leading to a more marked effect on depolarized tissue. It does not increase the Q-T interval. As an antiarrhythmic, it seems to be particularly effective in refractory arrhythmias. Amiodarone is primarily metabolized in the liver (desmethyl amiodarone). Renal function does not affect the elimination half-life of the drug.[49] The adverse side effects of the medication include bradycardia (minimum), prolonged Q-T interval at higher doses, and hypotension under general anesthesia (antiadrenergic effects) because of AV block, low cardiac output, or hypotension.[97] Furthermore, drugs such as halothane and lidocaine may exacerbate the effects of amiodarone by their decrease in automaticity of the S-A node. Amiodarone-induced arrhythmias may require ventricular pacing to improve cardiac output. Other side effects, including muscle weakness, tremor, and neuropathies have been reported.[41] A rare but significant complication is pulmonary fibrosis with decreased oxygen diffusion in alveoli.[66] In particular, patients with preexisting amiodarone-induced pulmonary toxicity can develop significant ARDS after surgery and cardiopulmonary bypass.[55] The pulmonary fibrosis seems to be an idiopathic reaction, and the risk factors are unknown. Chronic amiodarone therapy also may decrease thyroid function and in rare cases cause hyperthyroidism. Finally, microdeposits in the cornea have been noted but do not impair vision. If amiodarone is used in combination with digoxin, the free digoxin concentration may increase because of displacement of the digoxin from protein binding sites. Therefore, serum levels of digoxin should be carefully monitored.

### Class IV antiarrhythmic agents: calcium entry blockers

Calcium entry blockers (CEBs) selectively interfere with calcium ion movement into the cell.[21] The most frequently used calcium channel blockers in the clinical setting are verapamil, diltiazem, and nifedipine (Table 6–17). These agents block the inward movement of calcium across the cell membrane (Fig. 6–7). The slow calcium channel is the primary site of calcium influx. The extracellular (outer gate) membrane is a voltage-dependent gate that opens with depolarization of the cell. The intracellular (inner) gate modulates the calcium ion flux and is dependent on cyclic AMP. Cyclic guanosine monophosphate (GMP) will narrow the size of the gate. The CEBs discussed in this chapter

**Table 6–17** Characteristics of calcium entry blockers

| | Verapamil | Nifedipine | Diltiazem |
|---|---|---|---|
| **Dosage** | | | |
| Oral | 80-160 mg every 8 hours | 10-20 mg every 8 hours | 60-90 mg every 8 hours |
| Intravenous | 75-150 μg/kg$^{-1}$ | 5-15 μg/kg$^{-1}$ | 75-150 μg/kg$^{-1}$ |
| **Absorption (%)** | | | |
| Oral | >90 | >90 | >90 |
| Bioavailability | 10-20 | 65-70 | 40 |
| **Onset of effect (min)** | | | |
| Oral | <30 | <20 | 30 |
| Sublingual | | 3 | |
| Intravenous | 1-3 | 1-3 | 1-3 |
| **Protein binding (%)** | | | |
| **Clearance mechanisms** | | | |
| Renal (%) | 70 | 80 | 35 |
| Fecal (%) | 15 | <15 | 60 |
| **Active metabolites** | Yes | No | Yes |
| **Elimination** | | | |
| Half-time (h) | 6-12 | 2-5 | 3-5 |

From Antman EM, Stone PH, Muller JE, et al: Calcium channel blocking agents in the treatment of cardiovascular disorders I: basic and clinical electrophysiologic effects, *Ann Intern Med* 93:875, 1980.

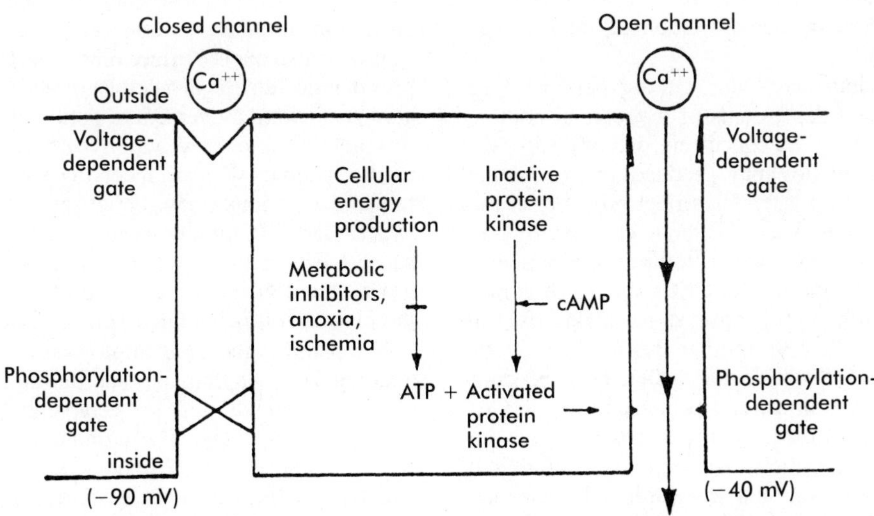


**Figure 6–7** Calcium channel blocking agents in the treatment of cardiovascular disorders part 1: basic and clinical electrophysiologic effects. (From Antman EM, Stone PH, Muller JE, et al: *Ann Intern Med* 93:875, 1980.)

**Table 6–18** Comparative effects of calcium entry blockers

| | Verapamil | Nifedipine | Diltiazem | Nicardipine |
|---|---|---|---|---|
| Blood pressure | – | – | – | – |
| Heart rate | – | +/NC | – | +/NC |
| Nodal conduction | – – | NC | – | NC |
| Myocardial contractility | – – | NC | – | NC |
| Peripheral vasodilation | – | – – | – | – – |

–, decrease; +, increase; NC, no change.
From Stoelting RK: *Pharmacology and physiology in anesthetic practice,* ed 2, Philadelphia, 1991, Lippincott.

selectively block the inward transfer of calcium through the outer gate. Verapamil may affect primarily on the inner gate; the others seem to affect the outer gate.

The CEBs affect the repolarization cycle of the cardiac action potential (phase II), which is due to inward calcium flux. Furthermore, calcium movement into the cell during this phase is responsible for cellular depolarization. Blocking these actions will result in several effects on the myocardium: (1) decreased contractility, (2) decreased heart rate, (3) decreased conduction through the AV node, and (4) relaxation of vascular smooth muscle resulting in vasodilation and lowering of blood pressure[85] (Table 6–18). CEBs are commonly used in the treatment of essential hypertension, supraventricular tachyarrhythmias, coronary vasospasms, cerebral artery vasospasm, myocardial protection, and cerebral protection. Because of the effect on calcium influx into the cell, CEB may interact synergistically or adversely with other pharmacologic agents. Drug interactions that affect not only the cardiovascular system but the neuromuscular system may produce specific problems for the anesthesiologist.

The calcium entry blockers are peripheral vasodilators and depressants of myocardial contractility. Therefore the concurrent use of CEBs with volatile anesthetics may produce an exaggerated hypotensive response. The effect probably is mediated by the blocking of calcium channels by both the CEBs and anesthetics.[71] When the patient is under general anesthesia, CEBs should be administered with caution; those at particular risk are patients with left ventricular dysfunction. In the absence of left ventricular dysfunction the combination of nifedipine and β-blockers is not associated with hypotension under narcotic anesthesia.[51] However, patients with left heart failure may show profound or mild myocardial depression.[11] The cautious and judicious use of intravenous verapamil under halothane anesthesia to treat cardiac dysrhythmias is associated with only transient hypotension and prolongation of the PR interval. In patients who have digitalis or β-adrenergic antagonists on board, verapamil should be used with caution because of the possibility of complete AV block. However, those who do not have preoperative conduction abnormalities usually tolerate CEBs quite well.[42] Furthermore, CEBs used in the presence of halothane may produce an exaggerated hypotension, but administration of halothane in the presence of a CEB may be associated with profound bradycardia. In particular, the combination of halothane with a CEB seems to entail significant risk. The administration of intravenous calcium to treat the hypotension is only partially effective.[67,80]

CEBs do not produce skeletal muscle relaxation. However, when used in combination with neuromuscular blockers,[22] the CEBs potentiate the action of the blockers. Furthermore, the inhibition of sodium flux through the fast sodium channels caused by verapamil may further exacerbate the neuromuscular blockade. Therefore, patients being treated with verapamil may be at greater risk and have a lower margin of safety with the use of neuromuscular blockade (e.g., patients with muscular dystrophy and otherwise compromised neuromuscular transmission).[114] Reversal of neuromuscular blockade also may be affected because of decreased presynaptic release of acetylcholine.[56] CEBs will slow the inward movement of potassium and therefore may be associated with hyperkalemia. In particular, patients who are receiving intravenous potassium infusions may be at greater risks for hyperkalemia.[80] Finally as mentioned earlier, because CEBs may reduce plasma clearance of digoxin, the digoxin level may actually increase in the plasma following CEB administration.

Verapamil is the CEB most commonly used for treatment of arrhythmias. The duration of action of an intravenous dose of verapamil is approximately 2 to 4 hours. The elimination half-life is approximately 4.5 to 12 hours. Verapamil is quite effective in the treatment of reentrant supraventricular tachydysrhythmias. Usually the drug is administered in a dose of 75 to 150 μg/kg IV infused over 3 minutes. This can be followed by a repeat IV bolus or by infusion at 5 μg/kg/min. Primary side effects of verapamil include an exaggerated

**Table 6–19** The pharmacology of digoxin

| | Digoxin | Digitoxin |
|---|---|---|
| Average digitalizing dose | | |
| Oral | 0.75-1.5 mg | 0.8-1.2 mg |
| Intravenous | 0.5-1 mg | 0.8-1.2 mg |
| Average daily maintenance dose | | |
| Oral | 0.125-0.5 mg | 0.05-0.2 mg |
| Intravenous | 0.25 mg | 0.1 mg |
| Onset of effect | | |
| Oral | 1.5-6 h | 3-6 h |
| Intravenous | 5-30 min | 30-120 min |
| Absorption from gastrointestinal tract | 75% | 90%-100% |
| Plasma protein binding | 25% | 95% |
| Route of elimination | Renal | Hepatic |
| Enterohepatic circulation | Minimal | Marked |
| Elimination half-time | 31-33 h | 5-7 days |
| Therapeutic plasma concentration | 0.5-2 $ng/ml^{-1}$ | 10-35 $ng/ml^{-1}$ |

Data from Hoffman BF, Bigger JT: Digitalis and allied cardiac glycosides. In Gilman AG, Goodman LS, Rall TW, Murad F, editors: *The pharmacological basis of therapeutics,* ed 7, New York, 1985, Macmillan.
From Stoelting RK: *Pharmacology and physiology in anesthetic practice,* ed 2, Philadelphia, 1991, Lippincott.

response of the AV blockade. The complete AV block is most likely in patients with preexisting conduction abnormalities. In addition, direct myocardial depression and reduced cardiac output can occur. Hypotension may occur because of verapamil peripheral vasodilation. When used in the presence of halothane, the anesthetic-related depression of the myocardium may be potentiated. Verapamil is the most commonly used calcium channel blocker in the treatment of arrhythmias. It blocks the inward flux of calcium in the myocardium and shortens the duration of cardiac action potential and repolarization. It is primarily eliminated in the kidneys (up to 70%).

***Digoxin.*** Digoxin (Table 6-19) and related digitalis compounds are commonly used in the treatment of cardiac tachyarrhythmias and congestive heart failure. In particular, supraventricular tachydysrhythmias such as PAT, PSVT, atrial fibrillation, or atrial flutter may respond well to digoxin therapy. Furthermore, in the presence of myocardial failure, these drugs may improve myocardial contractility and cardiac output. They usually are not effective in high cardiac output states.

The effects of digoxin and related compounds are exerted through direct and indirect action on the heart. A direct inotropic effect may be produced by the inhibition of the sodium potassium ($Na^+$ – $K^+$ ATPase) in cardiac muscle. The cardiac glycosides bind to the ATPases and interfere with outward sodium and calcium transport. The result is an increase in intracellular calcium concentration that may account for the inotropy (Fig. 6–5).

Digoxin can also affect the autonomic nervous system. Parasympathetic nervous activity may be increased because of sensitization of the carotid sinus and the vagotonic effects on the vagal neclei. The increased parasympathetic activity can lead to decreased S-A node activity and prolonged conduction time through the AV node. Thus, a slower heart rate can be seen with digitalis therapy, particularly in the case of atrial fibrillation or flutter. Digoxin is fairly rapidly absorbed through the GI tract (up to 75% bioavailability). IV administration of digoxin results in 100% bioavailability. The IV route permits achievement of therapeutic plasma concentrations within minutes (administration of up to 10 μg/kg over 30 minutes). Therapeutic concentrations of digozin can be maintained by repeated dosing according to each patient's needs, usually every 12 hours. The drug is primarily eliminated through the kidneys, with approximately a third excreted daily.

The principle cardiovascular effect of digoxin in patients with myocardial failure is a dose-related increase in myocardial contractility. This inotropic effect can be seen as increased stroke volume, decreased heart size and reduced LVEDP. In particular, the stroke volume can double from that of pretreatment levels. The improved cardiac output and renal perfusion will result in mobilization and excretion of edema fluid. The improvement in cardiac output can decrease systemic vascular resistance, further improving the hemodynamics. The heart rate is decreased, which also improves the relationship between $Mvo_2$ and myocardial blood flow.

The effect of digitalis on the cardiac conduction system is multifold. On ECG the changes observed include prolonged PR interval, a shortened Q-T interval because of rapid ventricular repolarization, ST-T depression from decreased phase III repolarization and diminished or inverted T waves. With therapeutic concentrations the PR interval is usually less than 0.25 second. The changes in ST-T segments are not dose related.

The therapeutic margin with digoxin is rather narrow. Toxic effects may occur at the higher therapeutic doses. The most common cause of the toxic effect is the inhibition of the $Na^+ - K^+$ ATPase system. Digoxin toxicity is most commonly seen in the presence of potassium depletion. Because of hypokalemia, the myocardial binding of digoxin and other cardiac glycosides may increase. Hypercalcemia and hypomagnesemia also can potentiate the toxicity. Patients with renal dysfunction will have decreased excretion of the digoxin and therefore are at risk for developing toxic levels of digoxin.

Early signs of digoxin toxicity include anorexia, nausea, and vomiting. This may progress to visual difficulties such as amblyopia and peripheral neuralgias. Changes seen on the electrocardiogram include increased automaticity resulting in atrial or ventricular arrhythmias, prolonged PR interval, AV block, and ventricular fibrillation. Although plasma digoxin concentrations are not diagnostic of toxicity, the levels may be useful in confirming the suspicion of digoxin toxicity. Plasma concentrations less than 0.5 ng/ml are not associated with toxicity. Therapeutic concentrations are between 0.5 and 2.5 ng/ml. Levels greater than 3 ng/ml are considered toxic. However, in infants and children, therapeutic levels may be as high as 2.5 to 3.5 ng/ml.

Treatment of digoxin toxicity includes correction of hypocalcemia, hypoxia, calcium, and magnesium levels. Drugs that depress cardiac automaticity, such as phenytoin and lidocaine, can be used. Atropine to increase S-A node and AV node activity also may be useful. A temporary pacemaker (transvenous cardiac pacing) may be necessary if complete AV block is present. Digoxin antibodies (Fab fragments) are also available to treat digoxin toxicity.[92] These antibodies bind to the digoxin, reducing the concentration of free drug in plasma. The Fab-digoxin complex is excreted through the kidneys.

## DIURETICS

Infants and children with congestive heart failure are frequently prescribed diuretics. The discussion here will focus on classes of the drugs rather than specific agents (Fig. 6–8 and the box at right).

Thiazide diuretics are usually administered orally. The drugs produce their diuretic effect by inhibiting sodium reabsorption and chloride reabsorption in the ascending loop of Henle and the proximal tubules.[70] Significant diuresis usually results in the loss of sodium as well as chloride and

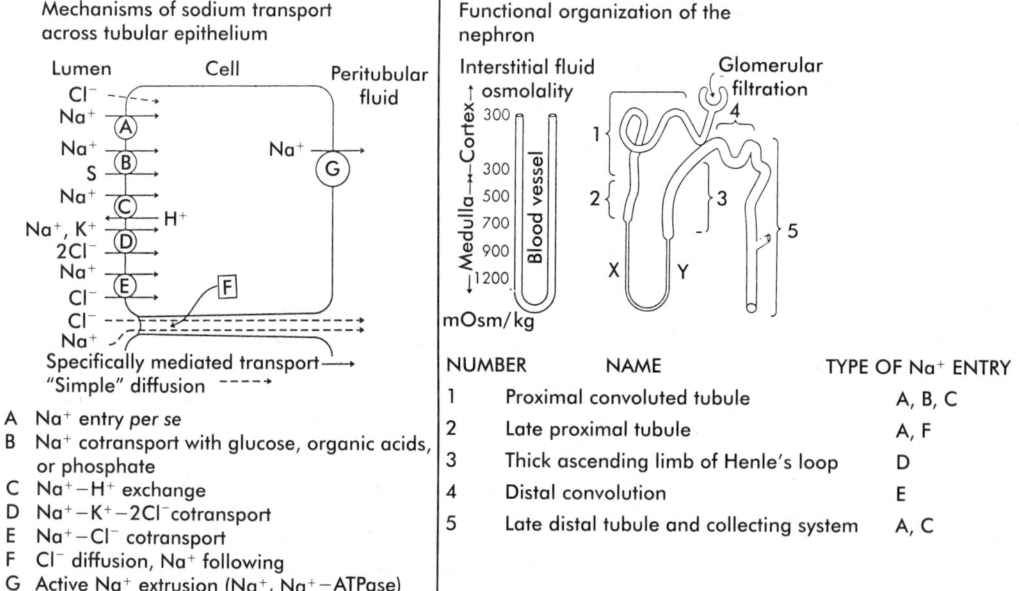


**Figure 6–8** Drugs affecting renal function and electrolyte metabolism. (From Weiner EM: Goodman LS and Gilman AG, editors: *The pharmacological basis of therapeutics,* ed 8, New York, 1990, Pergamon Press.)

bicarbonate ions. Potassium ions are also lost in the urine, and hypokalemia is a common side effect of thiazide diuretic therapy. The effect of loss of electrolytes, in particular sodium, is a reduction in extracellular fluid volume resulting in decreased cardiac output and lower blood pressure. The prolonged antihypertensive effect of thiazides may be due to peripheral vasodilation.

The principle side effects include electrolyte abnormalities (hypokalemia, hypochloremia, and metabolic alkalosis). In addition, patients may develop arrhythmias, skeletal muscle weakness, ileus, nephropathy, and potentiation of digoxin toxcity. Therefore, patients who are scheduled for surgery should be evaluated for electrolyte abnormality as well as intravascular depletion. The presence of orthostatic hypotension indicates intravascular volume depletion. Thiazides can induce significant hyperglycemia. In addition hyperuricemia occurs because of decreased urate secretion in the kidneys.

The classic loop diuretics are ethacrynic acid and furosemide. These agents inhibit reabsorption of chloride, and therefore sodium as well, in the medullary portion of the ascending loop of Henle.[70] The loop diuretics are useful in decreasing intravascular volume because of their profound diuretic effect. However, their prolonged use in the treatment of hypertension is questionable, as they do not have a sustained antihypertensive response. These drugs are quite useful in mobilizing edema fluid. When administered IV, furosemide first will result in peripheral vasodilation, soon followed by a diuresis. In patients with increased intracranial pressure, furosemide may decrease ICP because of mobilization of edema fluid in the brain.[16] Furosemide may also decrease production of CSF by inhibiting ion transport. The major untoward effects of loop diuretics include significant electrolyte abnormalities, that is, hypokalemia and hypochloremia. When used in the presence of digoxin, the hypokalemia can result in digitalis toxicity. Hypokalemia also potentiates the effects of neuromuscular blocking agents. Hyperuricemia may be seen but is rarely at the same level as that seen with thiazide diuretics. Effects on the kidney of loop diuretics include increased renal concentration of aminoglycosides, which can exacerbate the nephrotoxic effect of these drugs. Furosemide also reduces the excretion of calcium, producing hypercalcemia. High doses of furosemide lead to the accumulation of reactive metabolites that can produce ototoxicity. This side effect most probably is due to high plasma concentrations for long periods.

**CLASSIFICATION OF DIURETICS**

**Thiazide**
Chlorothiazide
Hydrochlorothiazide
Benzthiazide
Cyclothiazide

**Loop**
Ethacrynic acid
Furosemide

**Osmotic**
Mannitol
Urea

**Potassium sparing**
Triamterene
Amiloride

**Aldosterone antagonists**
Spironolactone

**Carbonic anhydrase inhibitors**
Acetazolamide

From Stoelting RK: *Pharmacology and physiology in anesthetic practice,* ed 2, Philadelphia, 1991, Lippincott.

***Potassium-sparing diuretics.*** Potassium-sparing diuretics are used in combination and occasionally alone to treat patients with congestive heart failure or with hypertension. Triamterene and amiloride act directly on renal tubular transport mechanisms of the distal convoluted tubule and act independently of aldosterone. The diuresis is produced by an increased secretion of sodium chloride and bicarbonate. The urine pH is elevated because of the bicarbonate loss. There is usually no change in serum or urinary potassium[100] because of the inhibition of potassium secretion into the distal tubule. These agents usually are used in combination with hydrochlorothiazide. The combination optimizes the diuretic effect of the drugs while sparing potassium. The primary side effect of the potassium-sparing agents is elevated serum potassium level. Therefore, supplemental potassium administration should be minimized and closely monitored.

Spironolactone is a competitive antagonist at aldosterone receptor sites in the renal collecting duct. The drug is effective only when aldosterone levels are high. Because aldosterone increases the tubular reabsorption of sodium and chloride and increases potassium in excretion, spironolactone exerts the opposite effect, that is, sparing potassium and producing a sodium and chloride diuresis. It can be used in combination with the thiazides to optimize the diuresis while minimizing potassium loss.

***Carbonic anhydrase inhibitors.*** Acetazolamide is the prototypical carbonic anhydrase inhibitor. The agent binds tightly and noncompetitively to carbonic anhydrase, primarily in the proximal tubule. This results in hydrogen ion excretion and a net loss of bicarbonate. Chloride is retained in the kidney, and sodium and potassium are excreted. The net effect is an alkaline urine, a progressive hyperchloremic metabolic acidosis, and mild diuresis. The drug is rarely used as routine treatment for hypertension or congestive failure. It is most commonly used to reduce intraocular pressure of glaucoma and to produce metabolic acidosis in children with epilepsy.

## ANTIHYPERTENSIVE DRUGS

Children with cardiovascular abnormalities and/or congestive heart failure also may require antihypertensive medication. The various classes of antihypertensive medications are listed in the box. For the purposes of this discussion we will focus on the drugs commonly used in pediatric patients, namely those that act on peripheral vascular smooth muscle and those that modulate the renin-angiotensin system.

Hydralazine, a thalazine derivative, is a direct smooth muscle relaxant. It may interfere with intracellular calcium ion transport in order to exert its effect. It has a greater effect on the arterioles than on veins. Coronary, cerebral, renal, and splanchnic vessels are affected to a greater extent than others. Hydralazine is absorbed well through the GI tract and undergoes significant first pass metabolism. It is acetylated and subsequently excreted in the urine. The elimination half-life is approximately 3 hours.

Hydralazine lowers blood pressure by decreasing systemic vascular resistance. The lower systemic vascular resistance leads to a reflex increase in heart rate and raises stroke volume and cardiac output. These effects occur slowly after administration of the drug and may take 15 to 20 minutes following an intravenous dose. Because of the vasodilation, significant hypotension may occur. A reflex increase in sodium and water retention will also occur. Common side effects include vertigo, diaphoresis, nausea, and tachycardia. The reflex tachycardia may result in increased $M\dot{V}O_2$. Less frequent side effects include fever, urticaria, polyneuritis, anemia, and pancytopenia. Patients who have received prolonged treatment with hydralazine may manifest with an idiosyncratic effect of the drug—a lupus erythematosus–like syndrome. The symptoms usually resolve when the drug is discontinued.

### PRINCIPAL SITE OF ACTION OF ANTIHYPERTENSIVE DRUGS

**Central nervous system**
Methyldopa
Clonidine
Reserpine
Guanabenz

**Peripheral vascular smooth muscle**
Hydralazine
Prazosin
Minoxidil
Trimazosin
Terazosin

**Peripheral sympathetic nervous system**
Guanethidine
Guanadrel

**Peripheral α- and β-adrenergic receptors**
Labetalol

**Angiotensin-converting enzyme**
Captopril
Enalapril

**Angiotensin II receptors**
Saralasin

**Tyrosine hydroxylase enzyme**
Metyrosine

From Stoelting RK: *Pharmacology and physiology in anesthetic practice,* ed 2, Philadelphia, 1991, Lippincott.

### α-I antagonists

Prazosin is a quinazoline derivative that causes hypotension by blockade of the postsynaptic α-I receptor.[44] The drug has no presynaptic α-II effects. As a selective peripheral vasodilator, prazosin is effective in lowering blood pressure by reducing afterload in patients with cardiac failure. Because of its specific site of action, it is also useful in the treatment of hypertension in pheochromocytoma. It is metabolized in the liver and eliminated through the urine within 3 hours. The reduction in systemic vascular resistance is not associated with a reflex tachycardia or increase in renin activity. Therefore, there is no concurrent increase in $M\dot{V}O_2$. The vascular tone is reduced in capacitance (venous) vessels as well, resulting in decreased venous return and thus decreased cardiac output. The principal side effects of prazosin are vertigo, fluid retention, and orthostatic hypotension. Gradual increase in the dose of prazosin to the desired daily maintenance dose will minimize these side effects.

Trimazosin is a weaker α-I antagonist than prazosin. The drug affects venules as well as arterioles. Terazosin is a long-acting α-I antagonist. Both have side effects similar to those of prazosin.

### Minoxidil

Minoxidil, an orally active antihypertensive, is a direct arteriolar smooth muscle relaxant.[10] It is quite effective in the treatment of hypertension associated with renal failure. The drug is readily absorbed from the GI tract and undergoes glucuronidation in the liver. The elimination half-life is approximately 4 hours.

Minoxidil causes arteriolar dilatation and resultant hypotension, which produces a reflex tachycardia and increased cardiac output. There is an associated increase in plasma norepinephrine and renin levels. Therefore, fluid retention and sodium retention are common side effects. A serious but infrequent side effect of minoxidil therapy is the development of pericardial effusion and cardiac tamponade.[46] ECG abnormalities include flattened or inverted T-waves and increased QRS voltage. Hypertrichosis of the face and arms may also occur during therapy.

### Captopril

Captopril is a competitive inhibitor of angiotensin I–converting enzyme (ACE),[107] the enzyme that converts inactive angiotensin I to active angiotensin II. The active form is responsible for aldosterone secretion by the adrenal cortex. This inhibitory action decreases circulating angiotensin II and aldosterone levels. There is a compensatory increase in renin and angiotensin I. The drug is quite effective in treating hypertension, particularly in patients with renovascular disease. Captopril also may increase the synthesis of prostaglandins and potentiate the effect of plasma kinins such as bradykinin.

The drug is administered via the GI tract, where it is well absorbed; the effects may be evident within 10 or 15 minutes. Approximately 50% of the drug is metabolized in the liver and 50% is excreted unchanged.

The antihypertensive effects of captopril result from a reduction in systemic vascular resistance (SVR) produced by decreased sodium and water retention. In addition, cerebral and coronary blood flow may decrease slightly because of decreased systemic blood pressure.[48] Furthermore, renal blood flow may decrease substantially. The reduction in blood pressure following captopril is usually not associated with alterations in cardiac output, and there is no compensatory tachycardia.[107]

Common side effects of captopril include a pruritic rash with fever and arthralgia.[46] Patients may develop proteinuria, and serum creatinine concentrations may increase because of reduced renal blood flow. Rarely neutropenia has been observed, Particularly in patients on immunosuppressive therapy. An extremely rare but potentially lethal side effect is angioedema produced by inhibition of bradykinin metabolism. Nonsteroid antiinflammatory drugs may attenuate the antihypertensive effects of captopril. Particular caution should be used in initiating captopril therapy, as the first dose may produce a severe fall in blood pressure. This most frequently occurs in patients who are intravascularly volume depleted.

Enalapril is an inhibitor of ACE with pharmacologic effects similar to those of captopril. It may be more useful than captopril because there are fewer side effects of rash and taste disturbance.

Saralasin and the related family of drugs are competitive inhibitors at angiotensin II receptors on vascular smooth muscle. The drug has a direct angiotension II–like effect with a potency 1% of that of angiotensin II. It is quite useful in treating patients with renovascular disease. Because of the direct action, patients with low normal plasma renin activity may actually manifest an elevated blood pressure after initial administration of saralasin.

### REFERENCES

1. Bailey PL: Timolol and postoperative apnea in neonates and young infants, *Anesthesiology* 61:622, 1984.
2. Baim DS, Colucci WS, Monrad ES et al: Survival of patients with severe congestive heart failure treated with oral milrinone, *J Am Coll Cardiol* 7:661, 1986.
3. Barnes PK, Thomas JE, Boyd I et al: Comparison of the effects of atracurium and tubocurarine on heart rate and arterial pressure in anesthetized man, *Br J Anaesth* 55:91S, 1983.
4. Basta SJ: Clinical selection of muscle relaxants. 38th annual refresher course, Lectures and Clinical Update Program, p 121. Presented Oct. 10-14, 1987, Georgia World Congress Center during Annual Meeting of American Society of Anesthesiologists.
5. Boudreaux JP, Schieber RA, Cook DR: Hemodynamic effects of halothane in the newborn piglet, *Anesth Analg* 63:731, 1984.
6. Bowdle TA, Freund PR, Slattery JT: Propranolol reduces bupivacaine clearance, *Anesthesiology* 66:36, 1987.
7. Brandom BW, Brandom RB, Cook DR: Uptake and distribution of halothane in infants: in vivo measurements and computer simulations, *Anesth Analg* 62:404, 1983.
8. Brandom BW, Rudd GD, Cook DR: Clinical pharmacology of atracurium in pediatric patients, *Br J Anaesth* 55:117s, 1983.
9. Brandom BW, Woelfel SK, Cook DR et al: Clinical pharmacology of atracurium in infants, *Anesth Analg* 63:309, 1984.
10. Campeese VM: Minoxidil: a review of its pharmacological properties and therapeutic use, *Drugs* 22:259, 1981.
11. Chew CYC, Hecht HS, Collett JT et al: Influence of severity of ventricular dysfunction on hemodynamic responses to intravenously administered verapamil in ischemic heart disease, *Am J Cardiol* 47:917, 1981.

12. Clotz MA, Nahata MC: Clinical uses of fentanyl, sufentanil, and alfentanil, *Clin Pharm* 10:581, 1991.
13. Collins G, Koren G, Crean P et al: Fentanyl pharmacokinetics and hemodynamic effects in preterm infants ligation of patent ductus arteriosus, *Anesth Analg* 64:1078, 1985.
14. Cook DR: Clinical use of muscle relaxants in infants and children, *Anesth Analg* 60:335, 1981.
15. Cook DR: Sensitivity of the newborn to tubocurarine, *Br J Anesth* 53:320, 1981.
16. Cottrell JE, Robustell A, Post K et al: Furosemide and mannitol-induced changes in intracranial pressure and serum osmolality and electrolytes, *Anesthesiology* 47:28, 1977.
17. DeBruijn N, Christian C, Fagraeus L et al: The effects of alfentanil on global ventricular mechanics, *Anesthesiology* 59:A33, 1983.
18. D'Hollander AA, Massaux C, Barvais L et al: Clinical evaluation of atracurium besylate requirement for a stable muscle relaxation during surgery: lack of age-related effects, *Anesthesiology* 59:237, 1983.
19. D'Hollander AA, Massaux F, Nevelsteen M et al: Age-dependent dose-response relationship of ORG NC45 in anesthetized patients, *Br J Anaesth* 54:563, 1982.
20. Duncan P, Gregory GA, Wade JA: The effects of nitrous oxide on the baroreceptor response of newborn and adult rabbits, *Can Anaesth Soc J* 18:339, 1981.
21. Durand P-G, Lehot J-J, Foex P: Calcium-channel blockers and anesthesia, *Can J Anaesth* 38:75, 1991.
22. Durant NN, Nugyen N, Katz R: Potentiation of neuromuscular blockade by verapamil, *Anesthesiology* 60:298, 1984.
23. Eger EL II, Smith NT, Cullen DJ et al: A comparison of cardiovascular effects of halothane, fluroxene, ether, and cyclopropane in man; a resume, *Anesthesiology* 34:25, 1971.
24. Eger EL II, Smith NT, Stoelting RK et al: Cardiovascular effects of halothane in man, *Anesthesiology* 32:396, 1970.
25. Gregory GA: The baroresponses of preterm infants during halothane anesthesia, *Can Anaesth Soc J* 29:105, 1982.
26. Filner BF, Karliner JS: Alterations of normal left ventricular performance by general anesthesia, *Anesthesiology* 45:610, 1976.
27. Fisher DM, Miller RD: Neuromuscular effects of vecuronium (ORG NC45) in infants and children during $N_2O$, halothane anesthesia, *Anesthesiology* 58:51, 1983.
28. Fragen, R, Shanks C, Molteni A et al: Effects of etomidate on hormonal response to surgical stress, *Anesthesiology* 61:652, 1984.
29. Friesen RH, Lichtor JL: Cardiovascular depression during halothane anesthesia in infants: a study of three induction techniques, *Anesth Analg* 61:42, 1982.
30. Gasser S, Cohen M, Aygen M: The effect of ketamine on pulmonary artery pressure, *Anesthesia* 29:141, 1974.
31. Ghonheim M, Yamanda T: Etomidate: a clinical and electroencephalographic comparison with thiopental, *Anesth Analg* 56:479, 1977.
32. Girard E, Shulman BJ, Thys DM et al: The safety and efficacy of esmolol during myocardial revascularization, *Anesthsiology* 65:157, 1986.
33. Goat VA, Feldman SA: The dual action of suxamethonium on the isolated rabbit heart, *Anaesthesia* 27:149, 1972.
34. Goldberg AH: Effects of halothane on force-velocity, length-tension, and stress-strain curves of isolated heart muscle, *Anesthesiology* 29:192, 1968.
35. Goldenberg IF, Cohn JN: New inotropic drugs for heart failure, *JAMA* 258:493, 1987.
36. Gooding J, Corssen G: Effects of etomidate on the cardiovascular system, *Anesth Analg* 56:717, 1977.
37. Gooding J, Weng J, Smith R et al: Cardiovascular and pulmonary responses following etomidate induction of anesthesia in patients with demonstrated cardiac disease, *Anesth Analg* 58:40, 1979.
38. Gootman PM, Gootman N, Buckley BJ: Maturation of central autonomic control of the circulation, *Fed Proc* 42:1648, 1983.
39. Grose RM, Strain JE, Bergman et al: Milrinone vs. dobutamine: a comparative study, *Circulation* 70:1, 1984.
40. Haefely W: The preclinical pharmacology of flumazenil, Eur J Anesthesiol 2:25, 1988.
41. Heger JJ, Prystowsky EN, Jackman WM et al: Amiodarone: Clinical efficacy and electrophysiology during long-term therapy for recurrent ventricular tachycardia or ventricular tachycardia or ventricular fibrillation, *N Engl J Med* 305:539, 1981.
42. Henling CE, Slogoff S, Kodali SV et al: Heartblock after coronary artery bypass: effect of chronic administration of calcium-entry blockers and β-blockers. *Anesth Analg* 63:515, 1984.
43. Hickey PR, Hansen DD, Cramolini GM: Pulmonary and systemic hemodynamic responses to ketamine in infants with normal and elevated pulmonary vascular resistance, *Anesthesiology* 61:A438, 1984.
44. Hoffman BF, Lefkowitz RJ: Adrenergic receptor antagonists. In Goodman LS, Gilman AG, editors: *The pharmacological basis of therapeutics,* ed 8, New York, 1990, Pergamon Press.
45. Horrow JC, Bartkowski RR: Pancuronium, unlike other nondepolarizing relaxants, retains potency at hypothermia, *Anesthesiology* 58:357, 1983.
46. Husserle FE, Messerle FH: Adverse effects of antihypertensive drugs, *Drugs* 22:188, 1981.
47. Iwatsuki N, Hashimoto Y, Amaha K et al: Inotropic effects of nondepolarizing muscle relaxants in osilated canine heart muscle, *Anesth Analg* 59:717, 1980.
48. Jensen K, Bunemann L, Ricsager S et al: Cerebral blood flow during anesthesia: influence of pretreatment with metoprolol or captopril, *Br J Anaesth* 62:321, 1989.
49. Kannan R, Nademannee K, Hendrickson JA et al: Amiodarone kinetics after oral doses, *Clin Pharmacol Ther* 31:438, 1982.
50. Kapur PA, Campos JH, Buchea OC: Plasma diltiazem levels, cardiovascular function, and coronary hemodynamics during enflurane anesthesia in the dog, *Anesth Analg* 65:918, 1986.
51. Kapur PA, Norel EJ, Dajee H et al: Hemodynamic effects of verapamil administration after large doses of fentanyl in man, *Can Anesth Soc J* 33:138, 1986.
52. Kaukinen S, Kataja J, Kaukinen L: Antagonism of benzodiazepine-fentanyl anesthesia with flumazenil, *Can J Anaesth* 37:40, 1990.
53. Keenan RL, Boyan CP: Cardiac arrest due to anesthesia, *JAMA* 253:2373, 1985.
54. Kupferberg HJ, Way EL: Pharmacologic basis for the increased sensivity of the newborn rat to morphine, *J Pharmacol Exp Ther* 141:105, 1963.
55. Kupferschmid JP, Rosengart TK, McIntosh CL et al: Amiodarone-induced complications after cardiac operation for obstructive hypertrophic cardiomyopathy, *Ann Thorac Surg* 48:359, 1989.
56. Lawson NW, Kraynack BJ, Gintautas J: Neuromuscular and electrocardiographic responses to verapamil in dogs, *Anesth Analg* 62:50, 1983.
57. LeDez KM, Swartz J, Strong A et al: The effect of age on the serum concentration of $\alpha_1$-acid glycoprotein in newborns, infants, and children, *Anesthesiology* 65:A421, 1986.
58. Leigh MD, Belton MK: *Pediatric anesthesiology,* ed 2, New York, 1960, MacMillan.
59. LeJemtel TH, Keung E, Ribner HS et al: Sustained ben-

eficial effects of oral amrinone on cardiac and renal function in patients with severe congestive heart failure, *Am J Cardiol* 45:123, 1980.

60. Leslie JB, Kalayjian RW, Sirgo MA et al: Intravenous labetalol for treatment of postoperative hypertension, *Anesthesiology* 67:413, 1987.
61. Lockhart CH, Nelson WL: The relationship of ketamine requirements to age in pediatric patients, *Anesthesiology* 40:507, 1974.
62. Lowenstein E, Hallowell P, Levine FH et al: Cardiovascular response to large doses of intravenous morphine in man, *N Engl J Med* 281:1389, 1969.
63. Lynn AM, Slattery JT: Morphine pharmacokinetics in early infancy, *Anesthesiology* 66:136, 1987.
64. MacCarthy EP, Bloomfield SS: Labetalol: a review of its pharmacology, pharmacokinetics, clinical uses, and adverse effects. *Pharmacotherapy* 3:193, 1983.
65. Marshall BE, Longnecker DE: General anesthetics. In Goodman LS, Gilman AG, editors: *The pharmacological basis of therapeutics,* ed 8, New York, 1990, Pergamon Press.
66. Mason JW: Amiodarone, *N Engl J Med* 316:455, 1987.
67. Maze M, Mason DM: Verapamil decreases the MAC for halothane in dogs, *Anesth Analg* 62:274, 1983.
68. McCammon RL, Hilgenberg JC, Stoelting RK: Effect of propranolol on circulatory responses to induction of diazepam–nitrous oxide anesthesia and endotracheal intubation, *Anesth Analg* 60:579, 1981.
69. Meistelman C, Benhamou D, Barre J et al: Effects of age on plasma protein binding of sufentanil, *Anesthesiology* 72:470, 1990.
70. Merin RG, Bastron RD: Diuretics. In: Smith NT, Miller RD, Corbascio AN, editors: *Drug interactions in anesthesia,* Philadelphia, 1986, Lea & Febiger.
71. Merin RG: Calcium channel blocking drugs and anesthetics: Is the drug interaction beneficial or detrimental? *Anesthesiology* 66:111, 1987.
72. Merin RG, Verdouw PD, de Jong JW: Dose-dependent depression of cardiac function and metabolism by halothane in swine (Ssus scrofa), *Anesthesiology* 46:417, 1977.
73. Meuldermans W, Hurkmans R, Heykants J: Plasma protein binding and distribution of fentanyl, sufentanil, alfentanil, and lofentanil in blood, *Arch Int Pharmacodyn Ther* 25:4, 1982.
74. Mishra P, Calvey TN, William NE et al: Intraoperative bradycardia and hypotension associated with timolol and pilocarpine eye drops, *Br J Anaesth* 55:897, 1983.
75. Morray JP, Lynn AM, Stamm SJ et al: Hemodynamic effects of ketamine in children with congenital heart disease, *Anesth Analg* 63:895, 1984.
76. Morris RB, Cahalan MK, Miller RD et al: The cardiovascular effects of vecuronium (Org NC 45) and pancuronium in patients undergoing coronary artery bypass grafting, *Anesthesiology* 58:438, 1983.
77. Moss IR, Conner H, Yee WFH, et al: Human β-endorphin in the neonatal period, *J Pediatr* 101:443, 1982.
78. Nicholas E, Deutschman CS, Allo M et al: Use of esmolol in the intraoperative management of pheochro mocytoma. *Anesth Analg* 67:1114, 1988.
79. Nicodemus HF, Nassiri-Rahimi C, Bachman L: Median effective dose ($ED_{50}$) of halothane in adults and children, *Anesthesiology* 31:344, 1969.
80. Nugent MK, Tinker JH, Moyer TP: Verapamil worsens rate of development and hemodynamic effects of acute hyperkalemia in halothane-anesthetized dogs: effects of calcium therapy, *Anesthesiology* 60:435, 1984.
81. Ostman PL, Chestnut DH, Robillard JE et al: Transplacental passage and hemodynamic effects of esmolol in the gravid ewe, *Anesthesiology* 69:738, 1988.
82. Philbin DM, Machaj VR, Tomichek RC et al: Hemodynamic effects of bolus injection of atracurium in patients with coronary artery disease, *Br J Anaesth* 55:131S, 1983.
83. Pollan S, Tadjziechy M: Esmolol in the management of epinephrine and cocaine induced cardiovascular toxicity, *Anesth Analg* 69:663, 1989.
84. Prielipp RC, McLean R, Rosenthal MH et al: Hemodynamic profiles of prostaglandin $E_1$, isoproterenol, prostacyclin, and nifedipine in experimental porcine pulmonary hypertension, *Crit Care Med* 19:60, 1991.
85. Reves JG, Kissin I, Lell WA et al: Calcium entry blockers: uses and implications for anesthesiologists, *Anesthesiology* 5757:504, 1982.
86. Reynolds RN: Halothane in pediatric anesthesia, *Int Anesthesiol Clin* 1:209, 1962.
87. Samuel IO, Unni N, Dundee JW: Peripheral vascular effects of morphine in patients without preexisting cardiac disease, *Br J Anaesth* 49:935, 1977.
88. Sarner JB, Brandom BW, Cook DR et al: Clinical pharmacology of doxacurium chloride (BW A938U) in children, *Anesth Analg* 67:303, 1988.
89. Saxena PD, Dhasmana KM, Prakash O: A comparison of systemic and regional hemodynamic effects of d-tubocurarine, pancuronium, and vecuronium, *Anesthesiology* 59:102, 1983.
90. Schieber RA, Namnoum A, Sugden A et al: Hemodynamic effects of isoflurane in the newborn piglet: comparison with halothane, *Anesth Analg* 65:633, 1986.
91. Singleton MA, Rosen JI, Fisher DM: Plasma concentrations of fentanyl in infants, children, and adults. *Can Anaesth Soc J* 34:152, 1987.
92. Smith TW, Butler VP, Haber E et al: Treatment of life-threatening digitalis intoxication with digoxin-specific Fab antibody fragments, *N Engl J Med* 307:1357, 1982.
93. Stiller RL, Brandom BW, Cook DR: Determinations of atracurium by high-performance liquid chromatography, *Anesth Analg* 64:58, 1985.
94. Stephen CR, Ahlgren AW, Bennett EJ: *Elements of pediatric anesthesia,* ed 2, Springfield IL, 1970, Charles C Thomas.
95. Stoelting RK: In *Pharmacology and physiology in anesthetic practice,* ed 2, Philadelphia, 1991, Lippincott.
96. Tanner GE, Angers DC, Barash PG et al: Effect of left-to-right shunts on inhalational anesthetic induction in children: a computer model, *Anesth Analg* 64:101, 1985.
97. Teasdale S, Downar E: Amiodarone and anesthesia. *Can J Anaesth* 37:151, 1990.
98. Thorne AC, Bedford RF: Esmolol for perioperative management of thyrotoxic goiter. *Anesthesiology* 71:291, 1989.
99. Todd MM, Chadwick HS, Shapiro HM et al: The neurologic effects of thiopental therapy following experimental cardiac arrest in cats, *Anesthesiology* 57:76, 1982.
100. Tonnesen AS: Clinical pharmacology and use of diuretics. In Hersey SG, Bumforth BJ, Zauder H, editors: *Review courses in anesthesiology,* Philadelphia, 1983, Lippincott.
101. Wallin JD, O'Neill WM: Labetalol, current research and therapeutic status, *Arch Intern Med* 143:485, 1983.
102. Wallin RF, Napoli MD: Sevoflurane, a new inhalational anesthetic agent, *Anesth Analg* 54:758, 1975.
103. Ward DS, Belville JW: Reduction of hypoxic ventilatory drive by dopamine, *Anesth Analg* 61:333, 1982.
104. Wear R, Robinson S, Gregory GA: The effect of halothane on the baroresponse of adult and baby rabbits, *Anesthesiology* 56:188, 1982.
105. Wechsler A: The effects of alfentanil on global ventricular mechanics, *Anesthesiology* 59:A33, 1983.
106. White PF, Shafer A, Boyle WA et al: Benzodiazepine antagonism does not provoke a stress response, *Anesthesiology* 70:636, 1989.

107. Williams ME, Rosa RM, Silva P et al: Impairment of extrarenal potassium disposal by α-adrenergic stimulation, *N Engl J Med* 311:145, 1984.
108. Woelfel SK, Brandom BW, Sarner JB et al: Potency of mivacurium chloride (BW B1090U) during halothanenitrous oxide anesthesia in children, *Anesth Analg* 67:S61, 1988.
109. Wood J, Wood AJJ: Changes in plasma drug binding and $\alpha$-$_1$ acid glycoprotein in mother and newborn infant, *Clin Pharmacol Ther* 29:522, 1981.
110. Wynn J, Malacoff RF, Benotti JR et al. Oral amrinone in refractory congestive heart failure, *Am J Cardiol* 45:1245, 1980.
111. Yamamura T, Haruda K, Okamura A et al: Is the site of action of ketamine anesthesia the N-methyl-D-aspartate receptor? *Anesthesiology* 72:704, 1990.
112. Yaster M: The dose response of fentanyl in neonatal anesthesia, *Anesthesiology* 66:433, 1987.
113. Zakwski M, Kaufman B, Berguson P et al: Esmolol use during resection of pheochromocytoma: report of three cases, *Anesthesiology* 20:875, 1989.
114. Zalman F, Perloff JK, Durant NW et al: Acute respiratory failure following intravenous verapamil in Duchenne's muscular dystrophy, *Am Heart J* 105:510, 1983.

# 7 Pacemakers

*James A. Johns*



With advances in pacemaker technology and an increasing number of patients surviving surgical repair of congenital heart disease, more and more infants, children, and young adults are undergoing pacemaker implantation.[2,3,14,25] In some of these patients the underlying arrhythmia is an isolated problem; in some it is a consequence of the natural history of structural congenital heart disease; and in others the arrhythmia is a complication of cardiac surgery.

## INDICATIONS FOR PACING

Bradycardia is the most common indication for pacing in children and young adults. This bradycardia may be the result of sinus node dysfunction, with an inadequate sinus rate, or it may be the result of atrioventricular (AV) node dysfunction, with failure of the AV node to conduct atrial impulses to the ventricles (AV block). The recommendations of a task force of the American College of Cardiology and the American Heart Association on indications for pacing in children are summarized in the box.[1]

In children without structural congenital heart disease, isolated sinus node dysfunction is uncommon. Pacing is generally needed in these children only if they have symptoms such as syncope that are clearly related to their bradycardia.[1] Sinus node dysfunction is common in children who have undergone extensive atrial surgery, such as the Mustard or Senning repair of transposition of the great arteries. In one series of patients following the Mustard operation, the number of patients with normal sinus rhythm declined to approximately 10% by 10 years after operation.[11] A number of these patients may have symptomatic bradycardia with syncope. Children with sinus node dysfunction following these operations may be at risk for sudden death, although it is not entirely clear that bradycardia is the cause of death. Bradycardia may increase the likelihood of tachyarrhythmias such as atrial flutter in some patients, and pacing may be helpful in preventing these tachyarrhythmias as well as bradycardia-related symptoms.[20] A number of pediatric cardiologists think pacing is indicated in children who have undergone atrial repair of transposition if there is a need for antiarrhythmic agents other than digoxin, since these drugs can exacerbate sinus node dysfunction.[7] Sinus node dysfunction resulting in junctional rhythm may have adverse hemodynamic consequences in patients with structural heart disease. In these patients atrial pacing may be indicated to improve their hemodynamics.

AV node dysfunction may be either congenital or acquired. Congenital AV block in children with structurally normal hearts is usually the result of maternal anti-Ro or anti-La antibodies, which are presumed to cross-react with the developing conduction system in utero.[17,23] The AV block in these children may progress from second degree block at birth to complete block later in infancy or childhood. Asymptomatic patients often do not require pacing unless their rates are quite slow (lower than 50 to 60 in infancy or 30 to 40 in childhood).[16,19] The most common cause of acquired AV block in children is injury to the AV node or His-Purkinje system at the time of cardiac surgery.[9] In children with surgical complete heart block lasting more than 2 weeks after the operation, pacemaker im-

### ACC/AHA TASK FORCE RECOMMENDATIONS FOR PERMANENT PACING IN CHILDREN

**Class I: Conditions for which there is general agreement that permanent pacemakers should be implanted**

Second or third degree AV block with symptomatic bradycardia
Advanced second or third degree AV block with moderate to marked exercise intolerance
External ophthalmoplegia with bifascicular block
Sinus node dysfunction with symptomatic bradycardia
Congenital AV block with wide QRS escape rhythm or with block below the His bundle
Advanced second or third degree AV block persisting 10 to 14 days after cardiac surgery

**Class II: Conditions for which pacemakers are frequently used but there is divergence of opinion with respect to the necessity of their insertion**

Bradycardia-tachycardia syndrome with need for an antiarrhythmic drug other than digitalis or phenytoin
Second or third degree AV block within the bundle of His in an asymptomatic patient
Prolonged subsidiary pacemaker recovery time
Transient second or third degree AV block that reverts to bifascicular block
Asymptomatic second or third degree AV block and a ventricular rate below 45 beats per minute when awake; complete AV block when awake, with an average ventricular rate below 50 beats per minute
Complete AV block with double or triple rest cycle length pauses or minimal heart rate variability
Asymptomatic neonate with congenital complete heart block and bradycardia in relation to age
Complex ventricular arrhythmias associated with second or third degree AV block or sinus bradycardia
Long QT syndrome

**Class III: Conditions for which there is general agreement that pacemakers are unnecessary**

Asymptomatic postoperative bifascicular block
Asymptomatic postoperative bifascicular block with first degree AV block
Transient surgical AV block that returns to normal conduction in less than 1 week
Asymptomatic type I second degree AV block
Asymptomatic congenital heart block without profound bradycardia in relation to age

From American College of Cardiology/American Heart Association Task Force on Assessment of Diagnostic and Therapeutic Cardiovascular Procedures (Committee on Pacemaker Implantation): Guidelines for implantation of cardiac pacemakers and antiarrhythmia devices, *Circulation* 84:455, 1991, and *J Am Coll Cardiol* 18:1, 1991.

plantation is generally required. Other causes of acquired AV block include infectious, inflammatory, and neuromuscular diseases.

## PACING SYSTEMS

Pacing systems consist of a pulse generator, which provides the electrical stimulus, and a lead system, which conducts the electrical stimulus to the myocardium. The generator may be a permanent implantable generator or a temporary external pacer. The lead system may be epicardial, in which the electrode is sewn onto or inserted into the epicardial surface of the heart, or it may be transvenous, in which the electrode is in contact with the endocardial surface of the heart. Like pulse generators, leads may be temporary, for short-term pacing, or permanent.

### Pulse generators

Pulse generators, whether temporary external pacers or permanent implantable generators, all carry out three basic functions. First, they supply the electrical pulse that stimulates the heart to beat. The amplitude of the pulse may be expressed either as current (in milliamperes) or as voltage (in volts). There is a linear relationship between current and voltage, with the ratio of voltage divided by current being impedance. Impedance is a characteristic of the lead, the heart, and the surrounding tissues. In general, pulse amplitude is expressed as voltage in implantable generators and as current in temporary external pacers. The energy delivered by a generator is a function of the pulse amplitude, the pulse duration, and the lead impedance. Pulse duration can be adjusted in most implantable generators but is fixed in most temporary pacers. It is important to note that energy increases with the square of the voltage or current but increases linearly with the pulse duration. Thus a doubling of the voltage or current will quadruple the energy, and a doubling of the pulse duration will double the energy. If the pulse energy is insufficient, failure to capture will occur; that is, the pulse will not result in depolarization of the myocardium and a mechanical contraction.

The second function of pulse generators is to sense the intrinsic activity of the heart. The sensitivity of both implantable and external generators can be adjusted. The sensitivity of a generator is the magnitude in millivolts of the smallest intrinsic signal that the pacemaker considers to be spontaneous activity of the chamber to which the lead is attached. Thus, a smaller numeric value for sensitivity results in the generator being more sensitive. For example, a setting of 2 mV is more sensitive than a setting of 5 mV, since a 3-mV spontaneous signal from the heart would be detected at the former setting but not at the latter. If a generator is set at too high a numeric sensitivity (too insensitive), it will fail to detect the spontaneous activity of the heart (failure to sense), and if it is set at too low a numeric sensitivity (too sensitive), it may sense skeletal muscle activity or activity of the other cardiac chambers (e.g., an atrial pacemaker may sense the ventricle). This condition is known as oversensing.

For a certain period after the pacemaker has paced a chamber, it will ignore any sensed events. This is the refractory period. It is desirable for a pacemaker to have a refractory period so that it will not mistake the P wave or QRS complex triggered by the pacing for spontaneous atrial or ventricular activity. For temporary pacemakers the refractory period is generally not adjustable, but for most implantable permanent pacemakers it can be programmed.

The third function of the pulse generator is to determine when to pace. Modern pacemakers contain sophisticated microcomputers that analyze the timing of previous sensed and paced events in determining when to pace the heart. The algorithm used by the pacemaker in controlling the timing of its output pulses depends on the pacing mode. The basic pacing mode is described by the first three letters of a code adopted by the North American Society of Pacing and Electrophysiology and the British Pacing and Electrophysiology Group,[4] as shown in Table 7–1. The first letter of the code indicates the chamber paced (A, atrium; V, ventricle; D, dual; or O, none). The second letter indicates the chamber sensed (A, V, D, or O), and the third letter indicates the response to sensed events (I, inhibit; T, trigger; D, dual; or O, none). Thus, for example, a ventricular demand pacemaker would be in VVI mode, pacing the ventricle, sensing the ventricle, and inhibiting after a sensed event. An asynchronous atrial pacemaker would be in AOO mode: pacing the atrium, sensing nothing, and having no response to sensed events.

In general, temporary pacemakers are AAI (atrial demand), VVI (ventricular demand), or DVI (dual chamber with sensing only of the ventricle). In either AAI or VVI mode, the pacer is set by the physician to a certain low rate. Figs. 7–1 and 7–2 show timing diagrams for VVI and AAI pacemakers. To understand pacemaker operation it is helpful to think in terms of intervals rather than rates. The pacing interval is determined by dividing 60,000 ms (1 minute) by the pacing rate in beats per minute. Thus, for a rate of 100 beats per minute, the pacing interval will be 600 ms. In VVI mode with a low rate of 100 beats per minute, if the pacer has not sensed spontaneous ventricular activity within 600 ms of the previous paced or sensed event, a pacing pulse will be delivered, and the timing circuit will be reset. If another 600 ms pass without sensed ventricular activity, another pacing pulse will be delivered, resulting in a paced rhythm at 100 beats per minute. If spontaneous ventricular activity is sensed, the output of the pacemaker will be inhibited, and the timing circuit will be reset. Thus, if the ventricle is beating spontaneously at intervals of less than 600 ms (i.e., at a rate greater than 100 beats per minute), the pacemaker's output will remain inhibited. If the sensitivity of the generator is set higher than the magnitude of the sensed intrinsic activity, the pacemaker will pace without regard to the intrinsic rhythm of the heart, which is asynchronous pacing (VOO in the case of an asynchronous ventricular pacemaker). For atrial pacemakers (AAI or AOO) the same algorithms are used except that it is the atrium that is paced and/or sensed.

For a dual chamber temporary pacemaker (DVI), the atrium and ventricle are both paced, only the ventricle is sensed, and the pacemaker output is inhibited by sensed ventricular activity. Fig. 7–3 shows the timing of a DVI pacemaker. In this

**Table 7–1** The NASPE/BPEG generic (NBG) pacemaker code

| Position<br>Category | I<br>Chamber(s) paced | II<br>Chamber(s) sensed | III<br>Response to sensing | IV<br>Programmability, rate modulation | V<br>Antitachycardia functions |
|---|---|---|---|---|---|
| | 0, None | 0, None | 0, None | 0, None | 0, None |
| | A, Atrium | A, Atrium | T, Triggered | P, Simple programmable | P, Pacing |
| | V, Ventricle | V, Ventricle | I, Inhibited | M, Multiprogrammable | S, Shock |
| | D, Dual (A + V) | D, Dual (A + V) | D, Dual (T + I) | C, Communicating | D, Dual (P + S) |
| | | | | R, Rate modulation | |

From Bernstein AD, Camm AJ, Fletcher RD et al: The NASPE/BPEG generic pacemaker code for antibradyarrhythmia and adaptive-rate pacing and antitachyarrhythmic-events, *PACE* 10:794, 1987.

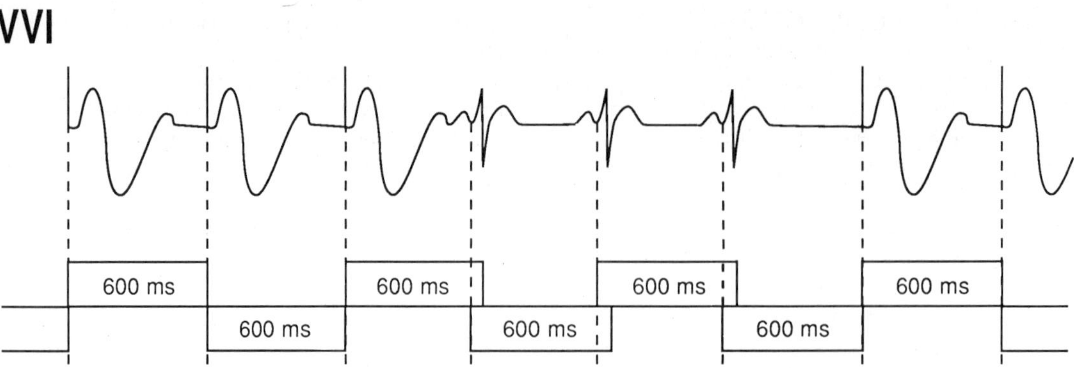


**Figure 7–1** Timing diagram for VVI (ventricular demand) pacing. The pacemaker is programmed at a rate of 100, corresponding to a pacing interval of 600 ms. After each of the first two ventricular paced beats *(VP),* no spontaneous activity is sensed within 600 ms so that a pacing stimulus is delivered 600 ms after the previous stimulus. After the third ventricular paced beat *(VP),* a spontaneous QRS is sensed *(VS).* The pacemaker output is inhibited, and another 600-ms interval is begun. Before the end of that interval, another QRS is sensed *(VS),* the pacer output is still inhibited, and another 600-ms interval begins. After the third sensed beat, 600 ms passes without a sensed event, and the pacing resumes. Note that each ventricular paced (VP) event is exactly 600 ms after the previous ventricular paced (VP) or sensed (VS) event.

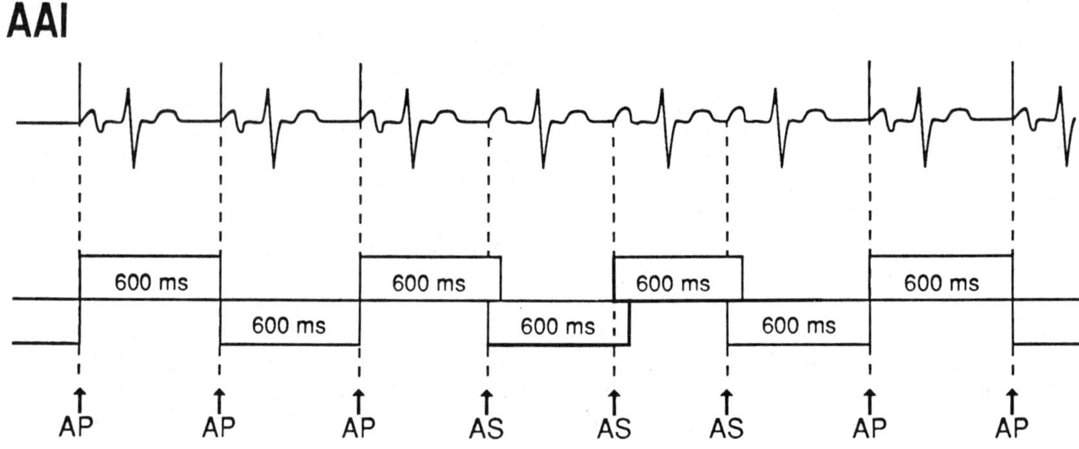


**Figure 7–2** Timing for AAI (atrial demand) pacing. The pacemaker is programmed to AAI pacing at 100. The timing is identical to that in Fig. 7–1 except that the atrium is paced and sensed.

mode, in addition to setting a low rate, the user must set an AV interval. Since the pacing interval consists of the AV interval plus the VA interval, the VA interval (the interval from the last ventricular event to the next atrial paced event) will be the difference between the pacing interval and the AV interval. For example with a low rate of 100 (600 ms pacing interval) and an AV interval of 150 ms the VA interval will be 450 ms. If no spontaneous ventricular beat is sensed within 450 ms after the last paced or sensed ventricular beat, the pacemaker will deliver an atrial pacing pulse. If no ventricular activity is sensed in the next 150 ms, a ventricular pacing pulse will be delivered. This mode of pacing will result in AV synchrony as long as the intrinsic atrial rate is lower than the programmed low rate of the pacemaker.

Many permanent implantable generators offer additional modes of pacing. The most common mode of dual chamber pacing is DDD, in which both the atrium and the ventricle are paced, both chambers are sensed, and sensed events may either

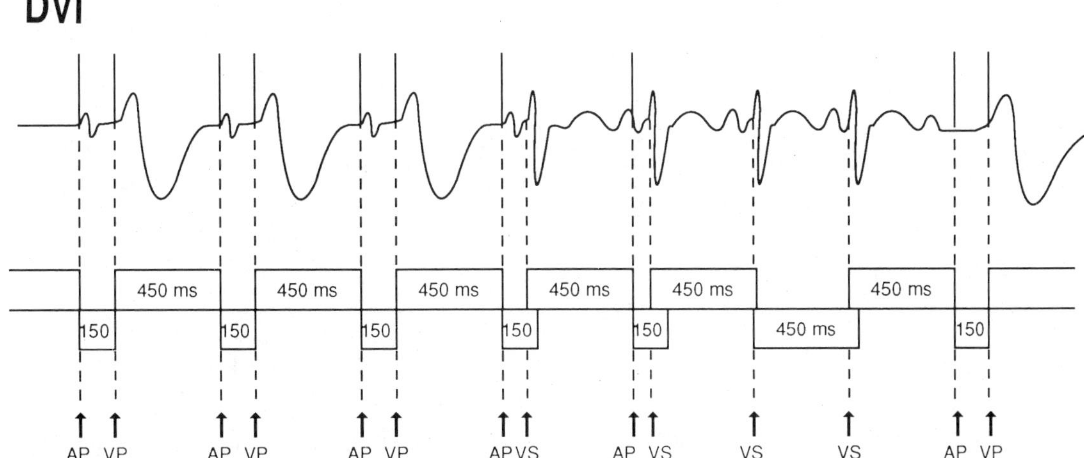


**Figure 7–3** Timing for DVI (AV sequential) pacing. The pacemaker is programmed to DVI mode with a low rate of 100 (a pacing interval of 600 ms) and an AV interval of 150 ms. The VA interval is 600 minus 150, or 450 ms. After the first atrial pacing stimulus *(AP)*, no ventricular activity is sensed within 150 ms, so a ventricular pacing stimulus *(VP)* is delivered and a VA interval begins. No ventricular activity is sensed within that 450-ms interval. At the end of that interval an atrial pacing spike is delivered and another AV interval begins. This process repeats itself several times. After the fourth atrial paced event *(AP)*, a spontaneous QRS is sensed *(VS)*, inhibiting the ventricular pacing and starting a new VA interval. Again, no spontaneous ventricular activity is sensed. Note that in DVI mode, atrial activity is never sensed, so that despite there having been a spontaneous P wave within the 450-ms VA interval, an atrial pacing spike is delivered. Again, a spontaneous QRS is sensed within the AV interval, ventricular pacing is inhibited, and another VA interval is initiated. During this interval a spontaneous QRS is sensed, and pacing of both the atrium and the ventricle is inhibited. Another VA interval is begun, and again a spontaneous QRS is sensed during this 450-ms interval. Thus, for atrial pacing to be inhibited with a DVI pacemaker, the spontaneous ventricular cycle length must be shorter than the VA interval. In this example the ventricular rate must be greater than 133 (a cycle length of 450 ms). After the third ventricular sensed *(VS)* event, no ventricular activity is sensed within the VA interval, so the atrium is paced *(AP)*, and no ventricular activity is sensed within the AV interval, so the ventricle is paced as well *(VP)*.

trigger or inhibit the pacemaker output. DDD pacing is shown in Fig. 7–4. This mode is similar to the DVI pacing described above except that an atrial sensed event will inhibit atrial pacing and may trigger ventricular pacing. If a spontaneous atrial contraction is detected prior to the end of the VA interval, the atrial pacing pulse will be inhibited. Either an atrial paced or an atrial sensed event will trigger the start of the AV interval; if no ventricular activity is sensed prior to the end of the AV interval, a ventricular pacing pulse will be delivered. In this mode patients with AV block and intact sinus node function will pace their ventricles at a rate determined by their own sinus nodes. This is the most physiologic mode, since it provides AV synchrony and allows variation of the pacing rate in response to changes in autonomic tone.

Some newer pacemakers can change rate in response to motion of the body, respiratory rate, blood temperature, or venous oxygen saturation. In patients in whom dual chamber pacing is not possible and in patients without normal control of the sinus rate, this rate-responsive pacing allows the heart rate to vary with activity. Rate-responsive pacing is denoted by an R as the fourth letter of the code: AAI-R, VVI-R, or DDD-R pacing.

Modern implantable generators are quite small, ranging in weight from 15 to 50 gm, with many dual chamber pacemakers weighing less than 30 gm. These generators are 25 to 50 mm in their largest dimension and 5 to 10 mm thick (Fig. 7–5). Implantable generators are generally programmable by radiofrequency signals from an external programmer and many can provide data to the programmer via telemetry. Such data may include the programmed parameters of the pacemaker, information on battery and lead voltage, current and resistance, and profiles of the patient's previous heart rate and activity. Some pacemakers can even provide recordings of the intracardiac electrograms detected by the lead. With modern battery tech-

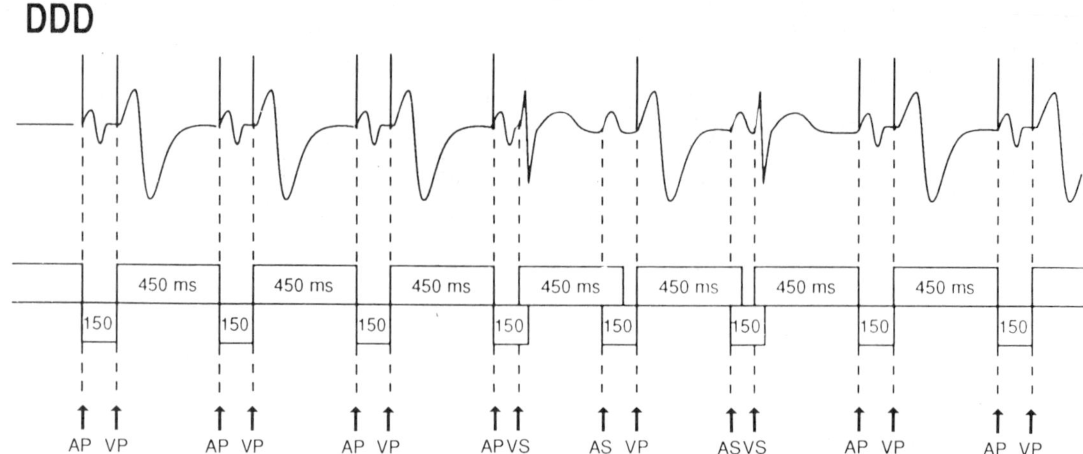


**Figure 7–4** Timing diagram for DDD pacing. Programmed settings are identical to those in Figure 7–3 except that the pacer is in DDD mode. The only difference between DVI and DDD mode is that the atrium is sensed in DDD mode. The pacemaker's behavior in the first four beats is identical to that in Fig. 7–3. After the first ventricular sensed event *(VS)* a spontaneous atrial event is sensed *(AS)* within the VA interval. This inhibits atrial pacing and begins an AV interval. Since no ventricular event is sensed during this interval, the ventricle is paced. In this mode the ventricular pacing can track the spontaneous atrial rate in patients with complete AV block.

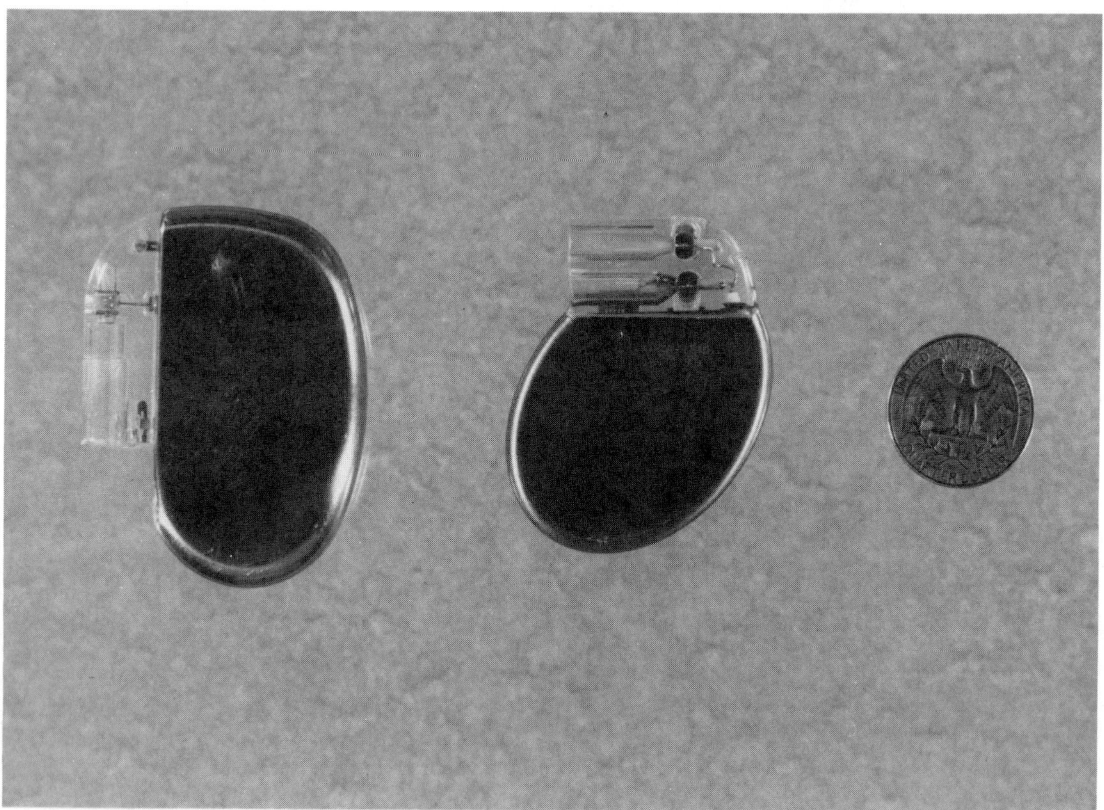

**Figure 7–5** Implantable pacemakers. At left is a single-chamber pace-maker from 1988. It weighs 40 gm and can sense vibration and adjust its rate in response to body motion. In the center is a DDD pacemaker from 1990. It weighs 26 gm and can record intracardiac electrograms, perform noninvasive programmed stimulation for diagnostic induction and termination of arrhythmias, and store histograms of the patient's heart rate for several months. A quarter is shown for scale. The pacemakers are approximately twice the diameter, five to eight times the weight, and 30,000 times the cost of the coin.

nology it is not unusual for an implantable pacemaker to have a battery life in excess of 10 years.

### Pacing leads

Pacing leads may be attached either to the outside of the heart (epicardial leads) or to the inside of the heart (transvenous endocardial leads). Epicardial leads require exposure of the epicardium for implantation via a sternotomy, a thoracotomy, or a subxiphoid approach. Transvenous leads may be implanted without entering the thorax. Epicardial and transvenous leads may be either temporary or permanent and may be either unipolar or bipolar. It is important not to confuse bipolar with dual chamber pacing. *Unipolar* and *bipolar* refer to the pacing configuration for a single chamber. In unipolar systems there is a single electrode in contact with the chamber being paced, and in bipolar systems there are two electrodes on each paced chamber. Bipolar pacing may be accomplished either with two separate leads attached to the same chamber, as is usual with epicardial bipolar pacing, or with a single lead having two electrodes and two conductors, as is the case in bipolar endocardial leads. Dual-chamber pacing systems may be either unipolar or bipolar, as may single-chamber systems. A dual-chamber bipolar system will actually have four electrodes in contact with the heart.

For any pacing system there must be a complete circuit for the current leaving the pulse generator to reach the heart and return to the generator. In the case of bipolar systems the path of the current is from the generator to one electrode, through the heart from one electrode to the other, and then back to the generator. In a unipolar system the current enters the heart through the electrode and returns by passing through the body tissues to an uninsulated portion of the pacemaker can. Unipolar pacing leads are simpler and often smaller but are more susceptible to sensing problems because of skeletal muscle activity.

The simplest epicardial leads are temporary wires either sewn to the heart or inserted into the myocardium. These are generally placed as a precaution at the time of open heart surgery. Two of these leads are generally attached to the atrium and/or the ventricle as a bipolar pair. Permanent epicardial leads are sewn to the heart, screwed into the heart, or plunged into the myocardium. In general, epicardial leads require higher energy to pace the heart than do transvenous endocardial leads, partly because of the development of scar tissue at the junction of the lead and the heart.[12] To minimize scarring, some epicardial leads include a small amount of corticosteroid in the tip of the electrode.[15,21] Early results suggest that these leads may have thresholds comparable with those of endocardial transvenous leads.[13] Epicardial leads may be used on the atrium, the ventricle, or both.

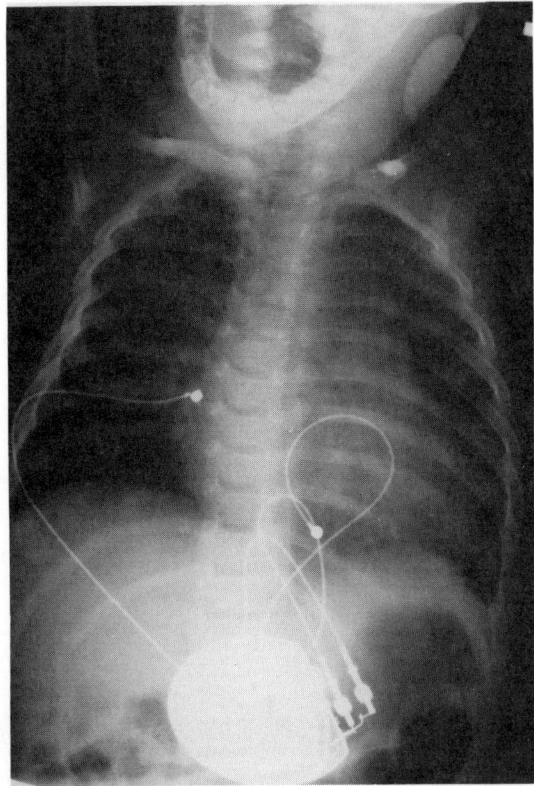

**Figure 7–6** Dual chamber epicardial pacing system. Unipolar atrial and ventricular epicardial steroid-eluting pacing leads were placed in this patient with congenital complete heart block and single ventricle when he was 3 months of age and weighed 4 kg. The generator is a dual-chamber generator identical to the one shown in Fig. 7–5.

Transvenous endocardial leads are inserted via the systemic veins and enter the atrium. Transvenous ventricular leads cross the AV valve to enter the ventricle. Transvenous endocardial leads may be passively held in place by tines projecting from the lead, or they may be screwed into the endocardium (active fixation). Atrial and ventricular leads are similar except for the preformed bend of atrial leads designed to aid in lodging the tip of the lead in the atrial appendage. Transvenous leads containing a small amount of corticosteroid in the tip are also available. Figs. 7–6, 7–7, and 7–8 show chest x-ray films of children with various lead configurations.

The decision whether to use epicardial or endocardial leads is based on the patient's size and anatomy. In general, endocardial transvenous leads have lower thresholds and greater longevity than epicardial leads,[12,18] but in some patients other fac-

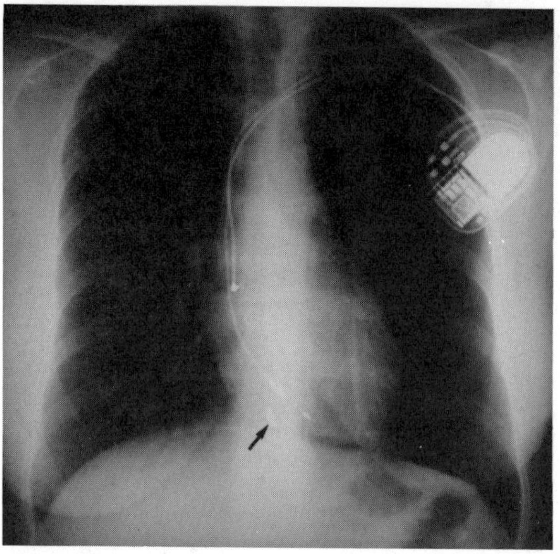

**Figure 7–7** Dual-chamber transvenous endocardial pacing system. Bipolar transvenous leads have been placed with their tips in the right atrial appendage and in the right ventricular apex. In early childhood this patient, who had congenital complete heart block without structural heart disease, underwent previous placement of a unipolar epicardial screw-in lead via a subxiphoid approach. That lead is also visible *(arrow).*

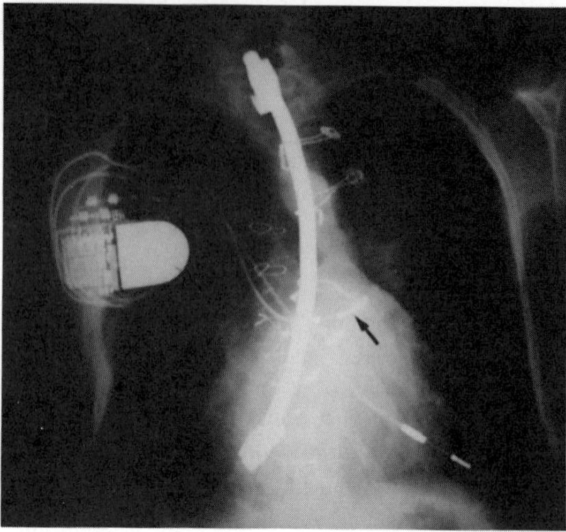

**Figure 7–8** Dual-chamber transvenous endocardial pacing system in a patient with transposition of the great arteries. This patient had undergone Mustard repair of transposition of the great arteries as well as a posterior spinal fusion for scoliosis. He has a bipolar screw-in transvenous lead fixed to the roof of the left atrium *(arrow)* and a bipolar lead in the apex of the left ventricle.

tors may favor epicardial pacing leads. In small children insertion of transvenous leads may be difficult because of the size of the veins. Furthermore, transvenous leads may cause problems with caval obstruction.[8] Caval obstruction is of particular concern in children who have undergone atrial repair of transposition of the great arteries, since these children are at risk for caval obstruction even without transvenous pacing leads.[10] Despite these concerns transvenous systems have been used successfully in many children smaller than 10 kg and in some children as small as 3 kg.[24,26] In most older children transvenous pacing systems are generally preferred to avoid a thoracotomy and because of better pacing thresholds. Younger children are likely to need pacing leads for many decades, and it may be preferable to use an epicardial system as the first system and to reserve the transvenous route for subsequent lead systems. In tiny infants the epicardial approach is clearly preferred. Epicardial lead systems are often used in patients who are undergoing concomitant corrective surgery for congenital heart disease at the time of lead implantation, since the additional morbidity of a thoracotomy or sternotomy to gain access to the epicardium is not an issue.

There are some patients whose cardiac anatomy or prior cardiac surgery precludes transvenous access, and in these patients epicardial pacing leads are needed. For example, following a Glenn shunt—anastomosis of the superior vena cava (SVC) to the right pulmonary artery—it is not possible to pass a transvenous lead from the SVC to the atrium or ventricle. In patients who have tricuspid atresia or prosthetic tricuspid valves or who have undergone right atrial to pulmonary artery anastomoses (Fontan operation), the transvenous route for ventricular pacing leads is not possible, and the use of epicardial leads is required.[22]

## IMPLANTATION TECHNIQUE

For permanent transvenous lead implantation a skin incision is made below the clavicle on the right or left. Through this incision a needle is placed in the subclavian vein in much the same manner as for placement of a percutaneous subclavian venous catheter. When the needle is in the proper position, blood should flow freely when aspirated with a syringe. A flexible guide wire is then inserted into the vein and advanced under fluoroscopic guidance to the heart, and the needle is removed. A dilator and sheath are inserted together over the guide wire, and the dilator is removed. If both atrial and ventricular leads are to be placed, a second guide wire can be placed to avoid the need for a second venous puncture. The pacing catheter is inserted into the vein through the sheath, and the sheath is removed either over the pacing catheter or in the

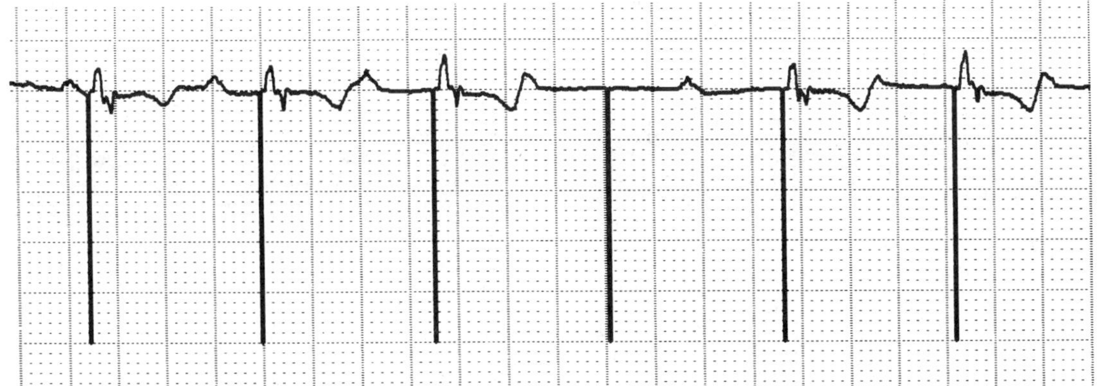

**Figure 7–9** VVI pacing with intermittent failure to capture. The pacemaker is programmed to VVI mode at a rate of 85. After the fourth pacing stimulus, there is no QRS (failure to capture).

case of peel-away sheaths, by separating the two halves of the sheath. Under fluoroscopic guidance the catheter is positioned in either the atrium or the ventricle. Most leads are supplied with stiff metal stylets to aid in positioning the tips in the desired location. Usually atrial leads are positioned with the tip in the right atrial appendage and ventricular leads with the tip in the right ventricular apex. In patients with congenital heart disease, anatomy may dictate the positioning of the leads in other locations. For example, in patients who have previously undergone atrial repair of transposition of the great arteries (Mustard or Senning repair), atrial leads are generally screwed into the roof of the left atrium, and ventricular leads are generally positioned in the apex of the left ventricle.

After the lead is in position, its electrical characteristics are tested (see discussion later in this section), and if they are not acceptable, it is repositioned. Once a satisfactory position for the lead has been found, it is secured to the tissue adjacent to entry of the vein. A pocket for the generator is then formed, either deep or superficial to the pectoralis major. The lead is connected to the generator, the generator is inserted into the pocket, and the incision is closed. The use of electrocautery should be avoided after insertion of the generator, since the electrical activity of the cautery may unintentionally reprogram the generator or revert it to its power-on settings.

Epicardial leads may be placed via a subxiphoid, thoracotomy, or sternotomy approach. The subxiphoid approach has the advantage of avoiding the need to enter the thorax. In this procedure a small incision is made below the xiphoid, and an area of the right ventricular diaphragmatic surface is exposed. Use of the subxiphoid approach for atrial leads is possible, but exposure is very limited. A left thoracotomy provides exposure to both the left atrium and the left ventricle. Right thoracotomy and median sternotomy are rarely used for epicardial lead placement except when other concomitant cardiac surgery requires them. Once an appropriate site is exposed, the lead is attached to the epicardial surface of the heart, either by suturing or by insertion of the lead into the myocardium, depending on the lead design. The electrical characteristics of the lead are tested and the lead is tunneled to the site of the generator pocket and attached to the generator.

Lead testing is performed using a pacing system analyzer. If the lead is unipolar, a grounding electrode must be inserted into the pocket and connected to the positive connector of the analyzer. A scalpel handle works well for this purpose. First the pacing threshold of the lead should be tested. To perform this test, the rate of the pacing system analyzer should be greater than the intrinsic rate of the chamber being paced. Usually a pulse width of 0.5 ms is used, and the amplitude of the pacing pulse is gradually decreased until there is loss of capture. The pacing threshold is the lowest voltage at which there is appropriate capture. For most leads a threshold of 1 volt at 0.5 ms is acceptable for the ventricle, and a threshold of 1.5 volts at 0.5 ms is acceptable for the atrium. Epicardial leads tend to have higher thresholds than endocardial leads. Fig. 7–9 shows an ECG from a patient with VVI pacing and intermittent failure to capture.

Next the ability of the lead to sense intrinsic activity of the heart is tested. The pacing rate must be lower than the intrinsic rate of the chamber to which the lead is attached. The peak-to-peak magnitude of the electrogram from the lead is measured. Usually a P-wave amplitude of 2 mV and an R-wave amplitude of 5 mV are desirable. Fi-

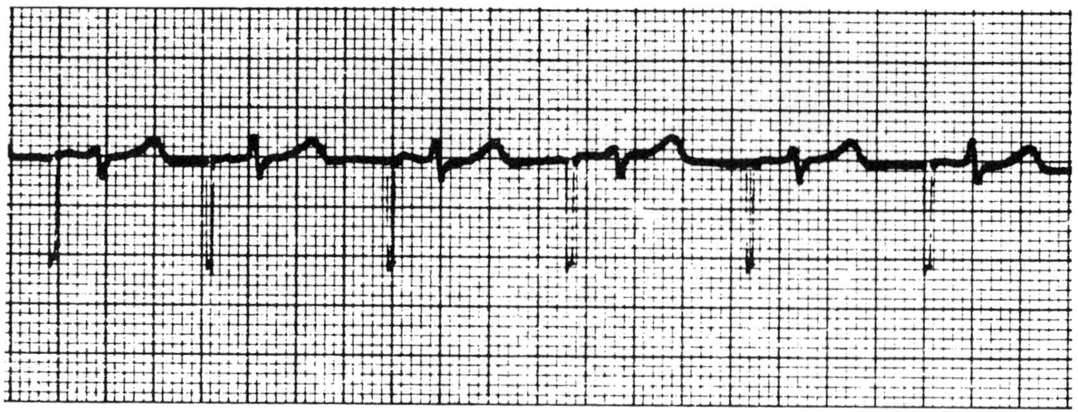

**Figure 7–10** AAI Pacing. An electrocardiogram of a patient with an AAI pacemaker programmed to a rate of 80. Although the paced P waves are difficult to see in this lead, they must be present, since the ventricle is beating spontaneously with a narrow QRS approximately 160 ms after each atrial pacing stimulus.

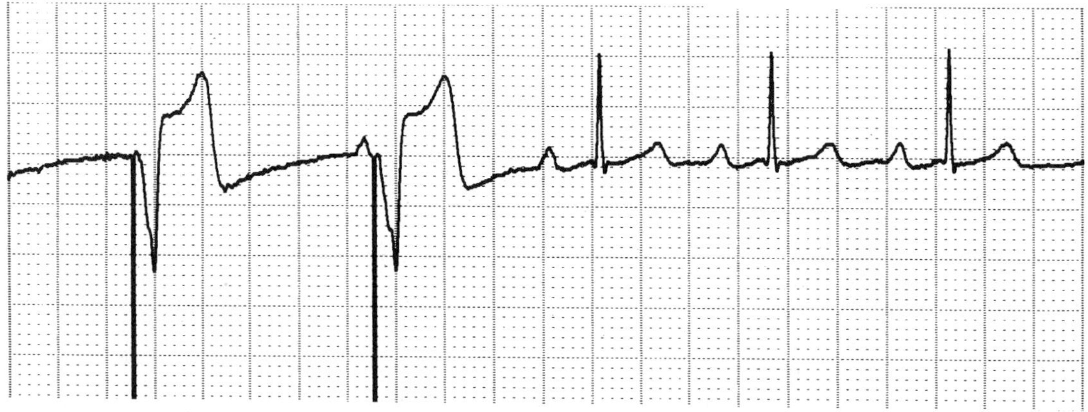

**Figure 7–11** VVI Pacing. An electrocardiogram of a patient with a VVI pacemaker programmed to a rate of 60 (pacing interval of 1000 ms). When the sinus rate exceeds 60 beats per minute, pacing is inhibited.

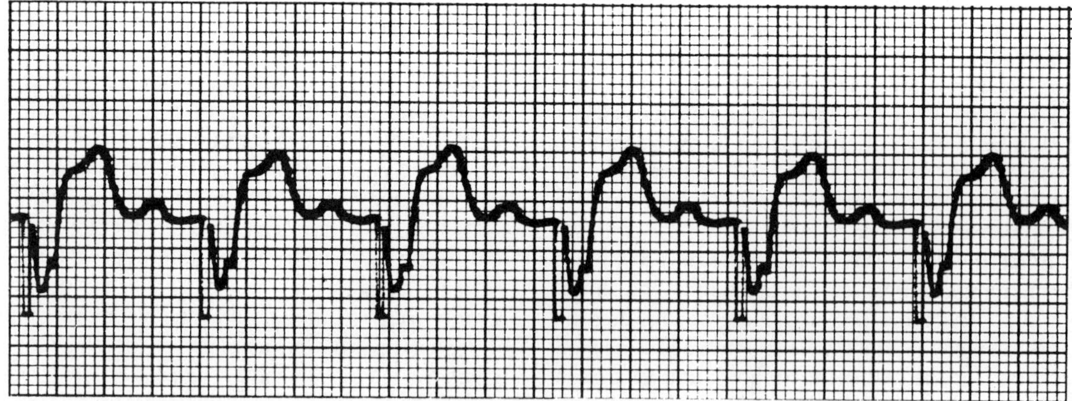

**Figure 7–12** DDD pacing. The pacemaker is sensing each spontaneous P wave and pacing the ventricle 200 ms after each sensed P wave. The atrial output is inhibited, since the atrial rate is faster than the programmed low rate of 60 beats per minute.

nally, the impedance of the lead is measured. The impedance varies according to the lead design, but most leads have impedances of 300 to 500 Ω. If any of these measured lead characteristics is not acceptable, the lead should be repositioned and the measurements repeated. Bear in mind that for most leads, the pacing and sensing characteristics worsen over time,[18] so if a lead is marginal at the time of implantation, it is likely to fail completely before long. Figs. 7–10 to 7–12 show ECGs of patients with AAI, VVI, and DDD pacemakers with normal function.

## SELECTION OF PACEMAKER SETTINGS

For most temporary pacemakers there are few adjustable parameters, and choice of settings is fairly straightforward. Most temporary pacemakers have a preset pulse width that cannot be changed. Thus the energy of the output pulse is determined only by the pulse amplitude. Generally in temporary pacemakers the pulse amplitude is expressed as the current in milliamps. To set the ventricular amplitude, set the rate higher than the intrinsic ventricular rate, the sensitivity to asynchronous, and the amplitude to the lowest setting. While watching the ECG, increase the amplitude until consistent capture of the ventricle is seen as a wide-complex QRS following every pacer spike. This amplitude is the pacing threshold. For an adequate safety margin set the amplitude at twice the threshold. For dual chamber pacing adjust the atrial amplitude in a similar fashion, with the threshold being the amplitude at which there are consistent P-waves after each atrial pacing spike. Note that to set the atrial amplitude the pacing rate must be greater than the intrinsic atrial rate. Selection of a relatively long AV interval will make it easier to see the paced P-waves, since a short AV delay will result in ventricular pacing superimposed on the end of the P-wave.

Next adjust ventricular sensitivity. Sensitivity is expressed in millivolts. Set the sensitivity at maximum (lowest numeric value) and the rate lower than the intrinsic ventricular rate. At this setting the pacemaker output should be inhibited, and the sense indicator on the pacemaker should flash with each QRS. Decrease the sensitivity (raise the numeric value) until the QRS is not consistently sensed, and occasional pacing pulses will be delivered. The sensing threshold is the lowest sensitivity (highest numeric value) at which there is consistent sensing of the QRS. Usually the sensitivity should be set at approximately half this numeric value, providing a 2:1 safety margin for sensing.

Finally, select the AV interval and rate. The AV interval must provide adequate time for ventricular filling after atrial pacing. This parameter is chosen empirically by observing the patient's blood pressure and perfusion. Usually an AV interval of 150 to 200 ms is optimum. The rate is also chosen empirically to provide adequate cardiac output without compromising filling times. Occasionally, in patients with a fairly rapid junctional rhythm, it is desirable to increase the rate of a dual chamber pacer to a rate faster than the junctional rate to provide AV synchrony and improve cardiac output.

Choice of permanent pacemaker parameters is slightly more complicated, since there are many more programmable parameters to set. The principles are the same as for temporary pacemakers. Atrial and ventricular pulse energies can be set by adjusting either the pulse width or the amplitude. Pulse width thresholds can be determined at several amplitudes. Initially, the pulse width is generally set to be approximately five times the threshold to allow an adequate safety margin if the threshold increases over time. It is not uncommon for implanting physicians to leave the amplitude and pulse width of a pacemaker at the factory preset values, but be sure that these settings give an adequate safety margin. Measure the sensing thresholds for the atria and ventricles and set sensitivities to provide at least a 2:1 safety margin. Pacing mode, rate, and AV interval are based on the patient's age, activity, and underlying cardiac abnormalities.

## ANTITACHYCARDIA PACING

Pacemakers with special circuitry to detect and terminate tachycardia are being used with increasing frequency as an alternative or adjunct to pharmacologic therapy for patients with supraventricular, and occasionally ventricular, tachycardia.[5,6] In addition to pacing for bradycardia as described above, these pacemakers can detect tachycardias using multiple criteria including high rate, sudden onset of tachycardia, lack of rate variability in tachycardia, and sustained high rate. Once tachycardia has been detected, the pacemaker can attempt to terminate it by overdrive pacing with bursts of paced beats at rates faster than the tachycardia rate. Multiple algorithms to terminate the tachycardia can be programmed. Fig. 7–13 shows an ECG of termination of atrial reentry tachycardia by an automatic implantable antitachycardia pacemaker. At present the only automatic antitachycardia pacemakers available are single chamber units designed for use in the atrium. Other pacemakers, both single and dual chamber units, can be temporarily programmed by the physician to terminate tachycardias. In addition, many of these generators can be used to perform programmed stimulation to induce tachycardias, allowing noninvasive electro-

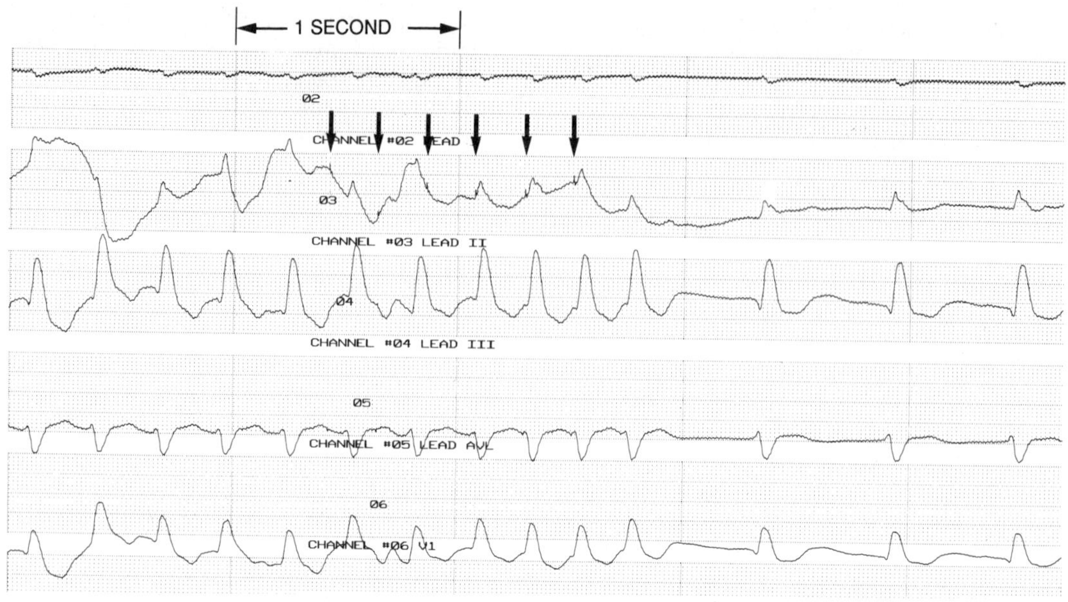


**Figure 7–13** Termination of intraatrial reentry tachycardia with an automatic antitachycardia pacemaker. This patient with single ventricle had undergone Fontan operation with good hemodynamic results but had recurrent tachycardia despite multiple antiarrhythmic medications. Five surface ECG leads are shown at a paper speed of 50 mm/sec. At left there is tachycardia at a rate of 210 beats per minute. The pacemaker has detected the tachycardia and delivers six atrial pacing stimuli *(arrows)* at 280 beats per minute. The pacing captures the atrium, and at the end of the pacing burst the tachycardia terminates.

physiologic testing in patients who have these generators. With the growing concern about proarrhythmic effects of antiarrhythmic agents, nonpharmacologic therapy of tachyarrhythmias using pacemakers becomes an increasingly attractive option.

## CONSIDERATIONS FOR ANESTHESIA

In general, anesthesia management of patients undergoing pacemaker implantation is fairly straightforward. Most adults and older children can have implantation of transvenous pacing systems under local anesthesia with sedation. In younger children, or for epicardial lead placement, general anesthesia is required.

Several aspects of the management of general anesthesia for pacemaker placement deserve special mention. Patients undergoing either initial pacemaker placement or replacement of a malfunctioning pacing system are at risk for severe bradycardia with the induction of general anesthesia. If severe bradycardia occurs, IV isoproterenol may increase the ventricular escape rate. Transcutaneous pacing using thoracic patches may also be effective. The use of neuromuscular blockade may be undesirable in patients having leads placed, since this may obscure phrenic or skeletal muscle pacing. Because of the proximity of the phrenic nerves to the heart, it is possible to stimulate the phrenic nerve with the pacing stimuli and thus pace the diaphragm. While not life threatening, diaphragmatic pacing is intolerable to most patients. With unipolar systems, pacing of skeletal muscle adjacent to the pacemaker is occasionally a problem, since the current must pass from the lead, through the myocardium, and back through the surrounding tissues to the generator. Placement of the insulated side of the generator toward the muscle minimizes but does not eliminate the risk of skeletal muscle pacing. Obviously it is desirable to recognize and correct diaphragmatic or skeletal muscle pacing at the time of implantation rather than after the patient awakens from anesthesia.

The increasing survival of children with congenital heart disease, both with and without surgery, has provided a growing number of patients with bradyarrhythmias requiring pacing. Antitachycardia pacing can be used to treat patients with poorly controlled tachyarrhythmias. Fortunately, advances in pacemaker and lead technology have increased the effectiveness and longevity of pacing systems in children. Still, it remains a challenge to provide effective pacing for a child over a life expectancy of many decades.

## REFERENCES


1. American College of Cardiology/American Heart Association Task Force on Assessment of Diagnostic and Therapeutic Cardiovascular Procedures (Committee on Pacemaker Implantation): Guidelines for implantation of cardiac pacemakers and antiarrhythmia devices, *Circulation* 84:455, 1991, and *J Am Coll Cardiol* 18:1, 1991.
2. Beder SD, Hanisch DG, Cohen MH et al: Cardiac pacing in children: a 15-year experience, *Am Heart J* 109:152, 1985.
3. Benrey J, Gillette PC, Nasrallah AT et al: Permanent pacemaker implantation in infants, children, and adolescents: long-term follow-up, *Circulation* 53:245, 1976.
4. Bernstein AD, Camm AJ, Fletcher RD et al: The NASPE/BPEG generic pacemaker code for antibradyarrhythmia and adaptive-rate pacing and antitachyarrhythmia events, *PACE* 10:794, 1987.
5. Case CL, Gillette PC, Zeigler VL et al: Successful treatment of congenital atrial flutter with antitachycardia pacing, *PACE* 13:571, 1990.
6. Fukushige J, Porter CJ, Hayes DL et al: Antitachycardia pacemaker treatment of postoperative arrhythmias in pediatric patients, *PACE* 14:546, 1991.
7. Garson A: Medicolegal problems in the management of cardiac arrhythmias in children, *Pediatrics* 79:84, 1987.
8. Gillette PC, Zeigler V, Bradham GB et al: Pediatric transvenous pacing: a concern for venous thrombosis? *PACE* 11:1935, 1988.
9. Goldman BS, Williams WG, Hill T et al: Permanent cardiac pacing after open heart surgery: congenital heart disease, *PACE* 8:732, 1985.
10. Graham TP Jr.: Hemodynamic residua and sequelae following intraatrial repair of transposition of the great arteries: a review, *Pediatr Cardiol* 2:203, 1982.
11. Hayes CJ, Gersony WM: Arrhythmias after the Mustard operation for transposition of the great arteries: a long-term study, *J Am Coll Cardiol* 7:133, 1986.
12. Henglein D, Gillette PC, Shannon C et al: Long-term follow-up of pulse width threshold of transvenous and myoepicardial leads, *PACE* 7:203, 1984.
13. Johns JA, Fish FA, Burger JD et al: Steroid-eluting epicardial pacing leads in pediatric patients: encouraging early results, *J Am Coll Cardiol* 20:395, 1992.
14. Kugler JD, Danford DA: Pacemakers in children: an update, *Am Heart J* 117:665, 1989.
15. Kugler JD, Fetter J, Fleming W et al: A new steroid-eluting epicardial lead: experience with atrial and ventricular implantation in the immature swine, *PACE* 13:976, 1990.
16. Pinsky WW, Gillette PC, Garson A et al: Diagnosis, management, and long-term results of patients with congenital complete atrioventricular block, *Pediatrics* 69:728, 1982.
17. Reed BR, Lee LA, Harmon C et al: Autoantibodies to SS-A/Ro in infants with congenital heart block, *J Pediatr* 103:889, 1983.
18. Serwer GA, Mericle JM, Armstrong BE: Epicardial ventricular pacemaker electrode longevity in children, *Am J Cardiol* 61:104, 1988.
19. Sholler GF, Walsh EP: Congenital complete heart block in patients without anatomic cardiac defects, *Am Heart J* 118:1193, 1989.
20. Silka MJ, Manwill JR, Kron J et al: Bradycardia-mediated tachyarrhythmias in congenital heart disease and responses to chronic pacing at physiologic rates, *Am J Cardiol* 65:488, 1990.
21. Stokes KB: Preliminary studies on a new steroid eluting epicardial electrode, *PACE* 11:1797, 1988.
22. Taliercio CP, Vlietstra RE, McGoon MD et al: Permanent cardiac pacing after the Fontan procedure, *J Thorac Cardiovasc Surg* 90:414, 1985.
23. Taylor PV, Taylor KF, Norman A et al: Prevalence of maternal Ro (SS-A) and La (SS-B) autoantibodies in relation to congenital heart block. *Br J Rheumatol* 27:128, 1988.
24. Till JA, Jones S, Rowland E et al: Endocardial pacing in infants and children 15 kg or less in weight: medium-term follow-up, *PACE* 13:1385, 1990.
25. Walsh CA, McAlister HF, Andrews CA et al: Pacemaker implantation in children: a 21-year experience, *PACE* 11:1940, 1988.
26. Ward DE, Jones S, Shinebourne EA: Long-term transvenous pacing in children weighing 10 kg or less, *Int J Cardiol* 15:112, 1987.

# 8 Perioperative Monitoring

***Sandra V. Lowe, Jayant K. Deshpande** and **Joseph D. Tobias***



Monitoring in the practice of pediatric anesthesia has become increasingly sophisticated and complex. However, the vigilance of the individual anesthesiologist remains the most important element in the safe conduct of pediatric cardiac anesthesia. The majority of pediatric patients requiring surgery are monitored noninvasively, but patients with congenital heart defects are often monitored invasively.

After the anesthesiologist's own sight, hearing, and touch, noninvasive monitors are the second line of defense against anesthetic mishap. In the past 20 years the noninvasive monitors have traditionally consisted of the precordial stethoscope, esophageal stethoscope, ECG, noninvasive blood pressure monitoring, pulse oximetry, temperature, and respiratory gas. Over the past decade continuous pulse oximetry and end tidal carbon dioxide analysis have made a significant impact on routine noninvasive monitoring.

## NONINVASIVE MONITORING IN THE PEDIATRIC CARDIAC PATIENT

In 1986 the American Society of Anesthesiology put forth its standards of monitoring, and many states have followed with specific requirements, such as for oximetry and capnometry, that are rapidly becoming de facto standards as well.

Monitoring standards must be age appropriate not only because of the size of the patient but also because of the specific physiologic factors of the child. To limit morbidity as much information as possible must be obtained from noninvasive monitors.

### Precordial and esophageal stethoscopes

Although not specifically required by the standards of intraoperative monitoring except by the American Society of Anesthesiologists, the precordial stethoscope fulfills one requirement for continuous monitoring of circulation and ventilation. The precordial stethoscope is the simplest modality for continuous monitoring of cardiorespiratory status during anesthesia. It is inexpensive and involves little risk. Although Harvey Cushing's anesthetist, Griffiths Davis, used a precordial stethoscope at Johns Hopkins Hospital in 1917 during neurosurgery, its use was forgotten until 1953, when Smith recommended that a precordial stethoscope be used throughout every pediatric anesthesia.[23,65] By 1959 Smith[67] advocated the use of a precordial stethoscope, small blood pressure cuffs, a temperature probe, and a heated water mattress to control the infant's body temperature. The ECG, he considered, was not essential for routine use but was most desirable for the patient with severe heart problems.

Esophageal stethoscopes have been used in anesthesia practice for over 3 decades.[66] The simplest ones are inexpensive and consist merely of a soft catheter with holes in its distal 2 to 3 cm, which are covered with a cuff. More sophisticated varieties incorporate thermistors or ECG electrodes or both. An esophageal stethoscope is commonly used when a precordial stethoscope is impractical because of the site of surgery or to facilitate temperature monitoring when a thermistor has been incorporated into the probe.

### Electrocardiogram

Continuous ECG monitoring should be used with all pediatric patients. When used appropriately the ECG provides valuable information regarding heart rate and rhythm and is essential in pediatric cardiac perioperative monitoring (Table 8–1).

Although there are distinct differences between infants and adults regarding cardiac depolarization, these differences have minimal impact on ECG monitoring in the operating room. The most significant difference that affects anesthesiologists is that in the infant the most pronounced R-wave will be seen in standard lead III as opposed to lead II in the adult. This results from the right axis shift seen in the neonatal ECG.[43]

The ECG allows the clinician to differentiate between normal sinus rhythm and other dysrhythmias such as heart block and the supraventricular tachycardias most commonly seen in children with congenital heart disease. Dysrhythmias such as premature atrial and ventricular contractions are usually benign in children. They often result from the interaction of either endogenous or exogenous epinephrine and the halogenated anesthetics. However, dysrhythmias should not be dismissed even in the absence of hypotension but should heighten suspicion for the existence of other problems, such as inadequate oxygenation or ventilation or early malignant hyperthemia.

Severe electrolyte disturbances may also be detected by using the ECG. Small infants requiring massive transfusion of stored banked blood are particularly prone to increases in serum potassium and decreases in serum calcium concentrations. These problems are commonly seen in children undergoing liver transplantation, craniofacial reconstruction, or removal of large vascular tumors and during surgery for the repair of congenital cardiac defects. Ischemic changes rarely occur in normal children. However, children with congenital heart disease may form a separate subset; whether these children are more susceptible to ischemia is controversial. Nonetheless, a recent study by Bell and colleagues[9] emphasizes that ischemic changes can occur in these children, and attention to ST segment analysis can be beneficial.

The ECG should always be used in conjunction with other monitors that detect changes in perfusion and blood pressure. An adequate heart rate does not imply adequate tissue perfusion. When used by itself the ECG will not detect significant reductions in cardiac output that can occur despite an adequate heart rate. Loss of sinus rhythm is a late finding in cardiac arrest, particularly when resulting from a high concentration of a halogenated agent.

**Table 8–1** Normal age-specific heart rates

| | Heart rate (beats/min) | |
|---|---|---|
| Age | Mean | Range |
| 0-24 h | 123 | 93-154 |
| 1-2 d | 123 | 91-159 |
| 3-6 d | 129 | 91-166 |
| 8-30 d | 148 | 107-182 |
| 1-2 mo | 149 | 121-179 |
| 3-5 mo | 141 | 106-186 |
| 6-11 mo | 134 | 109-169 |
| 1-2 y | 119 | 89-151 |
| 3-4 y | 108 | 73-137 |
| 5-7 y | 100 | 65-133 |
| 8-11 y | 91 | 62-130 |
| 12-15 y | 85 | 60-119 |

From Rowe PC, editor: *The Harriet Lane handbook*, ed 11, Chicago, 1987, Mosby.

### Noninvasive blood pressure monitoring

Pediatric anesthesiologists commonly state that the stroke volume of the infant heart is relatively fixed (Table 8–2), and therefore the cardiac output of the infant depends on the heart rate. Unfortunately, this relationship has led to the misconception that bradycardia in the infant results in hypotension and that restoration of heart rate means that the infant will be normotensive. As a result clinicians in anesthesia may be inclined to monitor heart rate only and not measure blood pressure.

Various methods are available for the noninvasive measurement of blood pressure in infants and children. These methods include the flush, the needle bounce, and the Riva-Rocci technique. In the flush technique the distal extremity is compressed so that blood will drain from it while an occluding cuff is inflated. As the cuff is deflated, the systemic systolic pressure is taken as the pressure at which

**Table 8–2** Range of normal blood pressure at various ages

| Age | Mean systolic blood pressure (± 2 SD) | Mean diastolic blood pressure (± 2 SD) |
|---|---|---|
| Newborn | 80 (16) | 46 (16) |
| 6 mo-1 yr | 89 (29) | 60 (10) |
| 1 yr | 96 (30) | 66 (25) |
| 2 yr | 99 (25) | 64 (25) |
| 3 yr | 100 (25) | 67 (23) |
| 4 yr | 99 (20) | 65 (20) |
| 5-6 yr | 94 (14) | 55 (9) |
| 6-7 yr | 100 (15) | 56 (8) |
| 7-8 yr | 102 (15) | 56 (8) |
| 8-9 yr | 105 (16) | 57 (9) |
| 9-10 yr | 107 (16) | 57 (9) |
| 10-11 yr | 111 (17) | 58 (10) |
| 11-12 yr | 113 (18) | 59 (10) |
| 12-13 yr | 115 (19) | 59 (10) |
| 13-14 yr | 118 (19) | 60 (10) |

SD, standard deviation
From Gregory GA: *Pediatric anesthesia*, ed 2, New York, 1989, Churchill/Livingstone.

the distal circulation returns, which is indicated by a flush as the arm turns pink. The needle bounce technique works best with a large aneroid manometer that can display a visible bounce as the cuff is deflated. The systolic pressure corresponds most clearly with the pressure at which the bounce is maximal. However, both techniques have been shown to be unreliable, especially in small vasoconstricted infants. In all three techniques the return of flow is noted as the systolic pressure.

Automated oscillometry has become increasingly popular over the past decade. With these devices the cuff acts as both an actuator and transducer. The cuff is automatically inflated above systolic pressure. One tube to the cuff results in its inflation, and the other transmits pressure to the transducer within the instrument housing. Because the cuff acts as a signal sensor of pressure oscillations involving the monitored limb, placement of the cuff directly over an artery is unnecessary. This ease of operation adds considerably to its popularity.

The automatic cuff is deflated in increments and compares two cardiac cycles with each deflation. If noise levels are low (lack of cuff movement during measurement), then deflation of the cuff continues. If noise is high, successive cardiac cycles are compared until two comparable cycles are recorded at a given inflation pressure. This accounts for the difference in time it can take for any given inflation cycle to measure blood pressure in the same patient. Averaged pairs of oscillations are then analyzed to determine systolic, diastolic, and mean pressures. Systolic pressure corresponds to the point of rapid increase in oscillations, mean pressure represents the maximum point of oscillation, and diastolic pressure is the point of rapid fade of sensed oscillation. The heart rate is determined by the median of all pressure pulse rates obtained during a given measurement cycle.

Accuracy of automated devices depends on several factors. Foremost is the use of an appropriately sized cuff. Recent studies have shown most accuracy using a cuff size determined by formulas based on the cross-sectional area of the mid-upper arm.[39,53] The cuff width should be 50% of the circumference or 120% of the diameter of the limb. A cuff that is too narrow may produce larger errors than one that is too wide. The manufacturers of most automated noninvasive blood pressure monitors recommend using the largest cuff that can be placed between the axilla and the antecubital fossa.

The accuracy of blood pressure measured by automated oscillometry as compared with pressures determined by Doppler and intraarterial catheters has been verified in children.[27] Additionally, these monitors have been shown to be accurate using either lower or upper extremities in children.[7] However, the accuracy of these devices in detecting hypotension in very low birth weight infants has been questioned.[18,25,73] These studies revealed that automatic oscillometry was accurate in very low birth weight infants when arterial pressure was above 40 mm Hg. For mean arterial pressure below 40 mm Hg, automated monitoring consistently gave readings above those determined by the intraarterial method. Note that in all age groups the diastolic pressures measured by these monitors are less accurate than the systolic and mean values.

Despite their noninvasive nature, automated cuffs are not without their hazards. The possibility of electric shock has been raised, although patients are usually isolated from the device by rubber or polyester tubing. Improper placement of the cuff can result in damage to nerves or extremities during inflation. This is particularly true during extensive cuff movement, when the cuff may stay inflated for an extended time to obtain an accurate measurement. In neonates automated cuffs with long inflation times and short intervals between measurements are best avoided; prolonged use under such circumstances leaves little time for perfusion of the limb.

### Pulse oximetry

Few technologic advances have had greater impact on the practice of anesthesia in the past decade than the introduction of the continuous pulse oximeter. Although pulse oximetry is not new, recent advances in technology have made its use feasible in nearly all anesthesia environments.

The origins of pulse oximetry are in the works of Nicolai,[51] who in 1931 applied the Beer-Lambert law to the transmission of light through the hand in an effort to study tissue oxygenation. With the same wavelength of light, oxygenated and deoxygenated blood absorbs different quantities of light proportional to their concentration or the percent saturation. In 1942 Millikan[45] coined the term *oximeter* when he developed a practical aviation ear oxygen meter. In 1974 Aoyagi noted that the difference in absorbance of red and infrared light transmitted through the tissue was related to arterial hemoglobin saturation.[49] This discovery eliminated the need to heat tissue to obtain an arterial saturation estimate. Measuring two wavelengths of light, one in the red (660 nm) and one in the infrared (940 nm) spectrum, could reveal the necessary data. Such an oximeter relies on the detection of a pulsatile signal and was called a pulse oximeter. Today's pulse oximeters incorporate plethysmography and oximetry in one instrument. Pulse oximeters compare the difference in light absorbance in the absence of a pulse wave form to that measured during the presence of a pulse wave form. Improvements in solid state electronics have resulted in pulse oximeters that have determined values within 2% of those measured in vitro and that require no calibration.[74]

Pulse oximeters are affected by dyes such as methylene blue, by nail polish, by carboxymethemoglobin, and most important, by ambient light and low signal to noise ratios. Fetal hemoglobin has no effect on the accuracy of pulse oximeters. Remember, however, that the arterial oxygen tension ($Pa{O_2}$) at a given arterial oxygen saturation ($Sa{O_2}$) is lower for hemoglobin F than for hemoglobin A.

Interference from ambient light is easily avoided by covering the oximeter probe with an opaque cover. Low signal to noise ratios and their management are often the most annoying for the anesthesiologist. Low flow states and motion artifact prevent accurate determination of pulsatile flow and thereby interfere with accurate measurement of arterial saturation. Most pulse oximeters have built-in mechanisms to minimize many of the causes of low signal to noise ratios. All these designs, however, interfere with the response time and accuracy of the monitor. Most pulse oximeters therefore provide a low signal strength error message or show a pulse wave form to confirm signal quality.

Pulse oximeters are capable of functioning over a wide range of pulse signals. As a result, they are relatively insensitive to flow. Never assume that the presence of an oximeter wave form and measurement of arterial saturation represent adequate tissue blood flow. Lawson and colleagues[41] showed that the pulse oximeter readings were present and accurate even when the blood flow was only 8.6% of the control.

During anesthesia for neonates and infants, it is not uncommon to lose an adequate wave form if the oximeter probe is placed on a finger or toe. This may occur especially during hypotensive anesthesia or cardiopulmonary bypass. This problem is easily avoided by placing a neonatal oximeter probe on the fleshy part of the hypothenar eminence of the hand or the lateral aspect of the foot. Alternatively, a flexible probe can gently be applied to the earlobe or tip of the tongue or around the external and internal surfaces of the cheek.

Because the use of the pulse oximeter involves placing a light-emitting diode (LED) on the skin or muscle surface, there is always a risk of electrical shock or burn injury. Probes should not be interchanged among various makes of oximeters. Electrical burns, for example, can result from the exchange of incompatible oximeter probes. To save money many anesthesiologists reuse disposable probes. These probes must be checked carefully to insure that the LED is intact and that no contact between the patient and exposed wires can occur. All oximeters should be electrically isolated.

To use the information provided by pulse oximetry, the anesthesiologist should be aware of two facts. First, pulse oximeters measure oxygen saturation and not arterial oxygen pressure. Large changes in arterial oxygen pressure can occur without a change in the oxygen saturation. The oximeter will read 100% until the arterial oxygen pressure is less than 95 mm Hg, assuming normal oxygen hemoglobin curve position. It should be appreciated that all oximeters are accurate only between 70% and 100% oxygen saturation. Second, measurements are not in real time. In experimental subjects desaturation half-times were between 24 and 35 seconds. Resaturation half-times were between 19 and 30 seconds.[63]

Coté and coauthors[22] have shown the value of pulse oximeters in pediatric anesthesia. In one randomized study they found that major hypoxic events (arterial oxygen saturation less than 85% for 30 seconds or longer) occurred in 35 of 152 patients; the majority of patients with major hypoxic events were under 2 years of age. Hypoxic events were twice as common in children when oximetry was not available.

### Temperature monitoring

Human regulatory responses to thermal disturbances are determined by the central and skin temperatures.[61] Intraoperative thermoregulatory responses can be measured by a change in central body temperature. This method is necessary in infants and children both to detect hypothermia, which readily occurs during surgical procedures, especially those involving body cavities, and to detect malignant hyperthermia. Central temperature monitoring is preferable to other types to determine the degree of heat loss.[17,20]

Hypothermia during general anesthesia usually develops in two distinct phases. During the initial 45 minutes after the induction of anesthesia, vasodilation cools peripheral blood and central temperature decreases relatively rapidly, by about 0.5° C.[37] In addition to vasodilation there is constant heat loss to the environment and a small decrease in metabolic heat production.[68] This initial hypothermic phenomenon is known as internal temperature redistribution. Skin surface insulation alone seldom prevents this immediate post-induction hypothermia.

By definition a thermal steady state occurs when metabolic heart production equals heat loss to the environment. Most of the metabolic heat is lost through skin, and a small fraction is lost through respiration.[10] The mechanisms of heat loss are based on the physical principles of radiation, convection, evaporation, and conduction.

### Thermometers

Recorded temperatures may deviate from actual temperatures because the temperature of the probe differs from that of the surrounding tissue or the temperature recorded by the probe differs from the temperature.[11] All thermometers are reasonably accurate near 0° C; the difficulty is in choosing the suitable tissue to measure. Also, there are many styles of thermometers, such as mercury in glass, thermistors, thermocouples, infrared thermometers, temperature-sensitive liquid crystals, and so on. Thermocouples, which measure a temperature-dependent bimetal electric potential, are by far the most commonly used in anaesthesia practice. They are inexpensive and come in a wide range of designs for the tympanic membrane, the pulmonary artery, the esophagus, the rectum, and the bladder. Temperature-sensitive liquid crystals can be used for the skin surface. Although inexpensive and convenient, crystals do not have the range or accuracy necessary for clinical use.[42]

### Temperature in monitoring sites

The tympanum has been suggested as the ideal monitoring site in that it represents hypothalamic temperature. However, there is no physiologic evidence that hypothalamic temperature represents central temperature.[21] It is now known that the hypothalamus integrates input from the entire body and then determines thermoregulatory responses. Consequently the correct approach to temperature monitoring is to recognize that different tissues may have different temperatures and that the physiologic and practical significance of such differences varies.

Although this is arbitrary, it is useful to categorize temperature measurement sites as central or core, peripheral or skin (Fig. 8–1). In general, core tissues contribute 80% to 90% of the thermal input to the thermoregulatory system.

Axillary temperatures are very useful, but only when the thermometer is carefully placed over the artery and the arm is abducted. The axil was reported to be as accurate for measuring central temperatures as were the tympanic membranes, esophagus, and rectum.[47]

Nasopharyngeal temperature is measured by positioning the probe in the nasal pharynx posterior

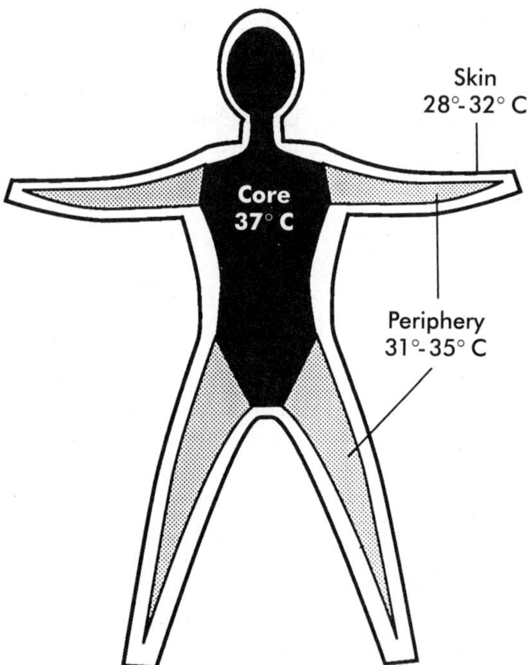


**Figure 8–1** Central compartment temperatures generally are higher than those of peripheral tissues. Vasodilation induced by anesthesia modifies the thermal balance between compartments. (From Bissonnette B: Temperature monitoring, *Int Anesthesiol Clin* 30[3]:67, 1992.)

to the soft palate. It should provide an estimate of the hypothalamic temperature. With the use of uncuffed endotracheal tubes in pediatric anaesthesia, however, this site is affected by leakage of air around the endotracheal tube and may yield inaccurate readings.

Esophageal temperature probes are usually incorporated into disposable esophageal stethoscopes. This system measures central temperature reliably when the probe is placed in the distal third of the esophagus at the point where maximum heart sounds are heard.[47] Infants and children have minimal thermal insulation between the tracheal bronchial tree and esophagus, so the effects of respiratory gas temperature on esophageal temperature may be pronounced.[47]

Traditionally, rectal probes have been used as a measure of core temperature despite problems such as insulation by feces, cool blood returning from the legs, and the influence of an open abdominal cavity. It has been shown that rectally measured temperature in infants and children is similar to that from other central temperature measurement sites.[47]

Bladder probes have been suggested as one of the most accurate means of measuring central temperature. It has been demonstrated that bladder temperature is identical to pulmonary artery temperature when urine flow is high.[35] It is not clinically useful in patients whose urine output is at or below normal levels.

Tympanic membrane and oral canal thermometers provide a reasonable approximation of central temperature. Early reports describe tympanic membrane perforation by these thermistors, but recently available probes are so soft and flexible that even vigorous insertion is unlikely to damage the ear.

Skin surface temperatures do not correlate well with central temperatures and therefore should not be considered a substitute for central temperature monitoring. In summary, the best single monitor of central temperature during pediatric anesthesia depends on the duration of the surgical procedure, the surgical site, the anesthesia technique, equipment, and cost. The most important factors are understanding the principles of temperature monitoring and being aware of the limitations of each site.

### Respiratory gas monitoring

The monitoring of carbon dioxide ($CO_2$) and other respiratory gases in pediatric patients was at first viewed skeptically because of limitations in obtaining accurate measurements.[60] In 1986 Swedlow[70] wrote that the anesthesiologist was unable to obtain good estimates of end tidal carbon dioxide values in very small infants and that the capnograph could be used only as a "monitor of cardiopulmonary and anaesthesia system integrity" in these patients. Fortunately, in the past 5 years, we have developed techniques that allow the accurate measurements of end tidal carbon dioxide tension and volatile agents in even the smallest patients. Capnometry is the measurement and numerical display of expired carbon dioxide, and capnography is the measurement and graphic display of expired carbon dioxide in real time. If the graphic display is calibrated, capnography includes capnometry. Therefore capnography is often used to indicate both capnography and capnometry. The use of capnometry without capnography may limit the clinician's diagnostic ability because capnography may be the only guide to the adequacy of gas sampling.

Respiratory gas for analysis may be aspirated from the airway or analyzed as it flows through a sensor in the breathing circuit. Gas can be measured from any location in the breathing circuit or tracheal tube. Respiratory gas may be measured by infrared analysis, mass spectrometry, acoustic spectroscopy, or Raman scattering.[50,72] In addition, if the capnometer is unavailable, gas for analysis of carbon dioxide in a blood-gas machine may be aspirated from the endotracheal tube using a needle and syringe during expiration while the fresh gas flow is discontinued.

In capnography, accuracy refers to the difference between the measured end tidal carbon dioxide values and alveolar end tidal values, which is essentially equivalent to arterial carbon dioxide pressure. Although a small physiologic difference may exist between the end tidal carbon dioxide tension and the arterial carbon dioxide pressure due to the effect of dead space ventilation, appropriately measured end tidal carbon dioxide tension approximates arterial carbon dioxide pressure in intubated children in the absence of significant lung disease or congenital cyanotic heart disease.[16] In the past accurate capnography was difficult in small infants ventilated through partial rebreathing circuits because the ratio of tidal volume to fresh gas flow was very small. As a result the exhaled gas was diluted, and the end tidal gas measurement was an underestimation of the true value. Recent advances such as proximal sampling have provided several methods to obtain accurate capnography in small infants.

Accurate capnography may be obtained with infrared analysis or mass spectrometry using proximal sampling in infants and children weighing more than 12 kg ventilated with a volume ventilator, in infants and children of all weights ventilated with a pediatric circle breathing system, and with a Bain circuit.[5]

A plateau on the capnographic wave form does

not always indicate that the end tidal carbon dioxide value reflects the arterial carbon dioxide pressure.[16] A flat plateau in the presence of a large arterial to end tidal difference may occur in patients with large dead space ventilation and in small infants when proximal sampling is used inappropriately.[4] When accurate sampling is available in anesthetized, intubated, ventilated healthy infants and children, the arterial to end tidal carbon dioxide pressure differences are small, negligible, or possibly of negative value.[4,5,72] These data suggest that dead space ventilation is minimal in these patients.

Some clinicians have suggested that capnography is accurate in the absence of a plateau phase. In one study distally sampled peak expired carbon dioxide pressure provided an estimate of arterial carbon dioxide pressure despite the lack of a plateau phase during expiration.[6] Peak expired carbon dioxide pressure was accurate in controlled and spontaneously ventilated critically ill neonates when the respiratory rate was less than 70 breaths per minute and when lung disease was not severe, that is, when expired oxygen (fractional inspired oxygen concentration) was less than 70%.[6] Other clinicians have reported anecdotally that peak expired carbon dioxide values may be low in rapidly and spontaneously ventilating infants and that peak expired carbon dioxide values increase markedly when carbon dioxide is manually compressed from the chest in these infants.

In infants and children with acyanotic heart disease, end tidal carbon dioxide pressure measurements are a reliable estimate of arterial carbon dioxide pressure.[16] However, in infants and children with cyanotic congenital heart disease, end tidal carbon dioxide pressure may not reliably estimate arterial carbon dioxide pressure.[16] In the latter group, both dead space ventilation and venous admixture ($\dot{Q}S/\dot{Q}T$) increase the difference between arterial and end tidal carbon dioxide pressure.[16] Increasing the $\dot{Q}S$ to $\dot{Q}T$ ratio increases the carbon dioxide pressure difference by shunting venous blood with a greater carbon dioxide pressure tension in the alveoli to the left side of the heart.

## INVASIVE MONITORING IN THE PEDIATRIC CARDIAC PATIENT

Invasive monitoring in anesthesia practice has become synonymous with the observation of cardiovascular variables. Medical and technical knowledge of invasive monitoring is rapidly expanding, with manufacturers being quick to correct equipment problems as they are identified for both commercial and legal reasons. This portion of the chapter describes the application of monitoring materials and techniques, including intraarterial monitoring, central venous pressure monitoring, pulmonary arterial catheter monitoring, transesophageal echocardiography, and transtracheal Doppler monitoring.

### Intraarterial monitoring

Direct monitoring of arterial blood pressure has been done for nearly three quarters of a century. Intraarterial monitoring became popular after advances in electronic and plastic technology in the 1950s. Today, new technology and the availability of high-quality narrow-gauge cannulas ensures that direct intraarterial monitoring is not only feasible but widely practiced in pediatric anesthesia.

***Indications.*** The indications for use of intraarterial pressure monitoring are primarily hemodynamic and pulmonary considerations. The individual patient's surgical factors and the risk to benefit ratio also play an important role in the decision to use this technique. The measured pressure is a function of blood volume, cardiac output, and peripheral vascular resistance.

Virtually all peripheral arteries have been used for direct monitoring; the most commonly used are the radial and femoral arteries.[29,32] Others include the ulnar, brachial, axillary, dorsalis pedis, posterior tibial, and superficial temporal vessels and the umbilical artery in newborns.[40,56]

***Material***

*Cannulas.* The size of the cannula is critical in pediatric patients, especially for the ease of insertion and withdrawal of samples, because of the risk of vessel thrombosis after removal of the cannula. A wide variety of cannula sizes are available. A 24-gauge cannula is recommended for infants weighing less than 3 kg. A 22-gauge catheter is usually appropriate for infants weighing 3 to 10 kg, and in all other cases a 20-gauge cannula is used. The shorter (3.2 cm) cannulas are suitable primarily for younger patients. The small-gauge nontapered nonpyrogenic (Teflon) cannulas are less thrombogenic than the polypropylene type, but those made of polyurethane are less rigid and potentially less traumatic.[8]

*Pressure transducers.* The fluid recommended for maintenance of arterial line patency is a solution of heparinized normal saline (1 USP unit/ml at 1 to 3 ml/hr).[52] Its use is not associated with an increase in the risk of hypernatremia, and it has the advantage over heparinized 5% dextrose solution that it permits access for blood-glucose measurement without confounding the result. Many commercial transducer sets incorporate an automatic pressurized continuous infusion and flush system.

Small dead-space stiff tubing should connect the arterial cannula to a strain gauge. The response time of the intravascular cannula, connecting tubing, and strain gauge must be rapid enough to allow accurate pressure wave transmissions at high heart rates. Ideally the internal volume of the tubing should be small (less than 0.5 ml) because it is thought that three times the volume of the line, catheter, and stopcock should be removed and discarded before the blood sample will accurately reflect the arterial pH, electrolytes, and blood gases.[14]

The accuracy and dynamic response of the newer disposable saline-filled transducer-tubing systems vary among manufacturers. There can be dramatic changes in dynamic response, depending on the length of tubing between the transducer and patient and the presence or absence of air bubbles in the system. Relatively long tubing or air bubbles can cause systolic overshoots or dampening of the arterial trace, but the extent of the alteration varies among manufacturers.

By convention the reference point of the transducer is at the level of the right atrium. However, the positioning of the transducer (zero, or reference point) should be at the most critical level in relation to perfusion—that is, at the level of the heart (mid axillary line) for the patient in a supine position or at the level of the brain (outer canthus of the eye) in neurosurgical procedures or in the head-up position.

***Insertion methods.*** The insertion technique is best determined by the skill and experience of the anesthesiologist. Percutaneous placement can be accomplished in several ways (Fig. 8–2). The most common is direct arterial puncture with the catheter

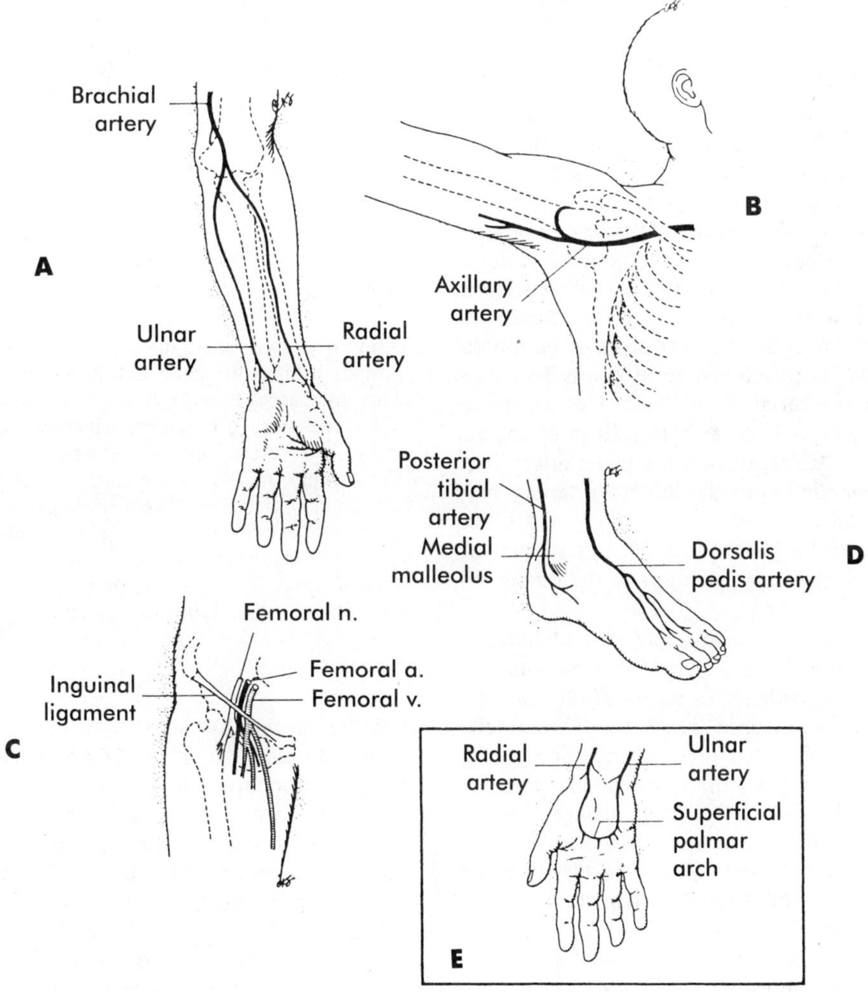


**Figure 8–2** Anatomic landmarks for sites commonly used for artery cannulation. **A,** Arterial suply of the arm and hand. **B,** Axillary artery. **C,** Femoral artery. **D,** Arterial supply of the foot. **E,** Arterial supply of the wrist and palm. (From Cohen NH, Brett CM: Arterial catheterization. In Benumof JL, editor: *Clinical procedures in anesthesiology and intensive care,* Philadelphia, 1992, Lippincott.

fed over the needle. In preparation for insertion the limbs should be immobilized, either manually by an assistant or by taping the limbs securely to a board. However, the Seldinger technique modified for small infants uses a 23-gauge butterfly needle from which the tubing has been removed and replaced by a 15-cm straight angiographic wire 0.4 mm in outer diameter.[62] The artery is punctured and the wire advanced; the needle is then removed and the cannula threaded over the wire and secured.

A surgical down cut may be preferred in patients in whom percutaneous placement is likely to be difficult or has failed previously. The incidence of vessel thrombosis is higher with the surgical down cut.[46] In difficult cases a Doppler flow transducer is occasionally useful for locating a pulsating artery that is hard to feel. In preterm and newborn infants the use of a cold (fiberoptic) light source shown through the wrist from below makes it possible to visualize the artery as it pulsates in the wrist.[54] This technique is most useful for inserting catheters in the radial, ulnar, and posterior tibial arteries.

Before insertion is attempted, an Allen's test for collateral circulation through the arteries at the wrist is recommended.[3] Other methods of assessing collateral circulation are available (e.g., finger plethysmography).[13] It may be difficult to perform an Allen's test on a very young or uncooperative patient. Percutaneous catheterization of peripheral arteries in the newborn can be difficult. To obtain access to the arterial circulation, a down cut is sometimes required for catheterization of the radial, posterior tibial, or dorsalis pedis artery. Remember, cannulation of the left radial artery may give preductal or postductal pressures and blood gases because the position of the left subclavian artery is variable to the position of the ductus arteriosus.

When access to the central arterial circulation is required, umbilical artery catheterization is usually performed. The catheter is inserted into the umbilical artery under sterile conditions. The catheter can usually be inserted directly into one of the umbilical arteries, particularly if cannulation is attempted shortly after birth.[71] If the catheter cannot be inserted directly, a down cut may be necessary. Most complications from umbilical artery lines are vascular because of thrombus formation, embolism, or trauma. The catheter will usually pass into the descending aorta but can migrate to other locations such as the renal arteries or celiac trunk. Many experts recommend placing the catheter in the lower aorta (T10), but there is still major disagreement about the ideal positioning of the tip of the umbilical artery catheter (Figs. 8–3 and 8–4). No matter where it is placed, the catheter position must be verified by radiographs. The more severe complications such as renal hypertension, necrotizing enterocolitis, and paraplegia are uncommon but tend to occur with the catheter in a high position at the midthoracic area. Less severe complications, which are more common, occur when the catheter is in the lower aorta (vascular spasm with reversible ischemia to the legs).[48] An indwelling cannula in the peripheral artery is often safer, and an umbilical arterial catheter should be removed as soon as possible or at the first sign of a complication.

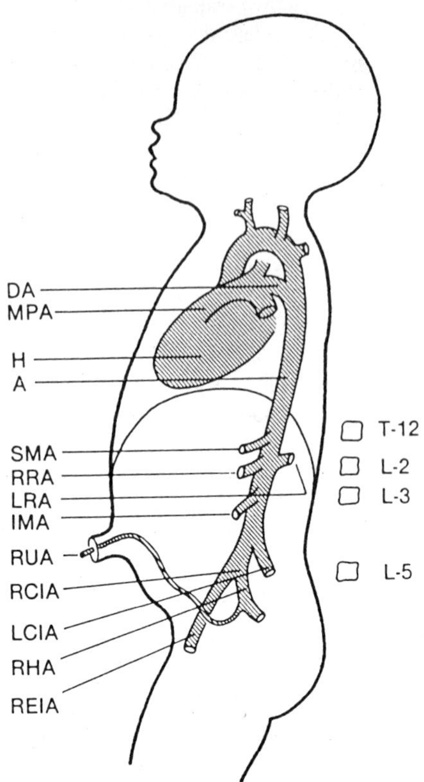


**Figure 8–3** Diagram of the newborn arterial system and its relationship to the spine. *DA,* ductus arteriosus; *MPA,* main pulmonary artery; *H,* heart; *A,* aorta; *SMA,* superior mesenteric artery; *RRA,* right renal artery; *LRA,* left renal artery; *IMA,* inferior mesenteric artery; *RUA,* right umbilical artery; *RCIA,* right common iliac artery; *LCIA,* left common iliac artery; *RHA,* right hypogastric artery; *REIA,* right external iliac artery. (From Cohen NH, Brett CM: Arterial catheterization. In Benumof JL, editor: *Clinical procedures in anesthesiology and intensive care,* Philadelphia, 1992, Lippincott.

### Central venous pressure monitoring

Although central venous cannulation was first described in 1733 by Steven Hales (as cited by Kalso),

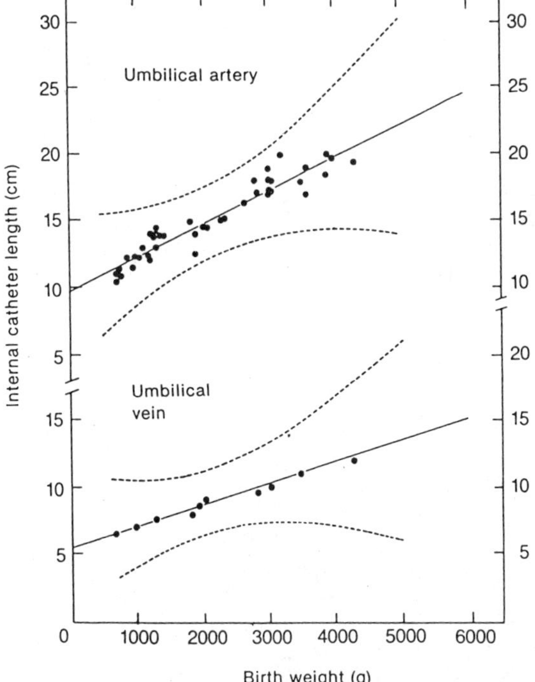


**Figure 8–4** Estimates of insertional length of umbilical catheters (umbilical artery catheter tip inserted between T-6 and T-10; umbilical vein catheter tip inserted above diaphragm in inferior vena cava near or in right atrium) based on birth weight *(BW)* (95% confidence intervals). Modified estimating equations using MW are as follows: umbilical artery length = 2.5 × BW + 5.6 (bottom), where BW is measured in kilograms and length in centimeters. (From Cohen NH, Brett CM: Arterial Catheterization. In Benumof JL, editor: *Clinical procedures in anesthesiology and intensive care,* Philadelphia, 1992, Lippincott.

it was not until the 1960s that the technique became popular for medical purposes.[38] Initially the femoral, antecubital, and external jugular venous routes to the central circulation were used. Today proximal routes such as the internal jugular and subclavian veins are the preferred sites in infants and children.

Central venous pressure is the venous blood pressure measured at the junction of the vena cava and the right atrium. Measurements are used to assess the status of the circulating blood volume and right atrial (RA) preload as well as the function of the right ventricle. The recorded value for CVP is usually quoted as a single mean figure at the end of expiration. As with adults, the trend is often more useful in the therapeutic management of children than is an absolute figure. It can be influenced by respiratory factors such as spontaneous or controlled ventilation, crying, position of the patient, and errors in the interpretation of the electrical signal.

The normal values for central venous pressure vary with age. A range of 5 to 10 cm $H_2O$ is acceptable for most healthy infants and young children. A truly high RA pressure (above 15 cm $H_2O$) may represent a relative volume overload, loss of RV function, or cardiac tamponade. Patients with right-sided obstructing lesions such as tetralogy of Fallot, pulmonic stenosis, or tricuspid atresia will have high RA pressures before correction.

***Site of insertion.*** Every insertion site that has been used in the adult has been used in the pediatric patient. The final choice of site depends on the indication for use of the central venous line and the skill of the operator.

Commonly, access to the central circulation is gained through the internal jugular (high, low, or posterior approach), external jugular, subclavian, femoral, basilic or axillary veins.[31,34] In newborns access may be gained through the umbilical vein. The placement during open cardiac surgery, of transthoracic intercardiac monitoring that lies directly in the right or left atrium has been described.[30] The final choice of site must take into consideration the degree of difficulty of insertion, the immediate risk of insertion, and the long-term complication rate. The comfort of the patient may also be an important factor.

***Insertion methods.*** The most common method used for successful placement of the CVP is the Seldinger technique, which can be used for insertion of single, double, and triple lumen catheters.[62] The use of real-time two-dimensional ultrasound to facilitate location of the internal jugular, subclavian, and femoral veins has been reported.[44] With this technique successful cannulation occurs more frequently with fewer needle thrusts and thus less risk of complications.

Identification of anatomic landmarks is necessary (Figs. 8–5 and 8–6). Infiltration of skin with local anesthetic is required in the awake child. A small sleeker needle (21 to 23 gauge) is used to identify the appropriate vessel. Correct needle placement is identified by the slight pop often felt as the vein is entered and is confirmed by aspiration of venous blood. Once the vein's position has been ascertained, either by blood aspiration or CVP transducer tracing, a larger introductory needle for the Seldinger guide wire is used. The guide wire and vein dilatator permit the insertion of a cannula of a suitable size, be it a large single-bore cannula, a double or triple lumen catheter, or a pulmonary artery catheter.

***Materials.*** Numerous types of CVP lines are available. The catheters vary in size, length, ratio

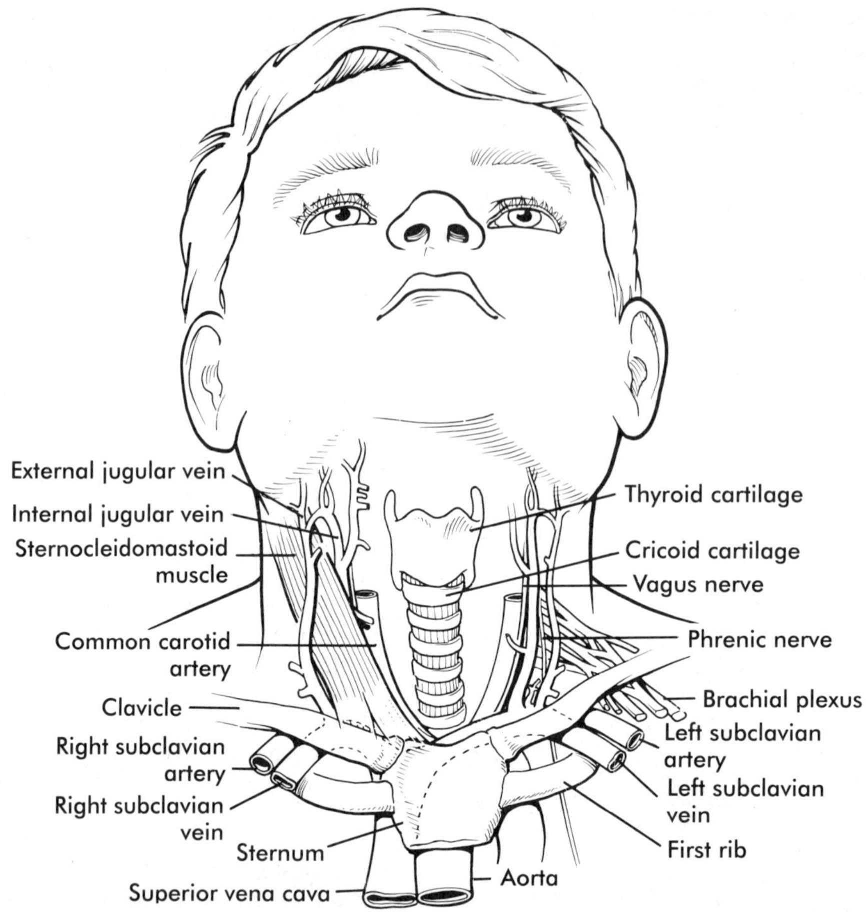


**Figure 8–5** The anatomy of the jugular and subclavian veins. (From: Mihm FG, Rosenthal MH: Central venous catheterization. In Benumof JL, editor: *Clinical procedures in anesthesiology and intensive care,* Philadelphia, 1992, Lippincott.)

of internal to external diameter, material composition, stiffness, and number of lumens. Selection is made on the basis of size and weight of the patient and the purpose of the catheter. The advantages and disadvantages of Teflon, polypropylene, and polyurethane catheters have been discussed in the section on Arterial Cannulas. Silicon rubber (Silastic) catheters are the least rigid available, and because of their lack of rigidity, they are the most difficult to insert and require special insertion sheaths. Most manufacturers provide heparin-bonded catheters and wires to reduce the incidence of thrombotic complications related to the catheter and its insertion.

***Fixation.*** Any of the numerous methods that prevent dislodgement of the CVP line is acceptable. Fixation can be achieved with tape or suture and a sterile dressing.

***Complications.*** Complications may be related to the placement or location of the CVP line (Fig. 8–7). Pneumothorax is perhaps the most severe complication, but there are many other complications to be considered. A recent study of neonates undergoing surgery reported a complication rate of 34%.[59] Sepsis, a particular problem, comprised almost 11% of the total complications. Infection rates were directly related to duration of catheter placement and inversely related to care given to the insertion site. Catheter-related colonization is frequent but may not lead directly to sepsis. However, its occurrence has been implicated as a causal factor.

In the small child fluid overload from repeated measurement with a fluid-filled column manometer or by continuous infusion through a constant flushing system is possible.

Malposition of the catheter can occur, especially in a peripheral site of insertion. The tip of the catheter may pass up into a neck vein from the subclavian route, antecubital fossa, or the femoral

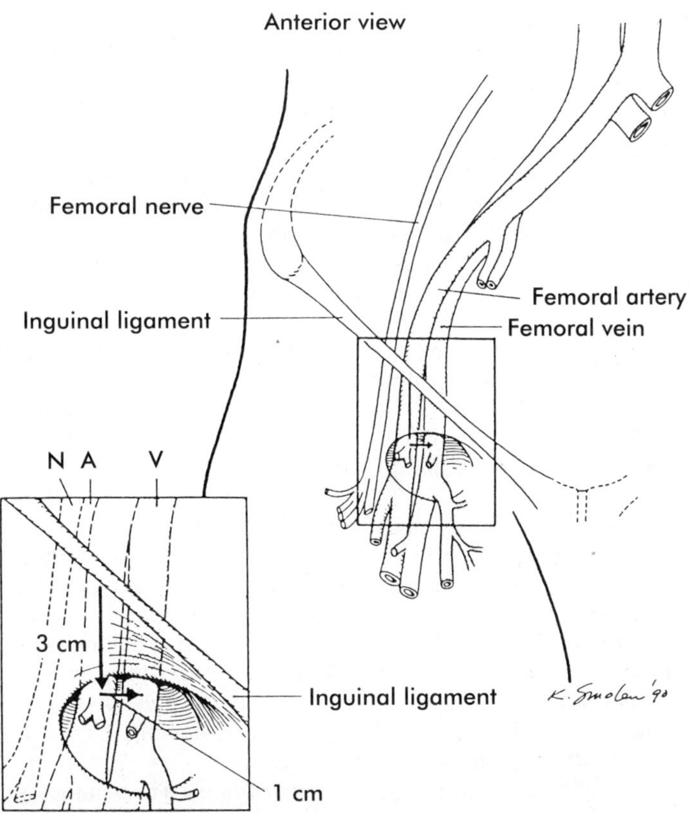


**Figure 8–6** Femoral vein catheterization. The leg should be positioned in external rotation and 30-degree abduction. The skin is entered at a 45-degree angle 3 cm below the inguinal ligament and 1cm medial to the maximal femoral artery pulsation. (From Mihm FG, Rosenthal MH: Central venous catheterization. In Benumof JL, editor: *Clinical procedures in anesthesiology and intensive care,* Philadelphia, 1992, Lippincott.)

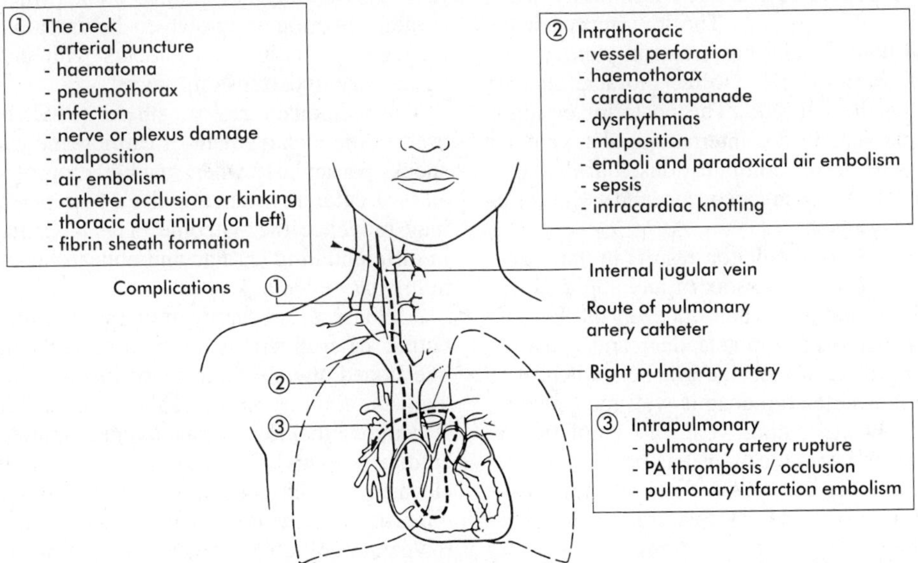


**Figure 8–7** Summary of complications associated with the insertion and use of central venous cannulas and pulmonary artery catheters. (From Miller CL et al: Invasive monitoring in the pediatric patient, *Int Anesthesiol Clin* 30[3]:99, 1992.)

vein (through the heart). A chest radiograph taken after insertion confirms position of the tip of the catheter and rules out pneumothorax.

The tip of a malpositioned catheter may rest against the endocardium and in time cause it to erode and perforate. Similarly, during insertion, perforation of the heart may lead to hemothorax and even cardiac tamponade. Dysrhythmias can arise from the passage of the wire or later from the catheter migrating through the tricuspid valve, which can irritate the myocardium and the conduction system. Microshock is also a recognized complication of the placement of an electrically conducted path directly into the heart.

Air embolism is a risk from insertion of a CVP line, especially in the patient who is breathing spontaneously, because of negative pressure in the thorax during inspiration. This risk can be obviated by the use of the Trendelenburg position and reduced by the use of positive pressure ventilation during insertion. Paradoxical air embolism is a real risk in children, particularly with right to left intracardiac shunt or with a patent foramen ovale if right arterial pressure exceeds left atrial pressure.

The following thrombotic complications have all been reported: deep vein thrombosis, thromboembolism, and dislodgement of neural thrombus and fibrin clot during guide wire placement of an indwelling CVP line.[36] Catheter occlusion, kinking, leaking, or thrombosis may require early removal of the catheter, all of which may be prevented by careful management of the line.

Injury to a nerve plexus in the vicinity of the catheter insertion is most likely to occur if the operator is inexperienced and lacks familiarity with the anatomy of the region. The low approach to the internal jugular vein may result in puncture of the carotid artery or injury to the thoracic duct if attempted on the left side. The posterior or high cervical approach to the internal jugular vein is associated with fewer complications, but damage to the sympathetic chain can occur, and a Horner's syndrome may result.

Subclavian vein cannulation results in the highest incidence of pneumothorax of any approach to the central circulation. When done on the left, it may also damage the thoracic duct and cause a chylothorax. Puncture of the trachea when the guide wire is inserted too deep is well recognized. With the use of the femoral vein for cannulation a rise in associated complications has been reported: 16% for thrombosis, 2% for emboli, 4% for phlebitis, 3% for sepsis, and 4% for direct or indirect cause of death.[15]

The umbilical vein has frequently been used as a site for intraoperative blood sampling and pressure monitoring in the newborn. Its use beyond the immediate newborn period is uncommon and will not be discussed here.

**Pulmonary artery pressure monitoring**

Pulmonary artery catheterization has been done for many years, but it was not until 1970, when Swan and colleagues[69] described the technique of placing a small balloon at the tip of the catheter to facilitate its positioning in the pulmonary artery tree that the procedure gained acceptance. It has provided an opportunity to quantify, monitor, and modify the hemodynamic status of the patient during therapeutic maneuvers.

The flow-directed pulmonary catheter is used in many different clinical situations because of advances in technology that allow the addition of thermistors, oximeters, and pacemakers. The application of these techniques in the treatment of children is much debated; their use depends on the clinical situation. In patients undergoing cardiac surgery, measurement errors are introduced by the complexities of shunting and anatomy, and the risks of improper placement are increased. Thus, the pediatric population is more commonly monitored using directly placed right and left atrial catheters.

***Indications.*** The pulmonary artery catheter may be indicated in the presence or anticipation of left ventricular dysfunction, but even then it has only limited pediatric application. In the pediatric cardiac patient these techniques are used to monitor pulmonary artery pressure. They are used in cardiac surgery for the manipulation of preload and afterload, with fluids or pharmacologic agents, and for the assessment of cardiac output when global cardiac function is known to be impaired. They may also be helpful in patients with underlying pulmonary hypertension.

The pulmonary artery catheter (PAC) has been used in the management of cardiogenic and septic shock, particularly when manipulation of stomach and vascular resistance and cardiac performance may influence the outcome. The PAC may assist in differentiating cardiac and noncardiac causes of pulmonary edema.

Although the accuracy of thermodilution cardiac output determinations in small infants has been questioned, there is value in the mixed venous oxygen saturation as an indicator of global perfusion. It is known that low arterial oxygen saturation, low cardiac output, low hemoglobin concentration, or elevated oxygen consumption will result in a decline in mixed venous oxygen saturation. Venous oxygen saturation can be measured by withdrawing a blood sample through the PAC distal port. Data must be interpreted in relation to the position of the hemoglobin-oxygen association curve as indicated by pH, carbon dioxide pressure, body temperature, and erythrocyte diphosphoglycerate concentration.

The normal venous oxygen saturation is 75%; a decrease of 5% to 10% is considered significant. Changes in saturation usually precede alterations and hemodynamic variables by a considerable time and so may well be a useful adjunct.

***Contraindications.*** Insertion of a pulmonary artery catheter is associated with a high risk of complications that can be fatal. Benefits must therefore be weighed against the risks. Contraindications may be absolute or relative and commonly must be interpreted in light of the clinical situation. An intracardiac or extracardiac defect may result in an aberrant catheter course, incorrect interpretation of the data, or an increased risk of systemic emboli.

The presence of coagulopathy or severe thrombocytopenia is only a relative contraindication; in these situations the use of a peripheral insertion site may be possible. Sepsis or broken skin at the site of insertion, however, is a more serious contraindication.

Dysrhythmias caused by the passage of the catheter through the heart may compromise the patient's condition. Children with preexisting conduction defects, for example a left bundle-branch block, may develop a complete heart block.

***Sites of insertion.*** The most commonly used sites for insertion of the pulmonary artery catheters are those used for central venous access, namely the internal jugular vein, the subclavian vein, and femoral or basilic vein for peripheral vein insertion. The internal jugular and femoral vein are used most commonly. Experience with a small child (less than 15 kg) shows that insertion of the sheath into the femoral vein is technically easier. Multilumen catheters capable of thermodilution come in two sizes, 5 and 7 French, with four options for intraluminal distance between the right atrium and pulmonary artery. Catheter recommendations are based on age. Double-lumen balloon-tipped catheters without a thermistor probe are available in 4 French (Table 8–3).

***Insertion methods.*** Insertion of a PAC is similar to that of a standard central venous catheter except that the PAC requires a large port of entry into the central vein, and dilation of the vein is often necessary.[55]

There are two methods of establishing placement of the catheter in the pulmonary vascular tree. The most common method is use of the pressure transducer to display wave forms, as is often done in adult practice. The distal lumen of the catheter should be connected to the pressure monitoring device, which displays the wave form continuously so that when the tip of the catheter is distal to the

**Table 8–3** Guidelines for the selection of correct pulmonary artery catheter size in pediatric patients

| Age (yrs) | Size (French) | CVP-PA port distance (cm) |
|---|---|---|
| Newborn-3 | 5 | 10 |
| 3-8 | 5 | 15 |
| 8-14 | 7 | 20 |
| >14 | 7 | 30 |

From Blitt CD: *Monitoring in anesthesia: critical care medicine*, ed 2, New York, 1990, Churchill Livingstone.

sheath, it will display the characteristic wave forms of the vessels and cardiac chambers through which it passes. When the child is small (less than 15 kg) or cardiac output is low, the use of fluoroscopy may be preferred.

A chest radiograph should be performed after every insertion to check the placement of the catheter and to exclude pneumothorax.

***Complications.*** Complications associated with pulmonary artery monitoring are numerous. Endocarditis, valve damage, and balloon rupture may be more specific to PAC; intercardiac tangles and knots have also been reported. Complications more common in children include misleading information, paradoxical systemic emboli, disruption of an intracardiac repair, and high-grade ventricular outflow tract obstruction due to the relatively large balloon diameter.[5]

## Transesophageal echocardiography

Transesophageal echocardiography (TEE) is a semiinvasive procedure used for both diagnosing and monitoring the cardiovascular system in anesthetized patients. A full discussion of TEE is beyond the scope of this chapter; interested readers may consult other sources.[24] First introduced for clinical use in 1976, the technology is now capable of producing M-mode, two-dimensional, and Doppler color-flow imaging; post-Doppler ultrasound; and continuous wave–mode Doppler ultrasound.[26]

TEE equipment design is based on the concept of the flexible gastroscope with a transducer monitor at the tip. The direction of the ultrasound beam may be manipulated by the TEE controls, as with the gastroscope.

It has been found that the biplane adult size probe is suitable for children who weigh more than 10 kg. The pediatric version is smaller, which allows its routine use in patients weighing as little as 2 kg. The technology necessary to produce these small probes allows only single-plane TEE with slightly decreased image resolution.[58]

TEE imaging permits continuous assessment of ventricular function through the short access view. With alteration of the direction of the ultrasound beam, it can provide superior views of the mitral valve and mitral valve function to those of other approaches.

Pediatric TEE facilitates intraoperative imaging of congenital cardiac malformations not visualized by standard transthoracic examinations and allows assessment of the adequacy of surgical intervention in newborns and small infants.

***Indications.*** Indications for the use of TEE in the operating room include evaluation of left ventricular function and regional wall motion (not restricted to cardiac patients), assessment of the adequacy of valve repair or replacement, examination for the presence of arterial thrombus or intracardiac air, examination for or evaluation of aortic dissection, and evaluation of intracardiac shunts and residual flow obstruction.[19] TEE monitoring can be used to provide continuous or intermittent intraoperative assessment of cardiac function and assess both the morphologic and functional state of the myocardium in children experiencing unexplained hemodynamic instability during surgery, whether or not they are cardiac patients.[57]

***Contraindications.*** Contraindications for TEE relate primarily to the size of the transducer probe relative to the size of the patient's esophagus. Such contraindications include unavailability of an appropriate size transducer probe and esophageal abnormalities such as strictures, fistulae, varices, and recent suture lines that may be disrupted by passage of the TEE probe. Whether the anesthesiologist or the cardiologist should be responsible for reading TEE images remains controversial. Because the cardiologist cannot be expected to remain in the operating room continuously, it is useful for the anesthesiologist to understand the cardiac imaging. Indeed, anesthesiologists frequently can make use of TEE for assessing cardiac function, and although a reasonable level of confidence in the use of the technique is mandatory for anesthesiologists, an on-call arrangement should be made with the cardiologist, for at times anatomic diagnoses or surgical decisions must be based on echocardiographic findings.

The disadvantages of using TEE on children are associated with the use of the smaller TEE probe necessary for patients weighing less than 10 kg and the resulting decreased image resolution. Esophageal probes are less maneuverable in small patients and therefore less capable of imaging certain aspects of the cardiac anatomy.[12]

The advantage of TEE is that superior views of certain cardiac structures are obtainable. The only limitation is that viewing the left pulmonary artery and the left ventricular outflow track from the esophagus may be difficult.[33]

### Transtracheal Doppler probe

Transtracheal Doppler sonography is designed to give continuous readings of ascending aortic blood flow and by extension cardiac output.[1] The ultrasound transducer is located at the tip of an endotracheal tube, and with the use of a special cuff it causes the probe to be held against the entry wall of the trachea. Transtracheal Doppler sonography was developed to overcome some of the problems associated with other probe locations, such as those encountered with transesophageal and standard transthoracic echocardiography.

Initial evaluation of the use of transtracheal Doppler sonography in adults showed good correlation of cardiac output measurement with standard thermodilution techniques,[1,2] but other studies have not confirmed these findings.[28,64] Experience with the probe in the pediatric population is limited, but miniature devices are becoming available. The disadvantages of transtracheal Doppler probe include its restriction to intubated patients and the fact that movement of the tube within the trachea coupled with the high angle of incidence of beam to aortic blood flow introduces air to the assessment of cardiac output.

The role of invasive monitoring techniques for the use of pediatric anesthesia is expanding. The skill and experience of the anesthesiologist in both insertion techniques and the interpretation of the data must be kept in mind when a particular monitor is selected. The complications and risk for the patient should be assessed on an individual basis, often in terms of the risk to benefit ratio.

## REFERENCES


1. Abrams JH, Weber RE, Holman KD: Transtracheal Doppler: a new procedure for continuous cardiac output measurement, *Anesthesiology* 70:134, 1989.
2. Abrams JH, Weber RE, Holman KD: Continuous cardiac output determination using transtracheal Doppler: initial results in humans, *Anesthesiology* 71:11, 1989.
3. Allen EV: Thromboangitis obliterans: methods of diagnosis of chronic occlusive arterial lesions distal to wrist with illustrative cases, *Am J Med Sci* 178:237, 1929.
4. Bagwell JM, McLeod ME, Lerman J et al: End-tidal $P_{CO_2}$ measurements sampled at the distal and proximal ends of the endotracheal tube in infants and children, *Anesth Analg* 66:959, 1987.
5. Bagwell JM, Heavner JE, May WS et al: End-tidal $CO_2$ monitoring in infants and children ventilated with either a rebreathing or non-rebreathing circuit, *Anesthesiology* 66:405, 1987.
6. Bagwell JM, Heavner JE: End-tidal carbon dioxide pres-

sure in neonates and infants measured by aspiration and flow-through capnography, *J Clin Monit* 7:285, 1991.

7. Baker MD, Marsels MJ, Marks KH: Indirect BP monitoring in the newborn: evaluation of a new oscillometer and comparison of upper and lower limits measurements, *Am J Dis Child* 138:775, 1984.
8. Bedford RF: Percutaneous radial-artery cannulation: increased safety using Teflon catheters, *Anesthesiology* 42:219, 1975.
9. Bell C, Rimar S, Barash P: Intraoperative ST segment changes with myocardial ischemia in the neonate: a report of three cases, *Anesthesiology* 71:601, 1989.
10. Bickler PE, Sessler DI: Efficiency of airway heat and moisture exchanges in anesthetized humans, *Anesth Analg* 71:415, 1990.
11. Bissonette B, Sessler DI: The thermoregulatory threshold in infants and children anesthetized with Isoflurane and caudal Bupivacaine, *Anesthesiology* 73:1114, 1990.
12. Bolger A, Czer L, Freidman A et al: Intraoperative transesophageal color Doppler imaging: advantages and limitations *J Am Coll Cardiol* 11:217, 1988, (abstract).
13. Brodsky JB: A simple method to determine patency of the ulnar artery intraoperatively prior to radial-artery cannulation, *Anesthesiology* 42:626, 1975.
14. Brown DR, Fenton LJ, Tsang RC: Blood sampling through umbilical catheters, *Pediatrics* 55:257, 1975.
15. Burri C, Ahnefeld FW: *Cava-Katheter.* Berlin, 1977, Springer.
16. Burrows FA: Physiologic dead space, venous admixture, and the arterial to end-tidal carbon dioxide difference in infants and children undergoing cardiac surgery, *Anesthesiology* 70:219, 1989.
17. Burton AC: Human calorimetry: the average temperature of the tissues of the body. *J Nutr* 9:261, 1935.
18. Chia F, Ang AT, Wong T: Reliability of the Dinamap noninvasive monitor in the measurement of blood pressure of ill Asian newborns, *Clin Pediatr* 29:262, 1990.
19. Clements FM: The evolution of the anesthesiologist-echocardiographer. In de Bruijn NP, Clements FM, editors: *Intraoperative use of echocardiography,* Philadelphia, 1991, Lippincott.
20. Colin J, Timbal J, Houdas Y et al: Consumption of mean body temperature from rectal and skin temperature. *J Appl Physiol* 31:484, 1971.
21. Cork RC, Vaughn RW, Humphrey LS: Precision and accuracy of intraoperative temperature monitoring, *Anesth Analg* 62:211, 1983.
22. Coté CJ, Goldstein EA, Coté MA et al: A single blind study of pulse oximetry in children. *Anesthesiology* 68:184, 1988.
23. Cushing H: Some principles of cerebral surgery, *JAMA* 52:186, 1909.
24. DeBruijn NP, Clements FM, editors: *Intraoperative use of echocardiography,* Philadelphia, 1991, Lippincott.
25. Diprose GK, Evens DH, Archer LN: Dinamap fails to detect hypotension in very low birth weight infants, *Arch Dis Child* 61:771, 1986.
26. Frazin L, Talano JV, Stephanides L et al: Esophageal echocardiography, *Circulation* 54:102, 1976.
27. Friesen RH, Lichtor JL: Indirect measurement of blood pressure in neonates and infants utilizing an automatic noninvasive oscillometric monitor, *Anesth Analg* 60:742, 1981.
28. Froese N, Friesen R: Measurement techniques: measurement of cardiac output—transtracheal Doppler versus thermodilution, *Can J Anaesth* 38:931, 1991.
29. Glenski JA, Beynen FM, Brady J: A prospective evaluation of femoral artery monitoring in pediatric patients, *Anesthesiology* 66:227, 1987.
30. Gold JP, Jonas RA, Lang P et al: Transthoracic intracardiac monitoring lines in pediatric surgical patients: a 10-year experience, *Ann Thorac Surg* 42:185, 1986.
31. Gouin F, Martin C, Saux P: Central venous and pulmonary artery catheterizations via the axillary vein, *Acta Anaesthesiol Scand* 29(suppl 81):27, 1985.
32. Graves PW, Davis AL, Maggi JC et al: Femoral artery cannulation for monitoring in critically ill children: prospective study, *Crit Care Med* 18:1363, 1990.
33. Greeley WJ, Ungerleider RM: Echocardiography during surgery for congenital heart disease. In de Bruijn NP, Clements FM, editors: *Intraoperative use of echocardiography,* Philadelphia, 1991, Lippincott.
34. Hermosura B, Vangas L, Dickey MW: Measurement of pressure during intravenous therapy (letter). *JAMA* 195:321, 1966.
35. Horrow JC, Rosenberg H: Does urinary catheter reflect core temperature during cardiac surgery? *Anesthesiology* 69:986, 1988.
36. Hoshal VL, Ause RG, Hoskins PA: Fibrin sleeve formation on indwelling subclavian central venous catheters, *Arch Surg* 102:353, 1971.
37. Hynson JM, Sessler DI: Comparison of intraoperative warming devices, *Anesth Analg* 72:S118, 1991.
38. Kalso E: A short history of central venous catheterization, *Acta Anaesthesiol Scand* 29(suppl 81):7, 1985.
39. Kimble KJ, Darnall RA, Yelderman M: An automated oscillometric technique for estimating mean arterial pressure in critically ill newborns, *Anesthesiology* 54:423, 1981.
40. Lawless S, Orr R: Axillary arterial monitoring of pediatric patients. *Pediatrics* 84:273, 1989.
41. Lawson D, Norley F, Karban G et al: Blood flow limits and pulse oximeter signal detection, *Anesthesiology* 67:599, 1987.
42. Leon JE, Bissonette B, Lermen J: Does liquid crystalline temperature monitoring estimate core temperature in anesthetized children? *Anesthesiology* 73:A419, 1990.
43. Liebman J: The normal electrocardiogram. In Liebman J, Plonsey R, Gilette PC, editors: *Pediatric electrocardiography,* Baltimore, 1982, Williams & Wilkins.
44. Mallory DL, McGee WT, Shawker TH et al: Ultrasound guidance improves the success rate of internal jugular vein cannulation: a prospective randomized trial. *Chest* 98:157, 1990.
45. Millikan GA: The oximeter, an instrument for measuring continuously the oxygen saturation of arterial blood in man, *Rev Scient Instruments* 13:434, 1942.
46. Miyasaka K, Edmonds JF, Conn AW: Complications of radial artery lines in the paediatric patient, *Can Anaesth Soc J* 23:9, 1976.
47. Moayeri A, Hynson JM, Sessler DI et al: Preinduction skin surface warming prevents redistribution hypothermia, *Anesthesiology* 75:A1004, 1991.
48. Mokrohisky ST, Levine RL, Blumhagen JD et al: Low positioning of umbilical-artery catheters increases associated complications in newborn infants, *N Engl J Med* 299:561, 1984.
49. Nakajima S, Hisa Y, Takase H et al: New pulsed-type earpiece oximeter, *Kokyu To Junkan* 23:41, 1975.
50. Neilsen J, Kahn T, Moller JT: Evaluation of the newly developed anesthetic agent monitors: Bruel and Kjaer anesthetic agent monitor 1304 and Dutex Ultima. *Anesthesiology* 73:A538, 1990.
51. Nicolai L, Uber Sichthormachung: Verlauf und cherusche knetik der Oxyhemoglobin Reduktion in lebender Gewebe, besonders in der merschlicher Haut. *Flugers Arch Gesante Physiol* 229:372, 1932.
52. Pais-Bahrami K, Karna P, Dolanski EA: Effect of fluids on life span of peripheral arterial lines, *Am J Perinatol* 7:122, 1990.

53. Park MK, Kawabori I: Need for an improved standard for blood pressure cuff size, *Clin Pediatr* 15:784, 1976.
54. Pearse PG: Percutaneous catheterization of the radial artery in newborn babies using transillumination, *Arch Dis Child* 53:549, 1978.
55. Pierce T, Woodcock T: How to insert a pulmonary arterial flotation catheter, *Br J Hosp Med* 42:484, 1989.
56. Prian GW, Wright GB, Rumack CM et al: Apparent cerebral embolization after temporal artery catheterization, *J Pediatr* 93:115, 1978.
57. Ritter S, Hillel Z, Narang J et al: Transesophageal real time Doppler flow imaging in congenital heart disease: experience with a new pediatric transducer probe, *Diagnostic Cardiovascular Imaging* 2:92, 1989.
58. Ritter SB, Thys SM: Pediatric transesophageal color flow imaging: smaller probes for smaller hearts, *Echocardiography* 6:431, 1989.
59. Roberts JP, Gollow IJ: Central venous catheters in surgical neonates. *J Pediatr Surg* 25:632, 1990.
60. Sasse FJ: Can we trust end tidal carbon dioxide measurements in infants? *J Clin Monit* 1:147, 1985.
61. Satinoff E: Neuronal organization and evaluation of thermal regulation in mammals, *Science* 201:16, 1978.
62. Seldinger SI: Catheter replacement of the needle in percutaneous arteriography, *Acta Radiol Diagnosis* 39:368, 1953.
63. Severinghaus JW, Naifeh KH: Accuracy of response of six pulse oximeters to profound hypoxia, *Anesthesiology* 67:551, 1987.
64. Siegel LC, Fitzgerald DC, Engstrom RH: Simultaneous intraoperative measurement of cardiac output by thermodilution and transtracheal Doppler, *Anesthesiology* 74:664, 1991.
65. Smith RM: Anesthesia for pediatric surgery. In Gross RE, editor: *Surgery of infants and children*, Philadelphia, 1953, Saunders.
66. Smith C: An endoesophageal stethoscope, *Anesthesiology* 15:566, 1954.
67. Smith RM: *Anesthesia for infants and children*, St Louis, 1959, Mosby.
68. Stevens WC, Cromwell TH, Halsey MJ et al: The cardiovascular effects of a new inhalation agent Forane in human volunteers at constant arterial carbon dioxide tension, *Anesthesiology* 35:8, 1971.
69. Swan HJC, Ganz W, Forrester J et al: Catheterization of the heart in man with use of a flow-directed balloon-tipped catheter, *N Engl J Med* 283:447, 1970.
70. Swedlow DB: Capnometry and capnography: the anesthesia disaster early warning system, *Semin Anesth* 5:194, 1986.
71. Symarsky MR, Fox HS: Umbilical vessel catheterization: indications, management and evaluation of the technique, *J Pediatr* 80:820, 1972.
72. Van Wagener RA, Westerskow DR, Brenner RE et al: Dedicated monitoring of anesthetic and respiratory gases by Raman scattering, *J Clin Monit* 2:215, 1986.
73. Wareham JA, Haugh LD, Yeager SB: Prediction of arterial blood pressure in the premature neonate using the oscillometric method, *Am J Dis Child* 141:1108, 1987.
74. Yelderman M, New W: Evaluation of pulse oximetry, *Anesthesiology* 59:349, 1982.

# 9 Preoperative Evaluation and Management

*James A. Johns*



Successful anesthetic and surgical management of infants and children with heart disease is critically dependent on recognition of cardiac and noncardiac malformations as well as their preoperative management. Specific aspects of the management of individual lesions are discussed in subsequent chapters. This chapter will focus on general principles of diagnosis and management.

## DETECTION OF CONGENITAL HEART DISEASE IN INFANTS AND CHILDREN

### Prenatal period

Congenital heart disease occurs in approximately 1% of live-born infants.[5] Although most often congenital heart disease is not suspected until after delivery, the frequency of prenatal diagnosis by fetal echocardiography is increasing. In some cases fetal echocardiography is performed because of a family history of congenital heart disease. Siblings of children with congenital heart disease have approximately a 2% to 3% incidence of congenital heart disease, and children of parents with congenital heart disease have approximately a 10% incidence.[9] It is important to bear in mind that even with congenital heart disease in a sibling or parent, the vast majority of infants will have normal hearts. If there is a family history of congenital heart disease, fetal echocardiography is often very reassuring. Fetal echocardiography may also be performed if there is a suspicion of congenital heart disease on a routine obstetric ultrasound. Most often it is a discrepancy in ventricular chamber sizes, fetal hydrops, or an irregularity of the fetal heartbeat that raises the suspicion of congenital heart disease.

If congenital heart disease is suggested by fetal echocardiography, the parents should be counseled by a physician with up-to-date knowledge of the management and prognosis of infants with congenital heart disease. Preparations should be made for the infant to be delivered at a center with the medical and surgical expertise and facilities to deal with heart disease in infants. In cases of severe cardiac malformations detected early in pregnancy, elective termination of the pregnancy may be considered by some parents. The advantages of prenatal diagnosis of congenital heart disease must be weighed against potential for false-positive or false-negative results as well as the psychologic trauma to the parents over the months prior to delivery. At present prenatal surgical correction of congenital heart disease is not possible, but this approach may become feasible in the next few years.

### Neonatal period

Most infants presenting with congenital heart disease in the neonatal period have a murmur, cyanosis, congestive heart failure (CHF) or shock. Often several of these manifestations occur together. Isolated murmurs do not necessarily indicate significant structural heart disease. Peripheral pulmonic stenosis caused by turbulence at the pulmonary artery bifurcation is a common functional murmur in infants. Transient tricuspid or mitral regurgitation after delivery, a small ventricular septal defect (VSD), a small patent ductus arteriosus (PDA), or mild aortic or pulmonic stenosis all may present with asymptomatic murmurs. None of these require immediate intervention, but all should be followed clinically.

Cyanosis is generally visible when the concentration of deoxyhemoglobin exceeds about 3 gm/dl. Thus in an anemic infant with a hemoglobin of 10 gm/dl cyanosis is not usually visible until the oxygen saturation is below 70%. In contrast, a polycythemic infant with a hemoglobin of 20 gm/dl will appear cyanotic with an oxygen saturation of 85%. One must distinguish between acrocyanosis of the extremities, which is common in normal infants, and true central cyanosis. With the frequent use of pulse oximeters in neonatal units, lesser degrees of cyanosis may be detected.

Lung disease may cause cyanosis by causing pulmonary venous desaturation. Often cyanosis caused by lung disease is responsive to an increase in the fractional inspired oxygen concentration ($Fio_2$), which may overcome the diffusion barrier. In most cyanotic congenital heart disease the pulmonary venous saturation is normal, and cyanosis is the result of right to left shunting of deoxygenated blood (from the systemic veins) out the aorta. Increasing the $Fio_2$ will not normalize the partial pressure of oxygen in arterial blood ($Pao_2$), since deoxygenated blood continues to enter the systemic arteries. One can use the hyperoxia test to take advantage of this difference between cyanosis caused by lung disease and that caused by cyanotic congenital heart disease. The infant is given oxygen at as close to an $Fio_2$ of 1.0 as possible. An arterial blood sample is obtained from the right radial artery, since it almost always arises proximal to the ductus arteriosus. If the $Pao_2$ rises above 150 torr, it is very unlikely that right to left intracardiac shunting accounts for the cyanosis. The partial pressure of carbon dioxide in arterial blood ($Paco_2$) can also be helpful in distinguishing heart disease from lung disease, since it is usually increased in lung disease but normal or decreased in cyanotic congenital heart disease.

Cyanotic congenital heart disease can be classified into three general types of lesions: right-sided obstructive lesions, lesions with preferential streaming of deoxygenated blood to the aorta, and complete mixing lesions. There is overlap between these groups. In right-sided obstructive lesions such as tetralogy of Fallot and critical pulmonary stenosis there is decreased pulmonary blood flow on chest radiographs. Because the pulmonary blood flow is less than the systemic blood flow, much of the systemic venous return reenters the systemic circulation by crossing either an atrial septal defect (ASD) or a VSD.

Complete transposition of the great arteries, with or without a VSD, comprises the second type of cyanotic lesion. In complete transposition the aorta arises from the right ventricle, which receives mostly systemic venous blood, and the pulmonary artery arises from the left ventricle, which receives mostly pulmonary venous blood. Thus there are two parallel circulations, with the deoxygenated blood returning to the body and the oxygenated blood returning to the lungs. Survival in patients with transposition physiology is dependent on communication between the two circulations at the atrial, ventricular, or great arterial levels; if there were no communication, there would be no way for oxygen to get from the lungs to the systemic circulation.

In patients with complete mixing lesions, such as single ventricle, truncus arteriosus, or atresia of any valve, all of the systemic and pulmonary venous blood mixes. In this type of lesion the amount of cyanosis depends on the relative amounts of pulmonary and systemic blood flow. The ratio of pulmonary to systemic blood flow is known as the $Q_p:Q_s$ ratio. If there is limited pulmonary blood flow, there may be profound cyanosis. For example, in a patient with pulmonary atresia or tricuspid atresia, there may be twice as much systemic as pulmonary blood flow (a $Q_p:Q_s$ ratio of 0.5:1). If the systemic venous saturation is 60% and the pulmonary venous saturation is 100%, then the saturation of the mixed blood is 73% (60 + 60 + 100)/3. In contrast, if there is excessive pulmonary blood flow, as may be the case in a patient with a single ventricle without pulmonic stenosis, there may be little or no cyanosis. For example, with the same assumptions as above but with a $Q_p:Q_s$ ratio of 3:1, the systemic saturation is 90% (60 + 100 + 100 + 100)/4, and there is no visible cyanosis.

A number of lesions may manifest as CHF and/or shock in the neonatal period. These include left-sided obstructive lesions, lesions with large left to right shunts, and severe AV valve insufficiency. Prolonged tachycardia, either supraventricular or ventricular, may also result in CHF in the neonatal period.

Left-sided obstructive lesions may occur at the level of the pulmonary veins (total anomalous pulmonary venous return with obstruction), left atrium (cor triatriatum, supravalvular mitral ring), mitral valve (mitral stenosis or atresia), aortic valve (aortic stenosis or atresia), or aortic arch (aortic coarctation or interrupted aortic arch). Lesions with obstruction proximal to the left ventricle generally cause CHF and pulmonary edema, and obstruction at the aortic valve or of the aortic arch often causes shock.

Left to right shunt lesions include atrial shunts (ASD or partial anomalous pulmonary venous return), ventricular shunts (VSD, complete AV septal defects, and single ventricle), and shunts at the level of the great arteries (PDA, aorticopulmonary window, and truncus arteriosus). Shunts at the great arterial level often cause heart failure early in the neonatal period, while ventricular level shunts usually present several weeks later, as the pulmonary vascular resistance falls. CHF often does not accompany atrial level shunts at all.

Severe insufficiency of the tricuspid valve (especially in Ebstein's anomaly) or mitral valve may also cause CHF in the neonatal period. (Ebstein's anomaly may also cause cyanosis when there is limited pulmonary blood flow.)

### Beyond the neonatal period

Most children with cyanotic heart disease present soon after birth. Children with tetralogy of Fallot may not manifest marked cyanosis until a few months of life, but most have murmurs soon after birth. A rare child with pulmonary atresia and multiple collaterals may also present later, as may children with single ventricle and pulmonic stenosis or tricuspid atresia without severe pulmonic stenosis. The majority of children presenting with congenital heart disease beyond the neonatal period have either asymptomatic murmurs or CHF.

A number of lesions may cause asymptomatic murmurs. These include aortic and pulmonic stenosis, insufficiency of any valve, ASD, VSD, and PDA. Coarctation may also cause an asymptomatic murmur, but more commonly there is upper extremity hypertension with decreased lower extremity pulses. There are specific features of the murmur and other aspects of the physical examination that provide clues to the diagnosis. These are discussed in the chapters on the individual lesions. It is important to remember that most children with murmurs do not have heart disease but rather have functional, or innocent, murmurs.

CHF may be the presenting sign of children with left to right shunt lesions, obstructive lesions, regurgitant lesions, or sustained tachycardia. As mentioned earlier, large VSD and AV septal defects typically cause heart failure at a few weeks of age. The reason for presentation at this age is probably related both to falling pulmonary vascular resistance and to physiologic anemia. It is unusual for aortic stenosis or coarctation to cause heart failure beyond about a month of age. Mitral stenosis, mitral insufficiency, and aortic insufficiency all can cause heart failure, particularly if they are acute in onset, such as the mitral insufficiency of acute rheumatic fever or the aortic insufficiency of acute bacterial endocarditis. Cardiomyopathy and myocarditis can cause CHF at any age, although both may also appear as arrhythmias.

## PREOPERATIVE EVALUATION

### History

As is true for any operation, it is important to take a complete history as a part of the preoperative evaluation of children undergoing heart surgery. Particular attention is focused on cardiovascular symptoms, including symptoms of arrhythmias (palpitations, tachycardia, syncope, etc.), CHF (dyspnea, sweating, poor growth, exercise intolerance), and cyanosis. One must ask the parents of children with cyanotic lesions, and tetralogy of Fallot in particular, about hypercyanotic spells. If there is a history of spells, great caution must be exercised in preoperative blood drawing and in induction of anesthesia, since spells in these settings can be disastrous. In critically ill infants and children it is important to determine whether there has been normal urine output, as prerenal azotemia and/or acute tubular necrosis can occur and complicate perioperative management. Any previous history of anesthetic-related problems in the patient or family members should be explored.

### Physical examination

A complete cardiovascular examination should be performed, including evaluation of precordial activity, the first and second heart sounds, murmurs, gallops, liver size, pulses, perfusion, clubbing, cyanosis, and edema. A thorough examination of the lungs and airway is essential. In addition to focusing on the specifics of the cardiac and respiratory examination, one must look for associated abnormalities of other systems. Congenital heart disease is often part of a complex of congenital anomalies.[7] Sometimes these anomalies are related to chromosomal abnormalities, as in the case of trisomy 21 (Down syndrome), trisomy 18, and trisomy 13. The latter two are almost universally fatal with or without surgical intervention, so repair of congenital heart defects in those patients is generally not undertaken. One must obtain blood for a karyotype in these patients prior to transfusion. In other syndromes such as VATER syndrome and CHARGE association the underlying abnormality has not yet been identified. Nonetheless, it is essential that the anesthesiologist, surgeon, and cardiologist all be aware of any associated noncardiac abnormalities. If there is a question of such anomalies, it is generally wise to delay any nonemergent operations until these questions have been resolved. Sometimes it is wise to assume that associated abnormalities are present until proven otherwise. For example, it is wise to treat infants with type B interrupted aortic arch as if they have DiGeorge sequence, since about half of infants with this cardiac abnormality have DiGeorge sequence.[3] Failure to irradiate blood products in this setting can result in graft versus host disease because of the associated immune deficiency.

***Electrocardiogram.*** ECG is helpful in several ways. First, it may screen for congenital heart disease. Although patients with any of a number of cardiac lesions may have normal ECG and patients with abnormal ECGs may not have heart disease, the presence of ECG abnormalities raises the index of suspicion. Second, the ECG may provide clues as to the specific form of congenital heart disease that is present. For example, left-axis deviation in a newborn is suggestive of tricuspid atresia if the infant is cyanotic and of some form of endocardial cushion defect if the child is not cyanotic. Third, the ECG may show abnormalities of cardiac rhythm. These may include AV block (common in congenitally corrected transposition), abnormal P-wave axis (common in abnormalities of atrial situs such as situs inversus or situs ambiguus), and Wolff-Parkinson-White syndrome (which can be seen in Ebstein's anomaly). Finally, the availability of a preoperative ECG may be immensely valuable for comparison if there are postoperative ECG abnormalities.

***Chest x-ray.*** A chest x-ray film should be taken on any infant or child with suspected heart disease. The lung parenchyma should be carefully examined for intrinsic pulmonary disease such as pneumonia or hyaline membrane disease, which may mimic heart disease by causing cyanosis. Pneumothorax may cause severe depression of cardiac output and is usually easily seen on x-ray film. The prominence of the pulmonary vascularity should be assessed. In lesions with large left to right shunts the pulmonary vascularity is increased, and in lesions with decreased pulmonary blood flow (including most cyanotic lesions), the vascularity is decreased on chest x-ray film. The presence of increased pulmonary vascularity in a patient with severe cyanosis suggests transposition of the great arteries or total anomalous pulmonary venous connection with obstructed pulmonary veins. In patients with left heart failure there may be signs of pulmonary edema, including increased alveolar densities as well as Kerley B lines and fluid in the major and minor fissures. In most forms of congenital heart disease the cardiac silhouette is enlarged. The bronchial morphology may provide clues to heterotaxia syndromes. In asplenia syndrome there is often bilateral right bronchial morphology (eparterial bronchi), and in polysplenia syndrome there is often bilateral left bronchial morphology (hyparterial bronchi). The presence of a right aortic arch raises the index of suspicion for congenital heart disease. Tetralogy of Fallot and truncus arteriosus are common in patients who have a right aortic arch.[8]

***Echocardiography.*** Based on physical examination, ECG and chest x-ray, it is usually possible to make a fairly specific diagnosis of congenital heart disease. With two-dimensional echocardiography it is possible to determine most of the anatomic details of the lesion noninvasively. Generally one can determine the sites of normal and abnormal systemic and pulmonary venous return, the size and relationship of the atria, the atrioventricular relations, the size and location of ASD or VSD, the relationship of the great arteries to the ventricles and to each other, and the size and branching pattern of the aorta and pulmonary arteries. By the application of the Bernoulli equation one can determine pressure gradients using pulsed and continuous-wave Doppler measurements of blood flow velocity. With Doppler one can measure gradients across stenotic valves, vessels, and orifices. Measurement of the velocity of mitral or tricuspid regurgitation often allows the echocardiographer to measure the systolic difference between right ventricular and right atrial pressure or between left ventricular and left atrial pressure. By making reasonable assumptions about right or left atrial pressure, one can estimate systolic ventricular pressure. Color Doppler flow mapping allows the detection of small jets of blood across an ASD, a VSD, or a PDA. It also allows a qualitative assessment of the severity of valvular regurgitation.

***Cardiac catheterization.*** Despite the advances in echocardiography, catheterization often must be performed in infants and children prior to cardiac surgery. In some patients it is performed to provide additional anatomic details that may be helpful to the surgeons. These details may include the coronary artery branching pattern, sites of pulmonary artery stenosis, and so on. In addition, catheterization can provide physiologic data not available by echocardiography. While Doppler echocardiography is reasonably good at determining pressure gradients, it cannot determine absolute pressures. Thus, to measure end diastolic pressures in the ventricle or absolute pulmonary artery pressures, catheterization is the gold standard. Although one can use echocardiography to estimate pulmonary and systemic flows by integrating flow velocity across a valve or in an artery and multiplying by the cross-sectional area, such estimates are not nearly so accurate as measurements at catheterization. When considering catheterization, one must weigh the value of the information to be obtained against the risks of the procedure. The risk of death or a serious complication from cardiac catheterization is approximately 1% in children and about twice that in neonates.[2,6]

In most infants and children cardiac catheterization is performed from a femoral approach. In neonates it is possible to perform cardiac catheterization using the umbilical artery and/or vein. In children with interrupted inferior vena cava or a previous Glenn shunt, it may be necessary to carry out venous catheterization from above, using an antecubital, axillary, subclavian, or internal jugular approach. I usually do not use general anesthesia for diagnostic catheterization, preferring sedation and local anesthesia. At some centers general anesthesia is routinely used. Usually the catheters can be introduced percutaneously using the Seldinger technique and vascular sheaths, but rarely cutdown is required. All of the last 500 pediatric cardiac catheterizations at Vanderbilt University Medical Center have been done percutaneously. I generally use flow-directed catheters such as Swan-Ganz catheters and Berman angiographic catheters for the venous side and pigtail catheters for the arterial side, with other catheter types being used under some circumstances.

The data obtained at catheterization include pressure, flow, and angiographic data. Pressure measurements are usually performed using fluid-filled catheters. Occasionally high-fidelity catheter-tip pressure transducers are used. Both right and left atrial pressures are obtained in most infants and in older children with a patent foramen ovale or an ASD. If the left atrium is not accessible, pulmonary artery wedge pressures provide a good estimate of left atrial pressures as long as there is no pulmonary vein stenosis. Right and left ventricular pressures are also measured in most patients. If there is an atrial communication, the left ventricular pressure can be measured using the venous catheter; otherwise, a retrograde arterial approach is used. Pulmonary artery pressures are usually obtained by crossing the pulmonic valve with the venous catheter. Occasionally it is necessary to approach the pulmonary artery from the SVC in patients who have had a Glenn shunt or from the arterial side in patients who have a systemic to pulmonary artery shunt.

Extreme caution should be exercised when crossing the ductus to enter the pulmonary artery in a patient with ductal-dependent pulmonary flow, since catheter manipulation may cause the ductus to close. Usually the risks of this approach outweigh the benefits. If it is not possible to measure the pulmonary artery pressure directly, one can obtain pulmonary vein wedge pressures using an end-hole catheter. Aortic pressures are usually measured with the arterial catheter, although it is sometimes possible to enter the aorta from the ventricle by crossing the aortic valve with the venous catheter. For measurement of pressure gradients the most useful pressures are those that are obtained either simultaneously, using two catheters, or in short succession by pullback of a single catheter from one structure to another. Ideally, one should obtain all pressure measurements prior to any angiography, since contrast administration may alter pressures. However, this principle is sometimes overridden by the principle of not making difficult catheter passes more than once. For example, in a patient with severe aortic stenosis one would obtain the pressure pullback across the aortic valve after the left ventriculogram rather than cross the valve twice. Normal intracardiac pressures are shown in Table 9-1.

Intracardiac shunting can be detected using oximetry. Normal intracardiac oxygen saturations are shown in Table 9–1. A pulmonary artery saturation that is more than 5% higher than the SVC saturation suggests a left to right shunt, and an aortic saturation that is lower than the pulmonary venous saturation suggests right to left shunting.

Flow measurements are usually made either by the thermodilution technique, if there is no intracardiac shunting, or the Fick method. For the Fick method oxygen consumption ($\dot{V}_{O2}$) can be either measured or estimated from patient size. To measure systemic flow ($Q_s$) one uses the aortic and mixed venous saturations to determine the $AV_{O2}$ difference across the systemic bed. The most accurate mixed venous saturation is the pulmonary artery saturation if there is no left to right shunting or the superior vena cava saturation if there is a left to right shunt. For measurement of pulmonary flow, the pulmonary artery and pulmonary venous saturations are used to determine the $AV_{O2}$ difference across the pulmonary bed. In the presence of right to left or left to right shunting one can calculate the effective pulmonary blood flow ($Q_{EP}$), which is defined as the amount of systemic venous blood that enters the pulmonary artery, using the mixed venous and pulmonary venous saturations. Knowing the systemic and pulmonary flows, one can determine the systemic and pulmonary vascular resistance. The pulmonary vascular resistance is of critical importance in many patients, since if it is elevated, the risk of operation may be markedly increased. The equations used in calculating flows, shunts, and resistances are shown in the box on p. 115.

Angiography is performed as part of most cardiac catheterizations in infants and children. Usually a nonionic contrast medium is used. One must

**Table 9–1** Normal cardiac catheterization data

| Pressures (in torr): | Newborns | Older children | $O_2$ saturations (%) |
|---|---|---|---|
| Superior vena cava | Same as right atrial pressure | | 65-75 |
| Inferior vena cava | Same as right atrial pressure | | 70-80 |
| Right atrium | | | 60-80 |
| a | 3-8 | 5-10 | |
| v | 2-6 | 4-8 | |
| mean | 0-4 | 2-6 | |
| Right ventricle | | | 65-75 |
| systolic | 65-80 | 15-25 | |
| end diastolic | 2-7 | 3-8 | |
| Pulmonary artery | | | 65-75 |
| systolic | 65-80 | 15-25 | |
| diastolic | 35-50 | 8-12 | |
| mean | 40-70 | 10-16 | |
| Pulmonary artery wedge | | | 95-100 |
| a | 6-10 | 8-14 | |
| v | 7-11 | 10-17 | |
| mean | 5-8 | 7-13 | |
| Left atrium | | | 95-100 |
| a | 4-7 | 6-12 | |
| v | 5-9 | 8-15 | |
| mean | 3-6 | 5-10 | |
| Left ventricle | | | 95-100 |
| systolic | 65-80 | 90-120 | |
| end diastolic | 3-7 | 5-12 | |
| Aorta | | | 95-100 |
| systolic | 65-80 | 90-120 | |
| diastolic | 45-60 | 60-75 | |
| mean | 55-65 | 70-90 | |
| **Flows** | | | |
| $Q_P$ | 3.5-5.0 L/min/$M^2$ | | |
| $Q_S$ | 3.5-5.0 L/min/$M^2$ | | |
| **Resistances** | | | |
| $R_P$ | 8-10 | 1-3 | Woods units × $M^2$ |
| $R_S$ | 10-15 | 15-30 | Woods units × $M^2$ |

Adapted from Rudolph AM: *Congenital diseases of the heart: clinical-physiologic considerations in diagnosis and management,* St Louis, 1974, Mosby.

always be careful to limit the amount of contrast material used to minimize the risk of contrast nephropathy. This is especially important in neonates in general and in neonates with aortic stenosis, coarctation, or interruption in particular, since renal perfusion may already by impaired. I try to limit the total dose of contrast to less than 4 ml/kg. Contrast is usually injected with a pressure injector, although in some circumstances hand injections may be preferable. Usually 1 to 2 ml/kg of contrast is adequate for ventriculography, and 0.5 to 1.5 ml/kg is adequate for aortography or pulmonary angiography. Angled views often provide more satisfactory visualization of the anatomy than straight frontal and lateral projections. The choice of cineangiograms depends on the specific anatomic questions for a particular patient.

## PREOPERATIVE MANAGEMENT

### General management

The most important aspect of preoperative management is meticulous attention to the cardiorespiratory status of the patient. One must be sure the patient is adequately ventilated; oxygenation should be optimized; pH should be kept near normal; and close attention should be paid to the heart rate, blood pressure, and perfusion. If there is either hypoventilation or acidosis, the patient should be intubated and mechanical ventilation begun. Even in patients with metabolic acidosis ventilation

## CALCULATIONS OF CATHETERIZATION DATA

**Flows**

$$Q_P = \frac{V_{O_2}}{(S_{PV}O_2 - S_{PA}O_2) \times Hgb \times 1.34 \times 10}$$

$$Q_S = \frac{V_{O_2}}{(S_{Ao}O_2 - S_{MV}O_2) \times Hgb \times 1.34 \times 10}$$

$$Q_{EP} = \frac{V_{O_2}}{(S_{PV}O_2 - S_{MV}O_2) \times Hgb \times 1.34 \times 10}$$

$Q_P$, pulmonary blood flow (L/min/m$^2$); $Q_S$, systemic blood flow (L/min/m$^2$); $Q_{EP}$, effective pulmonary blood flow (L/min/m$^2$); $V_{O_2}$, oxygen consumption (ml/min/m$^2$); $S_{Ao}O_2$, aortic oxygen saturation; $S_{MV}O_2$, mixed venous oxygen saturation; $S_{PA}O_2$, pulmonary artery oxygen saturation; $S_{PV}O_2$, pulmonary venous oxygen saturation; Hgb, is hemoglobin concentration (gm/dl); 1.34, oxygen carrying capacity of fully saturated hemoglobin (ml/gm); 10, conversion factor from deciliters to liters (dl/l). Saturations are expressed as decimal fraction, e.g., 0.95.

**Shunts**

$$Q_P/Q_S = \frac{S_{Ao}O_2 - S_{MV}O_2}{S_{PV}O_2 - S_{PA}O_2}$$

$$Q_{L\to R} = Q_P - Q_{EP} = \frac{V_{O_2} \times (S_{PA}O_2 - S_{MV}O_2)}{(S_{PV}O_2 - S_{PA}O_2) \times (S_{PV}O_2 - S_{MV}O_2) \times Hgb \times 1.34 \times 10}$$

$$Q_{R\to L} = Q_S - Q_{EP} = \frac{V_{O_2} \times (S_{PV}O_2 - S_{Ao}O_2)}{(S_{Ao}O_2 - S_{MV}O_2) \times (S_{PV}O_2 - S_{MV}O_2) \times Hgb \times 1.34 \times 10}$$

$$\%L\to R\ SHUNT = 100 \times \frac{Q_{L\to R}}{Q_P} = 100 \times \frac{S_{PA}O_2 - S_{MV}O_2}{S_{PV}O_2 - S_{MV}O_2}$$

$$\%R\to L\ SHUNT = 100 \times \frac{Q_{R\to L}}{Q_S} = 100 \times \frac{S_{PV}O_2 - S_{Ao}O_2}{S_{PV}O_2 - S_{MV}O_2}$$

$Q_{L\to R}$, left to right shunt flow; $Q_{R\to L}$, right to left shunt flow; other abbreviations as above.

**Resistances**

$$R_P = \frac{\overline{PAP} - \overline{LAP}}{Q_P}$$

$$R_S = \frac{\overline{AoP} - \overline{RAP}}{Q_S}$$

$R_P$, pulmonary vascular resistance; $R_S$, systemic vascular resistance; $\overline{PAP}$, mean pulmonary artery pressure; LAP, mean left atrial pressure; AoP, mean aortic pressure; RAP, mean right atrial pressure.

is helpful in minimizing the work of breathing. Since renal dysfunction is common, it is important to look for abnormalities of electrolytes. Although it is understandable to focus on the cardiac abnormalities, one must remember that other organ system problems can occur either as a result of the heart disease or as an associated finding. In particular, CNS abnormalities and infection should be kept in mind. In neonates hyperbilirubinemia is common, and necrotizing enterocolitis is an uncommon but life-threatening problem in sick infants. If children with congenital heart disease undergo noncardiac surgery, antibiotic prophylaxis for subacute bacterial endocarditis (SBE) should be provided. The recommendations of the American Heart Association are shown in the box on p. 116.

## AHA RECOMMENDATIONS FOR SBE PROPHYLAXIS

**Dental, oral, and upper respiratory procedures**

***Standard regimen***

Amoxicillin 50 mg/kg (maximum 3 g) PO 60 minutes prior to procedure, then 25 mg/kg (maximum 1.5 g) PO 6 hours later

***Standard regimen for amoxicillin- or penicillin-allergic patients***

Erythromycin ethylsuccinate 20 mg/kg (maximum 800 mg) PO 2 hours prior to procedure, then 10 mg/kg (maximum 400 mg) PO 6 hours later

OR

Erythromycin stearate 20 mg/kg (maximum 1 g) PO 2 hours prior to procedure, then 10 mg/kg (maximum 500 mg) PO 6 hours later

OR

Clindamycin 10 mg/kg (maximum 300 mg) PO 60 minutes prior to procedure, then 5 mg/kg (maximum 150 mg) PO 6 hours later

***Alternative regimen for patients who cannot take oral medications***

Ampicillin 50 mg/kg (maximum 2 g) IV or IM 30 minutes prior to procedure, then ampicillin 25 mg/kg (maximum 1 g) IV or IM 6 hours later

(Second dose may be given as PO amoxicillin; see standard regimen.)

***Alternative regimen for amoxicillin- or penicillin-allergic patients who cannot take oral medications***

Clindamycin 10 mg/kg (maximum 300 mg) IV 60 minutes prior to procedure, then 5 mg/kg (maximum 150 mg) IV or PO 6 hours later

***Alternative regimen for high-risk patients not candidates for standard regimen***

Ampicillin 50 mg/kg (maximum 2 g) IV or IM plus gentamicin 2 mg/kg (maximum 80 mg) IV or IM 30 minutes prior to procedure, then amoxicillin 25 mg/kg (maximum 1.5 g) PO 6 hours later (alternatively, may repeat parenteral regimen 8 hours later)

***Alternative regimen for amoxicillin- or penicillin-allergic patients considered high risk***

Vancomycin 20 mg/kg (maximum 1 g) IV over 1 hour, starting 1 hour before procedure (no repeat dose needed)

**GI or GU procedures**

***Standard regimen***

Ampicillin 50 mg/kg (maximum 2 g) IV or IM plus gentamicin 2 mg/kg (maximum 80 mg) IV or IM 30 minutes prior to procedure, then amoxicillin 25 mg/kg PO (maximum 1.5 g) PO 6 hours later (alternatively, may repeat parenteral regimen 8 hours later)

***Alternative regimen for ampicillin- or penicillin-allergic patients***

Vancomycin 20 mg/kg (maximum 1 g) IV over 1 hour, starting 1 hour before procedure, plus gentamicin 2 mg/kg (maximum 80 mg) IV or IM 1 hour before procedure. Doses may be repeated 8 hours later.

***Alternative oral regimen for low-risk patients***

Amoxicillin 50 mg/kg (maximum 3 g) PO 60 minutes prior to procedure, then 25 mg/kg (maximum 1.5 gm) PO 6 hours later

From American Heart Association Committee on Rheumatic Fever, Endocarditis and Kawasaki Disease: Prevention of bacterial endocarditis, *JAMA* 264:2919, 1990.

### Management of cyanotic heart disease in the neonate

Almost all cyanotic lesions are improved by maintaining ductal patency. In lesions with decreased pulmonary blood flow the ductus allows additional pulmonary flow, and in transposition it improves mixing. Thus in infants with severe hypoxemia prostaglandin $E_1$ should be considered as soon as cyanotic congenital heart disease is suspected. If cyanotic heart disease can be quickly ruled in or out by echocardiography, then it may be reasonable to wait a few minutes while the echocardiogram is performed. Otherwise prostaglandin $E_1$ should be begun. If an infant is to be transported to a distant referral center, one may wish to start prostaglandin even if the cyanosis is not yet severe, so as to prevent ductal closure. The usual starting dose of prostaglandin $E_1$ is 0.05 μg/kg/min given as a continuous IV infusion. Often after the ductus is open a lower dose will maintain ductal patency. The main side effect of prostaglandin $E_1$ is apnea, which is a dose-related side effect. Thus one should always be prepared to intubate and ventilate an infant who is given prostaglandin, and prophylactic intubation should be considered for infants who will be transported to a referral center in vehicles in which intubation is difficult. Supplemental oxygen is usually given, although in most cyanotic congenital heart disease it has little effect. If the supplemental oxygen is not helping, it should be weaned to a relatively nontoxic concentration ($FiO_2$ 0.3 to 0.4) as quickly as possible.

### Management of shock due to left-sided obstructive lesions in the neonate

Just as prostaglandin $E_1$ can be very helpful by improving pulmonary blood flow in cyanotic lesions, it can improve systemic blood flow in left-sided obstructive lesions such as aortic atresia, critical aortic stenosis, interrupted aortic arch, and coarctation of the aorta. In these lesions a PDA allows the right ventricle to provide flow to the aorta, improving systemic blood flow. The dose and side effects are the same as given earlier. Inotropic support with dobutamine 5 to 20 μg/kg/min is often helpful, and low-dose dopamine (3 to 5 μg/kg/min) can help maintain renal perfusion. Digoxin is not used in critically ill infants because of the risk of toxicity in a patient with tenuous renal perfusion. Intubation and ventilation are often helpful in decreasing the work of breathing.

### Management of congestive heart failure

In infants and children CHF requiring treatment is primarily left heart failure, with pulmonary edema and increased work of breathing. Usually CHF in this age group is the result of increased preloading of the ventricle such as in left to right shunt lesions or regurgitant lesions, or increased afterload, such as in left-sided obstructive lesions. Less commonly there is a primary abnormality of myocardial contractility like cardiomyopathy or myocarditis. In general, in patients with abnormal ventricular loading the ultimate therapy is surgical, and the goal of medical therapy is to allow the patient to grow or stabilize so as to decrease the risk of operation. In some situations medical therapy may obviate the need for operation. For example, some relatively large VSDs will close spontaneously, given time. Occasionally there is specific therapy for the problem, such as pharmacologic opening of the ductus as described above for left-sided obstructive lesions in the neonatal period. Usually medical therapy for CHF is palliative.

The primary goal of medical therapy is to lower the end diastolic pressure in the left ventricle while maintaining adequate systemic blood flow. The three types of therapy commonly used for CHF are inotropic agents, diuretics, and afterload-reducing agents. Digoxin has been used for CHF in infants and children for many years and is one of the mainstays of chronic oral therapy. Recent studies in adults have shown a beneficial effect of digoxin even in patients who are also receiving angiotensin converting enzyme (ACE) inhibitors.[11] The use of digoxin in critically ill patients has become less common, since there are other effective agents with shorter half-lives and less risk of toxicity in patients with impaired renal function. Dobutamine and isoproterenol are potent β-adrenergic agents that potently increase contractility and reduce afterload somewhat. Dobutamine is often preferred to isoproterenol, since it has less chronotropic effect. Dopamine in low doses has the additional benefit of improving renal blood flow through its dopaminergic action. Newer inotropic agents, including the phosphodiesterase inhibitors amrinone and milrinone, increase contractility through nonadrenergic mechanisms. Their long-term efficacy and safety are not fully known. In adults with CHF some of these agents may improve ventricular function but actually increase mortality.[10] Vesnarinone, a new agent with inotropic as well as antiarrhythmic properties, appears promising in adults with CHF.[4]

Diuretics act by decreasing total blood volume and decreasing left ventricular end diastolic volume. Loop diuretics such as furosemide and bumetanide are commonly used, as are thiazide diuretics, including hydrochlorothiazide and metolazone. All of these diuretics can cause potassium wasting and hypochloremic metabolic alkalosis, so one must pay close attention to the serum electrolytes. Often potassium supplementation is needed. Alternatively, agents that block the angiotensin/aldosterone pathway such as spironolactone or ACE inhibitors will decrease potassium excretion. Occasionally, in patients with refractory metabolic alkalosis, carbonic anhydrase inhibitors such as acetazolamide are used. Nephrocalcinosis can occur with loop diuretics as a result of their calciuretic effects, so one must be cautious with the chronic use of these agents in high doses.

Afterload reduction is an effective therapy for

patients with impaired ventricular function. In patients with left to right shunts afterload-reducing agents will reduce the shunt if they have a greater effect on the systemic resistance than on the pulmonary resistance. ACE inhibitors have been very effective in children and adults with CHF. In children captopril and enalapril are the most commonly used agents in this class. One must be very cautious in using these drugs in infants and children in whom coronary perfusion may be a problem, since lowering diastolic blood pressure may decrease coronary perfusion. Patients in whom this may be a problem include those with aortic stenosis or with already low diastolic pressures (e.g., patients with PDA or severe aortic insufficiency). In these patients coronary perfusion pressure may be low while myocardial oxygen demand is high, and pharmacologic reduction of systemic vascular resistance may result in myocardial ischemia.

Preoperative evaluation and management of infants and children with heart disease requires a team approach. With the cooperation of intensivists, neonatologists, pediatric cardiologists, cardiac surgeons, and anesthesiologists, close attention to preoperative management can markedly reduce perioperative and long-term morbidity and mortality.

## REFERENCES

1. American Heart Association Committee on Rheumatic Fever, Endocarditis, and Kawasaki Disease: Prevention of bacterial endocarditis, *JAMA* 264:2919, 1990.
2. Cassidy SC, Schmidt KG, Van Hare GF et al: Complications of pediatric cardiac catheterization: a 3-year study, *J Am Coll Cardiol* 19:1285, 1992.
3. Conley ME, Beckwith JB, Mancer KFK et al: The spectrum of the DiGeorge syndrome, *J Pediatr* 94:883, 1979.
4. Feldman AM, Bristow MR, Parmley WW et al: Effects of vesnarinone on morbidity and mortality in patients with heart failure, *N Engl J Med* 329:149, 1993.
5. Ferencz C, Rubin JD, McCarter RJ et al: Congenital heart disease prevalence at live birth: the Baltimore-Washington Infant Study, *Am J Epidemiol* 121:31, 1985.
6. Graham TP: Advances in invasive cardiac diagnosis and management, *Pediatr Clin North Am* 25:707, 1978.
7. Greenwood RD, Rosenthal A, Parisi L et al: Extracardiac abnormalities in infants with congenital heart disease, *Pediatrics* 55:485, 1975.
8. Knight L, Edwards J: Right aortic arch: types and associated abnormalities, *Circulation* 50:1047, 1974.
9. Nora JJ, Nora AH: Update on counseling the family with a first-degree relative with a congenital heart defect, *Am J Med Genet* 29:137, 1988.
10. Packer M, Carver JR, Rodeheffer RJ et al: Effect of oral milrinone on mortality in severe congestive heart failure, *N Engl J Med* 325:1468, 1991.
11. Packer M, Gheorghiade M, Young J et al: Withdrawal of digoxin from patients with chronic heart failure treated with angiotensin converting enzyme inhibitors, *N Engl J Med* 329:1, 1993.
12. Rudolph AM: *Congenital diseases of the heart: clinical-physiologic considerations in diagnosis and management,* Chicago, 1974, Year Book Medical.

# 10 Principles of Anesthesia for Children with Congenital Heart Disease

*Jay Kambam*



Certain congenital heart defects (CHDs), especially cyanotic CHDs, are likely to be detected and diagnosed earlier than others. Intensive studies have reported the incidence of CHD to be about eight per thousand live births (0.8%).[12,29,47] Of these patients 1 in 4, or 25%, will also have other congenital noncardiac defects, and many patients undergo both noncardiac and cardiac surgical procedures (box). Dramatic improvement in the overall survival rate of the children with CHDs may be attributed to a variety of factors. These include rapid advancement in diagnostic methods and understanding of the pathophysiology of CHDs, improvements in anesthesia, monitoring, and surgical techniques, and availability of an armamentarium of drugs, especially the prostaglandin E series. In addition to noncardiac and closed cardiac operations, each year more than 20,000 open heart operations are being performed in North America alone.[52] Overall surgical mortality has decreased to about 6% (compared with 23% 50 years ago) and anesthesia-related mortality to 0% (compared with

**SOME FACTS ABOUT CHD IN NORTH AMERICA**

Incidence: 0.8%.
Incidence of other noncardiac congenital defects: 0.2%.
Over 500,000 with CHD reached adulthood.
Over 20,000 open heart surgical procedures are performed per year in CHD patients.
Overall surgical mortality: 6%.
Anesthesia-related mortality: 0%.

10% 50 years ago).[27] For these reasons more and more infants with complex CHDs are undergoing early corrective surgical procedures, and as a result the role of palliative shunt procedures has diminished in recent years.

The anesthesiologist should apply the same principles of pediatric cardiac anesthesia whether a child with CHD is undergoing cardiac or noncardiac surgery. Thus this chapter contains a general discussion of anesthetic management of children with CHD for both cardiac and noncardiac surgery. Understanding the general principles and pathophysiology of various subgroups of CHD is essential for the management of a child with CHD for either type of surgery. The anesthesiologist also must understand thoroughly the effects of alterations of pulmonary vascular resistance (PVR), systemic vascular resistance (SVR), pressures (atrial, ventricular, aortic, and pulmonary), the contractile state of both the ventricles, heart rate changes, and volume status on various shunt lesions, obstructive lesions, and other miscellaneous lesions for safe management of these patients. This knowledge allows choice of an appropriate technique for induction and maintenance of anesthesia, including monitoring, ventilatory management, and postoperative care. A thorough knowledge of the management of a situation in which these hemodynamic parameters must be manipulated, either with ventilation or by use of various other methods, including cardiovascular drugs is also necessary. The desired hemodynamic parameters for optimal anesthetic management in commonly seen CHD and various factors that can alter these hemodynamic parameters are given in box (p. 121).

## PHYSIOLOGY

Cardiac output increases progressively during the first few weeks of extrauterine life. The neonatal heart increases cardiac output primarily by increasing heart rate rather than stroke volume. Although the neonatal heart follows the Frank-Starling relationship, its response to volume overload is distinctly more limited than in the adult.[7,32,56,68] The right ventricle is thicker than the left at birth, and it takes a few years for the left ventricle to become twice as heavy as the right ventricle (adult pattern). During the neonatal period both ventricles are about equal in size, and their relationship is such that any dysfunction with an increase in filling pressures in one ventricle rapidly affects the filling pressure of the other ventricle, thus leading to a biventricular dysfunction.[11,56] Since the ventricular compliance in the neonate is lower than in an adult, any increase in afterload is poorly tolerated by the neonate, leading to an increase in ventricular filling pressures and reversal of the circulatory pattern.[7,68] The functional closure of the foramen ovale occurs mainly because of the difference between the left and right atrial pressure, and this pressure difference is easily reversed by increasing afterload on the right side of the heart. The circulation of the newborn is thus transitional.

If stressed, the neonatal circulation will shift back to the fetal pattern, shunting through foramen ovale and/or patent ductus arteriosus (PDA). These factors may convert neonatal to fetal circulation:

1. Metabolic acidosis
2. Respiratory acidosis
3. Hypoxemia
4. Hypothermia
5. Hypoglycemia
6. Excessive airway pressure
7. Hypervolemia
8. Stress (awake intubation, cough, suction)
9. Drugs (prostaglandin E, etc.)

Fortunately, the neonate will revert to normal circulation if the stress is removed. Many stressful events such as hypoxemia, hypercarbia, hypoglycemia, metabolic acidosis, crying, straining, and excessive positive pressure to the airway can increase pulmonary vascular resistance and decrease pulmonary blood flow. For example, crying and straining are known to cause right to left shunting via the foramen ovale (FO) in about 50% of normal neonates.[54] In the healthy neonate the physiological closure of FO and PDA occur at about 8 and 24 hours, respectively, and anatomical closure of the FO and PDA is complete at about 1 year and 3 weeks, respectively (Table 10–1).

In the neonate with certain pathologic cardiac defects, persistence of flow across the FO and/or PDA is essential for survival (for example PDA and FO in TGA, and PDA in coarctation of the aorta and interrupted aortic arch). On the other hand, certain newborns with no cardiac defects, especially premature babies, are prone to have persistent fetal circulation or bidirectional shunts, especially via a PDA. Shunting is mainly from the

**Table 10–1** The times of occurrence of functional and anatomic closures of the foramen ovale and the patent ductus arteriosus[13,21,58]

| | Foramen ovale | PDA |
|---|---|---|
| Functional closure | 8-24 hours | 24-48 hours |
| Anatomic closure | 12 months | 2-3 weeks |
| Patent in 50% of the people | For 5 years | — |
| Patent in 25% of the people | More than 20 years | — |

right to the left side of the heart in the first few days after birth because of high pulmonary resistance. The right to left shunt will, however, be replaced with a left to right shunt as the pulmonary resistance is gradually decreased by the end of the neonatal period. Remember, noxious stimuli and hypoxemia can cause marked increases in vascular resistances in neonates. The increase in PVR is proportionately higher than that of SVR because of the presence of highly reactive pulmonary vasculature in neonates.[30,46] The box shows the causes of increase and decrease in both systemic and pulmonary vascular resistances.

## CLASSIFICATION OF CONGENITAL HEART DEFECTS

CHD can be conveniently classified into four major categories: (1) lesions with right to left shunt, (2) lesions with left to right shunt, (3) lesions with obstruction to the ventricles, and (4) miscellaneous lesions (see the left box on p. 122). In general lesions with left to right cardiac shunt are associated with an increased pulmonary blood flow and lesions with right to left shunt are associated with a decreased pulmonary blood flow (see the right box on p. 122).

## PHYSICS

The factors that determine the amount and direction of flow (shunting and obstruction of blood flow) across a defect are governed by two basic laws described in many textbooks of physics:

Ohm's law: $I = E \div R$
I, Flow; E, pressure difference; R, resistance

Modified Ohm's law:

$$\text{Flow (cardiac output)} = \frac{\text{Pressure difference (MP-CVP)}}{\text{Resistance (SVR)}}$$

$$\text{Flow (cardiac output)} = \frac{\text{Pressure difference (MP-PCWP)}}{\text{Resistance (PVR)}}$$

---

### CAUSES OF CHANGE IN VASCULAR RESISTANCE

**Increased pulmonary vascular resistance**

Hypoxemia
Hypercarbia
Acidosis
High mean airway pressure
Sympathetic stimulation (alpha)
Hypervolemia
Cough and laryngeal spasm
Crying and straining
$N_2O$ ? (in children with compromised myocardium)
Restriction of diaphragmatic movement from raised intra-abdominal pressure
Surgical manipulation of the heart and great vessels
Noxious stimuli

**Decreased pulmonary vascular resistance**

***Treatment of increased pulmonary vascular resistance***

Oxygenation
Hyperventilation
Alkalosis
Prostaglandins (PGE type)
α-Adrenergic antagonists
Vasodilators (nitroglycerin and nitroprusside)
β-2 stimulants (isoproterenol)
High $FIO_2$

**Increased systemic vascular resistance**

α-agonists
β-blockers
Cuff in the lower extremities
Increased intraabdominal pressure
Compression of the aorta

**Decreased systemic vascular resistance**

***Treatment of increased systemic vascular resistance***

Inhaled anesthetics
Vasodilators
- α-antagonists
- β stimulants
- $Ca^{++}$ channel blockers
- Nitroprusside
- Nitroglycerin
- Prostaglandins ($E_1$ and $E_2$)

---

MP, mean pressure; CVP, central venous pressure; PVR, pulmonary vascular resistance; SVR, systemic vascular resistance; PCWP, pulmonary capillary wedge pressure.

$$Q = \frac{P\Delta P \; \Pi \; r^4}{8 \; L \; n}$$

Q, blood flow (CO); PΔP, pressure difference; r, radius of the vascular conduit (heart defect); L,

### CLASSIFICATION OF CONGENITAL HEART DEFECTS

**Left to right shunts**

Patent ductus arteriosus
Atrial septal defects
Ventricular septal defects
Endocardial cushion defects

**Right to left shunts**

Truncus arteriosus
Tetralogy of Fallot
Transposition of great arteries
Anomalous pulmonary venous connection
Pulmonary stenosis and atresia with intact ventricular septum
Tricuspid atresia

**Obstructive lesions**

Coarctation of the aorta
Aortic stenosis and other lesions of left ventricular outflow obstruction
Pulmonary stenosis and other lesions of right ventricular outflow obstruction

**Miscellaneous deformities**

Double outlet right ventricle
Ebstein's anomaly
Anomalous systemic venous connection
Mitral valve prolapse syndrome
Coronary arterial anomalies

length of the vascular conduit; n, viscosity of the blood.

### Viscosity

According to Hagen-Poiseuille's law, viscosity increases vascular resistance and decreases the blood flow across the shunt. A variety of factors such as hematocrit, plasma proteins, and temperature increase viscosity.

***Hematocrit.*** The viscosity of blood is highly dependent on hematocrit. In large vessels an increase in hematocrit causes an appreciable increase in viscosity. However, in vessels smaller than 100 μm in diameter (arterioles, capillaries, and venules), the change in viscosity per unit change in hematocrit is much less than it is in large blood vessels. Plasma skimming may be the reason the hematocrit in these small resistance vessels is about 25% lower than the whole body hematocrit. The yield stress or tendency of blood to aggregate increases substantially with an increase in hematocrit. Viscosity doubles from 1.8 to 3.6 when hematocrit increases from 20% to 45%. The viscosity of blood increases substantially when hematocrit is above 40%.

***Plasma proteins.*** Proteins have less impact on viscosity than does hematocrit. Of all the plasma proteins only fibrinogen and γ-globulins significantly influence viscosity.

***Temperature.*** It is estimated that viscosity increases 5% for each 1° C decrease in temperature.

### CLASSIFICATION OF CONGENITAL HEART DEFECTS BASED ON THE CHARACTERISTICS OF PULMONARY BLOOD FLOW

**Increased pulmonary blood flow**

Atrial septal defect
Ventricular septal defect
Transposition of great arteries
Patent ductus arteriosus
AV canal
Single ventricle
Truncus arteriosus

**Decreased pulmonary blood flow**

Tetralogy of Fallot
Pulmonary atresia
Pulmonary stenosis
Ebstein's anomaly
Tricuspid atresia

## HYPOTHERMIA AND CONGENITAL HEART DISEASE

A decrease in body temperature in children with CHD is usually associated with an increase in arterial oxygen pressure and oxygen saturation. This is clearly desirable when deliberate cooling for heart surgery is executed. There are several reasons for increased oxygenation with cooling:

- Hypothermia reduces oxygen consumption.
- Hypothermia increases mixed venous oxygen tension as a result of decreased oxygen consumption; right to left shunt in turn will have less impact on arterial oxygen pressure when venous oxygen pressure is increased.
- Hypothermia shifts the oxygen dissociation curve, or P50, to the left (at any given oxygen pressure hemoglobin is saturated with more oxygen).
- Hypothermia increases systemic vascular resistance, which will reduce right to left shunt.

However, in the absence of adequate anesthesia and muscle paralysis oxygen consumption will actually increase and oxygen saturation and oxygen pressure will decrease because of increased metabolic

**PERIOPERATIVE COMPLICATIONS FROM HEMATOCRIT IN EXCESS OF 60%**[5,10,18,39,51,53,67,71]

Increased blood viscosity
Increased vascular resistance
Cerebral thrombosis and stroke
Renal and other organ thrombosis
Coagulopathies
Thrombocytopenia
Clotting of the shunts (grafts)

rate both from nonshivering and shivering mechanisms.

## HEMATOCRIT AND CONGENITAL HEART DISEASE

Monitoring of hematocrit levels is important in children with CHD. Both high and low hematocrit levels are frequently associated with certain neurologic complications ranging from minor headaches to major cerebrovascular accidents.[6,49,53] If the hematocrit exceeds 60%, phlebotomy and an exchange transfusion with a plasma substitute will improve cardiovascular status, reduce peripheral sledging, and improve the coagulation status of the patient perioperatively (box).[16,33,34,41,57,72] On the other hand, patients with a hematocrit below 30% are prone to develop signs of congestive heart failure as well as worsening of hypoxemia and acidosis.[6,49,53]

## CARDIAC DYSRHYTHMIAS

The etiology of cardiac dysrhythmias in children with CHD can be congenital, iatrogenic, or disease-induced (ischemic). Preoperative optimization of these dysrhythmias with appropriate antidysrhythmic agents or a pacemaker is important for the safe management of the patient. Maintenance of normal blood electrolyte levels is also essential for effective drug action and proper function of implantable pacemakers.

## PATHOPHYSIOLOGY OF CONGENITAL HEART DEFECTS

The correct diagnosis of the commonly occurring congenital heart defects such as patent ductus arteriosus (PDA), atrial septal defect (ASD), ventricular septal defect (VSD), and coarctation of the aorta may not be apparent in the first few days of life. Once the PVR is decreased and/or PDA is closed, the signs and symptoms of the CHD are revealed. When in doubt, especially when there are other associated systemic congenital anomalies, a pediatric cardiology consult and an echocardiographic evaluation of the heart are recommended.

A clear understanding of the pathophysiology of CHDs is very important for the optimal management of a child suffering these conditions. Experts in pediatric cardiac anesthesia believe that the pathophysiology of CHD is best clarified by classifying the lesions as simple shunt lesions, complex shunt lesions, and obstructive lesions.

### Simple shunt lesions

In general the amount and direction of shunting depend on the difference between the systemic and pulmonary vascular resistances, pressure difference across the two sides (atrial pressures in ASD, ventricular pressures in VSD, and pulmonary and aorta pressures in PDA), and the size (radius) of the defect. In cases of large cardiac defects (large ASD and VSD) a pressure gradient essentially does not exist, and shunting across the defect is primarily governed by the ratio of pulmonary and systemic vascular resistance. This is a nonrestrictive shunt. On the other hand, if the cardiac defect is smaller, the shunt across the defect is primarily influenced by the size of the lesion, and the ratio of PVR and SVR will play only a minor role. This is a restrictive shunt. The anesthetic management of children with nonrestrictive lesions is more difficult than with restrictive lesions, as anesthesia and surgery mainly influence the ratio of PVR and SVR and not the size of the lesion.

### Complex shunt lesions

In complex shunt lesions there is usually partial or complete obstruction of the outflow tracts in addition to the defect between the two chambers (e.g., ASD or VSD). The partial obstruction may be either dynamic or fixed. An example of a dynamic obstruction is tetralogy of Fallot, and an example of a fixed obstruction is pulmonary valvular stenosis. In these situations there is decreased pulmonary blood flow and a right to left shunt in spite of a low PVR. The pulmonary blood flow varies according to the extent of the obstruction. Finally, when there is complete obstruction in the outflow tracts (e.g., pulmonary atresia, tricuspid atresia, aortic atresia, interrupted aortic arch), flow through the defect (PDA, ASD, and VSD) depends primarily on the pressure difference across the defect. The ratio of PVR to SVR also influences the flow across the defect to a certain extent. This again depends on the size of the defect.

### Right to left shunt

Right to left shunting causes systemic hypoxemia and left ventricular volume overload. Cardiac shunting can occur at various levels of the heart and great vessels, including atrial level (foramen ovale or atrial septal defect), ventricular level (ventricular septal defect), and great arterial level (PDA or aortopulmonary window).

Shunting at all three levels can cause left ventricular volume overload. Shunting at the level of the great arteries only causes hypoxemia of the blood that goes to the lower body, thus sparing the heart, upper body, and brain. Slight to moderate hypoxemia is usually well tolerated by the neonate for short duration. Acute severe hypoxemia is usually not well tolerated because of the acidosis from inadequate oxygenation of the body organs, leading to cardiovascular collapse.[38] A child with a right to left shunt compensates for chronic hypoxemia mainly by a high hematocrit (oxygen carrying capacity), increased total blood volume, neovascularization, and hyperventilation. However, hematocrit in excess of 60% is known to cause an increased tendency toward renal and cerebral thromboembolic phenomena, increased blood viscosity and vascular resistance, increased incidence of coagulopathies, and decreased cardiopulmonary reserve.* It is generally recommended that surgery be postponed if the hematocrit is higher than 60% to correct to a lower level and avoid the perioperative complications.

### Left to right shunt

A left to right shunt causes volume overload not only to the right side of the heart but also to the left ventricle, leading to congestive heart failure. In addition, a left to right shunt can cause hypoperfusion of the vital organs leading to hypoxia and acidosis. Renal and hepatic perfusion may be compromised at times, leading to less than optimal handling of drug metabolism and excretion in these children. Gastrointestinal hypoperfusion is thought to be responsible for causing necrotizing enterocolitis in certain patients with a left to right shunt.[3,21] A diastolic steal of blood from the intestines to the pulmonary artery is also considered one of the mechanisms for necrotizing enterocolitis in patients with PDA.[44] Another effect of left to right shunt is decreased lung compliance and pulmonary reserve, and increased work of breathing. If uncorrected, a left to right shunt causes increased pulmonary blood flow and pulmonary hypertension resulting in pulmonary vascular obstructive disease (PVOD). Eventually this leads to reversal of the shunt (right to left shunt, or Eisenmenger's syndrome).

*References 5, 6, 10, 16, 18, 33, 39, 49, 51, 53, 67, 71, 72

**Table 10–2** Recommended induction doses of intravenous drugs and inhalational agents

| Agent | Dose/concentration |
|---|---|
| Ketamine (IM) | 4-6 mg/kg |
| Ketamine (IV) | 1-2 mg/kg |
| Sodium thiopental (IV) | 4-5 mg/kg |
| Midazolam (IV) | 25-75 μg/kg |
| Fentanyl (IV) | 7.5-15 μg/kg |
| Sufentanil (IV) | 5-10 μg/kg |
| Halothane | <1.5% |
| Sevoflurane | <2% |
| Nitrous oxide | <70% |

### Left ventricular outflow obstruction

Left ventricular outflow obstruction may be found as perivalvular aortic stenosis (at the valvular, subvalvular, or supravalvular level), coarctation of the aorta (at preductal, intraductal, or postductal level) or in severe cases as complete interruption in the aortic arch. Infants with left ventricular outflow obstruction may have signs and symptoms of low cardiac output syndrome (syncope and fatigue) or signs and symptoms of coronary ischemia (angina and dysrhythmias).[1] Chest x-ray film may reveal left ventricular enlargement, and ECG may show dysrhythmias and/or ischemic changes. These patients' left ventricular reserve is usually marginal, and they are particularly predisposed to ventricular fibrillation. They usually benefit from heavy premedication. Anesthetic management of these patients should consist of the measures that will decrease myocardial oxygen demand and increase oxygen supply. Detailed management of these patients is discussed in Chapters 24 and 25.

### Right ventricular outflow obstruction

Right ventricular outflow obstruction may result from either pulmonary atresia or perivalvular pulmonary stenosis. Infants with right ventricular outflow obstruction may have signs and symptoms of right ventricular hypertrophy, decreased pulmonary blood flow, hypoxemia, and acidosis. Chest x-ray film and ECG may reveal RV and LV enlargement and may show dysrhythmias and/or RV ischemic changes. RV reserve is usually very marginal in these patients, and they are particularly predisposed to acute RV failure. These patients usually benefit from adequate premedication. Anesthetic management should consist of the measures that will decrease PVR (see box on p. 121). Detailed management of the patients with particular malformations is discussed in Chapters 19 and 22.

**PREVENTION AND TREATMENT OF A HYPERCYANOTIC SPELL**

**Prevention**

A Prevent *a*cidosis
B Continue *b*eta blockers
C Avoid *c*rying and anxiety
D Avoid *d*rugs that decrease SVR
E Avoid *e*xcessive airway pressures
F Maintain adequate *f*luid status

**Treatment**

A *A*irway management
  Maintain the airway
  Hyperventilation
  Increase $FIO_2$
B *B*icarbonate to treat metabolic acidosis
C *C*ompression
  Abdomen before the commencement of surgery
  Aorta during the surgery
D *D*rugs
  Increase the depth of anesthesia
  Beta blockers
    propranolol (5-10 μg/kg, IV)
    esmolol (500 μg/kg, IV)
  Phenylephrine (1-2 μg/kg, IV)
E *E*liminate the stimulus
  Surgical compression of the PA or vena cava
  Stop surgery until adequately anesthetized
F *F*luids (maintain preload)

## OTHER CAUSES OF CYANOSIS

Worsening of hypoxemia in a patient with CHD need not necessarily result from the underlying heart lesion. These other causes must be kept in mind and should be systematically checked:

Endobronchial intubation
Obstruction in the endotracheal tube (Kink, secretions)
Pneumothorax (central line placement)
Pulmonary edema
Pulmonary embolism (air and other debris)
Airway spasm
Hypoventilation (restricted diaphragm)
Decreased cardiac output
Sudden change in vascular resistance
Drugs (inadvertent stoppage of prostaglandin drip)
Surgical interference or stimulation

For example, a right endobronchial intubation in a CHD patient undergoing a right thoracotomy could be calamitous. Endotracheal position could be extremely important in patients with CHD whose arterial oxygen pressure is already low. Once other causes are ruled out, the hypercyanotic spell should be promptly treated, as described in the box.

## PALLIATIVE OPERATIONS TO REGULATE PULMONARY BLOOD FLOW

Children with CHD who have inadequate pulmonary blood flow (lesions associated with pulmonary stenosis or atresia, tricuspid stenosis, or atresia) require palliative surgery in the form of a systemic to pulmonary shunt until corrective surgery can be performed. When there is excessive pulmonary blood flow, banding of the pulmonary artery can reduce its blood flow and may prevent PVOD. These operations (Fig. 10–1) are frequently performed to regulate pulmonary blood flow:

Blalock-Taussig shunt (classic BT shunt): right subclavian artery to right pulmonary artery
Modified Blalock-Taussig shunt: left subclavian artery to left pulmonary artery with Gore-Tex
Glenn shunt: superior vena cava to right pulmonary artery
Pott's shunt: descending aorta to left pulmonary artery
Waterston shunt: ascending aorta to right pulmonary artery
Blalock-Hanlon operation: creation of an ASD by surgical atrial septectomy
Brock procedure: pulmonary valvotomy
Pulmonary artery banding

The perioperative usage of prostaglandin $E_1$ and $E_2$ infusions (since the mid 1970s) has dramatically improved the survival and surgical mortality of these patients.[20,50,63]

## ANESTHESIA MANAGEMENT

### Preoperative assessment

Preoperative evaluation of a patient with CHD should include a thorough history, including past and present medications and physical examination; laboratory tests including chest x-ray film, ECG, echocardiogram, catheterization data, hemoglobin, glucose, and electrolyte status; any previous surgery; and pediatric cardiologist consult note (box on p. 127).

History and physical examination will reveal signs and symptoms of left to right shunt (congestive heart failure), right to left shunt (acute or chronic hypoxemia, and recurrent infections), or left ventricular outflow obstructive disease (poor exercise tolerance and failure to thrive). It is also important to evaluate cardiac and pulmonary reserves.

A chest roentgenogram reveals the size of the heart, any pleural effusions, signs of pulmonary congestion, or infection. An ECG gives information on rate and rhythm, conduction abnormalities,

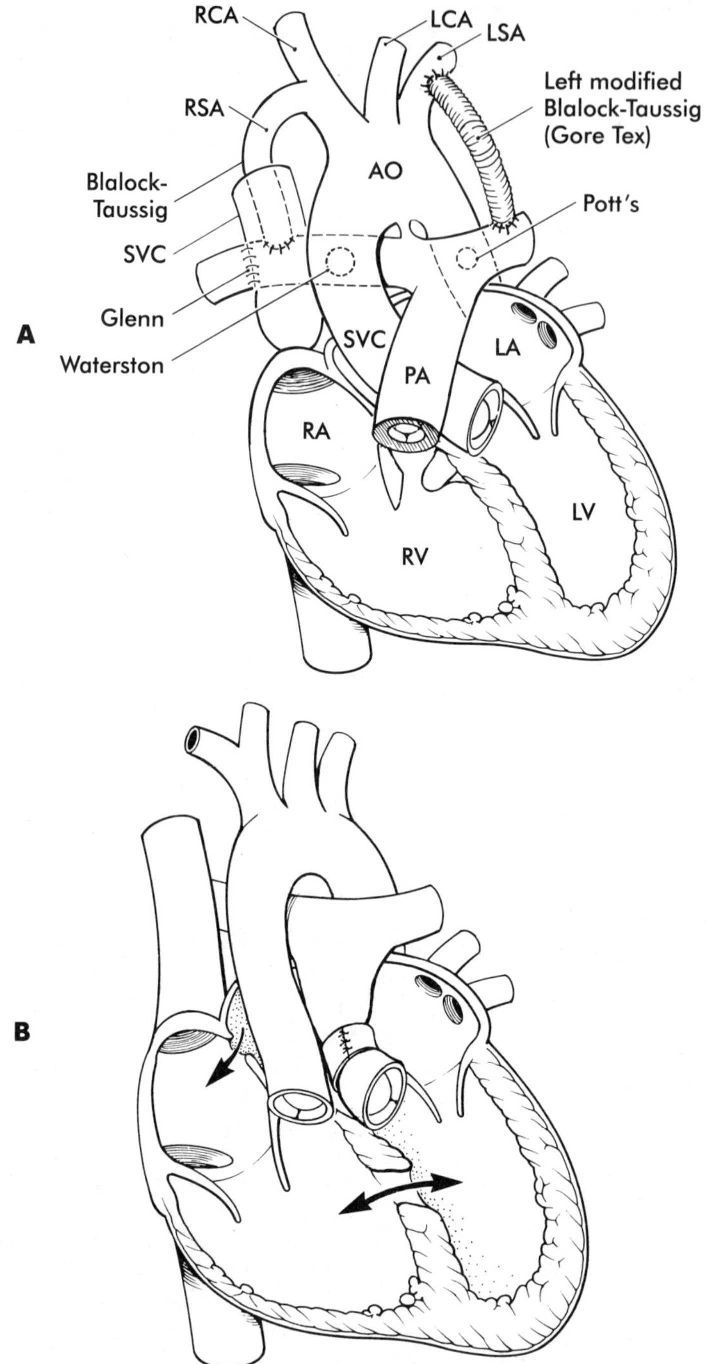


**Figure 10–1** **A,** Various palliative procedures that can be used in patients who have congenital heart disease with a decreased pulmonary blood flow. **B,** Pulmonary artery banding procedure to reduce the pulmonary blood flow.

**INFORMATION NECESSARY FOR THE OPTIMAL ANESTHETIC MANAGEMENT OF A PATIENT WITH CONGENITAL HEART DISEASE AND TO PREDICT THE PERIOPERATIVE RISKS**

Cardiac status
- Type of defect including history of palliative and/or corrective surgery
- Pressures and saturations in cardiac chambers and the great arteries
- Preload; SVR; PVR; HR; right and left ventricular inotropy
- Ventricular outflow pressure gradient

Status of other body systems

Type of shunt: right to left or left to right or poor mixing

Cardiac output
- Pulmonary blood flow ($Q_p$)
- Systemic blood flow ($Q_s$)
- Ratio of $Q_p$ to $Q_s$

Hematocrit and electrolytes

Antibiotic prophylaxis

Present and past medication

chamber hypertrophy, and coronary ischemia if any are present.

Echocardiogram and cardiac catheterization data will usually confirm the diagnosis or reveal new information. Both of these will provide information on ventricular function, on the amount and direction of shunt across the cardiac defect, and on the pressure and oxygen saturation gradients in all heart chambers and great arteries. The latter information usually identifies the children who are at increased risk for both cardiac and noncardiac surgery. Children with arterial oxygen saturation of less than 75%, hematocrit of more than 60%, ventricular outflow tract gradient of more than 50 mm Hg, pulmonary to systemic blood flow ratio of more than 2, or increased pulmonary vascular resistance are at high risk from surgery.[23]

### Prophylactic antibiotic therapy

Patients with CHD, with very few exceptions, should be given appropriate prophylactic antibiotic drugs to prevent infective bacterial endocarditis. A detailed discussion of this topic can be found in Chapter 9.

### Preoperative preparation

Based on the patient's history, the anesthesiologist should have a plan for induction, monitoring, maintenance, and postoperative management of a patient with CHD. Preparation of the drugs, including all the appropriate cardiac drugs and calculation of all the doses in advance are absolute necessities in all cases. Many of these drugs are routinely given by infusion. It is easy to make an error when calculating doses for small children. One way to remember how to calculate the infusion rate is as follows: the infusion rate in milliliters per hour is body weight in kilograms and the concentration of the drug in a bag or syringe in either micrograms or milligrams per milliliter.

Formulas for calculation of a drug infusion setting in milliliters per hour:

$$1\ \mu g/kg/min = \frac{\text{Body weight in kilograms} \times 60}{\text{Concentration of the drug in the bottle in } \mu g/ml}$$

$$1\ mg/kg/min = \frac{\text{Body weight in kilograms} \times 60}{\text{Concentration of the drug in the bottle in mg/ml}}$$

### Preoperative sedation

With a few exceptions, children with congenital heart defects should be brought to the operating room adequately sedated. The type of preoperative medication depends on the child's age, type of operation, and type of heart defect. In general for children under 6 months of age with noncardiac disease it is recommended not to give any preoperative medications. However, I frequently give preoperative medications even for children under 6 months of age who have cardiac defects because they frequently begin to cry vigorously as soon as they are brought into a cold operating room and feel the monitors being applied. Excessive crying, straining, hiccoughing, and breath holding at the time of induction can lead to an increase in pulmonary vascular resistance, an increased right to left shunt, and worsening of hypoxemia. In children with a ventricular outflow tract obstruction, excessive crying can also provoke a spasm leading to cyanosis or decrease in cardiac output. Cough and laryngeal spasm in unsedated children may lead to the use of excessive positive pressure ventilation, which in turn can cause increased pulmonary vascular resistance. Even in patients with left to right shunt, an increase in right-sided pressures can shift this shunt to a right to left shunt in these situations. At the same time, sedation to a point where ventilation and oxygenation are affected should be avoided. Once these children are sedated, close monitoring of their ventilation and oxygenation is essential. Sedation can best be performed in the intensive care unit or in the holding room, where monitoring is available several minutes before the scheduled operation time.

Other advantages of preoperative sedation of a child are that it helps reduce the dose requirement of an inhalational anesthetic, eases separation from

**Table 10–3** Times of onset and main routes of administration of some commonly used preoperative medicant drugs

| Drug | Recommended dose | Onset time (min) |
|---|---|---|
| Midazolam | | |
| Oral (mg/kg) | 0.50-0.75 | 15-20 |
| NTM (mg/kg) | 0.20-0.25 | 15-20 |
| Rectal (mg/kg) | 1.0-1.5 | 10-15 |
| Fentanyl | | |
| OTM (μg/kg) | 15-20 | 10-15 |
| Sufentanil | | |
| NTM (μg/kg) | 1.5-3.0 | 10-15 |
| Morphine | | |
| IM (mg/kg) | 0.10-0.15 | 30-45 |
| Meperidine | | |
| IM (mg/kg) | 1-2 | 30-45 |
| Methohexital | | |
| Rectal (mg/kg) | 20-25 | 10-15 |
| Ketamine | | |
| Oral (mg/kg) | 5-7 | 10-20 |
| Sodium thiopental | | |
| Rectal (mg/kg) | 30-35 | 15-20 |

OTM, oral transmucosal; NTM, nasal transmucosal; IM, intramuscular.

the child's parents, reduces induction time, and smooths induction of anesthesia.

The type and route of preoperative medicant vary widely from one hospital to another. Preoperative medication can be given via parenteral, oral, oral transmucosal, nasal transmucosal, and rectal routes (Table 10–3). Recently oral administration of benzodiazepines has gained popularity.

## Monitoring

The extent of perioperative monitoring should be based on a combination of factors including the child's overall physical status, the type of cardiac defect, and the type of surgical procedure proposed. Minimal basic monitoring in all children with CHD, irrespective of whether they are undergoing cardiac or noncardiac surgery, should include a noninvasive blood pressure device, ECG, temperature probe, pulse oximeter, and end tidal carbon dioxide pressure. A Foley catheter for monitoring urine output is routine for all open heart cases and certain closed and noncardiac procedures. In children undergoing noncardiac surgery the anesthesiologist should carefully consider more extensive invasive monitoring. The type of surgery and CHD should usually dictate necessary monitoring for a given patient. Remember that such children usually require multiple redo cardiac surgical procedures, and most of those procedures demand extensive invasive monitoring. In other words, the anesthesiologist should avoid placement of arterial and central lines by cut-down procedures where the lines are not absolutely necessary for the optimal management of a patient. However, if extensive invasive monitoring is necessary, as dictated by the combination of factors mentioned above, then an experienced person should place the lines to minimize the use of multiple sites in attempts at placement.

***Pulse oximeter.*** Monitoring of oxygen saturation with a pulse oximeter has become one of the standards of modern anesthesia practice. The site of monitoring can be influenced by the presence of a right to left shunt and by previous surgery involving aorta or subclavian arteries. For example, in patients with PDA and coarctation of the aorta or interrupted aortic arch, oxygen saturations in the left upper extremity and the rest of the lower body are different from those in right upper extremity and in cerebral and retinal saturations. I recommend placement of an oximeter probe in the right upper extremity in children who have PDA, who have undergone left Blalock-Taussig shunt procedure, or who are undergoing repair of coarctation of the aorta, PDA, or left Blalock-Taussig shunt. In children who are undergoing or have undergone right Blalock-Taussig shunt, one should not monitor oxygen saturation in the right upper extremity. Finally, in children who have undergone bilateral Blalock-Taussig shunts, one should not monitor oxygen saturation in either the left or right upper extremity. In children with cyanotic congenital heart disease a pulse oximeter reading may not be accurate, especially when the hemoglobin saturation is less than 80%.[60,69] The accuracy of an oximeter reading depends on the model of pulse oximeter and type of the patient's hemoglobin. For example, the presence of HbF overestimates the true hemoglobin saturation. Generally, in children with an excess of 30% right to left shunt, increasing inspired concentration of oxygen has very little effect on arterial oxygen pressure and saturation. An increase in cardiac output (provided the shunt fraction is unchanged) should increase arterial oxygen pressure and saturation. An increase in cardiac output increases venous oxygen pressure and venous saturation and thus increases arterial oxygen pressure and arterial saturation. A decrease in metabolic rate (anesthesia and hypothermia) will have the same effect on these saturations.

***End tidal $P_{CO_2}$.*** End tidal carbon dioxide pressure can give an accurate estimation of the arterial carbon dioxide pressure in children with acyanotic CHD. However, in children with cyanotic CHDs, end tidal carbon dioxide pressure underestimates the arterial carbon dioxide pressure.[4,37] A decrease in pulmonary blood flow and an increase in dead space ventilation is the reason for this underestimation in cyanotic CHD.

***Blood pressure.*** All children requiring cardiopulmonary bypass for their surgical procedure need an arterial line placement for pressure monitoring as well as for blood gas and other lab monitoring. But not all children with CHD undergoing noncardiac or closed cardiac surgical procedures necessarily need an arterial line placement. The location of monitors can be important in patients with certain CHDs. Follow the guidelines described in the section on the pulse oximeter for their placement in children with CHD. Place the blood pressure cuff on the right arm or insert an arterial cannula into the right radial or right temporal artery for pressure monitoring and sampling of blood gases in a patient with PDA, with or without coarctation of the aorta. On the other hand, do not use the right arm for blood pressure monitoring in children who have undergone or in patients who are undergoing a right BT shunt.

***Central venous lines.*** All patients undergoing cardiac surgery with cardiopulmonary bypass should have a central line placed. This line will be used both for monitoring central pressures and for drug infusions (isoproterenol, epinephrine, etc.). It requires sound judgment, based on all the facts available, to determine whether or not a central line is necessary for patients undergoing a closed cardiac or noncardiac surgical operation. Do not approach CVP line placement by a subclavian stick on the proposed side for the palliative shunt because a subclavian hematoma may make the operation technically troublesome.

***Arterial blood gases.*** Frequent arterial blood gas evaluations to verify proper ventilation and oxygenation and to treat metabolic acidosis are essential in the management of many pediatric heart patients undergoing corrective surgical procedures. Metabolic acidosis results from a decrease in cardiac output or an increase in right to left shunt with hypoxemia and hypoxia of various body organs. If uncorrected, severe metabolic acidosis will cause further deterioration and cardiac collapse. As with the pulse oximeter, the site of placement of the arterial line is important both for pressure monitoring and for measurement of arterial blood gases.

***Glucose, electrolytes, and hematocrit.*** Along with blood gases, frequent hematocrit, glucose and electrolyte determinations are necessary in the safe management of children with CHD, especially the sicker neonates.

## Fluid and blood replacement

More information on fluid and ventricular contractility status is available during a cardiac operation than during any other surgical procedure. One can directly see the chamber sizes and the contractile state of the individual ventricles In addition, the surgeon can feel the pressures in the pulmonary artery and aorta. Various invasive monito[illegible] oratory values, and urine output are readily a[illegible] able for continuous evaluation of fluid and electro[illegible] lyte balance and contractile status of the heart. In spite of all these monitoring devices, it is easy to fluid-overload a patient with CHD because of the body size and the drugs, infusions, blood, and blood products that are involved with most complex procedures. Any extra burden to an already compromised heart may be very deleterious. Fresh banked blood is always preferable in children with CHD, as fresh blood is less acidotic and less hyperkalemic and has higher P50 values than old banked blood.

In general, in smaller and sicker children, 5% or 10% dextrose in electrolyte solution is recommended for maintenance. A balanced electrolyte solution without glucose can be used in children over 1 month old. Excessive blood levels of glucose may be harmful to the cerebral function if there are periods of hypoperfusion to the brain. There is evidence to suggest that hyperglycemia will worsen neurologic outcome in animal models associated with complete or near-complete ischemia.[2,48,55,61]

## General precautions

***Bradycardia.*** In contrast to adults, children with CHD usually display bradycardia in response to many perioperative common insults such as hypoxemia, hypercarbia, metabolic acidosis, and hypotension with a decreased cardiac output. In these infants bradycardia is a grave warning sign that may herald cardiac arrest if not corrected promptly.

***Blood and fluid warmer.*** Blood should be administered via some kind of warming device. A rapid push of blood (especially cold blood) or blood products into a small neonate whose left ventricular end diastolic volume is only about a few milliliters can cause bradycardia, decreased inotropy, ischemia, and dysrhythmias. This is especially true if the banked blood is not fresh, as the older the blood gets, the more acidotic and hyperkalemic it becomes.

***Air bubbles.*** In all cases of communication between the right and left sides of the heart, it is absolutely essential that all intravenous tubings be free of air bubbles. In addition, use extra caution not to push any air bubbles when injecting drugs or blood and blood products through an IV line. Air bubbles can reach cerebral, coronary, and other vital organs as emboli and can cause organ dysfunction. There is great need of some kind of effective air filter to prevent this problem.

***Blood filters.*** Routine use of blood filters is also recommended whenever a child with CHD receives transfusion of blood or its products, as microaggregates and other particulate matter can travel he circulation. Just like air s can lodge in vital organs ise organ dysfunction and

***ion.*** In patients who will e in temperature is allowed ... of bypass. A decrease in temperature not only decreases oxygen consumption and systemic hypoxemia but also increases SVR. An increase in SVR may be beneficial, especially in patients with right to left shunt, as this will reduce the shunt. However, once these children are weaned from ECC, it is important to maintain body temperature near normal levels to avoid postoperative coagulation problems.

## NITROUS OXIDE AND CHD

Data from several studies in adult patients suggest that nitrous oxide when used in combination with narcotics produces myocardial depression, a decrease in cardiac index and systemic blood pressure, and an increase in pulmonary vascular resistance.[9,28,36,40,42,43,45,59] These studies also show that increases in PVR in adult patients will vary according to the baseline PVR. It is concluded from these studies that nitrous oxide produces a slight increase in PVR in adult patients with a normal baseline PVR and a large increase in patients with elevated baseline PVR. In contrast, Hickey et al[24] have shown in children with CHD that pulmonary arterial pressure and PVR were not significantly changed by administration of 50% nitrous oxide in either the group with normal PVR or the group with elevated PVR.[24] Although nitrous oxide does not have adverse hemodynamic effects in children with CHD, many pediatric cardiac anesthesiologists are using it less frequently in children with CHD for the fear of causing expansion of any accidentally introduced intravascular air bubbles. Also, nitrous oxide is contraindicated in children with severely compromised myocardium because it depresses myocardium to a much greater extent in these children.[43]

## KETAMINE AND CHD

Ketamine is known to increase heart rate, systemic blood pressure, and PVR in adult patients.[14,62,66,70] It is concluded from the studies conducted during catheterization as well as during the early postoperative period that hemodynamic alterations, especially pulmonary vascular resistance index, are small in infants with CHD regardless of their baseline PVR.[26] Because ketamine produces favorable hemodynamic effects in children with CHD, it is frequently used (both intramuscularly and intravenously) as an induction agent in these children.

## IMPLICATIONS FOR ANESTHESIA IN A PATIENT WITH RIGHT TO LEFT SHUNT

Avoid factors that increase pulmonary vascular resistance in the presence of a right to left shunt. Also, pay utmost attention to ventilation and oxygenation along with the other measures mentioned in the box on p. 121, which may be necessary to reduce the PVR and right to left shunt. The correct placement of the endotracheal tube is very important in these patients. Since their oxygen status is marginal to start with, it is absolutely necessary to make sure that the tracheal tube is not advanced too far down into one of the bronchi. Also, I routinely reintubate the trachea if it has been intubated for more than 12 hours, as many tubes gradually block with mucus during the operation. Recent data from several investigators suggest in general that a number of induction techniques such as IM and IV ketamine, IV narcotics, and halothane with or without nitrous oxide can be used safely in the management of a child with cyanotic CHD (Tables 10–2 and 10–4).* Unlike in adult patients, both nitrous oxide and ketamine have been shown to have no adverse effects on the pulmonary vasculature in young children with CHD. However, choose an optimal technique for a particular cardiac defect based on the preoperative evaluation. For example, in a patient with right to left shunt in whom a decrease in SVR may further increase shunt, use of isoflurane as a main anesthetic agent may not be unsafe but at the same time is not optimal. In general, for quite sick children with poor ventricular function, induction with IV ketamine and/or IV narcotics has been shown to be safe and effective. In these children all inhalational agents, including nitrous oxide, have been shown to depress myocardium and reduce systemic blood pressure to a greater degree than ketamine or narcotics.[22,73] An anesthesiologist should have a thorough knowledge of the pathophysiology of all the cardiac lesions and should be able to predict the effects of various anesthetics and ventilation techniques on the hemodynamic stability of these patients. Then only can he or she select a technique that is optimal for a particular patient.

### Effect of right to left shunt on uptake, distribution, and induction of inhaled anesthetics

Uptake and distribution of inhaled anesthetic agents are influenced by ventilation, cardiac output, blood gas partition coefficient of the anesthetic agent, presence of a right to left shunt ($Q_s$), and other

---

*References 15, 17, 19, 22, 24, 25, 35, 73

**Table 10–4** Recommended doses of narcotics and concentrations of inhalational anesthetic agents for cardiac and noncardiac surgery

| Agent | Maintenance dose (total dose for narcotics) | | |
|---|---|---|---|
| | Cardiac (bypass) | Cardiac (closed) | Noncardiac |
| Fentanyl (μg/kg) | 75-100 | 10-50 | 10-50 |
| Sufentanil (μg/kg) | 25-30 | 5-15 | 5-15 |
| Morphine (mg/kg) | 1.5-2.0 | – | – |
| Halothane (%) | | | |
| Alone | 0.75-1.00 | 0.75-1.00 | 0.75-1.00 |
| As an adjuvant | 0.25-0.50 | 0.25-0.50 | 0.25-0.50 |
| Isoflurane (%) | | | |
| Alone | 1.0-1.5 | 1.0-1.5 | 1.0-1.5 |
| As an adjuvant | 0.50-0.75 | 0.50-0.75 | 0.50-0.75 |
| Enflurane (%) | | | |
| Alone | 1.0-1.5 | 1.0-1.5 | 1.0-1.5 |
| As an adjuvant | 0.50-0.75 | 0.50-0.75 | 0.50-0.75 |
| Desflurane (%) | | | |
| Alone | 4-6 | 4-6 | 4-6 |
| As an adjuvant | 1-3 | 1-3 | 1-3 |
| Sevoflurane (%) | | | |
| Alone | 1.5-2.0 | 1.5-2.0 | 1.5-2.0 |
| As an adjuvant | 0.50-0.75 | 0.50-0.75 | 0.50-0.75 |
| Nitrous oxide (%)* | <70 | <70 | <70 |

*Always used as an adjuvant to either narcotic or inhalational anesthetic agent.

factors. While ventilation and cardiac output have a remarkable effect on the uptake of soluble anesthetic agents, they have only limited effect on the uptake of insoluble anesthetic agents. On the other hand, a right to left shunt should theoretically prolong the uptake and induction time of insoluble anesthetics (nitrous oxide, desflurane, and sevoflurane) and shorten the onset of intravenous anesthetics. The least effect should be seen with the most soluble anesthetics (diethyl ether and cyclopropane) and intermediate results with the intermediate soluble anesthetics (isoflurane, halothane, and enflurane).[8,64] These conclusions were made from a dog study in which a 50% $Q_s$ was assumed. However, many patients, including children with CHD who come for surgery and anesthesia, have less than 30% $Q_s$. Clinical data to support this theory have not yet been presented, but the computerized models somewhat support it.[31,65] Kambam and King[31] have used a simple computer program to determine the effects of up to 90% of $Q_s$ on the uptake of various inhaled anesthetic agents, including the least soluble agents, nitrous oxide, desflurane, and sevoflurane; most soluble agent, diethyl ether; and the intermediately soluble agents, isoflurane, enflurane, and halothane. Table 10–5 shows the results of this computer model. These computer-derived results show that in the presence of up to 30% $Q_s$ there should be a minimal overall effect on the speed of induction of general anesthesia with intermediate and least soluble agents, and with up to 60% $Q_s$ there should be negligible effects with a most soluble agent. Many pediatric cardiac anesthesiologists believe a right to left shunt slightly delays the induction time with commonly used inhaled anesthetics and is of little practical concern in the clinical setting.

**Table 10–5** Effect of right to left shunt on the uptake of various inhaled anesthetics

| | Uptake expressed as normalized percent | | | | |
|---|---|---|---|---|---|
| $Q_s$, % | N/D/S | I | E | H | DE |
| 0 | 100 | 100 | 100 | 100 | 100 |
| 10 | 93 | 96 | 96 | 97 | 99 |
| 20 | 85 | 91 | 92 | 93 | 98 |
| 30 | 77 | 85 | 87 | 89 | 97 |
| 40 | 69 | 78 | 81 | 83 | 95 |
| 50 | 60 | 71 | 74 | 77 | 93 |
| 60 | 49 | 62 | 65 | 69 | 90 |
| 70 | 39 | 51 | 54 | 59 | 85 |
| 80 | 27 | 38 | 41 | 45 | 77 |
| 90 | 14 | 21 | 24 | 27 | 59 |

N/D/S, nitrous oxide/desflurane/sevoflurane; E, enflurane; I, isoflurane; H, halothane; DE, diethylether.

**CONDITIONS THAT ARE KNOWN TO INCREASE LEFT TO RIGHT SHUNT**

Low hematocrit
Increased SVR
Decreased PVR
Hyperoxemia
Hyperventilation
Negative airway pressure

### Effect of right to left shunt on induction time of intravenous anesthetics

Theoretically, a right to left shunt should slightly accelerate the onset of intravenous anesthetics. Again there are really no clinical data to support or contradict this theory.

### Effect of dead space ventilation on induction time

Right to left intracardiac shunts are associated with an increase in dead space ventilation and a decrease in end tidal carbon dioxide pressure for a given arterial carbon dioxide pressure. In other words, in children with right to left shunts with a decreased pulmonary blood flow and increased dead space ventilation, there is a widening of the difference between arterial and end tidal carbon dioxide pressure. As long as adequate ventilation is maintained, an increase in dead space ventilation has no effect on the uptake and induction time of the inhaled anesthetics.[8] However, when dead space ventilation is increased and alveolar ventilation is inadequate as a result of an increased right to left shunt (decreased pulmonary blood flow), the induction time of most soluble anesthetics will be delayed, and intermediate and least soluble anesthetics will be least effected.

## IMPLICATIONS FOR ANESTHESIA IN A PATIENT WITH LEFT TO RIGHT SHUNT

In general, management of a patient with a left to right shunt is less of a problem than with right to left shunt. Again one should pay a great deal of attention to ventilation and oxygenation of these patients (box).

Hyperventilation and hyperoxemia should be avoided, as these can reduce pulmonary vascular resistance, leading to an increase in left to right shunt. On the other hand, hypoventilation and hypoxemia should also be avoided, as these can acutely revert a left to right shunt to a right to left shunt in a neonate. An increase in systemic vascular resistance can cause more shunting to the right side. One should also take air bubble and other embolism prevention measures, as left to right shunt can become a bidirectional shunt with anesthesia and operative manipulations.

**Table 10–6** Effects of shunts on uptake and induction time of halothane, enflurane, and isoflurane and onset time of sodium pentothal and ketamine[31,65]

| | Anesthesia induction time | |
|---|---|---|
| | **Inhaled** | **Intravenous** |
| **Right to left shunt** | | |
| Theoretic | Slow | Fast |
| Clinical concern | No | No |
| **Left to right shunt** | | |
| Theoretic | No | Slow |
| Clinical concern | No | No |
| **Mixed shunt** | | |
| Theoretic | Slightly prolonged | Slightly faster |
| Clinical concern | No | No |

### Effect of left to right shunt on uptake, distribution, and induction time of inhaled and intravenous anesthetics

A left to right shunt should not theoretically change the uptake and induction time of any inhaled anesthetics and should slightly prolong the onset of intravenous anesthetics (Table 10–6). Again there are really no clinical data to support or contradict this theory. Many pediatric cardiac anesthesiologists believe a left to right shunt is of little practical concern in the clinical setting when they use either type of anesthetic (Table 10–6).

## OBSTRUCTIVE LESIONS

Potent inhaled anesthetics may actually benefit patients with certain types of dynamic outflow obstructive defects (tetralogy of Fallot and idiopathic hypertrophic subaortic stenosis [IHSS]) because a slight decrease in myocardial contractility would actually increase the blood flow through the defect. Hypovolemia, light anesthesia, direct-acting inotropic drugs, and low SVR should be avoided in dynamic obstructive lesions, as these conditions aggravate the obstruction.

The same principles of pediatric cardiac anesthesia apply whether a child with CHD undergoes cardiac or noncardiac surgery. Understanding of pathophysiology, anatomy of CHD and cardiovascular pharmacology and last but not least experience with clinical pediatric cardiac anesthesia are essential for optimal anesthetic management of children with CHDs for either type of surgery.

## REFERENCES


1. Adams FH, Emmanouilides GC, Reimenschneider TA: *Moss' heart disease in infants, children and adolescents,* Baltimore, 1989, Williams & Wilkins.
2. Baughman VI, Hoffman WF, Thomas C et al: Neurologic outcome in aged rats after incomplete cerebral ischemia, *Anesth Analg* 67:677, 1988.
3. Bhat R, Fisher E, Raju TN et al: Patent ductus arteriosus: recent advances in diagnosis and management, *Pediatr Clin North Am* 29:1117, 1982.
4. Burrows FA: Physiological dead space, venous admixture, and the arterial to end-tidal carbon dioxide difference in infants and children undergoing cardiac surgery, *Anesthesiology* 70:219, 1989.
5. Colo-Otero G, Gilchrist GS, Holcomb GR et al: Preoperative evaluation of hemostasis in patients with congenital heart disease, *Mayo Clin Proc* 62:379, 1987.
6. Cottrill CM, Kaplan S: Cerebral vascular accidents in cyanotic congenital heart disease, *Am J Dis Child* 125:484, 1973.
7. Downing SE, Talner NS, Gardner TH: Ventricular function in the newborn lamb, *Am J Physiol* 208:931, 1964.
8. Eger EI: Uptake of inhaled anesthetics: The alveolar to inspired anesthetic difference: effect of ventilation/perfusion abnormalities. In Eger EI, editor: *Anesthetic Uptake and Action.* Baltimore, 1974, Williams & Wilkins.
9. Eisele JH, Smith NT: Cardiovascular effects of 40% nitrous oxide in man, *Anesth Analg* 51:956, 1972.
10. Ekert H, Gilchrist GS, Stanton R, et al: Hemostasis in cyanotic congenital heart disease, *J Pediatr* 76:221, 1970.
11. Emery JL, Mithal A: Weights of cardiac ventricles at and after birth, *Br Heart J* 23:313, 1961.
12. Fyler DC: Report of the New England regional infant cardiac program, *Pediatrics* 65:375, 1980.
13. Gentile R, Stevenson G, Dooley T et al: Noninvasive determination of time of ductal closure in normal newborn infants, *Pediatr Cardiol* 1:177, 1979.
14. Gooding JM, Dimick AR, Tavakoli M, et al: A physiologic analysis of cardiopulmonary responses to ketamine anesthesia in noncardiac patients, *Anesth Analg* 56:813, 1977.
15. Greeley WJ, Bushman GA, Davis DP et al: Comparative effects of halothane and ketamine on systemic arterial oxygen saturation in children with cyanotic congenital heart disease. *Anesthesiology* 65:666, 1986.
16. Gross S, Keffer V, Leibman J: The platelets in cyanotic congenital heart disease. *Pediatrics* 42:651, 1968.
17. Hansen DD, Hickey PR: Anesthesia for hypoplastic left heart syndrome: use of high-dose fentanyl in 30 neonates, *Anesth Analg* 65:127, 1986.
18. Henriksson P, Varendh G, Lundstrom N-R: Hemostasis defects in cyanotic congenital heart disease, *Br Heart J* 41:23, 1979.
19. Hensley FA, Larach DR, Martin DE et al: The effect of saturation in cyanotic heart disease, *Journal of Cardiothoracic Anesthesiology* 1:289, 1987.
20. Heymann MA, Rudolph AM, Silverman NH: Closure of the ductus arteriosus in premature infants by inhibition of prostaglandin synthesis, *N Engl J Med* 295:530, 1976.
21. Heymann MA: Patent ductus arteriosus. In Adams FH, Emmanouilides GC, editors: *Heart disease in infants, children and adolescents,* ed 3, Baltimore, 1968, Williams & Wilkins.
22. Hickey PR, Hansen DD, Wessel DL et al: Blunting of stress responses in the pulmonary circulation of infants, *Anesth Analg* 64:1137, 1985.
23. Hickey PR, Streitz S: Preoperative assessment of the patient with congenital heart disease. In Mangano DT, editor: *Preoperative cardiac assessment,* Philadelphia, 1990, JB Lippincott.
24. Hickey PR, Hansen DD, Straford M et al: Pulmonary and systemic effects of nitrous oxide in infants wit normal and elevated pulmonary vascular resistance, *Anesthesiology* 65:374, 1986.
25. Hickey PR, Hansen DD, Wessel DL et al: Pulmonary and systemic hemodynamic responses to fentanyl in infants, *Anesth Analg* 64:483, 1985.
26. Hickey PR, Hansen DD, Cramolini GM et al: Pulmonary and systemic hemodynamic responses to ketamine in infants with normal and elevated pulmonary and vascular resistance, *Anesthesiology* 62:287, 1985.
27. Hickey PR, Hansen DD, Norwood WI et al: Anesthetic complications in surgery for congenital heart disease, *Anesth Analg* 63:657, 1984.
28. Hilgenberg JC, McCammon RL, Stoelting RK: Pulmonary and systemic vascular responses to nitrous oxide in patients with mitral stenosis and pulmonary hypertension, *Anesth Analg* 59:323, 1980.
29. Hoffman JIE, Christianson R: Congenital heart disease in a cohort of 19,502 births with long-term follow-up, *Am J Cardiol* 42:641, 1978.
30. James LS, Rowe RD: The pattern of response of pulmonary and systemic arterial pressures in newborn and older infants to short periods of hypoxia, *J Pediatr* 51:5, 1957.
31. Kambam JR, King P: Effect of right to left cardiopulmonary shunt on the uptake and distribution of inhaled anesthetics. *Int J Clin Monit Comput* 8:169, 1991 (abstract).
32. Kirkpatrick SE, Pitlick PT, Naliboff J et al: Frank-Starling relationship as an important determination of fetal cardiac output, *Am J Physiol* 231:495, 1976.
33. Komp DM, Sparrow AW: Polycythemia in cyanotic heart disease: a study of altered coagulation, *J Pediatr* 76:231, 1980.
34. Kontras SB, Bodenbender JG, Cranen J et al: Hyperviscosity in congenital heart disease, *J Pediatr* 76:214, 1970.
35. Laishley RS, Burrows FA, Lerman J et al: Effect of anesthetic induction regimens on oxygen saturation in cyanotic congenital heart disease. *Anesthesiology* 65:673, 1986.
36. Lappas DG, Buckley MJ, Laver MB et al: Left ventricular performance and pulmonary circulation following administration of nitrous oxide during coronary artery surgery, *Anesthesiology* 43:61, 1975.
37. Lazzell VA, Burrows FA: Stability of the intraoperative arterial to end-tidal carbon dioxide partial pressure difference in children with congenital heart disease, *Can J Anaesth* 38:859, 1991.
38. Lee JC, Halloran KH, Taylor JFN et al: Coronary flow and myocardial metabolism in newborn lambs: effects of hypoxia and acidemia, *Am J Physiol* 224:1381, 1973.
39. Linderkamp O, Klose HJ, Betke K et al: Increased blood viscosity in patients with cyanotic congenital heart disease and iron deficiency, *J Pediatr* 95:567, 1979.
40. Lunn JK, Stanley TH, Eisele J et al: High dose fentanyl anesthesia for coronary artery surgery: plasma fentanyl concentrations and influence of nitrous oxide on cardiovascular responses, *Anesth Analg* 58:390, 1979.
41. Maurer HM, McCue CM, Robertson LW et al: Correction of platelet dysfunction and bleeding in cyanotic congenital heart disease by simple red cell volume reduction, *Am J Cardiol* 35:831, 1975.
42. McDermott RW, Stanley TH: The cardiovascular effects of low concentration of nitrous oxide during morphine anesthesia, *Anesthesiology* 41:89, 1974.
43. Meretoja OA, Takkunen O, Heikkila H et al: Haemody-

namic response to nitrous oxide during high-dose fentanyl pancuronium anaesthesia, *Acta Anaesthesiol Scand* 29:137, 1985.

44. Mikhail M, Lee W, Toeros W et al: Surgical and medical experience with 734 premature infants with patent ductus arteriosus, *J Thorac Cardiovasc Surg* 83:349, 1982.
45. Moffitt EA, Scovil JE, Barker RA et al: The effects of nitrous oxide on myocardial metabolism and hemodynamics during fentanyl or enflurane anesthesia in patients with coronary disease, *Anesth Analg* 63:1071, 1984.
46. Moss AJ, Emmanouilides GC, Rettori O et al: Postnasal circulatory adjustments in normal and distressed premature infants, *Biol Neonate* 8:177, 1964.
47. Nadas AS, Fyler DDC: *Pediatric cardiology,* ed 3, Philadelphia, 1972, Saunders.
48. Nakakimura K, Fleischer JE, Drummond JC et al: Glucose administration before cardiac arrest worsens neurologic outcome in cats, *Anesthesiology* 72:1005, 1990.
49. Newburger JW, Sibert AR, Buckley LP et al: Cognitive function and age at repair of transposition of the great arteries in children, *N Engl J Med* 310:1495, 1984.
50. Olley PM, Coceani F, Bodach E: E type prostaglandins: a new emergency therapy for certain cyanotic heart malformations. *Circulation* 53:728, 1976.
51. Perloff JK, Rosove MH, Child JS et al: Adults with cyanotic congenital heart disease: hematologic management, *Ann Intern Med* 109:406, 1988.
52. Perloff JK: Congenital heart disease after childhood: an expanding patient population, *J Am Coll Cardiol* 18:311, 1991.
53. Phornphutkul C, Rosenthal A, Nadas AS et al: Cerebrovascular accidents in infants and children with cyanotic congenital heart disease, *Am J Cardiol* 32:329, 1973.
54. Prec KJ, Cassels DE: Oximeter studies in newborn infants during crying, *Pediatrics* 9:756, 1952.
55. Pulsinelli WA, Waldman S, Rawlinson D et al: Moderate hyperglycemia augments ischemic brain damage: a neuropathologic study in the rat, *Neurology* 32:1239, 1982.
56. Romero T, Covell J, Friedman WF: A comparison of pressure volume relations of the fetal, newborn and adult heart. *Am J Physiol* 222:1283, 1972.
57. Rosenthal A, Nathan DG, Marty AT et al: Acute hemodynamic effects of red cell volume reduction in polycythemia of cyanotic congenital heart disease, *Circulation* 42:297, 1970.
58. Scammon RE, Norris EH: On the time of the postnatal obliteration of the fetal blood passages (foramen ovale, ductus arteriosus, ductus venosus), *Anat Rec* 15:165, 1918.
59. Schulte-Sasse U, Hess W, Tarnow J: Pulmonary vascular responses to nitrous oxide in patients with normal and high pulmonary vascular resistance, *Anesthesiology* 57:9, 1982.
60. Severinghaus JW, Naifeh KH: Accuracy of response of six pulse oximeters to profound hypoxia, *Anesthesiology* 67:551, 1987.
61. Sieber FE, Smith DS, Traystman RJ et al: Glucose: a reevaluation of its intraoperative use, *Anesthesiology* 67:72, 1987.
62. Spotoft H, Korshin JD, Sorensen MB et al: The cardiovascular effects of ketamine used for induction of anesthesia in patients with valvular heart disease, *Can Anaesth Soc J* 26:463, 1979.
63. Starling MB, Elliott RB: The effects of prostaglandins, prostaglandin inhibitors, and oxygen on the closure of the ductus arteriosus, pulmonary arteries, and umbilical vessels in vitro, *Prostaglandins* 8:187, 1974.
64. Stoelting R, Longnecker DE: Effect of right-to-left shunt on rate of increase in arterial anesthetic concentration, *Anesthesiology* 365:352, 1972.
65. Tanner GE, Angers DG, Barash PG et al: Effect of left-to-right, mixed right-to-left, and right-to-left shunts on inhalational anesthetic induction in children: a computer model, *Anesth Analg* 64:101, 1985.
66. Tarnow J, Hess W, Schmidt D et al: Narkoseeinleitung bei Patienten mit koronarer Herzkrankheit: Flunitrazepam, Diazepam, Ketamine, Fentanyl, *Anaesthetist* 28:9, 1979.
67. Territo MC, Rosove MH: Cyanotic congenital heart disease: hematologic management, *J Am Coll Cardiol* 18:320, 1991.
68. Thornberg KL, Morton MJ: Filling and atrial pressures as determinants of RV stroke volume in the sheep fetus, *Am J Physiol* 244:H656, 1983.
69. Tremper KK, Barker SJ: Pulse oximetry, *Anesthesiology* 70:98, 1989.
70. Tweed WA, Minuck M, Mymin D: Circulatory responses to ketamine anesthesia, *Anesthesiology* 37:613, 1972.
71. Wedemeyer AL, Edson Jr, Krivit W: Coagulation in cyanotic congenital heart disease, *Am J Dis Child* 124:656, 1972.
72. Wells R: Syndrome of hyperviscosity, *New Engl J Med* 283:183, 1980.
73. Wessel DL, Hickey PR, Hansen DD: Pulmonary and systemic hemodynamic effects of hyperventilation in infants after repair of congenital heart disease, *Anesthesiology* 67:A526, 1987.

# 11 Management of Perioperative Coagulation Function

*Jay Kambam*



## HISTORY

Heparin and protamine are two of the most important drugs in extracorporeal circulation during cardiac surgery. However, as with many other drugs, both heparin and protamine are sometimes associated with certain adverse effects. The anticoagulation and coagulation actions of both these drugs were discovered accidentally. Friedrick Miescher in 1868 identified a nitrogenous base that was coupled to the acidic nuclear material of Rhine salmon sperm; this coupled material is now called protamine.[2] Kossel in 1896 isolated protamines from various kinds of fish and suggested naming each protamine according to the species of fish from which it was isolated, for example, salmine from salmon, scombrine from mackerel, and clupeine from herring.[2] In 1916 a medical student, Jay Mclean, accidentally discovered heparin's anticoagulant property while volunteering his own tissue extracts toward the advancement of science.[26] Hagedorn and associates[15] in the 1930s demonstrated that protamine can delay the absorption of subcutaneously administered insulin and thus prolong its action. This important achievement stimulated several investigators to look at the effect of protamine in prolonging the absorption of other compounds. Heparin was one of the compounds examined at that time. It is said that while Best in Toronto was testing long-acting insulin in depancreatized dogs, Jaques was working on heparin chemistry in the adjacent room. One evening in the 1930s, when Jaques and his colleague McCutcheon mixed protamine with heparin, a precipitate that resembled a plastic (the so called heparin-protamine complex) appeared.[16,19] At about the same time, in 1937-38, Chargoff and Olson[7] discovered heparin's antidote, again quite by accident, when they were trying to develop a long-acting heparin by adding protamine to heparin. Anaphylactic reactions to protamine were first reported by Walther and Ammon[34] in 1939. They reported that three guinea pigs had died of pulmonary edema after receiving intracardiac protamine. In the 1940s Jaques extensively studied the toxic effects of protamine, including its adverse circulatory effects.[18] In 1973 Jacques[19] developed the heparin-protamine titration test (Table 11–1).

## HEPARIN

Heparin can be found in the lungs, liver, intestinal mucosa, and in the mast cells of the reticuloendothelial system. Heparin is one of the strongest acids in the body, primarily because of its heavily sulfated polyanionic mucopolysaccharide structure. The molecular weight of heparin ranges from 6,000 to 25,000 daltons. It is a long polymeric chain of acid groups. Heparin and nucleic acids are very similar in structure. In nucleic acids the

**Table 11–1** Historical achievements involving heparin and and protamine

| Date | Achievement |
|---|---|
| Miescher (1868) | Discovered protamine in salmon gonads |
| Kossel (1896) | Isolated protamines from various kinds of fish |
| McLean (1916) | Discovered heparin's anticoagulant action |
| Hagedorn (1930's) | Made long-acting insulin with protamine |
| Jaques and McCutcheon (1930s) | Produced heparin-protamine complex |
| Chargoff and Olson (1937-38) | Discovered heparin's antidote |
| Walther (1939) | Reported protamine's adverse effects |
| Jaques (1949) | Pioneered study of protamine's toxic effects |
| Hersley (1966) | Developed ACT test |
| Jaques (1973) | Developed heparin-protamine titration test |

**Table 11–2** Heparin source comparison

| | Porcine mucosal | Bovine lung |
|---|---|---|
| Cost | Less | More |
| Molecular weight (daltons) | 5000-20,000 | 6000-30,000 |
| Chemical structure | Shorter chains | Longer chains |
| Platelet aggregation | More | Less |
| Thrombin inhibition | Less | More |
| Factor aX inhibition | More | Less |
| Postoperative bleeding | More | Less |
| Protamine requirement | Less | More |
| Delayed thrombocytopenia | Less | More |

acid groups are phosphates, and in heparin they are sulfates. Protamines maintain the integrity of DNA in chromosomes by their interactions with the phosphate groups in nucleic acids. This same property of protamine neutralizes the anticoagulant activity of heparin (Table 11–2).

## Mechanism of coagulation

Heparin induces anticoagulation by inhibiting four coagulation-activating factors (aII, aIX, aX, and aXI). In sufficient concentrations heparin binds to a β-globulin, antithrombin III, and potentiates its attraction to several substrates participating in the coagulation cascade. In particular, the heparin–antithrombin III complex inhibits the thrombogenic actions of activated thrombin (aII) and factor X (aX).

The anticoagulation action of heparin begins immediately after systemic administration and peaks in 2 to 5 minutes. The small volume of distribution strongly implies that heparin distributes exclusively into the plasma compartment. However, recent animal data suggest that there is also uptake into the reticuloendothelial system.

Most normothermic patients maintain adequate anticoagulation during cardiopulmonary bypass for 60 to 90 minutes after receiving 3 to 4 mg/kg of heparin. However, under hypothermia this action of heparin is markedly prolonged.

## Resistance

Heparin resistance is the state of patients in whom the administration of standard heparin doses produces a negligible effect on coagulation. Some of the suggested causes for heparin resistance include ongoing active coagulation, antithrombin III deficiency, prolonged heparin therapy, drug interactions (oral contraceptives and nitroglycerin), Prinzmetal's angina, advanced age, and septicemia.[1,10,12,29]

## Side effects

The usual side effects of heparin may not manifest for several days to weeks. The acute side effects seen during cardiovascular surgery are vasodilation secondary to a decrease in systemic vascular resistance (about 15%) and heparin rebound, or the recurrence of heparin's anticoagulant effect following adequate protamine neutralization.

## Monitoring of anticoagulant action of heparin and reversal by protamine

No single test can reliably be used alone to test the anticoagulation action of heparin. There are at least two accepted tests being used to monitor the state of anticoagulation during cardiopulmonary bypass. The first method, a qualitative one, estimates the effect of heparin by using an activated clotting time (ACT). The second method, a quantitative one, measures the actual concentration of circulating heparin. ACT has been widely used during cardiovascular surgery to monitor the effects of circulating heparin. ACT measures the clotting time of fresh whole blood activated by surface contact through the detection of fibrin formation. ACT measures the anticoagulation effect but fails to provide quantitative data essential for safe heparinization and its reversal. Measuring circulating heparin concentration or ACT alone does not guarantee that a patient is optimally anticoagulated with heparin. Both qualitative (ACT) and quantitative (heparin assay) tests are essential for safe heparinization and its reversal with protamine. The ACT test is influenced by hypothermia, hemodilution, and any other factors that affect the intrinsic clotting mechanism.[4,13]

There are three heparin assays that do not rely on functional or qualitative tests, one direct and two indirect. The activated factor aX assay permits direct measurement of plasma heparin concentration. The two indirect methods are titration of heparin activity with protamine or protamine-like substance, and dye binding, in which the spectral properties of the dye change when it binds to heparin. Of the two indirect methods, titration with protamine is by far the more common. Titration with protamine generally uses clot formation as the end point of the test. The dye-binding test monitors the change in special characteristics of the dye and relates these findings to the concentration of heparin.

Hepcon/System A-10 (HemoTec) and Hepcon/System Four (HemoTec) offer semiautomated procedures for heparin-protamine titrations (HPT). Hepcon/System Four (HemoTec) offers an ACT and a heparin dose response (HDR) using the same ACT methodology. Hemochron system also offers the ACT test.

Bull and colleagues[4,5] in 1975 demonstrated in several patients that heparin therapy is associated with wide variations both in effect and duration. They recommended a protocol for heparin titration during extracorporeal circulation. Although they suggested maintaining ACT between 300 and 480 seconds, every institution has developed its own protocol.[20,36] At Vanderbilt University Medical Center my colleagues and I maintain ACT between 480-600 seconds. There is little information on heparin administration in small children during cardiopulmonary bypass. At our institution we give 2 to 3 mg/kg heparin for children during hypothermic procedures and 1 to 2 mg/kg during profound hypothermia.

## PROTAMINE

Protamine is prepared from salmon gonads by a crude extraction and filtration process using alcohol and sodium chloride. Protamine is available both as powder and as 1% solution (protamine sulfate; protamine chloride; protamine phosphate). The sulfate is used because of its stability, and protamine chloride (not available in the United States) is used because it is thought to be less prone to heparin rebound.

Protamines are composed primarily of basic and neutral amino acids. Protamine is a highly alkaline polycationic compound with a molecular weight of about 10,000 daltons. It is very alkaline because approximately 70% of the amino acid composition of protamine is arginine. The multiple positive charges on protamine in conjunction with negatively charged phosphate groups on DNA form the nucleoprotamine of sperm. Protamines are similar in structure to histones, which are found in the nuclei of all cells. Both protamines and histones are believed to help maintain the integrity of DNA in chromosomes. This is accomplished through interactions with the phosphate groups in nucleic acids (box).

**PROTAMINE**

**Structure**

Highly alkaline
Polycationic peptide
Molecular weight, 8000 to 10,000 daltons
Arginine rich

**Uses**

Reverses anticoagulation
Prolongs insulin absorption
Converts fine VF to coarse VF
Antineoplastic
Diagnostic test for disseminated intravascular coagulation

### Uses

Protamine is used primarily to reverse anticoagulation induced by heparin. It also prolongs the absorption of subcutaneously administered insulin preparations, namely PZI (protamine zinc insulin) and isophane, or NPH (neutral protamine Hagedorn) insulin. Protamine was once used to convert fine ventricular fibrillations to coarse ventricular fibrillations. It is now being seriously investigated as an antineoplastic agent.[32,35] Since protamine's biologic function is associated with DNA, its role in cellular processes in general is being examined. Laboratory studies have shown that both protamine and heparin inhibit angiogenesis and tumor growth.[32] However, clinical trials have produced unsatisfactory results thus far.[35] Protamine has been used in a diagnostic test for soluble fibrinogen monomers, which are indicative of an intravascular coagulation process. Protamine at moderate concentrations in plasma induces paracoagulation precipitating protamine and various fibrinogen breakdown products.

### Mechanism of termination of heparin's action

Heparin, a polyanionic mucopolysaccharide, induces anticoagulation by inhibiting four coagulation activating factors, aII, aIX, aX, and aXI. The most noticeable effect of heparin is activation of antithrombin III. When protamine, a polycationic peptide, is added to heparin, ionic forces form a stable precipitate (heparin-protamine complex), neutralizing heparin's anticoagulant action.

### Adverse reactions

Adverse side effects of protamine fall into the four categories shown in the box.

Protamine is a protein derived from fish sperm and is thus immunogenic. Administration of protamine is frequently associated with adverse hemodynamic effects. Certain patients have been reported to have anaphylactic reactions (box).[6,24,27] IgE antibodies to protamine have also been demonstrated in these patients. Although investigators have demonstrated the presence of antibodies in patients who have undergone vasectomies, except for one questionable case report, to date there is no documented case of anaphylactic reaction to protamine in postvasectomy patients. Protamine, if used in excessive amounts, can have an anticoagulation effect (box).[8,19]

### Treatment

Treatment of protamine reactions can be divided into two types (box), prophylactic and therapeutic.

***Prophylaxis.*** Even though investigators have reported that prophylactic treatment with certain drugs attenuates some of the adverse effects of protamine, these prophylactic measures do not reliably prevent all adverse effects. Nevertheless, they seem to help some patients. Aspirin and indomethacin have been reported as preventing thromboxane and other prostaglandin release. My studies show that prophylactic treatment with $H_1$ and $H_2$ receptor blockers seems to prevent some of the reactions caused by protamine administration.[21] The efficacy of prophylaxis with steroids and calcium chloride is uncertain. Other measures that can be used to prevent some of the side effects of protamine include slow (longer than 3 minutes) administration; peripheral rather than central administration; and beef heparin (beef heparin is claimed to be superior to pork heparin in patients with pulmonary hypertension). Fresh protamine has been shown to have no significant difference from prepacked protamine.

***Therapy.*** Hypotension related to rapid administration of protamine is usually due to transient release of histamine from mast cells. This reaction can be treated with a fluid bolus and calcium chloride administration (50 to 75 mg/kg). In these situations protamine should be administered slowly after the volume status of the patient is rectified. True anaphylactic reactions are rare and are not usually related to the rapidity of administration of protamine. Depending on the severity of the reaction, fluids, antihistamines, steroids, and epinephrine are used. Catastrophic pulmonary vasoconstriction (CPVC) should be treated promptly

---

**FACTORS IN THE USE OF PROTAMINE**

**Adverse reactions**

Hypotension related to rapid administration of protamine. This is usually transient and requires no major therapy. It is believed to result from minimal to moderate release of histamine from pulmonary circulation.

Anaphylactic and anaphylactoid reactions.

Catastrophic pulmonary vasoconstriction, usually in patients with a history of pulmonary hypertension.

Miscellaneous side effects
- Calcium chelation
- Negative inotropy
- Anticoagulation-related effects secondary to depression of certain coagulation factors
- Hypoxemia secondary to inhibition of HPVC (hypoxic pulmonary vasoconstriction)
- Heparin-protamine complex–related phenomena
- Noncardiogenic pulmonary edema
- Thrombocytopenia from platelet activation followed by inactivation
- Bradycardia
- Neutropenia
- Protein (fibrinogen) precipitation
- Leaky biologic membranes

**Risk factors for adverse effects**

Protamine-containing insulin therapy
Previous exposure to protamine or protamine-containing insulins
History of vasectomy
History of allergy to fish
History of protamine reaction

**Mechanisms of the anticoagulation effect**

Thrombocytopenia
Impaired aggregation of platelets
Competes with anti thrombin III for thrombin
Inhibits thrombin activity
Depletes fibrinogen

**Treatment of adverse effects**

Prophylaxis
- Drug therapy
- Other

Therapy
- Stop protamine administration
- Drugs for anaphylaxis
- Drugs for CPVC
- $H_2$ receptor antagonist

---

with nitroglycerin and isoproterenol. Prostaglandin $E_1$ should also be helpful in treating CPVC. In patients who develop CPVC the mortality rate is very high. In certain patients who develop anaphylactoid reactions and do not respond to conventional therapy, $H_2$ receptor blocker (cimetidine 5 mg/kg, slow IV push) seems to attenuate effectively the adverse hemodynamic effects.[22]

One can avoid adverse reactions to protamine by not giving it. These are alternatives to its use:

1. Eliminate the need for anticoagulation by constructing bypass circuits with materials that do not activate platelets or coagulation cascade.
2. Anticoagulate with preparations that do not require neutralization with protamine: ancrod, an enzyme found in the venom of the Malayan pit viper, acts by destroying fibrinogen. Its main drawback is that all currently used tests of anticoagulation—ACT, PT, PTT, and TT—require the presence of fibrinogen, and thus the adequacy of anticoagulation can not be determined in the presence of ancrod.
3. Allow spontaneous recovery from heparin.
4. Reverse with other than protamine; that is, give platelet factor 4, which neutralizes heparin's anticoagulant activity. However, it is not available in quantities large enough to be considered a true alternative (box).

**ALTERNATIVES TO PROTAMINE**

No protamine (spontaneous recovery)
Platelet concentrates
Heparinase
Toluidine blue
No heparin
Snake venom
Special circuits
Prostaglandins
Platelet factor 4

### Incompatibilities

Protamine usage is considered to be incompatible with certain antibiotics, including cephalosporins and penicillins.

## DESMOPRESSIN

Desmopressin (1-deamino-8-D-arginine vasopressin, or DDAVP) is a synthetic analogue of arginine vasopressin, the naturally occurring human antidiuretic hormone. In addition to its diuretic action, it increases levels of factor VIII and von Willebrand's factor (vWf) in individuals with hemophilia A or type III von Willebrand's disease. DDAVP has also been found useful in combating postoperative bleeding problems in bypass patients. The vWf, required for platelets' adhesiveness, is reduced during extracorporeal circulation, primarily by adhering to the surface of the extracorporeal circuit. Consequently, factor VIII levels also decrease. DDAVP is also known to improve the platelet function, which is depressed in patients with uremia, and from drug therapy such as acetylsalicylic acid. Anaphylactoid reactions from the use of DDAVP have been reported. The recommended dose after coming off bypass is 0.3 μg/kg IV, which should be diluted and given slowly over about 5 minutes.

## PERIOPERATIVE EXCESSIVE BLEEDING

Once the patient has been successfully weaned from extracorporeal circulation and heparin's anticoagulant function has been reversed with protamine, excessive postoperative bleeding can occur for several reasons. The common causes of bleeding, their testing, and suggested management are given in Table 11–3.

Causes of excessive bleeding range from the effects of mechanical trauma to hypothermia during the surgical procedure. Blood components can be traumatized by the mechanical forces of the cardiopulmonary bypass pump and pump suction, resulting in various types of bleeding and coagulation abnormalities in the postoperative period.* The cardiopulmonary bypass pump is known to cause platelet aggregates, which are usually sequestrated in the liver. In addition, the adhesiveness of platelets may be diminished.

Both protamine and heparin-protamine complex are known to cause diminution of platelet aggregation.[3,11,17] Occasionally, a few other drugs that are being administered to the patient can cause platelet dysfunction.[30] Circulating fibrinolysins are sometimes associated with postoperative bleeding.

Hypothermia is often used during pediatric cardiac surgery. However, it frequently causes bleeding diathesis during the postbypass period, as hypothermia has been attributed to the reduction of platelet count,[23,25,33] fibrinogen activity,[28,31] and other enzymatic elements.[14] Altered platelet count and function are thought to be due to hypothermia-induced abnormal function of the liver, spleen, and bone marrow.

If bleeding and coagulation abnormalities are ruled out as the cause of persistent postoperative bleeding, then a diagnosis of surgical bleeding

*References 9, 14, 23, 25, 28, 31, 33.

**Table 11–3** Postoperative bleeding: causes, testing, and suggested management

| Causes | Tests | Suggested management |
|---|---|---|
| Incomplete reversal of heparin | ACT, heparin-protamine titration test, PTT* | Additional protamine |
| Platelet abnormality (function or count)<br>Dilutional<br>Hypothermia induced<br>Pump induced<br>Pump suction induced<br>Heparin induced<br>Protamine induced<br>Other drug induced | Bleeding time, platelet count | Desmopressin, platelet transfusion |
| Denaturation of coagulation factors | PT, PTT† | FFP |
| Fibrinolysis | TEG, clot liquefication test, fibrinogen | Hematology consult |
| Surgical bleeding | Negative lab tests | Reoperation for hemostasis |

*PTT is prolonged, but PT will be normal in case of incomplete reversal of heparin.
†Both PT and PTT are prolonged if bleeding is due to deficit of coagulation factors.
PT, Prothrombin time; PTT, partial thromboplastin time; TEG, thromboelastogram.

must be made and the patient should be reoperated upon for effective hemostasis. In general surgeons tend to use excessive blood components to treat postoperative bleeding for fear of pericardial tamponade and also to avoid the risks of reoperation.

## REFERENCES


1. Anderson EF: Heparin resistance prior to cardiopulmonary bypass, *Anesthesiology* 65:504, 1986.
2. Ando T, Yamasaki M, Suzuki K: Protamines. In Klienzeller A, Springer GF, Wittman HG, editors: *Molecular biology, biochemistry and biophysics,* vol 12, Berlin, 1973, Springer-Verlag.
3. Bjoraker DG, Ketcham TR: In vivo platelet response to clinical protamine sulfate infusion, *Anesthesiology* 57:A7, 1982.
4. Bull BS, Huse WN, Brauner FS et al: Heparin therapy during extracorporeal circulation II: the use of a dose-response curve to individualize heparin and protamine dosage, *J Thorac Cardiovasc Surg* 69:685, 1975.
5. Bull BS, Korpman RA, Huse WN et al: Heparin therapy during extracorporeal circulation I: problems inherent in existing heparin protocols, *J Thorac Cardiovasc Surg* 69:674, 1975.
6. Caplan SN, Berkman EM: Protamine sulfate and fish allergy (letter), *N Engl J Med* 295:172, 1976.
7. Chargoff F, Olson KB: Studies on the chemistry of blood coagulation VI: studies on the action of heparin and other anticoagulants: the influence of protamine on the anticoagulant effect in vivo, *J Biol Chem* 122:153, 1937-1938.
8. Cobel-Gerd RJ, Hassouna HI: Interaction of protamine sulfate with thrombin, *Am J Hematol* 14:227, 1983.
9. Deleval MR, Hill JD, Mielke CG et al: Blood platelets and extracorporeal circulation, *J Thorac Cardiovasc Surg* 69:144, 1975.
10. Ellison N, Beatty CP, Blake DR et al: Heparin rebound, studies in patients and volunteers, *J Thorac Cardiovasc Surg* 67:723, 1974.
11. Ellison N, Edmunds LH, Colman RW: Platelet aggregation following heparin and protamine administration, *Anesthesiology* 48:65, 1978.
12. Esposito RA, Culliford AT, Colvin SB et al: Heparin resistance during cardiopulmonary bypass, the role of heparin pretreatment, *J Thorac Cardiovasc Surg* 84:346, 1983.
13. Fiser WP, Read RC, Wright FE et al: A randomized study of beef lung and pork mucosal heparin in cardiac surgery, *Ann Thorac Surg* 35:615, 1983.
14. Foldes FF: *Enzymes in anesthesiology,* New York, 1978, Springer-Verlag.
15. Hagedorn HC, Jensen BN, Krarup NB et al: Protamine insulinase, *JAMA* 106:177, 1936.
16. Horrow JC: Protamine: a review of its toxicity, *Anesth Analg* 64:348, 1985.
17. Horrow JC: Thrombocytopenia accompanying a reaction to protamine sulfate, *Can Anaesth Soc J* 32:49, 1985.
18. Jaques LB: A study of the toxicity of the protamine, salmine, *Br J Pharmacol* 4:135, 1949.
19. Jaques LB: Protamine: antagonist to heparin, *J Can Med Assoc* 1087:1291, 1973.
20. Jobes DR, Schwartz AJ, Ellison N et al: Monitoring heparin anticoagulation and its neutralization, *Ann Thorac Surg* 31:161, 1981.
21. Kambam JR, Merrill W, Smith BE: The beneficial role of histamine$_2$ receptor blocker in the treatment of protamine-related anaphylactic reactions: two case reports, *Can J Anaesth* 36:463, 1989.
22. Kambam JR, Meszaros R, Smith BE et al: Effect of histamine$_1$ and histamine$_2$ receptor blockers in the prevention of protamine reactions, *Can J Anaesth* 37:420, 1990.
23. Kendall AG, Lowenstein L: Alterations in blood coagulation and hemostasis during extracorporeal circulation, part 1, *Can Med Assoc J* 87:786, 1962.
24. Knape JTA, Schuller JL, de Haan P et al: An anaphylactic reaction to protamine in a patient allergic to fish, *Anesthesiology* 55:324, 1981.
25. Marin HM: Hemostasis mechanism in extracorporeal circulation, *Arch Surg* 88:988, 1964.

26. McLean J: The thormboplastic action of cephalin, *Am J Physiol* 41:250, 1916.
27. Moorthy SS, Pond W, Rowland RG: Severe circulatory shock following protamine (an anaphylactic reaction), *Anesth Analg* 59:77, 1980.
28. Ollendorf P, Strom O, Rygg I et al: Activation of the thromboplastic and the fibrinolytic system during extracorporeal circulation, *Acta Chir Scand* 122:217, 1961.
29. Pifarre R, Babka R, Sullivan HJ et al: Management of postoperative heparin rebound following cardiopulmonary bypass, *J Thorac Cardiovasc Surg* 81:378, 1981.
30. Radegran K, McAshlan C: Circulatory and ventilatory effects of induced platelet aggregation and their inhibition by acetylsalicylic acid, *Acta Anaesthesiol Scand* 16:76, 1972.
31. Samama M, Weiss M, Yver J et al: Coagulation et circulation extracorporéal avec hypothermie profonde, *Ann Chir Thorac Cardiovasc* 1:633, 1962.
32. Taylor S, Folkman J: Protamine is an inhibitor of angiogenesis, *Nature* 297:307, 1982.
33. Villaloboo TJ, Adelson E, Riley P: The effect of hypothermia on platelets and white cells in dogs, *Proc Natl Acad Sci* 451:186, 1956.
34. Walther G, Ammon R: Anaphylaktischer Shock nach Protamine, *Klin Wochenschr* 18:288, 1939.
35. Wright JEC: Clinical trial of protamine in the treatment of malignant diseases, *Br J Cancer* 22:415, 1968.
36. Young JA, Kisker CT, Doty DB: Adequate anticoagulation during cardiopulmonary bypass determined by activated clotting time and the appearance of fibrin monomer, *Ann Thorac Surg* 26:231, 1978.

# 12 Postoperative Care

*Joseph D. Tobias, Jayant K. Deshpande, and Sandra V. Lowe*



Even with improved surgical technique, the postoperative care of the pediatric cardiac patient represents an integral step in the correction and palliation of congenital heart defects. The initiation of this transition begins with the safe transport of the patient from the operating room to the intensive care unit. Extreme vigilance is necessary during this critical time, and continued monitoring of vital signs and invasive hemodynamic parameters is required. Recent advances in transport monitor technology allow the cassette or module used to monitor the patient in the operating room to be removed and inserted into a transport module. This also allows storage of intraoperative data such as blood pressures and filling pressures in case later review of this information is necessary. If such equipment is not available, then a separate transport monitor capable of continuous ECG, oxygen saturation, and invasive hemodynamic monitoring should be used. Additionally, resuscitation medications and equipment must be carried with and readily available to those transporting the patient. This is especially relevant when transport involves significant times and distances.

On arrival in the intensive care unit, thorough communication and cooperation are required to ensure the safe transition from the intraoperative to the postoperative period. Regardless of the service primarily responsible for the patient's care, a multidisciplinary approach involving several medical and surgical specialties as well as the nursing and respiratory therapy staff is required for the postoperative care of these patients. This chapter will discuss the postoperative care of the pediatric cardiac patient by dealing with each specific organ system and the issues that may arise during the postoperative period.

## INITIAL ASSESSMENT

The assessment of the pediatric cardiac patient begins with a systematic review of the preoperative history, the intraoperative course, and the surgical procedure. Particular attention should be paid to the length of cardiopulmonary bypass and difficulties encountered following its discontinuation. The initial assessment should follow the ABC's of resuscitation with observation of adequate chest excursion with ventilation and auscultation for bilateral breath sounds. This is followed by a preliminary assessment of perfusion and cardiac output. Once initial stabilization is achieved, a more thorough assessment should be undertaken to evaluate each organ system.

The initial assessment begins with a careful physical examination and evaluation of baseline vital signs. Aside from routine vital signs of heart rate, blood pressure, and respiratory rate, measurement of core temperature is an important part of the initial assessment of the child following cardiac surgery. Although hypothermia is an integral part of cerebral protection during cardiopulmonary bypass and circulatory arrest, inadvertent hypothermia following the cessation of bypass or during closed heart procedure can have significant deleterious effects on the pediatric patient.

Several factors contribute to the high incidence of hypothermia in the pediatric patient. Heat loss occurs through four basic mechanisms: evaporation, conduction, convection, and radiation. Children and especially neonates have a larger surface to volume ratio, which increases heat loss to the environment. Regulation of body temperature and correction of hypothermia have significant implications in the postsurgical patient. Hypothermia has several deleterious physiologic effects including cardiac arrhythmias, depression of myocardial contractility, altered drug metabolism, decreased glomerular filtration rate, and a leftward shift of the oxyhemoglobin dissociation curve.[17] As such hypothermia can severely compromise oxygen delivery to tissues through several different mechanisms. General anesthetic agents further aggravate hypothermia by inhibition of thermoregulation.[95,104] Measures to prevent hypothermia include humidification and warming of inspired gases, external heating by warming lights or a radiant warmer, and the warming of fluids and blood products. With such measures, rewarming of patients can usually be accomplished within the first 4 to 6 postoperative hours.

## CARDIOVASCULAR SYSTEM

Evaluation of the cardiovascular system begins with an assessment of cardiac output. Although the placement of invasive hemodynamic monitors such as a pulmonary artery catheter allows the direct measurement of cardiac output, its use in the pediatric cardiac patient may be limited by size constraints and the presence of residual cardiac shunts and malformations. Invasive hemodynamic monitoring such as PA (pulmonary artery) catheters and left atrial lines may be used in certain situations (i.e., following the Fontan procedure or in patients at risk for pulmonary vasospasm), but the postoperative assessment of cardiac function must rely on physical assessment and laboratory values. Cardiac output can be assessed through peripheral perfusion, capillary refill, peripheral pulses, and blood pressure. Peripheral vasoconstriction may maintain blood pressure in the normal range despite a low cardiac output state, which makes arterial blood pressure a relatively poor reflection of cardiac output. Mental state may also be an indicator of cardiac output, but its use in the immediate postoperative period is limited by residual anesthetic agents. Additional tools used in the assessment of cardiac status include urine output and acid-base status. Although several factors may play a role in oliguria, especially following cardiac surgery, urine output is one end-organ measure of cardiac output. Additionally, metabolic acidosis with elevated lactate levels suggests inadequate tissue perfusion with anaerobic metabolism.

In the immediate perioperative period cardiorespiratory failure is the primary cause of mortality. Several etiologies may play a role in perioperative myocardial failure, including preoperative myocardial dysfunction, intraoperative events such as damage due to cardiopulmonary bypass, and residual cardiac lesions and shunts. Shortly after the introduction of cardiopulmonary bypass (CPB), it became apparent that low cardiac output was the primary cause of early postoperative death. Taber and associates[105] were the first to document scattered areas of myocardial necrosis in patients dying after CPB. In that same year, Najafi and colleagues[71] suggested that the diffuse myocardial necrosis was the result of damage related to CPB. Although various cardioplegia solutions have been investigated, none have been totally successful in preventing myocardial necrosis and the resultant postbypass myocardial dysfunction.

Concerns regarding myocardial preservation may be particularly relevant in the neonate, since it has been suggested that the neonatal myocardium is particularly vulnerable to ischemic injury and that methods of protection used in adult patients may be ineffective in the pediatric population.[15,121] This increased sensitivity may be related to the limited glycogen stores and rapid intracellular lactate accumulation. In the perioperative period part of the dysfunction may be reversible, and prevention of imbalances in myocardial oxygen demand and delivery may prevent further cardiac decompensation.

The balance of myocardial oxygen delivery and consumption may be precarious in the immediate postoperative period, and alterations in various parameters (e.g., heart rate) may not only increase oxygen demand but also limit delivery. Myocardial oxygen consumption is determined primarily by heart rate, left ventricular end diastolic pressure (LVEDP), afterload, and contractility. Although the use of inotropic agents is frequently necessary, agents such as epinephrine that increase heart rate and systemic vascular resistance may increase myocardial oxygen consumption and lead to increased myocardial damage.[69,80] However, improved myocardial contractility and decreased LVEDP with the use of such agents may decrease oxygen consumption.

Aside from limiting increases in oxygen consumption, improvement in oxygen delivery may also limit myocardial necrosis. Oxygen delivery occurs primarily during diastole, so the importance of control of heart becomes readily apparent, since increases not only increase oxygen consumption but also limit diastolic time and oxygen delivery. The other determinant of myocardial oxygen delivery is the difference between diastolic pressure and LVEDP. Therefore, alterations in LVEDP not only affect consumption but may also decrease delivery. Such imbalances may be of particular relevance in patients with systemic to pulmonary shunts (either surgical or medical with prostaglandin administration), since diastolic runoff may lead to significant decreases in diastolic pressure. Abnormalities of oxygen delivery and consumption may be further aggravated by anatomic abnormalities of the coronary vasculature.

With such concerns, maintenance of adequate cardiac output and tissue oxygen delivery should be the primary goal in the immediate postoperative period. As in any other clinical situation, cardiac output is determined by the product of heart rate and stroke volume. Although alterations in heart rate may be of little clinical significance in older patients, bradycardia can lead to significant decrease in cardiac output in the neonate and infant. Alterations in rhythm and asynchrony of the atria and ventricles may also impair cardiac output. Although the atrial kick is responsible for only 10% to 15% of the cardiac output in the healthy person, alterations in ventricular compliance may leave the ventricle dependent on atrial contraction to ensure adequate ventricular preload. In such instances loss of the synchrony between atrial and ventricular contraction may lead to significant decreases in cardiac output. Such alterations in ventricular compliance, leaving it dependent on atrial contraction for filling, are common in the postbypass period. In addition to alterations in rhythm related to CPB, dysrhythmias may be related to the surgical procedure and are commonly seen following closure of atrial septal defects (sinus venosus type) and following atrial shunt procedures (Mustard and Senning procedures). The treatment of dysrhythmias is discussed in Chapter 13.

Aside from heart rate, cardiac output is dependent on stroke volume, which is determined by left ventricular end diastolic volume (preload), afterload, and contractility. In the immediate postoperative period, assessment of rhythm and these three factors allow for pharmacologic and fluid management to optimize the hemodynamic status of the patient. Immediately following CPB and in the postoperative period maintenance of sinus rhythm is of prime importance to ensure adequate ventricular preload. Postsurgical atrioventricular (AV) block may be due to surgical damage during repair but is most likely a transient residual effective of cardioplegia. Temporary AV sequential pacing via epicardial leads may be required. Permanent pacemaker placement is generally deferred for 7 to 14 days.[74] The immediate treatment of tachyarrhythmias is mandatory. Pharmacologic treatment is acceptable if the patient is hemodynamically stable, but cardioversion is indicated if cardiac decompensation occurs. Aside from dysrhythmias sinus node dysfunction with bradycardia may be temporarily present following CPB. Low dose isoproterenol (0.01 to 0.05 μg/kg/min) may be required to maintain an acceptable heart rate. Once a sinus rhythm or AV synchrony with a normal heart rate for age are obtained, manipulation of cardiac function depends on alterations in stroke volume.

In the patient with acute decompensation mechanical difficulties such as tension pneumothorax and cardiac tamponade should be ruled out. Once these factors are ruled out, fluid and inotropic management to improve cardiac output are indicated. Fluid management should be guided by measurement of filling pressures via invasive monitoring when available. Although the CVP can be used to estimate right ventricular preload, its use to assess left ventricular preload is limited. This is especially true in the patient with alterations in ventricular function and elevated pulmonary vascular resistance. Elevated ventricular preload may be required in the patient with compromised cardiac function. As such, left atrial pressures (PCWP) of 10 to 14 mm Hg may be required. Direct measurement of cardiac output and afterload is generally not available in the pediatric cardiac patient. Residual intracardiac shunts and the small size of many patients preclude the use of thermodilution measurements of cardiac output and calculation of afterload.

Aside from systemic vascular resistance, respiratory function may also affect afterload. In the healthy awake state spontaneous ventilation leads to an increase in ventricular filling and increased cardiac output with little or no increase in afterload. However, in the patient with respiratory distress, large negative increases in interpleural pressure may significantly increase afterload and decrease cardiac output. Therefore, an acute decompensation of cardiac output may respond most quickly to endotracheal intubation and the resultant decrease in afterload.

In patients without invasive hemodynamic monitoring, fluid and inotropic administration are titrated by clinical responses such as improvements in perfusion, capillary refill, urine output, and peripheral temperature. Once an adequate volume status is reached, the administration of inotropic agents is indicated to optimize cardiac contractility and manipulate systemic vascular resistance. Agents used to improve contractility act to increase intracellular calcium availability by increasing calcium release from the sarcoplasmic reticulum, which leads to increased muscle fibril cross-linking and contraction. Three basic choices are available: (1) exogenous administration of calcium, (2) drugs that act through activation of adrenergic receptors, and (3) the newest class of agents that inhibit phosphodiesterase.

Exogenous calcium administration improves contractility by increasing the transmembrane concentration, hence increasing intracellular accumulation when calcium channels are opened during action potential propagation.[61] Although some evidence links increases in intracellular calcium with subsequent neuronal damage, several factors in the immediate postoperative period may lead to decreased serum ionized calcium. They include the administration of citrate-preserved blood or of protamine and alterations in parathyroid function in the chronically ill patient. Therefore, calcium administration is indicated to achieve normal serum levels. The choice of agent, calcium chloride versus calcium gluconate, is somewhat controversial. It is generally accepted that the administration of equimolar concentrations of either agent will normalize serum calcium.

The adrenergic agonists interact with specific cell receptors. Although several subclasses of the receptors exist, three are of predominant importance for inotropic administration. α-Receptors are located primarily on vascular tissue, although recent evidence has also documented their presence on myocardial cells. Stimulation of these receptors leads to vasoconstriction. $\beta_1$-Receptors are located on myocardial cells. Stimulation leads to increased force of contraction (inotropy), increased heart rate (chronotropy), and increased speed of impulse conduction along the conduction pathways (dromotropy). $\beta_2$-Receptor stimulation, present on vascular tissue, causes vasodilatation.

Much controversy remains over the optimal inotropic agent following CPB.[56,107] Proponents of going directly with potent agents such as epinephrine believe that quick and prompt correction of the low cardiac output state is mandatory to prevent further cardiac decompensation and necrosis.[107] Epinephrine with equal effects at the α and $\beta_2$ receptors will improve contractility with little or no change in SVR when used in doses of 0.05 to 0.2 μg/kg/min. However, venoconstriction may increase filling pressures, and a venodilator such as nitroglycerin may be needed to offset this effect. A second approach is the combination of norepinephrine with a vasodilator (phentolamine or nitroprusside). With these two agents, the potent inotropic effects of norepinephrine may be achieved while minimizing its deleterious effects on SVR.

Although many centers use dopamine or dobutamine initially and then switch to epinephrine if these agents fail, adult studies suggest that the dose-response curve to both dopamine and dobutamine are flat following CPB.[103] Additionally, the use of an indirect agent that relies on the release of endogenous catecholamines such as dopamine may be ineffective in a patient who has been chronically stressed and whose endogenous stores are depleted. Regardless of the agents chosen, serial measurements of cardiac output (when available) or repeated evaluation of cardiac output on clinical examination should be used to guide the administration of fluid and inotropic agents.

The newest class of inotropic agents in clinical practice are the phosphodiesterase inhibitors (amrinone). These agents inhibit phosphodiesterase in cardiac cells, thereby increasing cyclic adenosine monophosphate (AMP) levels, which results in an increase in the availability of intracellular calcium. The final common pathway of inotropic agents is an increase in intracellular cyclic AMP levels. Since these agents bypass the adrenergic receptors, they may be useful in patients chronically receiving adrenergic agents who have alterations in receptor number and function. The prototype of these agents, amrinone, is administered as a bolus (1 to 2 mg/kg) followed by a continuous infusion of 10 to 20 μg/kg/min. Cardiovascular effects include increased inotropy and vasodilatation. These effects combine to decrease filling pressures and afterload, thereby improving cardiac output and favorably affecting myocardial oxygen demand and delivery. Further clinical studies are needed to define the role of these agents in the immediate postoperative period.

Regardless of the inotropic agents chosen, progressive myocardial dysfunction may lead to progressive cardiogenic shock. In such instances mechanical support of the circulation may be an option to maintain the circulation and prevent further myocardial damage while allowing time for myocardial recovery. Alternatives include extracorporeal membrane oxygenation (ECMO),[87] ventricular assist devices,[11,63] and the intraaortic blood pump (IABP).[116] ECMO was originally introduced as salvage therapy for progressive respiratory failure. However, with arteriovenous ECMO, flow (cardiac output) is provided by the roller pump, and the circulation can be supported. The technique involves the placement of a venous cannula that drains blood into a reservoir. From there blood is pumped through a membrane oxygenator and then returned to the patient via the arterial cannula. This support may be instituted through the sternotomy incision with cannulas placed directly in the right atrium and aorta or with percutaneous cannulas. The venous cannula may be placed percutaneously into either the internal jugular or femoral vein, and the arterial cannula is generally placed into the ascending aorta through the carotid artery. The major disadvantage of this technique is carotid artery obstruction during the process and the resultant risk of neurologic complication. However, studies in neonatal ECMO have shown a very low risk of neurologic sequelae.

Ventricular assist devices have recently been used to support the failing heart in children.[11,63] These devices drain blood from either the right atrium or right ventricle and return it through a cannula in the aorta. The third option for mechanical assist is the IABP. Although it is most commonly used in adults, a recent report[116] documents its efficacy in children. The device is placed through the femoral artery and positioned in the first part of the descending aorta, distal to the left subclavian artery. The balloon inflates during diastole and deflates prior to systole. This reduces afterload and improves flow during diastole. The improvement in diastolic flow augments myocardial perfusion. Although systolic pressure is generally slightly lowered, mean arterial pressure and cardiac output increase. Despite the reported success in one pediatric series,[13] mechanical problems with the device are particularly common in children. The small size of many patients precludes its use, and the general elasticity of the child's artery limits the IABP's ability to decrease afterload and augment diastolic flow. Additionally, the relatively rapid heart rate of children makes the timing of inflation and deflation more difficult. Complications inherent in the use of any of the mechanical devices include bleeding from heparinization, thromboembolic events, infection, hemolysis, and vascular compromise related to cannulas.

## RESPIRATORY SYSTEM

Respiratory failure is second to cardiac failure as a cause of death in the immediate postoperative period. The initial assessment following auscultation for breath sounds includes examination of the postoperative chest x-ray film for endotracheal tube placement and to rule out residual pneumothoraces. Following this, initial ventilator settings should be determined. Virtually all patients will receive conventional volume-controlled ventilation with tidal volumes of 10 to 12 ml/kg. Initial respiratory rate should be appropriate for age (30 to 40 breaths per minute for a neonate and 10 to 14 for an adolescent) with subsequent increases or decreases based on analysis of arterial blood gases.

The optimal duration of mechanical ventilation in the postoperative pediatric cardiac patient remains controversial. Twenty to 30 years ago, mechanical ventilation was arbitrarily continued for 24 to 48 hours in all patients.[60] However, later reports documented the safety of early (less than 12 hours) extubation.[82] Additionally, early extubation permitted earlier discharge from the ICU. Prospective randomized studies have also documented the benefits of early extubation.[83] With this approach, morbidity related to endotracheal intubation such as mucus plugging, atelectasis, pulmonary infections, and tracheal trauma may be decreased. Additionally, the deleterious hemodynamic effects of positive pressure ventilation may be avoided. Although these studies were performed in adults following coronary artery bypass grafting, the feasibility of early extubation for selected pediatric patients has also been demonstrated. Heard and co-workers[45] demonstrated a correlation of the duration of CPB with the probability of early extubation (within 6 hours). Correlation with CPB time is not surprising, since histologic studies show interstitial and intraalveolar edema, perivascular and intraalveolar hemorrhage, and miliary atelectasis after prolonged CPB.[18,25] Early extubation appears appropriate for most patients undergoing relatively simple procedures such as repair of atrial or ventricular septal defects and coarctation of the aorta.

Neonates and those with more complex lesions may require a more prolonged course of mechanical ventilation. In fact, as many as 40% of neonates undergoing cardiac surgery require prolonged ventilation. The etiologies for this postoperative respiratory dysfunction are both controversial and most likely multifactorial. Furthermore, physical examination and laboratory findings do not differentiate infants who will tolerate early extubation from those who will require prolonged ventilation.

When an infant requires prolonged ventilation, an organized approach to the possible mechanism(s) of the respiratory failure is helpful. This can be categorized into one of four groups: CNS dysfunction, airway problems, neuromuscular weakness, and pulmonary parenchymal disease. CNS dysfunction may be related to residual anesthetic effects, ongoing administration of sedative drugs, metabolic derangements, or damage related to CPB and episodes of hypoperfusion. The evaluation of the infant who fails to wake up following surgery is discussed later. Following a careful physical examination, metabolic work-up including serum electrolytes, calcium, magnesium, glucose, and ammonia will rule out many of the metabolic causes of altered mental status. Computed tomography (CT) electroencephalogram (EEG) may also be indicated. Airway problems include postextubation stridor and airway edema. This is particularly common in patients with trisomy 21.[98] Measures to minimize airway edema include use of an appropriate size tube (uncuffed in patients less than 8 years of age) and adequate sedation during mechanical ventilation to prevent excessive movement. For patients with prolonged courses of ventilation without an audible leak around the endotracheal tube, the administration of corticosteroids (dexamethasone 1 mg/kg/day divided every 6 hours) may be beneficial in decreasing the incidence of postextubation stridor.[21] Additionally, the use of an oxygen-helium mixture may decrease the work of breathing in infants with a compromised airway, allowing time for resolution of subglottic edema. If such measures fail and prolonged ventilation is required due to airway problems, direct laryngoscopy may be indicated to rule out vocal cord paralysis. This is especially true following surgical procedures involving the arch and great vessels, since inadvertent damage to the recurrent laryngeal nerve may occur.

Neuromuscular weakness also may compromise postoperative respiratory function. Aside from the residual effects of neuromuscular blocking agents, several metabolic derangements including hypokalemia, hypomagnesemia, and hypophosphatemia may lead to generalized muscle weakness. Such derangements are particularly common in infants maintained on parenteral alimentation. Diuretics (furosemide) and aminoglycoside antibiotics may have neuromuscular blocking properties as a side effect, and their role in muscle weakness should be considered.

Inadequate cardiovascular function may also affect respiratory function. Poor cardiac output may lead to easy fatigue of the diaphragm and respiratory failure. In such instances inotropic support and improvement of cardiovascular function may permit weaning from mechanical ventilation. Additionally, diaphragmatic dysfunction may be related to phrenic nerve damage during surgical manipulation. If such concerns are entertained, fluoroscopic examination of both diaphragms during spontaneous ventilation is required to be sure that diaphragmatic movement is normal. Ultrasound evaluation may be possible in the smaller infant and neonate. The advantage of the latter technique is that it may be done in the ICU.

In the immediate postoperative period one must also consider the deleterious effects of pain, including decreased tidal volume, functional residual capacity, and forced expiratory volume.[22,66] These changes, combined with decreased cough effort and the residual effects of anesthetic agents, lead to ventilation-perfusion mismatch, postoperative hypoxemia, and respiratory failure.

The primary cause of postoperative respiratory dysfunction remains confined to the pulmonary parenchyma itself. This is a collection of processes resulting in increased lung water and increased work of breathing. Inspissated secretions, alterations in airway reactivity, and recurrent pulmonary infections may affect postoperative respiratory function. Periodic examination of chest x-ray films and tracheal aspirates may be helpful in guiding diuretic therapy and the need for antibiotics to clear pulmonary infections. Edema of the chest wall or pulmonary interstitium may also lead to respiratory failure. In addition, cardiac dysfunction with engorgement of pulmonary and bronchial veins may impinge on the airway space. Most important, residual cardiac shunts and increased pulmonary flow may lead to postoperative edema. Therefore, postoperative echocardiography or catheterization may be needed to define the presence of a shunt and its effect on cardiorespiratory function.

When an infant requires prolonged ventilation, an assessment of the four components (CNS, airway, neuromuscular system, and pulmonary parenchyma) should be pursued to evaluate the cause of the respiratory failure. In many cases optimization of cardiovascular function and the judicious use of diuretics to decrease lung water allow for a gradual wean from mechanical ventilation. The other component of muscle weakness that should be aggressively addressed is nutrition. Many of these infants and neonates have little or no nutritional reserve. This, compounded by a prolonged postoperative course, can have significant deleterious effects on the patient.

Aside from concerns regarding gas exchange, alterations in pulmonary vascular resistance and the development of pulmonary vasospasm can have significant implications during the postoperative period. Since the first report of pulmonary hypertension in 1897 by Eisenmenger, it has become increasingly clear that prevention and treatment of pulmonary hypertension can alter postoperative outcome. Although it is impossible to identify all patients at risk for postoperative pulmonary vasospasm, patients with high flows through the pulmonary vascular bed (preoperative $Q_p/Q_s$ greater than 2 : 1 to 3 : 1) or those with obstruction to venous return (anomalous pulmonary venous return with obstruction) are to be considered at risk. Patients with trisomy 21 appear to be at risk for developing pulmonary vascular changes despite low to moderate shunt ratios ($Q_p/Q_s$ 1 : 1 to 2 : 1). Although additional information may be gained from the preoperative cardiac catheterization, it should be remembered that pulmonary vascular resistance may be affected by the type and degree of sedation administered during the procedure.

Once the patients most at risk are identified, prevention of pulmonary vasospasm is particularly important in the immediate postoperative period, since the use of CPB may increase the chances of developing pulmonary hypertension. Several factors play a role in the propensity to develop pulmonary vasospasm following CPB. These include alterations in pulmonary endothelial function with decreased synthesis of endothelial dependent relaxing factor (EDRF) and alterations in platelet and leukocyte function with release of thromboxanes and leukotrienes.

Prevention of pulmonary vasospasm is easiest with early detection. This requires invasive hemodynamic monitoring, including intraoperative placement of pulmonary artery and left atrial lines. Treatment and prevention include both ventilator and pharmacologic management. Ventilator management includes modest hyperventilation with arterial carbon dioxide pressure of 25 to 30 mm Hg and arterial oxygen pressure above 80 mm Hg. Hyperventilation is continued for 2 to 3 days and slowly weaned as tolerated. In addition, metabolic acidosis and hypothermia should be aggressively treated, since either condition may lead to vasospasm. Likewise, adequate sedation and analgesia are of utmost importance. Uncontrolled pain and release of endogenous catecholamines can lead to irreversible episodes of pulmonary vasospasm and death. Fentanyl appears to be particularly advantageous, since it provides analgesia with relative cardiovascular stability while having beneficial effects on the reactivity of the pulmonary vasculature. Initial doses of 3 to 6 μg/kg should be followed with a continuous infusion of 2 to 4 μg/kg/hour and increased as needed.

In patients who develop episodes of pulmonary vasospasm, vasodilator therapy may be helpful. Available pharmacologic agents include nitroglycerin, nitroprusside, tolazoline, prostacyclin, and isoproterenol. Although it has been suggested that some of these agents may be more specific for the pulmonary vascular bed, all of them will also cause some degree of peripheral vasodilatation. Most recently inhaled nitric oxide has been used in experimental studies to treat pulmonary hypertension.[35,79] Nitric oxide, recently identified as EDRF, is synthesized in pulmonary endothelial cells and leads to smooth muscle relaxation through interactions with the intracellular cyclic GMP system. The exogenous administration of inhaled nitric oxide (40 to 60 ppm) leads to selective pulmonary vasodilatation, since the agent is immediately inactivated by hemoglobin when it reaches the blood stream. Early studies suggest that it may have many therapeutic uses, including the treatment of pulmonary hypertension following cardiac surgery.

## CENTRAL NERVOUS SYSTEM

Although dysfunction of the cardiorespiratory system may have the greatest effect on mortality in the immediate perioperative period, CNS damage may have more prolonged consequences for the patient. CPB and surgery for congenital heart disease pose several embolic and hemodynamic threats to neurologic function. Despite several ongoing areas of research in the field, pharmacologic manipulation to prevent post-CPB neurologic dysfunction is still limited to the laboratory. For the most part hypothermia and limitation of circulatory arrest time remain the mainstay of measures to prevent postoperative neurologic dysfunction.[23]

Although the incidence of CNS complications following CPB has decreased in the past 20 years, little or no change has occurred in the past 10 years. The difference from 20 years ago has been attributed to the use of filters in the extracorporeal part of the circuit, which limits the risk of embolic events.[58] Despite the accepted risks of CNS dysfunction following CPB, few if any preoperative or intraoperative events or risk factors have been shown to correlate with CNS damage. However, CNS effects are more commonly seen following open than closed heart procedures.

In the perioperative period the first suggestion that some CNS event occurred may be that the patient does not wake up following surgery. In such cases the residual effects of anesthetic agents should be ruled out. This may include either intravenous agents (opioids and benzodiazepines) or neuromuscular blocking agents. Peripheral nerve stimulation with a standard train-of-four is helpful in evaluating residual neuromuscular blockade. The effects of residual anesthetic agents are more difficult to evaluate. Although reversal agents exist for both narcotics (naloxone) and benzodiazepines (flumazenil), their use in the perioperative period is not recommended because of the risks of precipitating acute withdrawal symptoms and cardiovascular effects of hypertension and tachycardia.

Following a thorough physical examination, laboratory evaluation of the patient should include a search for metabolic causes of altered mental status, including serum electrolytes, blood urea nitrogen, glucose, calcium, magnesium, and ammonia. Further investigation may include CT of the head to rule out ischemic, hemorrhagic, or thrombotic damage. However, changes may not be present for 3 to 5 days on CT scan following thrombotic or embolic events.

A second adverse neurologic event seen following CPB and especially circulatory arrest is the onset of seizures. The incidence of seizures increases with the length of circulatory arrest and is greatest in patients with arrest times longer than 60 minutes. Although circulatory arrest with deep hypothermia is generally well tolerated in infants and neonates with little or no impairment of long-term outcome,[8] perioperative seizures may occur in 1% to 2% of patients.[29] These generally occur within the first 48 hours of the surgery and do not require long-term anticonvulsant therapy. Once metabolic causes of seizures are ruled out, therapy should be started with a single agent, either phenobarbital or phenytoin. Anticonvulsants should be continued for 4 to 6 weeks but can be discontinued at that time in patients with a normal EEG and no further evidence of seizure activity.

## GASTROINTESTINAL AND HEPATIC CONSIDERATIONS

Several issues concerning both the GI system and the liver affect perioperative care. Few topics have gathered as much controversy as the role of various agents in the prevention of stress ulceration in the ICU patient. The first controversy is who needs prophylaxis. There is little or no information about whether all or none of the patients require GI prophylaxis following cardiac surgery. If one decides to treat all patients, further controversy exists over which agent to use. Choices to prevent GI bleeding include $H_2$ antagonists, sucralfate, antacids, omeprazole, and prostaglandin agonists. These latter two agents have just recently been introduced, and their role in the care of the postsurgical patient is yet to be determined. GI ulceration in the critically ill patient is thought to occur not only from increased acid secretion but also from alterations in the normal protective barrier of the stomach. Agents such as the prostaglandins increase the protective mucus layer of the stomach, and omeprazole blocks acid secretion through inhibition of the $Na^+/H^+$ pump.

Recent concern with the use of $H_2$ antagonists has centered on an increased incidence of nosocomial pneumonia.[1,27] It is postulated that alterations in gastric pH allow the growth of gram-negative enteric organisms in the GI tract. This leads to retrograde colonization of the pharynx with aspiration of the pathogenic bacteria into the respiratory tree. Aside from limiting the risk of GI ulceration without altering pH, sucralfate may have some antimicrobial properties.[112] Further studies are needed to define the true significance of these findings and the effects of the newer agents (omeprazole and prostaglandin analogues) on the incidence of nosocomial pneumonia.

A second question on the use of $H_2$ antagonists is which agent to use. Three agents (cimetidine, ranitidine, and famotidine) are available for clinical use. The major advantage of famotidine is a prolonged half-life allowing for an every 12-hour dosing schedule. The first $H_2$ antagonist released, cimetidine, can have significant cardiovascular effects including bradycardia and hypotension.[50] Such effects are uncommon with ranitidine.[39] Additional adverse effects described with cimetidine include CNS alterations including somnolence and altered mental status and alterations in drugs metabolized by the P-450 system. With such effects in mind, the newer $H_2$ antagonists seem preferable. Options for ranitidine include either an 8-hour dosing schedule (1 to 1.5 mg/kg) or a continuous infusion. In either case doses should be increased as needed to maintain a gastric pH above 4.

With the recent information concerning the increased incidence of pneumonia in intubated patients receiving $H_2$ antagonists, it has become apparent that alterations of the flora of the GI tract may have significant impact on the host. It has been suggested that alterations in gut flora may prevent morbidity and mortality in the ICU patient.[10,114,117] These studies have used various combinations of nonabsorbable oral antibiotics to eradicate pathogenic bacteria in the GI tract. The eradication of such bacteria may not only prevent colonization of the pharynx and aspiration in the respiratory system but may also prevent bacterial translocation. This event is thought to occur when ischemia or hypoperfusion leads to alterations in the integrity of the GI tract. The alteration in the GI barrier allows the escape of these pathogenic bacteria and endotoxin into the circulation and may be one factor responsible for multisystem organ failure in the ICU patient. The role of these processes in morbidity and mortality following pediatric cardiac surgery and the impact of selective gut decontamination remains to be determined.

Of a more practical nature is the issue of nutrition in the perioperative period. Nutritional concerns are not of paramount importance for the majority of patients with a brief postoperative course; however, these issues have significant impact on patients with prolonged postoperative courses, especially neonates and patients who were malnourished preoperatively. When oral feedings cannot be administered for more than 3 to 5 days, parenteral nutrition should be started. Although parenteral nutrition sustains the patient when enteral feeds are not possible, our approach is to use enteral feeds whenever possible. Therefore, once cardiovascular stability is achieved and the patient has evidence of gastrointestinal activity, enteral feeds are started. A very cautious increase in enteral feeds is mandatory for patients with recent bouts of cardiovascular compromise that might have led to gut ischemia. Such patients may develop necrotizing enterocolitis if feeds are advanced too quickly. Further restrictions of feedings may be imposed by the need for fluid restriction. In such cases the use of calorie-rich formulas (30 calories/ounce) may provide adequate calories within the guidelines of the fluid restriction. The increase in caloric density should be achieved with the use of both carbohydrate and lipid. The overzealous administration of carbohydrate may lead to feeding intolerance and diarrhea due to carbohydrate malabsorption. Additionally, the increased carbon dioxide production from carbohydrate metabolism as opposed to fat metabolism may lead to hypercarbia and respiratory failure. Other factors, including pancreatic injury following CPB[30] and alterations in GI motility due to narcotic administration, may affect the success of enteral feedings. The latter problem may respond to metoclopramide administration.

Several factors also impact on hepatic function in the perioperative period. Preoperative drug therapy and abnormalities in cardiac output may leave the patient with compromised GI and hepatic function prior to surgery, which may be further complicated by the stress of CPB. Hepatic function may be further affected by infection (cytomegalovirus, Epstein-Barr virus, hepatitis B and non-A, non-B) and parenteral nutrition. Therefore, periodic monitoring of hepatic function and the coagulation profile are suggested. Treatment of hepatic dysfunction is supportive, with blood products to correct abnormalities of coagulation and treatment of hyperammonemia in severe hepatic failure.

Histologic examination of patients with hepatic failure due to alterations in cardiac output reveals centrilobular necrosis. The patients at greatest risk include those with prolonged periods of hypoperfusion requiring inotropic support, especially in the setting of elevated right-sided filling pressures.[53]

## ELECTROLYTE AND FLUID CONSIDERATIONS

Several factors in the perioperative period impact on fluid and electrolyte balance. Alterations in cardiovascular function, residual effects of CPB on pulmonary capillary integrity, and ongoing fluid shifts and losses make close monitoring of fluid status imperative. Although filling pressures (CVP and left atrial pressures) may be used to guide fluid administration, periodic physical examination and measurement of urinary output are also helpful.

Initial fluid management generally includes the administration of hypotonic crystalloid (half normal saline with 5% glucose) at half-maintenance. Periodic monitoring of serum sodium and glucose are recommended. Avoidance of both hypoglycemia and hyperglycemia is important. Seizures, altered mental status, and permanent neurologic damage may result from prolonged hypoglycemia. On the other hand, hyperglycemia may also adversely affect neurologic outcome. Neurologic outcome may be worse following episodes of hypoxemia or hypoperfusion during hyperglycemia. This is thought to result from increased lactic acid production during anaerobic metabolism in the presence of hyperglycemia.

Full maintenance fluids are generally required on postoperative day 2 or 3. Patients on preoperative diuretics or those with residual shunts or mixing lesions will generally require postoperative diuretic administration. For most patients, furosemide is an effective diuretic in a dose of 1 to 2 mg/kg every 8 to 12 hours. However, some patients, in particular those requiring larger preoperative doses, may become resistant. Several options are available in the diuretic-resistant patient, including furosemide by continuous infusion,[100] another loop diuretic (bumetidine or ethacrynic acid), and the addition of oral metolazone.[94]

Diuretic administration can lead to electrolyte disturbances, including hyponatremia, hypokalemia, hypochloremic alkalosis, and hypercalciuria. The issue of hypercalciuria is more a long-term problem; however, significant nephrocalcinosis and impairment of renal function may occur with the prolonged administration of loop diuretics. Periodic monitoring of the urinary calcium to creatinine ratio and the substitution of thiazide diuretics for loop diuretics are indicated.

In our experience hyponatremia may be a problem when switching from parenteral to enteral nutrition. Most parenteral nutrition solutions contain anywhere from 30 to 60 mEq/l of sodium, and most formulas contain only 4 to 8 mEq/l. Therefore, periodic monitoring of serum sodium is recommended, especially when switching from enteral feeds. In some patients sodium supplementation may be required.

Hypokalemia can be corrected with either potassium supplementation or the addition of spironolactone to the diuretic regimen. Spironolactone may be administered alone or in a fixed combination with a thiazide-type diuretic. A major advantage of the thiazide diuretics is the prevention of excessive urinary losses of calcium, thereby limiting the risks of nephrocalcinosis. Hypochloremia may also arise from excessive urinary losses. This is accompanied by a metabolic alkalosis. Although it is generally of little clinical significance, some patients may have impaired respiratory drive and develop a respiratory acidosis with hypercarbia to compensate for the alkalosis. The mainstay of treatment is chloride supplementation; however, the addition of a carbonic anhydrase inhibitor (acetazolamide) will increase urinary losses of bicarbonate and provide a quicker resolution of the electrolyte imbalance.

Alterations in other serum anions and cations such as calcium, phosphorus, and magnesium may also follow cardiac surgery. Several factors may affect serum calcium, including dilution with CPB fluid and the administration of large quantities of blood. Additionally, impairment of parathyroid activity with an inability to mobilize calcium from bone may be seen in the neonate, the stressed infant, and following asphyxia. Treatment consists of calcium supplementation with either calcium chloride or calcium gluconate. Either agent will increase serum calcium to the same extent provided equivalent doses of the calcium cation are administered (0.1 ml/kg of calcium chloride or 0.3 ml/kg of calcium gluconate). Addition of calcium to the intravenous fluids may be required to maintain calcium in the normal range.

Recent interest has been directed toward magnesium and its effects on cardiovascular function.[123] Magnesium losses are increased by the administration of loop diuretics and aminoglycoside antibiotics. Although magnesium is required for parahormone synthesis and release, it has effects on cardiovascular function separate from those of the calcium ion. Hypomagnesemia may occur in up to 60% of patients following CPB leading to decreased cardiac contractility and ventricular arrhythmias.

Several physiologic effects have been ascribed to hypophosphatemia, including impaired cardiac contractility, muscle weakness, respiratory failure, and leftward shift of the oxyhemoglobin dissociation curve with impaired oxygen delivery at the tissue level. Diuretic therapy with increased urinary losses, nasogastric drainage, dilution during CPB, and inadequate replacement in parenteral nutrition solutions are common causes of hypophosphatemia. Periodic monitoring of the above serum cations and anions and appropriate replacement therapy are indicated in the perioperative period.

## HEMATOLOGIC CONCERNS

Cardiac surgery and CPB can have significant effects on all three formed elements of the bone marrow: platelets, erythrocytes, and leukocytes. These effects include alterations not only in numbers but also in function of the formed elements. Of primary concern in the immediate postoperative period are effects on platelet numbers and function. Such effects may lead to severe postoperative hemorrhage and further complicate the postoperative course.

Thrombocytopenia in the immediate postoperative period has many possible causes. A drop in the platelet count occurs during the initiation of bypass. Other effects include mechanical damage to platelets and adherence to the surface of the oxygenator and tubing. Such effects are less with the use of membrane than with bubble oxygenators. Damage to platelets may also lead to alterations in platelet function without a decrease in number. These coagulation disturbances may be aggravated by other causes of postoperative coagulopathy, including incomplete reversal of heparin or protamine overdose.

Persistent postoperative bleeding requires immediate evaluation including platelet count, PT/PTT, and fibrinogen. Although a thorough evaluation of coagulation status is indicated in patients with persistent bleeding, inadequate surgical hemostasis may also cause persistent hemorrhage. In such cases repeated surgical intervention is the only answer. However, every attempt should be made to correct coagulation abnormalities when time permits. A normal PT with a prolonged PTT suggests heparin overdose and may be corrected with incremental doses of protamine (0.1 to 0.2 mg/kg) given by slow intravenous infusion. Prolongation of both the PT and PTT suggests alterations in coagulation factors because of dilution, consumption, or inadequate hepatic synthesis. Correction with fresh frozen plasma (10 ml/kg) is indicated. Thrombocytopenia generally responds to platelet infusion (0.2 units/kg). One additional approach in the treatment of bleeding related to platelet dysfunction has been the administration of DDAVP, a synthetic analogue of posterior pituitary hormone. This agent acts by increasing levels of factor VIII antigen and thereby improving platelet function. Prospective controlled studies are still needed to define the exact role of this agent in the perioperative period. Adverse effects related to DDAVP include hypotension due to systemic vasodilatation and hyponatremia due to its antidiuretic hormone actions.

Anemia is also a common problem in the postoperative period. Dilution from CPB, ongoing losses through chest tubes, repeated phlebotomy for diagnostic laboratory investigation, and mechanical damage to erythrocytes all contribute to the problem. Measurement of hematocrit every 4 to 6 hours is indicated in the immediate postoperative period. Although there is much controversy concerning the optimal hematocrit, our general practice is to keep it above 30% in patients with acyanotic lesions and above 40% in cyanotic lesions. Higher hematocrits may also be indicated in patients with compromised cardiovascular status to optimize oxygen delivery to the tissues. In the immediate postoperative period this may require daily transfusions, especially in infants and small children. Once enteral feeds are started, the addition of iron to the formula may limit the need for transfusions. An additional intervention that may find some role in the perioperative period is the administration of synthetic erythropoietin. This may be especially important for patients with religious objections to the use of blood products.

Hemolysis may also contribute to the drop in hematocrit following CPB. Damage to erythrocyte membrane due to contact with the oxygenator leads to decreased erythrocyte life span. These effects are more common with bubble oxygenators than with the newer membrane oxygenators. Erythrocyte damage and hemolysis may also be seen with prosthetic devices such as heart valves or with high velocity flow through shunts or septal defects. Treatment includes repeated transfusions to maintain an acceptable hematocrit and repair of the defect if the hemolysis persists.

## INFECTIOUS DISEASE

Alterations in both number and function of leukocytes have been described in the immediate postoperative period. These factors, compounded by the need for intravascular devices, places these patients at risk for nosocomial infections and sepsis. Outside of the immediate postoperative period infectious complications remain one of the primary causes of delayed morbidity and mortality.[81]

Adult studies have shown that CPB leads to complement activation, leukopenia, and alterations in both humoral and cellular immune function.[113] Hauser and associates[44] demonstrated similar alterations in immune function (both cellular and humoral) in children following open heart surgery. Alterations in complement and immunoglobulin levels persisted for 2 to 7 days following surgery, as did changes in T cell counts and lymphocyte transformation to antigenic stimulation. Such studies further document alterations not only in numbers but also in function of several components of the immune system, including leukocytes and lymphocytes. These effects may be especially deleterious in neonates, since their immune function is immature and significantly less efficient than in adults. Further studies are needed to investigate various means of modulating the immune system such as the perioperative administration of cytokines and/or immunoglobulins.

Regardless of the various factors leading to immunodepression, an aggressive search for the cause of fever is required in the postoperative cardiac surgery patient. The appearance of more subtle signs such as mild cardiovascular instability, thrombocytopenia, or neutropenia should be considered as sepsis until proven otherwise. Blood, urine, and tracheal aspirates should be obtained and sent for routine and fungal cultures. Broad-spectrum antibiotic coverage should be instituted until cultures are negative. We generally begin antibiotic coverage with a combination of vancomycin and a third-generation cephalosporin. Our preference is ceftazidime, since it provides coverage for *Pseudomonas* in addition to other gram-negative organisms. Antibiotic coverage may have to be tailored to the resistance pattern in the particular hospital.

For patients already on antibiotics the addition of imipenem or tobramycin may be indicated to cover for resistant organisms. Persistent fever despite appropriate antibiotic coverage may indicate invasive fungal disease. Ophthalmologic examination as well as CT or ultrasonography of the liver, spleen, and kidneys may identify occult fungal disease. In such patients the empiric administration of amphotericin B may be indicated until cultures are negative.

## RENAL CONCERNS

Alterations in renal function are common in the perioperative period. Drug therapy, alterations in hemodynamic status, and changes in renal blood flow during CPB all affect renal function. The etiology of renal insufficiency in the perioperative period is generally multifactorial, and control of several factors is needed to ensure proper renal function. Of prime importance are limiting the use of nephrotoxic drugs and close monitoring of renal function when such drugs are administered. Commonly used medications that may be nephrotoxic include antibiotics (especially aminoglycosides and amphotericin B), diuretics, and dyes used during cardiac catheterization.

The onset of oliguria should prompt a thorough investigation into the cause. Prerenal, renal, and postrenal (obstructive) factors may contribute to postoperative oliguria. The judicious use of inotropic agents and fluid administration while following hemodynamic parameters is required to maintain adequate renal blood flow. When oliguria develops, the calculation of the fractional excretion of sodium may be useful in separating prerenal from renal causes. Ultrasonography of the kidneys will rule out obstructive causes.

Although the early and aggressive restoration of cardiac output will restore renal function in most patients, this is easier said than done in the postoperative cardiac patient. Persistent low output may lead to acute tubular necrosis and renal insufficiency. In such cases support of the patient with external devices may be required. The initial treatment of renal insufficiency is directed at amelioration of metabolic abnormalities. Fluid restriction and withholding of exogenous potassium should be the first steps. Fluids should be limited to insensible losses plus urinary output. Insensible losses are generally 20% to 40% of maintenance fluids but may be higher for patients with fever, increased respiratory losses due to tachypnea, or nasogastric or chest tube losses. Indications for dialysis include fluid overload, hyperkalemia, hyperphosphatemia, severe hyponatremia (serum sodium less than 120 mEq/l) and profound metabolic acidosis.

Although hemodialysis was previously the most commonly used means of supporting the oliguric or anuric patient, other options include peritoneal dialysis and hemofiltration. Continuous arteriovenous hemofiltration allows the removal of an ultrafiltrate composed of plasma, water, and non–protein bound small and middle weight molecules. The system uses the patient's own blood pressure to drive the blood through an exogenous system with a semipermeable membrane. This allows the removal of excessive fluid without hemodialysis. Recent alterations in this system include the use of a pump to move the blood through the system, obviating the need for arterial access and allowing a better control of flow through the system. Additionally, the infusion of dialysis fluid in a countercurrent direction across the membrane permits the more rapid removal of solutes including blood urea nitrogen and potassium. The latter system is known as continuous arteriovenous or venovenous hemodiafiltration. These techniques may totally replace hemodialysis or more likely decrease its use.

For some patients either peritoneal dialysis or hemodialysis will also be required. Hemodialysis may be unsuitable in the perioperative period because of its deleterious effects on cardiovascular function. Additionally, peritoneal dialysis may be more efficacious in children because of the relatively large surface area of the peritoneum. Recovery of renal function generally occurs in 3 to 10 days following acute tubular necrosis (ATN). The onset may be heralded by a polyuric phase, during which close attention to fluid and electrolyte replacement is required.

## POSTOPERATIVE ANALGESIA AND SEDATION

There are several options for the provision of postoperative analgesia following thoracic surgery, including systemic narcotics (administered as needed or by a patient-controlled analgesia device), intercostal nerve blocks, epidural local anesthetics or narcotics, and intrathecal narcotics. Of these options, systemic narcotics remain the most frequently used because of the ease of administration and limited requirement for experienced personnel.

The administration of parenteral narcotics necessitates three choices: the route of administration, the narcotic to be used, and the method of administration (continuous versus intermittent). Options for route of administration include intravenous, intramuscular, subcutaneous, oral, and transmucosal (sublingual, buccal, intranasal, rectal). However, intravenous administration remains the primary route in the immediate postoperative period because of variability in absorption and uptake with the other routes. Furthermore, several investigators[90,102] have demonstrated superior analgesia with intravenous administration.

Therefore, intravenous administration appears to be the most feasible and readily accessible means of narcotic administration for the majority of patients. For most patients continuous infusion supplemented with intermittent intravenous bolus doses appears to provide the best level of analgesia. Although studies with children are limited, adult studies suggest that a continuous narcotic infusion provides superior analgesia and fewer adverse effects than either as needed or fixed-interval dosing.[72,77] Lynn and associates[64] evaluated the respiratory effects of continuous morphine infusion in children following cardiac surgery. They found that morphine infusions of 10 to 30 μg/kg/hour resulted in serum concentrations of 10 to 22 ng/ml, provided adequate analgesia, and did not impair weaning from mechanical ventilation. One disadvantage of the continuous infusion of narcotics is that tolerance may occur more quickly with continuous than with intermittent dosing.

A second alternative to continuous infusion or intermittent intravenous administration is the use of a PCA (patient-controlled analgesia) pump. This device allows the patient or bedside nurse to administer a preset amount of narcotic at preselected intervals. This technique requires an awake, cooperative patient who is able to comprehend the purpose of the machine and push the button when additional analgesia is required, so its use in the immediate postoperative period is limited. However, it may be an effective means of providing analgesia once the residual effects of general anesthesia have dissipated. Advantages of PCA include improved analgesia with decreased total narcotic use.[3,37,38] Although its use in children following cardiac surgery has not been investigated, it has proved successful following major orthopedic and abdominal procedures and appears to be applicable to children as young as 6 to 8 years of age.

Although parenteral narcotic is the most commonly chosen postoperative analgesic regimen, regional anesthetic techniques may provide more effective postoperative analgesia and prevent pulmonary dysfunction while avoiding the risks of respiratory depression due to parenteral narcotics.[55,70] Regional anesthetic techniques for the alleviation of pain following thoracic surgery include interpleural analgesia, intercostal nerve blocks, and epidural analgesia.

Intercostal nerve blocks can be performed either intraoperatively under direct vision or immediately postoperatively. These blocks provide effective analgesia, alleviate postoperative pain, decrease narcotic requirements, and improve postoperative pulmonary function and arterial blood gases.[24,32] Reported complications include sympathetic blockade with hypotension, total spinal block due to inadvertent dural puncture, pneumothorax, and intravascular absorption of local anesthetic.[20,67] Furthermore, because of their short duration of action (8 to 12 hours even when long-acting local anesthetics such as bupivacaine are used), they must be repeated postoperatively to provide continuous analgesia. This is not only time consuming, requiring skilled personnel, but also causes pain and discomfort to the patient. A newer approach to decrease provider time and obviate the need for repeated injections involves the placement of an intercostal catheter as the thoracotomy incision is closed.[75] However, this provides analgesia only for that individual intercostal space and not for the chest tube insertion site or the posterior spinal ligaments and muscles, which are involved in the genesis of postthoracotomy pain. Spinal ligaments and muscles are innervated by the posterior primary ramus, which branches from the intercostal nerve proximal to the site of intercostal blocks.

Epidural analgesia uses local anesthetics, narcotics, or a combination of the two. The deposition of local anesthetic in the thoracic epidural space results in multiple bilateral intercostal blocks. This technique also effectively blocks the posterior primary rami. The major disadvantage of thoracic epidural with local anesthetics is that it requires the placement of the needle or catheter in close proximity to the level of the incision. This may require considerable time and skill. Other disadvantages of thoracic epidural analgesia with local anesthetics include bilateral sympathetic blockade leading to hypotension, partial or complete lower extremity motor blockade that may limit postoperative ambulation, inadvertent intravascular injection of local anesthetic with cardiovascular and central nervous sytem toxicity, and inadvertent dural puncture resulting in total spinal block or trauma to the spinal cord. Most important, because of the rich vasculature of the epidural space and the risks of epidural hematoma, this technique is contraindicated in patients with coagulation disturbances. This is especially important in the cardiac surgery patient who requires anticoagulation for cardiopulmonary bypass.

Information concerning the safety of catheter placement before or after anticoagulation is limited. In a series of adult patients undergoing lower extremity revascularization, Rao and El-Etr[84] found no cases of epidural hematoma formation in 3164 patients. In this study the epidural catheter was placed prior to heparinization and heparin was administered to prolong the activated clotting to only twice baseline. Therefore, the safety of this technique in patients with full anticoagulation and CPB has not been investigated. Additionally, anecdotal reports document spinal epidural hematoma following lumbar puncture in patients who receive anticoagulation.[78]

The use of thoracic epidural anesthesia in children is further limited to experienced pediatric anesthesiologists because of the techniques required for catheter placement. Recently, to avoid these problems, the placement of a catheter into the thoracic epidural space through a caudal approach has been described.[6] However, this technique, which involves threading the catheter up the spinal axis for a considerable distance, can be technically difficult. During threading, the catheter may kink, double back on itself, or pass through a vertebral foramina and down a dural root sheath, leading to an incomplete block.

Although the use of local anesthetics necessitates their placement near the dermatomes to be anesthetized, the use of epidural or intrathecal narcotics does not. Lumbar epidural morphine has been shown to be as effective as thoracic epidural morphine in providing postoperative analgesia following thoracic and upper abdominal procedures.[59] Following the spinal administration of narcotics, diffusion into the cerebrospinal fluid and cephalad spread along the spinal axis occurs. Therefore, the caudal or lumbar administration of spinal narcotics provides analgesia along the entire spinal axis regardless of the site of administration.[110] An additional advantage of caudal administration over lumbar administration is to avoid the epidural vasculature and thereby limit the risk of epidural hematoma formation. Rosen and Rosen[88] evaluated the safety and efficacy of caudal epidural morphine following cardiac surgery in children. They found that caudal epidural morphine (0.075 mg/kg) administered at the completion of the surgical procedure decreased pain scores and lowered intravenous morphine requirements, without hemorrhagic complications.

Although the use of epidural opioids has been limited in cardiac surgery patients, at least three reports address the administration of intrathecal opioids in this patient population.[31,54,115] Jones and associates[54] were among the first investigators to report the use of intrathecal morphine in children. In their study 56 children received either 0.03 mg/kg (27 patients) or 0.02 mg/kg (29 patients) of morphine in the lumbar intrathecal space prior to the start of surgery. Although no formal pain scoring system or control group was used, they found that 67% of the patients required no additional analgesic agents during the first 22 postoperative hours. Additionally, they found no difference in length of analgesia between the two doses of morphine. Fitzpatrick and Moriarty[31] evaluated the efficacy of intrathecal morphine following coronary revascularization surgery in adults. The patients were randomized to receive either morphine 30 mg intravenously or one of two doses of intrathecal morphine (1 or 2 mg) following the induction of anesthesia and prior to the start of surgery. Mean overall pain scores and postoperative supplemental morphine requirements were significantly lower in both of the intrathecal groups than in the intravenous morphine group. Also, peak expiratory flow rates were significantly improved in both of the intrathecal groups. Although there was no significant difference in the quality of analgesia when comparing the patients who received 1 mg of intrathecal morphine with those who received 2 mg, there was a significant increase in the arterial carbon dioxide pressure in the patients who received 2 mg. The third study evaluating the efficacy of intrathecal morphine was also performed following coronary revascularization surgery in adults.[115] Patients were randomized to receive either intrathecal morphine 0.5 mg or a placebo injection. Patients who received intrathecal morphine required significantly less supplemental intravenous morphine during the first 24 hours and significantly less nitroprusside to control postoperative hypertension. No hemorrhagic complications occurred in any of these three studies despite the fact that lumbar puncture was performed prior to heparinization.

The advantages of spinal narcotics in contrast to local anesthetics is that they provide a selective sensory blockade without effects on either the sympathetic or motor nerves while providing a prolonged duration of action (up to 24 hours with morphine). As with narcotics by any route, the epidural or intrathecal administration can lead to respiratory depression. However, in contrast to intravenous or intramuscular administration, respiratory depression can be delayed for up to 24 hours following the dose.[41] Additional adverse effects associated with spinal narcotics include pruritus, urinary retention, and vomiting.[41] Current practice for epidural analgesia generally includes a continuous infusion with a combination of dilute local anesthetic (bupivacaine) and narcotic (fentanyl).[109]

In summary, several options exist for the provision of analgesia following cardiac surgery in children. To date the majority of experience resides in the use of parenteral narcotics. When this route is chosen, the initial use of a continuous infusion of either morphine or fentanyl supplemented with intermittent bolus doses seems to be the optimal modality. Fentanyl appears to be the most appropriate choice in patients with cardiovascular instability and in patients at risk for episodes of postoperative pulmonary hypertension.[47,48] The use of a PCA device may improve analgesia and is indicated in patients who are awake enough and old enough to understand the device. In many circumstances regional anesthetic techniques such as epidural anesthesia may provide better analgesia than parenteral narcotics. This is especially true in patients not requiring CPB and anticoagulation. When anticoagulation is required, the safety of epidural anesthesia remains unproved. However, preliminary evidence does support the safety and efficacy of caudal epidural and lumbar intrathecal morphine.

Besides pain, several situations may require sedation or amnesia and not necessarily analgesia. In the doses commonly used to provide postoperative analgesia, opioids can be expected to provide sedation but not amnesia. However, several classes of agents other than narcotics provide amnesia and anxiolysis. Early trials included the use of etomidate and inhaled nitrous oxide. Although etomidate resulted in improved cardiovascular stability, prolonged administration resulted in suppression of adrenocortical function. Nitrous oxide was abandoned because of suppressive effects on bone marrow activity related to interference with methionine synthetase function and resultant megaloblastic anemia.

Today opioids and benzodiazepines (diazepam, midazolam, and lorazepam) are the most commonly used drugs for sedation in the intensive care unit.[42] Although diazepam can be expected to provide adequate sedation, disadvantages include a long elimination half-life and a hypnotically active metabolite (n-desmethyldiazepam),[120] and prolonged sedation may occur after its discontinuation. Several investigators have documented the efficacy of the continuous infusion of midazolam for sedation following cardiac surgery.[5,62,99] Midazolam is an imidazobenzodiazepine with a rapid onset of action, short elimination half-life, and no active metabolites. Additional benefits include cardiovascular stability with limited effects on respiratory function when administered by itself.[33] In line with the advent of PCA for the delivery of opioids, Egan and co-workers[28] have recently described the delivery of midazolam by a PCA device for sedation in the ICU.

Although its short half-life is an advantage when considering recovery time once the infusion is discontinued, this necessitates its use by continuous infusion for sedation. When intravenous access is limited, the administration of the longer-acting agent lorazepam may be preferred. Midazolam and lorazepam have relatively low cardiorespiratory effects and no active metabolites when they are administered alone. Both agents may cause significant respiratory and cardiovascular depression if administered concurrently with opioids.[122] Additionally, benzodiazepines possess no analgesic properties,[89] and supplemental analgesic agents should be administered when the patient is in pain.

As with narcotics, the prolonged administration of benzodiazepines may result in physical dependence, and an abstinence syndrome may develop if these agents are abruptly discontinued after prolonged administration.[4,34] This can be prevented by slowly tapering them off. An alternative is switching from intravenous midazolam to an orally active agent with a longer half-life, such as lorazepam, to obviate the need for intravenous access.

Over the years, adverse effects associated with the use of narcotics and benzodiazepines have led to the trial of various other agents for sedation in the ICU. Of particular value would be an agent that provided sedation without significantly altering cardiorespiratory function. Although the narcotic fentanyl and the benzodiazepines are generally well tolerated, significant adverse effects on cardiorespiratory function may necessitate switching to another agent. In such situations ketamine may be an effective alternative.[108]

Ketamine is an intravenous anesthetic agent, chemically related to phencyclidine, first described for use in clinical anesthesia by Domino and colleagues[26] in 1965. It produces dissociative anesthesia, an electrophysiologic break between the limbic and thalamoneocortical systems.[19] Although it was initially used for the induction of general anesthesia, later studies documented its efficacy by continuous infusion for intraoperative anesthesia[52,85] and postoperative sedation.[14,51,97] Of prime importance is the ability of ketamine to produce both amnesia and analgesia.

Commercially available ketamine is a racemic mixture of equal concentrations of the two enantiomers (+, −). Metabolism occurs primarily by hepatic N-methylation to norketamine. The metabolite retains anesthetic properties of roughly one third that of the parent compound. Further metabolism is carried out by hydroxylation and urinary excretion. As the primary route of metabolism is hepatic, doses should be reduced in patients with hepatic dysfunction.

The major advantage of ketamine lies in its relative cardiovascular stability. Ketamine produces a dose-related increase in heart rate and blood pressure. Although the exact mechanisms accounting for this phenomenon have not been clearly delineated, it is thought to be mediated through the sympathetic nervous system and the release of endogenous catecholamines.[12,91] Evidence for this mechanism has been offered by Chernow and associates,[12] who demonstrated increased urine, plasma, and cerebrospinal fluid epinephrine levels following ketamine administration. This indirect sympathomimetic effect generally overshadows ketamine's direct negative inotropic properties. However, unstable patients may become hypotensive following ketamine administration.[118] It is postulated that in these patients ketamine's direct negative inotropic properties predominate either because chronic illness depletes endogenous catecholamine stores or sympathetic stimulation is already maximal.

An issue of utmost importance in the child with congenital heart disease is the possible effects of ketamine on pulmonary vascular resistance (PVR). Increased PVR has been reported in adults, and avoidance of ketamine has been recommended in patients with pulmonary hypertension.[40,101] However, further analysis has attributed the alterations in PVR to changes in respiratory function. These previous studies were performed in spontaneously breathing patients without consideration for alterations in arterial carbon dioxide pressure. Conflicting results have been found in children. Morray and associates[68] found statistically significant increases in pulmonary artery pressure (20.6 to 22.8 mm Hg) and PVR during cardiac catheterization in spontaneously breathing patients after ketamine administration. In contrast, Hickey and colleagues[46] found no change in PVR in intubated infants with minimal ventilatory support (4 breaths per minute and $FiO_2$ of 0.4). This latter study included 14 patients, 7 with normal baseline PVR and 7 with elevated baseline PVR. Pending further studies ketamine should be used cautiously in patients with pulmonary hypertension, especially during spontaneous ventilation.

Respiratory function is generally well maintained during ketamine administration. Mankikian and co-workers[65] demonstrated that functional residual capacity, minute ventilation, and tidal volume were unchanged following ketamine administration. Furthermore, ketamine improves pulmonary compliance and relieves bronchospasm.[49] These effects are also attributed to the release of endogenous catecholamines, since they can be blocked by β-antagonist administration.[49] Although ventilation is generally well maintained, elevations in arterial carbon dioxide pressure and a shift to the right of the carbon dioxide response curve does occur.[7]

Ketamine increases salivary and bronchial glands secretion through stimulation of central cholinergic receptors.[57] Therefore, the administration of an antisialogogue such as atropine or glycopyrrolate is recommended. Controversy exists over ketamine's effects on protective airway reflexes. Although clinical use and experimental studies[57] suggest that these reflexes are maintained, aspiration has been reported following ketamine administration.[106]

Ketamine may also increase intracranial pressure (ICP) and therefore should be avoided in patients at risk for intracranial hypertension.[96] Alterations in ICP are a consequence of cerebral vasodilatation, mediated directly through central cholinergic receptors and not secondary to alterations in cerebral metabolic rate or changes in arterial carbon dioxide pressure.[36,76,86]

The adverse effect of ketamine that receives the most attention is emergence phenomena, or hallucinations. Emergence phenomena, most common in older patients, are dose-related, and their incidence can be decreased by the preadministration of a benzodiazepine.[119] These emergence reactions have been postulated to be due to ketamine's depression of auditory and visual relay in the inferior colliculus and the medical geniculate nucleus.[73] This effect may lead to misinterpretation of visual and auditory stimuli.

Due to its favorable effects on cardiorespiratory function, ketamine may be quite useful in patients who do not tolerate narcotics or benzodiazepines, and it provides both analgesia and amnesia. Therefore it may be quite useful in bolus administration (1 to 2 mg/kg) prior to painful procedures such as central line placement. For continuous infusion for sedation, we generally start with a bolus dose of 1 to 2 mg/kg followed by a continuous infusion of 0.5 to 1.0 mg/kg/hour and increase this as needed.[108]

Additional options for sedation include the barbiturates and the new intravenous anesthetic agent, propofol. However, due to their depressant effects on cardiovascular function (negative inotropic properties combined with systemic vasodilatation), the use of barbiturates in the child with congenital heart disease is limited.

Propofol (Diprivan) is an intravenous anesthetic agent that is chemically unrelated to barbiturates and other commonly used anesthetic agents.[93] Due to its rapid onset and quick recovery time following discontinuation, it has become a popular agent for sedation in the ICU.[2,43] However, like the barbiturates, propofol may be associated with hemodynamic instability attributed to its negative inotropic properties.[9] Although well tolerated in patients with adequate cardiac reserve, in hemodynamically unstable patients it is not recommended. Additionally, several reports have described unusual neurologic manifestations following its use including opisthotonic posturing, generalized twitching, and convulsions.[16,92,111] These effects limit its use in the immediate postoperative period, especially following cardiopulmonary bypass and/or circulatory arrest.

In summary, several options exist for sedation in children following cardiac surgery. We generally use the continuous infusion of either fentanyl or midazolam. In patients with limited vascular access the intermittent administration of a longer acting benzodiazepine may be advantageous. When adverse effects occur following narcotic or benzodiazepine administration, ketamine may be an effective alternative. Because of its amnestic and analgesic properties, it may be particularly useful by bolus dosing for brief invasive procedures.

## REFERENCES


1. Apte NM, Karnad DR, Medhekar TP et al: Gastric colonization and pneumonia in intubated critically ill patients receiving stress ulcer prophylaxis: a randomized control trial, *Crit Care Med* 20:590, 1992.
2. Beller JP, Pottecher T, Lugnier A et al: Prolonged sedation with propofol in ICU patients: recovery and blood concentration changes during periodic interruptions infusions, *Br J Anaesth* 61:583, 1988.
3. Berde CB, Lehn BM, Yee JD et al: Patient-controlled analgesia in children and adolescents: a randomized prospective comparison with intramuscular administration of morphine for postoperative analgesia, *J Pediatr* 118:460, 1991.
4. Bergman I, Steeves M, Bruckart G et al: Reversible neurologic abnormalities associated with prolonged intravenous midazolam and fentanyl administration, *J Pediatr* 119:644, 1991.
5. Booker PD, Beechey A, Lloyd-Thomas AR: Sedation of children requiring artificial ventilation using an infusion of midazolam, *Br J Anaesth* 58:1104, 1986.
6. Bosenberg AT, Bland BAR, Schulte-Steinberg O et al: Thoracic epidural via caudal route in infants, *Anesthesiology* 69:265, 1988.
7. Bourke DL, Malit LA, Smith TC: Respiratory interactions of ketamine and morphine, *Anesthesiology* 66:153, 1987.
8. Brunberg JA, Reilley EI, Doty DB: Central nervous system consequences in infants and children with cyanotic congenital heart disease, *Circulation* 50(suppl 2):60, 1974.
9. Brussel T, Theissen JL, Vigfusson G et al: Hemodynamic and cardiodynamic effects of propofol and etomidate: negative inotropic properties of propofol, *Anesth Analg* 69:35, 1989.
10. Cerra FB, Maddaus MA, Dunn DL et al: Selective gut decontamination reduces nosocomial infections and length of stay but not mortality or organ failure in surgical intensive care unit patients, *Arch Surg* 127:163, 1992.
11. Chang AC, Hanley FL, Weindling SN et al: Left heart support with a ventricular assist device in an infant with acute myocarditis, *Crit Care Med* 20:712, 1992.
12. Chernow B, Laker R, Creuss D et al: Plasma, urine, and cerebrospinal fluid catecholamine concentrations during and after ketamine sedation, *Crit Care Med* 10:600, 1982.
13. Christensen DW, Veasy G, McGough J et al: Intraaortic balloon counterpulsation in children: a review of 29 patients, *Crit Care Med* 19:S75, 1991.
14. Clausen L, Sinclair DM, Van Hasselt CH: Intravenous ketamine for postoperative analgesia, *S Afr Med J* 49:1437, 1975.
15. Coles JG, Watanabe T, Wilson GJ et al: Age-related differences in the response to myocardial ischemic stress, *J Thorac Cardiovasc Surg* 94:526, 1987.
16. Collier C, Kelly K: Propofol and convulsions: the evidence mounts, *Anaesth Intensive Care* 19:573, 1991.
17. Coniam SW: Accidental hypothermia, *Anaesthesia* 34:250, 1979.
18. Connell RS, Page US, Bartley TD et al: The effect of pulmonary ultrastructure of Dacron wool filtration during cardiopulmonary bypass, *Ann Thorac Surg* 65:425, 1973.

19. Corssen G, Miyasaka M, Domino EF: Changing concepts in pain control during surgery: dissociative anesthesia with CI-581, *Anesth Analg* 47:746, 1968.
20. Cottrell WM, Schick LM, Perkins HM et al: Hemodynamic changes after intercostal block with bupivacaine-epinephrine solution, *Anesth Analg* 57:492, 1978.
21. Couser RJ, Ferrara TB, Falde B et al: Effectiveness of dexamethasone in preventing extubation failure in preterm infants at increased risk for airway edema, *J Pediatr* 121:591, 1992.
22. Craig CB: Postoperative recovery of pulmonary function, *Anesth Analg* 60:46, 1981.
23. Crittenden MD, Roberts CS, Rosa L et al: Brain protection during circulatory arrest, *Ann Thor Surg* 51:942, 1991.
24. Delikan AE, Lee LK, Yong NK: Postoperative local analgesia for thoracotomy with direct bupivacaine intercostal blocks, *Anaesthesia* 28:561, 1973.
25. DiCarlo JV, Raphaely RC, Steven JM et al: Pulmonary mechanics in infants after cardiac surgery, *Crit Care Med* 20:22, 1992.
26. Domino EF, Chodoff P, Corssen G: Pharmacologic effects of CI-581, a new dissociative anesthetic in man, *Clin Pharmacol Ther* 6:279, 1965.
27. Driks MR, Craven DE, Celli BR et al: Nosocomial pneumonia in intubated patients given sucralfate as compared with antacids or histamine$_2$ blockers, *N Engl J Med* 317:1376, 1987.
28. Egan KJ, Ready LB, Nessly M et al: Self-administration of midazolam for postoperative anxiety: a double-blind study, *Pain* 49:3, 1992.
29. Ehyai A, Fenichel GM, Bender HW Jr: Incidence and prognosis of seizures in infants after cardiac surgery with profound hypothermia and circulatory arrest, *JAMA* 252:3165, 1984.
30. Fernandez-Del Castillo C, Harringer W, Warshaw AL et al: Risk factors for pancreatic cellular injury after cardiopulmonary bypass, *N Engl J Med* 325:382, 1991.
31. Fitzpatrick GJ, Moriarty DC: Intrathecal morphine in the management of pain following cardiac surgery, *Br J Anaesth* 60:639, 1988.
32. Fleming JH, Sarafian LB: Kindness pays dividends: the medical benefits of intercostal nerve blocks following thoracotomy, *J Thoracic Cardiovasc Surgery* 74:273, 1977.
33. Fragen RJ, Meyers SN, Barresi V et al: Hemodynamic effects of midazolam in cardiac patients, *Anesthesiology* 51:172, 1979.
34. Freda JJ, Bush HL, Barie PS: Alprazolam withdrawal in a critically ill patient, *Crit Care Med* 20:545, 1992.
35. Frostell C, Fratacci M, Wain JC et al: Inhaled nitric oxide: a selective pulmonary vasodilator reversing hypoxic pulmonary vasoconstriction, *Circulation* 83:2038, 1991.
36. Gardner AE, Dannemiller FJ, Dean D: Intracranial cerebrospinal fluid pressure in man during ketamine anesthesia, *Anesth Analg* 151:741, 1972.
37. Gaukroger PB, Omkins DP, Van Der Walt JH: Patient-controlled analgesia in children, *Anaesth Intensive Care* 17:264, 1989.
38. Gillespie JA, Morton NS: Patient-controlled analgesia for children: a review, *Pediatric Anaesthesia* 2:51, 1992.
39. Goelzer SL, Farin-Rush C, Coursin DB: Ranitidine produces minimal hemodynamic depression in stable intensive care unit patients: a double-blind prospective study, *Crit Care Med* 16:8, 1988.
40. Gooding JM, Dimick AR, Travakoli M et al: A physiologic analysis of cardiopulmonary responses to ketamine anesthesia in noncardiac patients, *Anesth Analg* 56:813, 1977.
41. Gustaffson LL, Schildt B, Jacobsen K: Adverse effects of epidural and intrathecal opiates: report of a nationwide survey in Sweden, *Br J Anaesth* 54:479, 1982.
42. Hansen-Flaschen JH, Brazinsky S, Basile C et al: Use of sedating drugs and neuromuscular agents in patients requiring mechanical ventilation for respiratory failure, *JAMA* 266:2870, 1991.
43. Harris CE, Grounds RM, Murray AM et al: Propofol for long-term sedation in the intensive care unit: a comparison with papveretum and midazolam, *Anaesthesia* 45:366, 1990.
44. Hauser GJ, Chan MM, Casey WF et al: Immune dysfunction in children after corrective surgery for congenital heart disease, *Crit Care Med* 29:874, 1991.
45. Heard GG, Lamberti JJ, Park SM et al: Early extubation following surgical repair of congenital heart disease, *Crit Care Med* 13:830, 1985.
46. Hickey PR, Hansen DD, Cramolini GM et al: Pulmonary and systemic hemodynamic responses to ketamine in infants with normal and elevated pulmonary vascular resistance, *Anesthesiology* 62:287, 1985.
47. Hickey PR, Hansen DD, Wessel DL et al: Pulmonary and systemic hemodynamic responses to fentanyl in infants, *Anesth Analg* 64:483, 1985.
48. Hickey PR, Hansen DD, Wessel DL et al: Blunting of stress response in pulmonary circulation of infants by fentanyl, *Anesth Analg* 64:1137, 1985.
49. Hirshman CA, Downes H, Farbood A et al: Ketamine block of bronchospasm in experimental canine asthma, *Br J Anaesth* 51:713, 1979.
50. Iberti TJ, Pzluch TA, Helmer L et al: The hemodynamic effects of intravenous cimetidine in intensive care unit patients: a double-blind prospective study, *Anesthesiology* 64:87, 1986.
51. Ito Y, Ichivanagi I: Postoperative pain relief with ketamine infusion, *Anaesthesia* 29:222, 1974.
52. Jastak JT, Goretta C: Ketamine as a continuous drip anesthesia for outpatients, *Anesth Analg* 52:341, 1973.
53. Jenkins JG, Lynn AM, Wood AE et al: Acute hepatic failure following cardiac operation in children, *J Thorac Cardiovasc Surg* 84:865, 1982.
54. Jones SEF, Beasley JM, Macfarlane DWR et al: Intrathecal morphine for postoperative pain relief in children, *Br J Anaesth* 56:137, 1984.
55. Kambam JR, Shanta TR: Interpleural analgesia in the management of pain, *Pain Digest* 2:18, 1992.
56. Kapur PA: Con: epinephrine and norepinephrine are the inotropes of choice: an opposing view, *J Cardiothor Anes* 3:259, 1987.
57. Lanning CF, Harmel MH: Ketamine anesthesia, *Annu Rev Med* 26:137, 1975.
58. Larmi TKI, Karkola P, Kairaluoma MI et al: Calcium microemboli and microfilters in valve operations, *Ann Thorac Surg* 21:412, 1976.
59. Larsen VH, Iversen AD, Christensen P et al: Postoperative pain treatment after upper abdominal surgery with epidural morphine at thoracic or lumbar level, *Acta Anaesthesiol Scand* 29:566, 1985.
60. Lefemine AA, Harken DE: Postoperative care following open-heart operations: routine use of controlled ventilation, *J Thorac Cardiovasc Surg* 52:207, 1966.
61. Lindemann JP, Bailey JC, Watanabe AM: Potential biochemical mechanisms for regulation of the slow inward current: theorectical basis for drug action, *Am Heart J* 103:746, 1982.
62. Lloyd-Thomas AR, Booker PD: Infusion of midazolam in paediatric patients after cardiac surgery, *Br J Anaesth* 58:1109, 1986.
63. Louis PT, Bricker JT, Frazier OH et al: Nonpulsatile left

ventricular support in pediatric patients, *Crit Care Med* 20:704, 1992.

64. Lynn AM, Opheim KE, Tyler DC: Morphine infusion after pediatric cardiac surgery, *Crit Care Med* 12:863, 1984.
65. Mankikian B, Cantineau JP, Sartene R et al: Ventilatory and chest wall mechanics during ketamine anesthesia in humans, *Anesthesiology* 65:492, 1986.
66. Marshall BE, Wyche MQ: Hypoxia during and after anesthesia, *Anesthesiology* 37:178, 1972.
67. Moore MC, Reitan JA: Sudden total spinal block after intraoperative intercostal injections: a case report, *Anesth Rev* 8:36, 1978.
68. Morray JP, Lynn AM, Stamm SJ et al: Hemodynamic effects of ketamine in children with congenital heart disease, *Anesth Analg* 63:895, 1984.
69. Mueller HS, Evans R, Ayres SM: Effect of dopamine in hemodynamics and myocardial metabolism in shock following acute myocardial infarction in man, *Circulation* 57:361, 1978.
70. Muneyuki M, Ueda Y, Urabe N et al: Postoperative pain relief and respiratory function in man: comparison between intermittent intravenous injections of meperidine and continuous lumbar epidural analgesia, *Anesthesiology* 29:304, 1968.
71. Najafi H, Henson D, Dye WS et al: Left ventricular hemorrhagic necrosis, *Ann Thorac Surg* 88:423, 1969.
72. Nayman J: Measurement and control of postoperative pain, *Ann R Coll Surg Engl* 61:419, 1979.
73. Nelson SR, Howard RB, Cross RS et al: Ketamine alters regional glucose utilization in the rat brain, *Anesthesiology* 52:330, 1980.
74. Nishimura RA, Callahan MJ, Homes DR et al: Transient atrioventricular block after open-heart surgery for congenital heart disease, *Am J Cardiol* 53:198, 1984.
75. Olivet RT, Nauss LA, Payne WS: A technique for continuous intercostal nerve block analgesia following thoracotomy, *J Thorac Cardiovasc Surg* 80:308, 1980.
76. Oren RE, Rasool NA, Rubinstein EH: Effect of ketamine on cerebral cortical blood flow and metabolism in rabbits, *Stroke* 18:445, 1987.
77. Orr IA, Keenan DJM, Dundee JW: Improved pain relief after thoracotomy: use of cryoprobe and morphine infusion, *Br Med J* 283:945, 1981.
78. Owens EL, Kasten GW, Hessel EA: Spinal subarachnoid hematoma after lumbar puncture and heparinization, *Anesth Analg* 65:1201, 1986.
79. Pepke-Zaba J, Higenbottam TW, Dinh-Xuan AT et al: Inhaled nitric oxide as a case of selective pulmonary vasodilatation in pulmonary hypertension, *Lancet* 338:1171, 1991.
80. Pisctelli RL, Fox LM: Myocardial injury from epinephrine overdose, *Am J Cardiol* 21:735, 1968.
81. Pollock EMM, Ford-Jones EE, Rebeyka I et al: Early nosocomial infections in pediatric cardiovascular surgery patients, *Crit Care Med* 18:378, 1990.
82. Prakash O, Jonson B, Meij S et al: Criteria for early extubation after intracardiac surgery in adults, *Anesth Analg* 59:703, 1977.
83. Quasha AL, Leober N, Feeley TW et al: Postoperative respiratory care: A controlled trial of early and late extubation following coronary-artery bypass grafting, *Anesthesiology* 52:135, 1980.
84. Rao TLK, El-Etr AA: Anticoagulation following placement of epidural and subarachnoid catheters, *Anesthesiology* 55:618, 1981.
85. Rees DI, Howell ML: Ketamine-atracurium by continuous infusion as the sole anesthetic for pulmonary surgery, *Anesth Analg* 65:860, 1986.
86. Reicher D, Bhalla P, Rubinstein EH: Cholinergic cerebral vasodilator effects of ketamine in rabbits, *Stroke* 18:445, 1987.
87. Rogers AJ, Trento A, Siewers RD et al: Extracorporeal membrane oxygenation for postcardiotomy cardiogenic shock in children, *Ann Thorac Surg* 47:903, 1989.
88. Rosen KR, Rosen DA: Caudal epidural morphine for control of pain following open heart surgery in children, *Anesthesiology* 70:418, 1989.
89. Rosland JH, Hole K: 1,4-Benzodiazepines antagonize opiate-induced antinociception in mice, *Anesth Analg* 71:242, 1990.
90. Rutter PC, Murphy F, Dudley HAF: Morphine: Controlled trial of different methods of administration, *Br Med J* 280:12, 1980.
91. Saegusa K, Furukawa Y, Ogiwara Y: Pharmacologic analysis of ketamine-induced cardiac actions in isolated, blood-perfused canine atria, *J Cardiovasc Pharmacol* 8:414, 1986.
92. Saunders PRI, Harris MNE: Opisthotonic posturing and other unusual neurological sequelae after outpatient anesthesia, *Anaesthesia* 47:552, 1992.
93. Sebel PS, Lowdon JD: Propofol: a new intravenous anesthetic, *Anesthesiology* 71:260, 1989.
94. Segar JL, Robillard JE, Johnson KJ et al: Addition of metolazone to furosemide in infants with bronchopulmonary dysplasia, *J Pediatr* 120:966, 1992.
95. Sessler DI, Rubinstein EH, Maoyeri A: Physiologic responses to mild perianesthetic hypothermia in humans, *Anesthesiology* 75:594, 1991.
96. Shapiro HM, Wyte SR, Harris AB: Ketamine anesthesia in patients with intracranial pathology, *Br J Anaesth* 44:1200, 1972.
97. Sheref SE: Ketamine and bronchospasm, *Anaesthesia* 40:701, 1985.
98. Sherry KM: Postextubation stridor in Down's syndrome, *Br J Anaesth* 55:53, 1983.
99. Silvasi DL, Rosen DA, Rosen KR: Continuous intravenous midazolam infusion for sedation in the pediatric intensive care unit, *Anesth Analg* 67:286, 1988.
100. Singh NC, Kissoon N, Mofada S et al: Comparison of continuous versus intermittent furosemide administration in postoperative pediatric cardiac patients, *Crit Care Med* 20:17, 1992.
101. Spotoft H, Korshin JD, Sorensen MB et al: The cardiovascular effects of ketamine used for induction of anesthesia in patients with valvular heart disease, *Can Anaesth Soc J* 26:463, 1979.
102. Stapleton JV, Austin KL, Mather LE: A pharmacokinetic approach to postoperative pain: continuous infusion of pethidine, *Anaesth Intensive Care* 7:25, 1979.
103. Steen PA, Tinker JH, Pluth JR et al: Efficacy of dopamine, dobutamine, and epinephrine during emergence from cardiopulmonary bypass in man, *Circulation* 57:378, 1978.
104. Stoen R, Sessler DI: The thermoregulatory threshold is inversely proportional to isoflurane concentration, *Anesthesiology* 72:822, 1990.
105. Taber RE, Morales AR, Fine G: Myocardial necrosis and the postoperative myocardial necrosis syndrome, *Ann Thorac Surg* 4:12, 1967.
106. Taylor PA, Towey RM: Depression of laryngeal reflexes during ketamine administration, *Br Med J* 2:688, 1971.
107. Tinker J: Pro: strong inotropes (i.e. epinephrine) should be drugs of first choice during emergence from cardiopulmonary bypass, *J Cardiothor Anes* 3:256, 1987.
108. Tobias JD, Martin LD, Wetzel RC: Ketamine by contin-

uous infusion for sedation in the pediatric intensive care unit, *Crit Care Med* 18:819, 1990.
109. Tobias JD, Oakes L, Rao B: Continuous epidural anesthesia for postoperative analgesia in the pediatric oncology patient, *Am J Pediatr Hematol Oncol* (in press).
110. Tobias JD, Deshpande JK, Wetzel RC et al: Postoperative analgesia: Use of intrathecal morphine in children, *Clin Pediatr* 29:44, 1990.
111. Trotter C, Serpell MG: Neurological sequelae in children after prolonged propofol infusions, *Anaesthesia* 47:340, 1992.
112. Tryba M, Mantey-Stiers F: The antibacterial activity of sucralfate, *Am J Med* 83(suppl 3B):125, 1987.
113. Utley JR: The immune response to cardiopulmonary bypass. In Utley JR, editor: *Pathophysiology and technique of cardiopulmonary bypass,* vol 1, Baltimore, 1982, Williams & Wilkins.
114. Van Saene HKF, Stoutenbeek CC, Stoller JK: Selective decontamination of the digestive tract in the intensive care unit: current status and future prospects, *Crit Care Med* 20:691, 1992.
115. Vanstrum GS, Bjornson KM, Ilko R: Postoperative effects of intrathecal morphine in coronary artery bypass surgery, *Anesth Analg* 67:261, 1988.
116. Veasy LG, Webster HF, McGough EC: Intraaortic balloon pumping: adaptation for pediatric use, *Crit Care Clin* 2:237, 1986.
117. Wainer S, Cooper PA, Funk E et al: Prophylactic miconazole oral gel for the prevention of neonatal fungal rectal colonization and systemic infection, *Pediatr Infect Dis J* 11:713, 1992.
118. Wayman K, Shoemaker WC, Lippmann M: Cardiovascular effects of anesthetic induction with ketamine, *Anesth Analg* 59:355, 1980.
119. White PR, Way WL, Trevor AJ: Ketamine: its pharmacology and therapeutic uses, *Anesthesiology* 56:119, 1982.
120. Willatts SM: Intravenous sedation by infusion on the intensive therapy unit, *Br J Parent Ther* 1:13, 1985.
121. Wittnich C, Peniston C, Ianuzzo D et al: Relative vulnerability of neonatal and adult hearts to ischemic injury, *Circulation* 76:156, 1987.
122. Yaster M, Nichols DG, Deshpanbe JK et al: Midazolam-fentanyl intravenous sedation in children: case report of respiratory arrest, *Pediatrics* 86:463, 1990.
123. Yurvati AHO, Sanders SP, Dullye LJ et al: Antiarrythmic response to intravenously administered magnesium after cardiac surgery, *So Med J* 85:714, 1992.

# 13 Perioperative Disturbances in Cardiac Rhythm

*Frank A. Fish and James A. Johns*



Perioperative rhythm disturbances may occur in a number of settings among patients undergoing either cardiac or noncardiac operation. These dysrhythmias may be a direct consequence of the operation itself or may reflect an underlying predisposition to the dysrhythmia that has been exacerbated by the stress of the procedure, the withholding of chronic antiarrhythmic therapy, or direct manipulation of the heart.

Less commonly, dysrhythmia may represent an adverse reaction to the anesthesia itself or to associated metabolic or ventilatory derangements. These include profound hypothermia, malignant hyperthermia, cocaine or lidocaine toxicity, hyperkalemia or hypocalcemia due to massive transfusions, and unrecognized extubation. While such iatrogenic causes should always be considered, they will not be directly addressed in this discussion.

## BASIS

Bradyarrhythmias include sinus bradycardia, sinus pauses, and various types of AV block. All except for high-grade or complete AV block may represent normal physiologic variants due to high resting vagal tone. However, unrelenting and profound sinus bradycardia or repeated long pauses (longer than 3 or 4 seconds) are rarely normal. Particularly in young infants, hypoxia should always be considered as a cause for any severe bradyarrhythmia.

In children, sinus node dysfunction is usually seen in the setting of previous cardiac surgery, most notably atrial repair of transposition. The proportion of these children developing nonsinus rhythm increases with time after operation, often eventually manifesting the full tachycardia-bradycardia syndrome (sick-sinus syndrome). It is often unclear whether this represents direct damage to the S-A node or adjacent tissue, nerve inputs to the sinus node, or damage to the S-A node artery. In the vast majority of cases sinus node dysfunction develops late after operation and rarely constitutes an acute perioperative problem.

AV block is characterized as first degree (PR prolongation without actual block), second degree (intermittent AV conduction), or third degree (complete failure of AV conduction). Second degree can be further divided into Mobitz I (intermittent block preceded by progressive PR prolongation) or Mobitz II (abrupt loss of conduction), or when at least every other beat fails to conduct, by the ratio of atrial to ventricular depolarizations. Mobitz II and high-grade second degree block (greater than 3:1 AV block except during tachycardia) along with third degree block indicate AV conduction system disease or damage, but milder forms may occur either pathologically or as a consequence of vagal tone. (Note that 2:1 AV block does not constitute either Mobitz I or Mobitz II block.)

In the setting of cardiac surgery acute AV block may be a consequence of either irreversible interruption of specialized conduction tissue or transient inflammation and edema due to adjacent trauma or suture lines. Long-standing AV block usually reflects either fibrosis and scarring of the AV node and/or the His bundle or complete discontinuity of the conduction system due to abnormal atrioventricular relations (commonly L-transposition of the great arteries or heterotaxia syndromes).[24] Congenital AV block in the absence of structural heart disease is usually associated with maternal connective tissue disease, though functional 2:1 AV block is occasionally the first manifestation of congenital long QT syndrome in infants.[25,31]

The most common preexisting dysrhythmias encountered in pediatric patients without underlying heart disease are supraventricular tachycardias (SVT) (with or without associated Wolff-Parkinson-White syndrome) and frequent ventricular premature beats (VP).[21,39] Though it is usually recognized before the operation, susceptible patients occasionally experience their first recognized episode of tachycardia during a cardiac or noncardiac operation (Fig. 13–1).

Most SVT in children fit the clinical phenotype of paroxysmal supraventricular tachycardias (PSVT). The *clinical diagnosis* is usually due to either of two *reciprocating mechanisms:* AV recip-

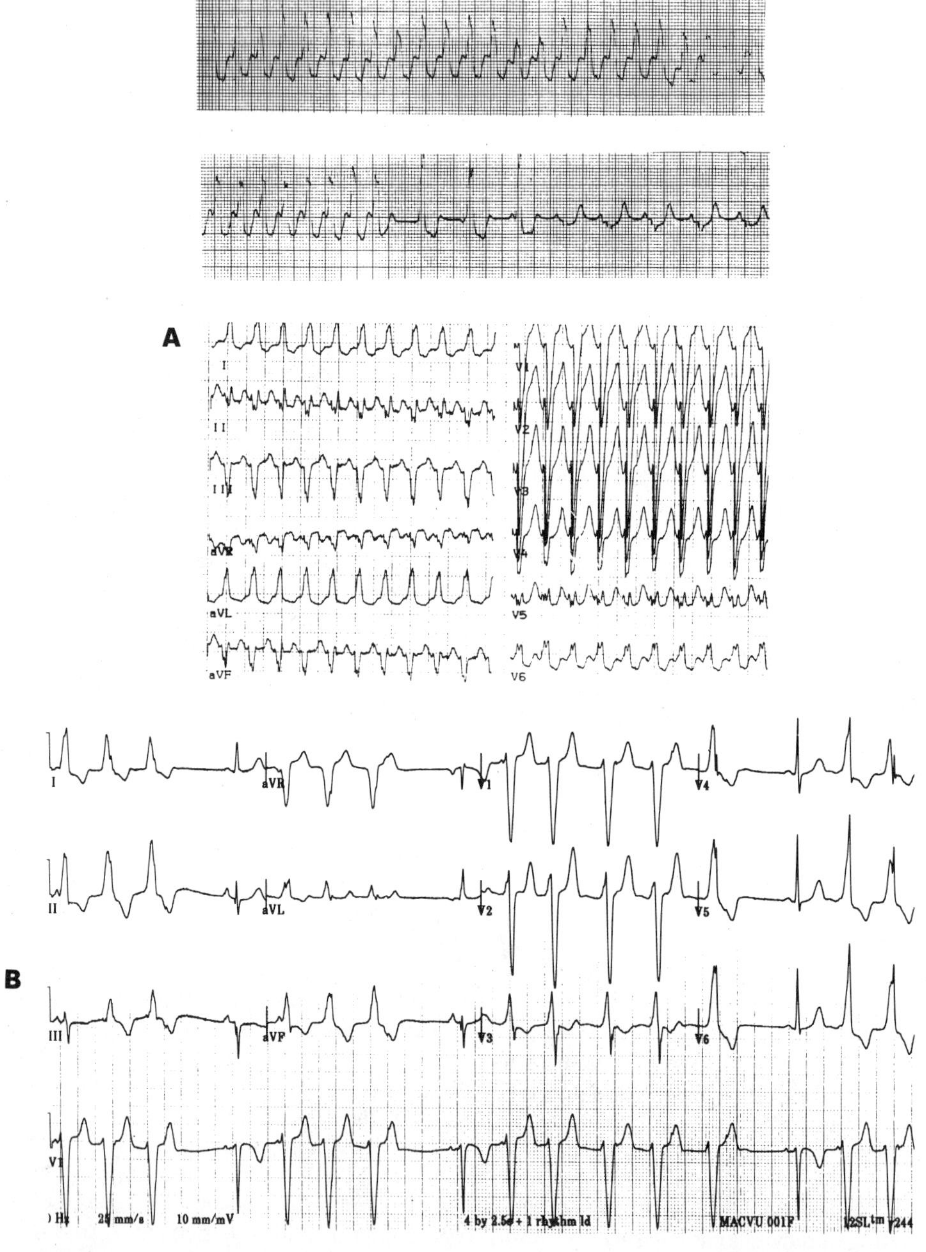


**Figure 13–1 A,** Wide QRS tachycardia. First noted in a patient undergoing elective tonsillectomy. Electrophysiology study revealed tachycardia due to Mahaim fiber. **B,** Repetitive monomorphic tachycardia. First noted in a patient undergoing elective orchiopexy. Electrophysiology study and MRI revealed arrhythmogenic right ventricular dysplasia.

rocating tachycardia or AV node reentrant tachycardia.[21] Reciprocating tachycardias are a consequence of antegrade conduction from atria to the ventricles, which is immediatley followed by retrograde conduction from ventricles to atria, in turn followed by alternating antegrade and retrograde conduction, and so on. Since the antegrade limb of the circuit is refractory to immediate retrograde conduction, this pattern requires two discrete limbs over which antegrade and retrograde conduction traverse separately.

Prior to adulthood AV reciprocating tachycardias (AVRT) predominate, particulary in infancy.[21] In AVRT an accessory AV connection (also called the bundle of Kent) serves as one of the conducting limbs (most commonly retrograde). When antegrade conduction is also carried over the accessory connection during sinus rhythm, the diagnosis of Wolff-Parkinson-White syndrome (WPW) is made. Though AVRT and WPW are commonly associated, many accessory connections conduct only retrograde (i.e., during tachycardia) and do not result in WPW during sinus rhythm.

In AV node reentry (AVNRT), both antegrade and retrograde conduction are carried over electrophysiologically (and probably anatomically) discrete limbs of the AV node, both of which converge distally with the His bundle. Both AVRT and AVNRT usually result in the classic ECG features of PSVT and cannot be distinguished with certainty according to the surface ECG. However, they share sufficient mechanistic similarities to allow a common approach to acute therapy. The substrates for both AVRT and AVNRT usually occur in the absence of other structural heart disease, though accessory AV connections and WPW are unusually prevalent in patients with Ebstein's anomaly (both with normal cardiac relations and in corrected or L-transposition of the great arteries).[15,28]

While other SVTs are less common in children, patients with underlying heart disease are much more likely to have primary atrial tachycardias than either AVRT or AVNRT. This diverse group of SVT includes tachycardia due to intraatrial reentry (and the closely related atrial flutter), atrial fibrillation, and automatic ectopic atrial tachycardia.[2] Each may at times fulfill some or all of the ECG characteristics of PSVT. However, regardless of the specific mechanism, all primary atrial tachycardias differ from the reciprocating tachycardias in that the rhythm disturbance is exclusive to the atria, with neither the AV node nor the ventricles required for perpetuation of the tachycardia. This distinction has important diagnostic and therapeutic implications.

Cardiac lesions predisposing to primary atrial tachycardias include cardiomyopathies (hypertrophic and dilated) and severe AV valve dysfunction (regurgitation or stenosis). Operations involving large suture lines in the atria or damaging the sinus node are particularly likely to result in both acute and chronic atrial dysrhythmias.[5] The classic examples of these are Mustard's and Sennings's operations for D-transposition of the great arteries and Fontan-type operations for single ventricle-type lesions, but atrial dysrhythmias may even follow repair of anomalous pulmonary venous connections or ASD.[35]

Ventricular tachycardias (VT) almost always reflect underlying functional or structural heart disease. Unlike in adults (in whom ischemic heart disease prevails), structural congenital heart disease (preoperative and postoperative) and the cardiomyopathies account for most VT in children (Fig. 13–1, *B*). In contrast, isolated VPs are relatively common in otherwise healthy children (particularly adolescents), and unless exacerbated during anesthesia itself are unlikely to pose a particular risk to the patient in whom no underlying heart disease is evident.[39]

While virtually any heart disease may predispose to ventricular tachycardias, certain situations may be particularly dangerous. Lesions such as tetralogy of Fallot and complicated VSDs requiring a ventriculotomy may result in a fixed scar that serves as the basis for reentrant arrhythmias. While these appear to predominate during late follow-up, perioperative ventricular tachycardias in this setting are relatively uncommon unless related to prior damage or surgical procedures.

In contrast, perioperative ventricular dysrhythmias are more likely to be either iatrogenic or ischemic in origin. Left ventricular outflow obstruction as in severe aortic stenosis and hypertrophic cardiomyopathy may predispose to myocardial ischemia and resulting arrhythmias (Fig. 13–2). While atherosclerotic coronary artery disease is uncommon except in severe familial hyperlipidemias, coronary artery stenosis, obstruction of coronary artery ostia, and anomalous origin of the coronaries are occasionally seen and may predispose to cardiac arrest or sudden death. The most common of these are anomalous origin of the left coronary artery from the pulmonary artery, left coronary artery arising from the right coronary artery, and ventricular-coronary sinusoids commonly seen in pulmonary atresia with an intact septum. Unrecognized origin of the left anterior descending coronary from the right coronary artery may also lead to inadvertent damage during repair of tetralogy of Fallot. Acute ischemic and reperfusion arrhythmias may be particularly malignant. They do not appear to be due to reentrant mechanism and may instead

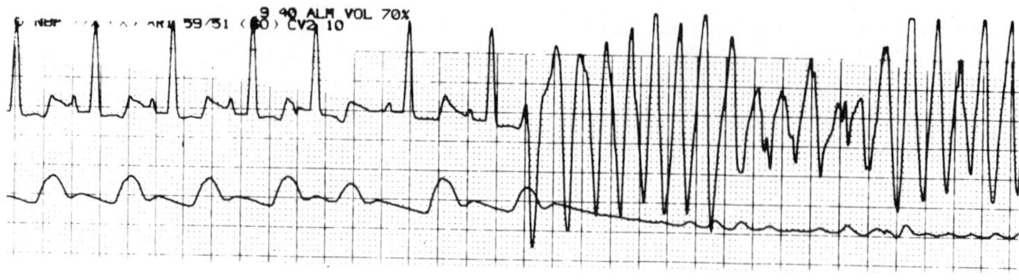

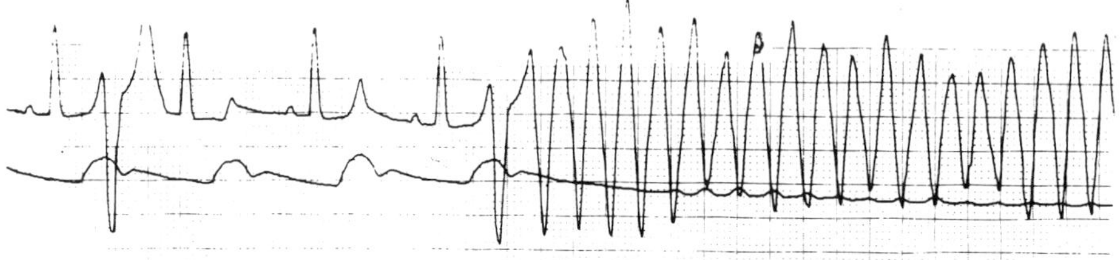

**Figure 13–2** Rapid polymorphic VT following aortic valvotomy. Dependence on slow rates supports reperfusion-related triggered activity as presumed mechanism.

display characteristic-rate dependence suggesting a triggered mechanism.

Inadvertent digoxin or catecholamine toxicity can lead to particularly refractory arrhythmias, especially a characteristic bidirectional tachycardia that alternates between two distinct QRS axes with each consecutive complex.[4,7,12] Finally, treatment with various QT-prolonging antiarrhythmic agents such as procainamide and quinidine may lead to acquired long QT syndrome and torsades de pointes; associated bradyarrhythmias and perioperative electrolyte disturbances (hypokalemia, hypocalcemia, and hypomagnesemia) may further predispose to these lethal dysrhythmias.[29]

Junctional ectopic tachycardia (JET) is a poorly understood but well recognized dysrhythmia that is uncommonly seen except immediately after cardiac surgery in young patients. Though sometimes associated with obvious trauma to the proximal AV conduction tissue it may occasionally follow cardiac operations where the nature of the insult is more obscure (Fig. 13–3). The tachycardia behavior is consistent with an automatic rather than reentrant focus but fortunately is self-limited, usually resolving within the first 24 to 48 hours postoperatively.[17]

## DIAGNOSIS

The recognition and diagnosis of all dysrhythmias begins with the surface ECG, which should be scrutinized *in order* for the following features:

1. Ventricular rate (too fast, too slow, or appropriate for given setting)
2. QRS duration and morphology (normal QRS, prolonged QRS, morphology same or different from morphology during sinus rhythm, varying morphology)
3. Regularity of ventricular depolarization (regular, irregular in recurring fashion, or irregularly irregular)
4. Atrial rate and relationship of atrial depolarizations to ventricular depolarizations (1:1 conduction, intermittent conduction, completed absence of conduction)
5. Morphology of P waves (if evident) relative to P waves during sinus rhythm

While adherence to the above algorithm will lead to an appropriate differential diagnosis, additional measures are often necessary to establish a diagnosis. The most important of these include running a hard copy of any dysrhythmia in multiple ECG leads to allow careful inspection for hidden P waves or differences in QRS morphology, which may be evident only in certain leads. Whenever feasible, this should include a full 12-lead ECG to compare with preoperative findings.

If temporary epicardial pacing wires are in place on the atrium, these may be used to record atrial activity and identify atrial depolarizations that might otherwise be obscured. The easiest means is to record a unipolar atrial electrogram by connecting a precordial (V) lead to the atrial wire, with the

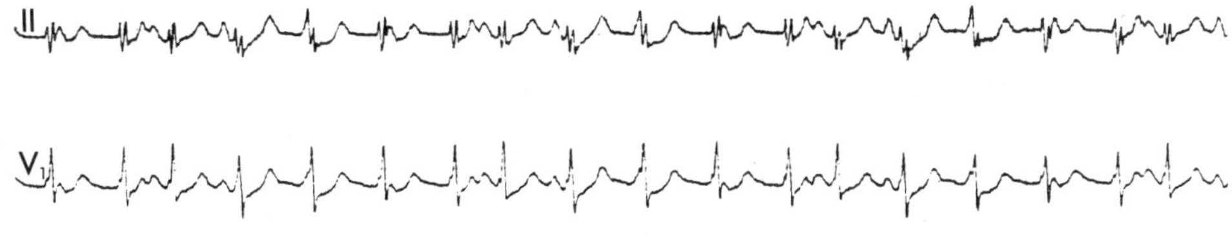

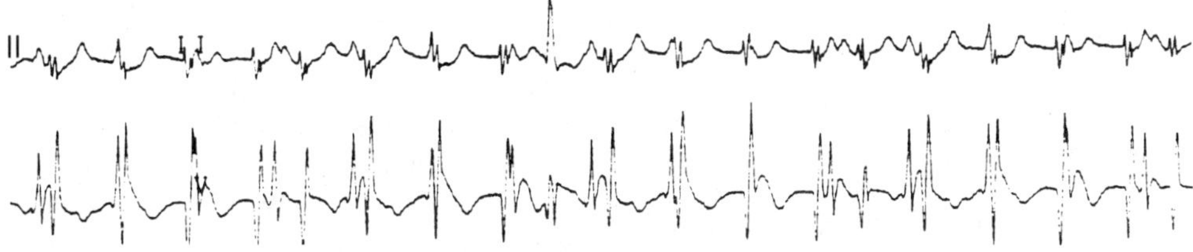

**Figure 13–3** Postoperative junctional ectopic tachycardia following fontan procedure. Rate is sufficiently slow that no intervention is warranted, though suppressed with atrial pacing at faster rate.

Wilson Central Terminal serving as the ground; atrial and ventricular activation in this configuration can be differentiated by comparison with other surface ECG leads (Fig. 13–3). When atrial wires are not available, an esophageal lead may be placed for both diagnostic and therapeutic purposes.[3]

Response of a tachycardia to maneuvers that affect AV node conduction is an excellent means for quickly establishing a tachycardia mechanism when 1:1 AV conduction appears to be present. *It is essential to run a continuous ECG strip during any of these maneuvers to document the transient changes that result.* When the AV node is an integral part of the circuit, as in AVRT or AVNRT, such interventions (carotid massage, ice applied to face, edrophonium, adenosine) should immediately terminate the tachycardia. When the AV node is not integral to the tachycardia, interruption of AV conduction will alter the AV relationship without interrupting tachycardia, allowing primary atrial or ventricular tachycardias to be identified. IV verapamil or β-adrenergic blockade should be avoided in the perioperative setting, particularly when the diagnosis is in question, because of the potential for profound and even lethal hemodynamic effects.

Description of a rhythm as "AV dissociated" is imprecise and inadequate to characterize the appropriate course of action. Ventricular tachycardias, JET, complete AV block (with narrow or wide QRS escape), and accelerated junctional or ventricular rhythms may all display AV dissociation. *In complete AV block, the atrial rate exceeds the ventricular rate;* in all others the ventricular rate is faster. When the junctional or ventricular rate exceeds 100 to 120 beats per minute, it usually represents an actual tachycardia rather than simply accelerated rhythm, though the specific rate criteria for defining tachycardia depend both on age and on clinical situation.

A similar situational evaluation is useful in distinguishing sinus tachycardia from SVT. When the rate is faster than expected or appropriate for the clinical situation, a nonsinus tachycardia is usually present, and the ECG should be carefully inspected for hidden P waves or transient interruption of AV conduction. Unfortunately, it is sometimes difficult to distinguish an *appropriate sinus tachycardia* in response to *impaired hemodynamics* or pain from a poorly tolerated SVT *resulting in hemodynamic embarrassment.*[14] A high index of suspicion is therefore required for prompt recognition of SVT simulating sinus tachycardia.

Care must always be taken to avoid misdiagnosis or VT for SVT with aberrancy. While the latter is common, the distinction often requires detailed electrophysiologic evaluation, and erroneous treatment of VT with measures appropriate for SVT (such as IV verapamil) might be disastrous. The QRS duration should be considered relative to norms for both age and rate, but preexisting conduction delays must also be taken into account.

Occasionally the appropriate diagnosis can be made only by inference or in retrospect. *Any tachycardia with prolonged QRS duration should always be presumed to represent VT until proven otherwise.*

As noted above, the diagnostic evaluation for any bradyarrhythmia should include a review for any correctable iatrogenic causes, particularly digoxin toxicity, antiarrhythmic drug therapy, electrolyte disturbances, hypoxia, acidosis, and direct mechanical stimulation of the myocardium due to improperly positioned mediastinal tubes or indwelling catheters.

## TREATMENT

The acute treatment of perioperative bradyarrhythmias (box) is often facilitated by the availability of temporary epicardial pacing wires placed during cardiac operations to allow temporary atrial, ventricular, or AV sequential pacing. When such wires are not available, pharmacologic agents (isoproterenol, epinephrine, atropine) should usually be administered, but only long enough to establish more reliable means for maintaining the rate (transcutaneous or transvenous pacing). Even before any of these maneuvers, *CPR should always be initiated immediately for any dysrhythmia without an adequate pulse or blood pressure,* whether ventricular or supraventricular in origin.

Atrial bradycardias due to S-A node dysfunction usually do not require pacing beyond the immediate postoperative period unless associated with symptoms (syncope, exercise intolerance) or atrial tachycardias (tachycardia-bradycardia or sick sinus syndrome). When AV conduction is intact, atrial pacing is often preferred to preserve the benefits of AV synchrony. Otherwise, ventricular or dual chamber pacemakers maintain an adequate atrial rate while protecting from the possible development of subsequent AV block. Various pacing modes are available to preserve appropriate rate response even in the absence of an adequately functioning AV node. The details of chronic pacing therapy and implantation are discussed in Chapter 7.

### MANAGEMENT OF PERIOPERATIVE DYSRHYTHMIAS

**Bradycardias**

***Bradycardia without associated AV block***

- If pacing wires available
  - Atrial pacing
  - Ventricular pacing
- If pacing wires unavailable
  - Atropine 0.01 to 0.02 mg/kg or Isoproterenol 0.02 to 0.2 μg/kg/min
  - Transcutaneous or transvenous pacing.

***Bradycardia with associated AV block***

- If pacing wires available
  - Ventricular pacing
- If pacing wires unavailable and stable escape rhythm
  - Isoproterenol 0.02 μg/kg/min
  - Transvenous pacing
- If pacing wires unavailable and inadequate escape rhythm
  - CPR
  - Transcutaneous pacing
  - Transvenous pacing (Permanent pacing if longer than 1 to 2 weeks)

**Tachycardias***

***Supraventricular tachycardia***

- Hemodynamically stable
  - Vagal maneuvers, ice to face
  - Adenosine 0.05 to 0.2 mg/kg
  - Atrial or transesophageal pacing if no termination with above
  - Procainamide 10 to 15 mg/kg over 15 minutes
  - DC cardioversion
- Hemodynamically unstable
  - DC cardioversion 0.25 to 1 J/kg
  - Atrial or transesophageal pacing for recurrences.

***Atrial flutter and intraatrial reentrant tachycardia***

- Atrial or transesophageal pacing
- DC cardioversion if pacing unsuccessful or unavailable
- Digoxin, procainamide, diltiazem

***Atrial fibrillation***

- DC cardioversion
- Digoxin, procainamide, diltiazem

***Junctional ectopic tachycardia***

- Moderate hypothermia (32° to 35° C).
- Atrial pacing to achieve 2:1 AV block; paired ventricular pacing
- ? Intravenous amiodarone, procainamide

***Ventricular tachycardia and fibrillation*****

- DC cardioversion or defibrillation 2 J/kg
- Lidocaine, procainamide, bretylium, amiodarone (IV)
- Ventricular pacing (especially for Torsades de Pointes, polymorphic VT).

*Whenever possible, attempt to record atrial electrogram.

**If Wide QRS (different from sinus), treat as presumed ventricular tachycardia.

AV block acquired at the time of cardiac surgery often recovers within 1 to 2 weeks, and pacemaker implantation should usually be delayed beyond this period until adequate time is allowed for conduction to return.[11,26] The need for acute pacing does not reflect the need for chronic pacing, though limited pacing maneuvers at the bedside (for example measurement of the pacemaker recovery time) may be helpful in determining the integrity of AV conduction and subsidiary pacemakers.

The treatment of apparent PSVT (PSVT is usually defined as abrupt-onset narrow QRS tachycardia without evident P waves or with P waves immediatley following the QRS) can usually be delayed for a short period until appropriate diagnostic equipment and medications can be readied. However, if acute hemodynamic compromise is present, DC cardioversion should be employed promptly. The most appropriate choice for acute treatment of PSVT is ice to the face (to elicit the dive reflex) or adenosine (0.1 to 0.3 mg/kg/day adminstered rapidly) to block antegrade or retrograde conduction over the AV node.[7] When repeated terminations are necessary within a short time, pace termination from a transesophageal catheter or temporary atrial wires may be employed.[3] This approach has been advocated for perioperative management of patients with known PSVT for whom chronic therapy has been withheld preoperatively.[32]

When a primary atrial tachycardia is identified, the choices of treatments include DC cardioversion, acute therapy to limit AV node conduction, and pace termination. Pharmacologic conversion with procainamide (10 to 15 mg/kg over 15 to 30 minutes followed by 30 to 40 μg/kg/min) is occasionally employed (especially for atrial fibrillation or recurrent nonsustained atrial arrhythmias). Adenosine infrequently terminates primary atrial tachycardias,[7] though transient termination followed by reinduction may be missed when an ECG strip is not run during administration. *Likewise, failure to run a strip may lead to the erroneous conclusion that a reciprocating mechanism is operative because tachycardia was terminated.* However, most will be primary atrial tachycardia due to intraatrial reentry, thus amenable to pace termination using temporary epicardial pacing wires, transesophageal pacing, or occasionally transvenous pacing as an alternative to acute pharmacologic therapy. A critically coupled and short burst of impulses is delivered to the atria, enabling interruption of the tachycardia. Often, pace termination of primary atrial tachycardia due to reentry is preceded by a brief period of atrial fibrillation or acceleration of the atrial rate. Since either of these may increase the rate of ventricular response to the new atrial rate, appropriate equipment for resuscitation and emergency DC cardioversion must be immediately available.[16,18] When recurrences warrant pharmacologic treatment, procainamide can be given IV and later switched to an oral regimen.

Any presumed VT (i.e., any tachycardia with prolonged QRS) requires prompt intervention. Usually this is with DC cardioversion, though limited diagnostic maneuvers can be occasionally employed when there is a high likelihood for a SVT (such as known WPW or previous SVT). The role of IV antiarrhythmic agents such as lidocaine, propafenone, and amiodarone is more to prevent reinitiation or recurrences than to accomplish acute termination. The role for low-dose β-adrenergic blockade in acute postoperative VT is not well established in this population, though extrapolation from acute postinfarction arrhythmias suggests a potential beneficial role.[38]

Occasionally ventricular arrhythmias prove to be bradycardia dependent, so that augmenting the heart rate with atrial or ventricular pacing prevents the triggering event from initiating without directly addressing the underlying cause for the dysrhythmia. However, extreme caution should be taken to avoid asynchronous pacing, which might result in inadvertent R on T wave phenomenon and induction of ventricular fibrillation.

The issue of chronic therapy for supraventricular or ventricular arrhythmias is usually made independent of the need for perioperative therapy. Occasionally empiric postoperative therapy is reasonable, with follow-up electrophysiology study a few weeks later serving as the basis for long-term therapeutic strategies. One of the few exceptions is the patient with asymptomatic or minimally symptomatic WPW for whom cardiac surgery is being planned. Previously, electrophysiologic study was recommended prior to the operation with possible surgical ablation performed at the same time as the planned operation. In the current era of radiofrequency catheter ablation, preoperative study and RF ablation of the accessory connection are usually warranted to avoid the potential for perioperative dysrhythmias, which might not be tolerated well in the postoperative setting (Fig. 13–4).

A specific exception to the acute therapeutic approaches outlined above is taken when JET is recognized. This dysrhythmia is often poorly tolerated as a consequence of rapid rate, loss of AV synchrony, and the immediacy with which it tends to follow major cardiac surgery. Traditional antiarrhythmic therapy (including digoxin, propranolol, and verapamil) is of little benefit for this dysrhythmia. Potent antiarrhythmics such as IV propafenone and amiodarone have been used sparingly

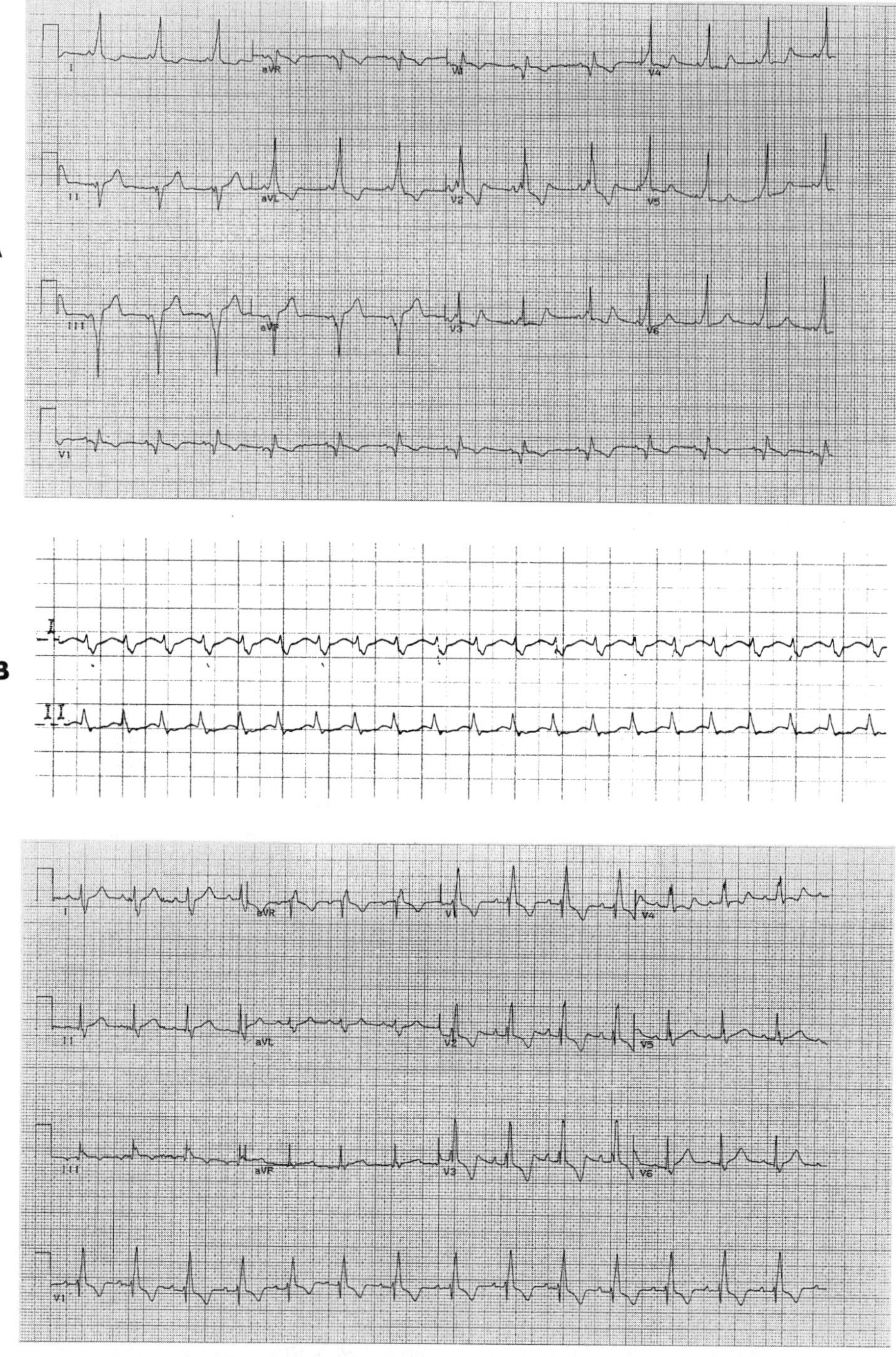


**Figure 13–4** Symptomatic WPW-associated sinus venosus ASD with PAPVC. **A,** ECG prior to ablation. No tachycardia or palpitations appear prior to catheterization, but elective catheterization with electrophysiology is recommended preoperatively. **B,** Sustained SVT induced during hemodynamic catheterization. Multiple episodes are induced with catheter manipulation and pacing. Accessory pathway is mapped and RF ablation performed. **C,** ECG following ablation. There is no perioperative tachycardia at time of routine repair of ASD and anomalous draining right upper pulmonary vein.

under investigational protocols and showed promise. However, reduction in the patient's body temperature to 94° to 95° F appears to slow the tachycardia and hasten its eventual disappearance.[1,7] Often even smaller reductions are adequate. Occasionally overdrive atrial pacing at a faster rate may slow the ventricular response by resulting in 2:1 AV block. However, in young patients experiencing this arrhythmia, AV conduction may be quite good, and multiblock (2:1 or greater) may be difficult to achieve. Another alternative occasionally employed is paired ventricular pacing, rendering the ventricle refractory to incoming junctional depolarizations. However, there is a substantial risk for precipitating ventricular fibrillation by this technique, whereas the risk of fibrillation with mild cooling appears to be low.[36]

## ABLATION THERAPY OF CARDIAC ARRHYTHMIAS

As the knowledge that many dysrhythmias persist indefinitely is coupled with the increasing awareness of proarrhythmic response to therapy, there is an ever-increasing emphasis on curative ablation procedures over chronic antiarrhythmic therapy. These include surgical ablation and more recently various catheter ablation techniques, the most important currently being radiofrequency catheter ablation.

Surgical ablation was first described for WPW and related accessory AV connections,[9] and the technique has subsequently been extended to the treatment of virtually all supraventricular dysrhythmias, including atrial fibrillation, atrial flutter, and many ventricular tachycardias, particularly incessant ventricular tachycardia in infants and young children.[8,10,16,19,27] The anesthesia approach to these patients is similar to that for any open cardiac operation with only a few exceptions.

The types of dysrhythmias the patient has been documented as having should be reviewed along with doses of medications (particularly isoproterenol) that may be requested by the electrophysiologist and surgeon. *The patient should not receive any antiarrhythmic medication* except adenosine prior to beginning the mapping procedure itself.

After sternotomy is made, epicardial pacing is performed to confirm the results of preoperative endocardial mapping and to guide the surgeon's incision. The patient is placed on bypass, and the appropriate surgical ablation is performed in the area indicated by mapping. Once ablation is completed, the heart is reperfused and assessed for residual conduction properties and any evidence of persisting dysrhythmias. Sometimes it is necessary to return to bypass several times before the arrhythmia substrate is adequately eliminated. Epicardial wires are left in place not only to assess residual conduction but to allow emergency pacing for recurrent tachycardia or delayed AV block.

More common now than surgical ablation, radiofrequency catheter ablation is becoming the treatment of choice for a variety of tachyarrhythmias.[20] This technique is an extension of the standard electrophysiology mapping study, during which precise location of the offending tissue is determined. This may represent an automatic focus in automatic atrial tachycardia, accessory connection AV connection in WPW, or critical zone of slow conduction in atrial flutter or even some ventricular tachycardias.[13,33,34,37] After localization of the ablation target, filtered RF energy (usually 350 to 500 kHz) is delivered to the site, creating a very discrete injury lesion. When this is successful, the tachycardia is cured, usually without any extraneous damage to other tissues (conduction tissue or otherwise). Life-threatening complications to the patient are uncommon, but careful hemodynamic monitoring for evidence of perforation and cardiac tamponade is necessary.[20] In young patients general anesthesia is usually advisable to facilitate the controlled application of RF energy.[30]

Acute postablation ECG abnormalities and dysrhythmias are uncommon, except when AV node reentry is accomplished by ablation of the fast pathway rather than the slow pathway of the AV node. Fast AV node modification carries a slightly higher incidence of acute AV block than does slow pathway ablation or modification.[23] Since slow pathway ablation appears to provide a success rate equivalent to that of fast pathway ablation but at lower risk of inadvertent AV block, slow pathway modification has gained general acceptance as the preferred approach to treating PSVT due to reentry over the AV node.[22]

Because proper disposal of inhaled anesthetic agents may not be available in the catheterization laboratory, IV anesthesia with an agent such as fentanyl may be advisable. The anesthesiologist, due to proximity to the fluoroscopy beam, should also take appropriate precautions to minimize radiation exposure.[6]

## REFERENCES

1. Bash SE, Shah JJ, Albers WH et al: Hypothermia for the treatment of postsurgical greatly accelerated junctional ectopic tachycardia, *J Am Coll Cardiol* 10:1095, 1987.
2. Benditt DG, Benson DW, Dunnigan A et al: Atrial flutter, atrial fibrillation, and other primary atrial tachycardias, *Med Clin North Am* 68:895, 1987.
3. Benson DW Jr, Dunnigan A, Benditt DG et al: Transesophageal cardiac pacing: history, application, technique, *Clin Prog Pacing Electrophys* 2:360, 1984.
4. Benson DW Jr, Gallagher JJ, Sterba R et al: Catecholamine induced double tachycardia: case report in a child, *PACE* 3:96, 1980.

5. Butto F, Dunnigan A, Overholt ED et al: Transesophageal study of recurrent atrial tachycardia after atrial baffle procedures for complete transposition of the great arteries, *Am J Cardiol* 57:1356, 1986.
6. Calkins H, Niklason L, Sousa J et al: Radiation exposure during radiofrequency catheter ablation of accessory atrioventricular connections, *Circulation* 84:2376, 1991.
7. Camm AJ, Garratt CJ: Adenosine and supraventricular tachycardia, *N Engl J Med* 325:1621, 1991.
8. Case CL, Crawford FA, Gillette PC et al: Management strategies for surgical treatment of dysrhythmias in infants and children, *Am J Cardiol* 63:1069, 1989.
9. Cobb FR, Blumenschein SD, Sealy WC et al: Successful surgical interruption of the bundle of Kent in a patient with Wolff-Parkinson-White syndrome, *Circulation* 38:1018, 1968.
10. Cox JL, Boinneau JP, Schuessler RB et al: A review of surgery for atrial fibrillation, *J Cardiovasc Electrophysiol* 2:541, 1991.
11. Daicoff GR, Aslami A, Tobias JA et al: Management of postoperative complete heart block in infants and children, *Chest* 66:639, 1974.
12. Dolara A, Manetti A, Pozzi L et al: Bidirectional tachycardia, *Cardiology* 55:302, 1970.
13. Feld GK, Fleck P, Chen P-S et al: Radiofrequency catheter ablation for the treatment of human type I atrial flutter: identification of a critical zone in the reentrant circuit by endocardial mapping techniques, *Circulation* 86:1223, 1992.
14. Fisher DJ, Gross DM, Garson A Jr: Rapid sinus tachycardia: differentiation from supraventricular tachycardia, *Am J Dis Child* 137:164, 1983.
15. Follath F, Hallidie-Smith KA: Unusual ECG changes in Ebstein's anomaly, *Br Heart J,* 34:513, 1972.
16. Garson A Jr, Smith RT, Moak JP et al: Incessant ventricular tachycardia in infants: myocardial hamartomas and surgical cure, *J Am Coll Cardiol* 10:619, 1987.
17. Grant JW, Serwer GA, Armstrong BE et al: Junctional tachycardia in infants and children after open heart surgery for congenital heart disease, *Am J Cardiol* 59:1216, 1987.
18. Guarnerio M, Furlanello F, Del Greco M et al: Transesophageal atrial pacing: a first-choice technique in atrial flutter therapy, *Am Heart J* 117:1241, 1989.
19. Guiradon GM, Klein GJ, Gulamhusein SS et al: Total disconnection of the right ventricular free wall: surgical treatment of right ventricular tachycardia associated with right ventricular dysplasia, *Circulation* 67:463, 1983.
20. Jackman WM, Xunzhang W, Friday KJ et al: Catheter ablation of accessory atrioventricular pathways (Wolff-Parkinson-White syndrome) by radiofrequency current, *N Engl J Med* 324:1605, 1991.
21. Ko JK, Deal BJ, Strasburger JF et al: Supraventricular tachycardia: mechanisms and their age distribution in pediatric patients, *Am J Cardiol* 69:1028, 1992.
22. Langberg JJ, Leon A, Borganelli M et al: A randomized, prospective comparison of anterior and posterior approaches to radiofrequency catheter ablation of atrioventricular nodal reentry tachycardia, *Circulation* 87:1551, 1993.
23. Lee MA, Morady F, Kadish A et al: Catheter modification of the AV junction with radiofrequency energy for control for AV nodal reentry tachycardia, *Circulation* 83:827, 1991.
24. Lev M: Pathogenesis of congenital AV block, *Prog Cardiovasc Dis* 15:145, 1972.
25. Litsey SE, Noonan JA, O'Connor WN et al: Maternal connective tissue disease and congenital heart block, *N Engl J Med* 312:90, 1985.
26. Nishimura RA, Callahan MJ, Holmes DR et al: Transient AV block after open-heart surgery for congenital heart disease, *Am J Cardiol* 53:198, 1984.
27. Ott DA, Garson A, Cooley DA et al: Cryoablative techniques in the treatment of cardiac tachyarrhythmias, *Ann Thorac Surg* 43:138, 1987.
28. Porter CJ, Holmes DR: Preexcitation syndromes associated with congenital heart disease. In Benditt DG, Benson DW Jr, editors: *Cardiac preexcitation syndromes,* Boston, 1986, Martinus Nijhoff.
29. Roden DM, Thompson KA, Hoffman BF et al: Clinical features and basic mechanisms of quinidine-induced arrhythmias, *J Am Coll Cardiol* 73A, 1986.
30. Saul JP, Hulse JE, De W et al: Catheter manipulation for ablation of accessory AV pathways in young patients: use of long vascular sheaths, the transseptal approach, and the left posterior end run, *J Am Coll Cardiol* 21:571, 1993.
31. Scott W, Dick M: 2 : 1 AV block in infants with congenital long QT syndrome, *Am J Cardiol* 60:1409, 1987.
32. Stevenson GW, Kross J, Schuster J et al: The use of transesophageal pacing for perioperative control of neonatal tachydysrhythmia, *Can J Anaesth* 672-674, 990.
33. Stevenson WG, Nademanee K, Weiss JN et al: Treatment of catecholamine-sensitive right ventricular tachycardia by endocardial catheter ablation, *J Am Coll Cardiol* 16:752, 1990.
34. Van Hare GF, Lesh MD, Scheinman M et al: Percutaneous radiofrequency catheter ablation for supraventricular arrhythmias in children, *J Am Coll Cardiol* 17:1613, 1991.
35. Vetter VL, Horowitz LN: Electrophysiologic residua and sequelae of surgery for congenital heart defects, *Am J Cardiol* 50:588, 1982.
36. Waldo AL, Krongard E, Kupersmith J et al: Ventricular paired pacing to control rapid ventricular heart rate following open heart surgery, *Circulation* 53:176, 1976.
37. Walsh EP, Saul JP, Hulse JE et al: Transcatheter ablation of ectopic atrial tachycardia in young patients using radiofrequency current, *Circulation* 86:1138, 1992.
38. Wolfe CL, Nibley C, Bhandari A et al: Polymorphous ventricular tachycardia associated with acute myocardial infarction, *Circulation* 84:1543, 1991.
39. Yabek SM: Ventricular arrhythmias in children with an apparently normal heart, *J Pediatr* 119:1, 1991.

# *PART TWO*

# **Particular Malformations**

# Section A LEFT-TO-RIGHT SHUNTS

# 14 Patent Ductus Arteriosus (Botallo's Duct)

*Jay Kambam*



Patent ductus arteriosus (PDA) was first described by Aranzio in 1564 and Carcano in 1593.[4] A persistent PDA as an isolated lesion occurs in about one in 2500 full term live births, accounting for 10% to 15% of all congenital malformations of the heart.[2] Premature infants have a much higher incidence of PDA.[7] There is good evidence to suggest that the presence of PDA is inversely related to the maturity of the infant.[31] Diseases such as congenital rubella syndrome or a genetic predisposition may increase the incidence of PDA.[12] At higher altitudes the incidence exceeds that at sea level by about 30 times, even among full-term neonates.[1] Females are more commonly affected than males at a ratio of about 3:1.[33] PDA is the most comon familial anomaly among siblings.

## EMBRYOLOGY

The first major intraembryonic vessels appear as a pair of dorsal aortas that run along the axis of the embryo and form the continuation of the endocardial heart tubes. Between the fifth and sixth weeks of gestation, the aortic arch system develops as six paired arches proliferating from the apex of the truncus arteriosus. These arches develop successively and are never all present at the same time. The first pair of the aortic arches appears at the cranial portions of the dorsal aortas at about 3 weeks of gestational age. The junction of the first aortic arches with the truncus arteriosus, which is somewhat dilated, is called the aortic sac. It is from this aortic sac that the subsequent five pairs of aortic arches are formed as the heart and aortic sac undergo a caudal displacement.

The sixth pair of aortic arches participates in the formulation of pulmonary arteries. The proximal portions on the right and left sides become the proximal segments of the right and left pulmonary arteries, respectively. The distal portions communicate with the corresponding aortas. When pulmonary vascularization is established, the communication with the right dorsal aorta is totally regressed and the communication with the left dorsal aorta persists until after birth as the ductus arteriosus, or Botallo's duct (Fig. 14–1).

## ANATOMY

The ductus arteriosus is a short vessel that makes a connection between the aorta and pulmonary artery during fetal life. PDA is a persistence of this

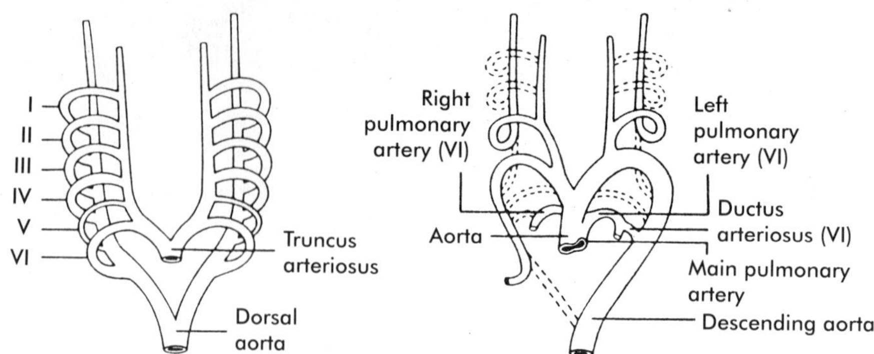


**Figure 14–1** Diagrammatic representation of the development of the aortic arch system as it relates to the ductus arteriosus. Note that the left pulmonary artery and the ductus arteriosus were the embryonic sixth arch. (From Fink BW, editor: *Congenital heart disease: a deductive approach to its diagnosis,* ed 3, St Louis, 1991, Mosby.)

connection between the aorta and pulmonary artery after birth. PDA usually has a diameter of 5 to 15 mm and length of 2 to 15 mm. The ductus arises from the left of the bifurcation near the origin of the left pulmonary artery. Ductus is inserted into the lesser curvature of the aorta (anterolateral aspect) slightly distal to and opposite from the origin of the left subclavian artery. The ductus is related to the left main bronchus posteriorly and vagus nerve anteriorly. The left recurrent laryngeal nerve encircles the ductus and ascends behind the aortic arch into the neck (Fig. 14–2). The pulmonary end of the ductus is covered by a reflection of pericardium. In small children the wall of the ductus is relatively thick and strong. In older children the wall is thin and friable, particularly in those with pulmonary hypertension. In older patients and in cases associated with pulmonary hypertension, calcifications may be found in the wall of the ductus and sometimes spreading into the aortic wall.

The most common anatomic types of PDA are (1) cylindrical, (2) funnel-shaped, (3) window, and (4) aneurysmal. There are two types of aneurysms of the ductal arteriosus, spontaneous and acquired secondarily by mycotic infection, trauma from surgical interruption, or hypertension.

## PHYSIOLOGY

### Fetal circulation

There are two umbilical arteries and one umbilical vein. The two umbilical arteries carry relatively unoxygenated and hypoglycemic blood to the placenta, whereas a single umbilical vein carries relatively oxygenated blood with a higher glucose concentration from the placenta to the fetus. About 40% to 60% of this umbilical venous blood enters the portal vein to supply the liver. The remainder of the umbilical venous blood travels through the ductus venosus into the inferior vena cava. The ductus venosus connects the umbilical vein to the

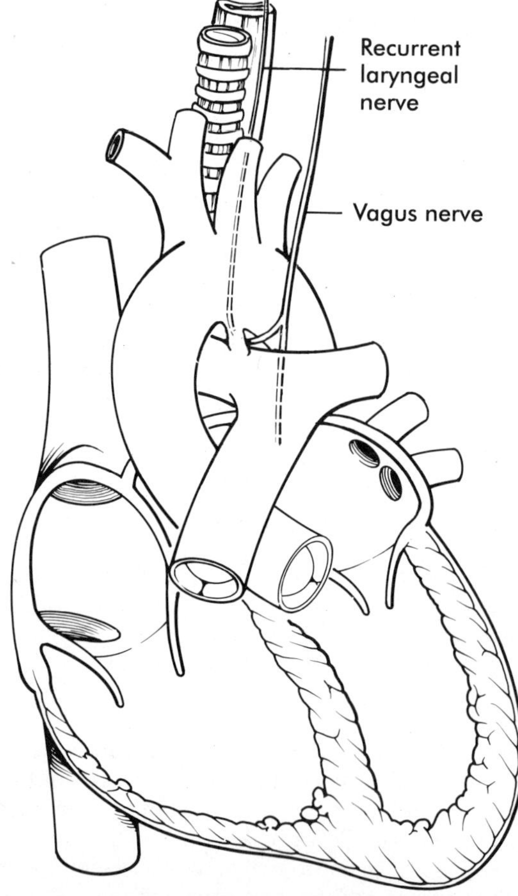


**Figure 14–2** Anatomy of the PDA. Note its close relationship to the left recurrent laryngeal nerve.

inferior vena cava near the junction of the hepatic veins. About one third of the blood from the inferior vena cava (mostly umbilical venous blood) is deflected across the foramen ovale into the left atrium as it enters the right atrium, and the remainder enters the right ventricle via the tricuspid valve. Almost all the blood from the superior vena cava enters the right ventricle and only about 2% to 3% of the blood enters the left atrium via the foramen ovale. The right ventricle pumps about 65% and the left ventricle about 35% of the cardiac output. Right ventricular blood is largely shunted to the systemic circulation via the ductus arteriosus, although 7% to 20% reaches the pulmonary circulation. There is now considerable evidence to suggest that ductal patency during fetal life is actively maintained by prostaglandin $E_2$ as a result of its continuous production both within the vessel wall and from the other sources.[24] The synthesis of prostaglandins starts with arachidonic acid with the help of cyclooxygenase enzymes.[30]

### Neonatal circulation

After birth, once the umbilical cord is tied, an increase in systemic vascular resistance results from elimination of the low-resistance placental circulation. Pulmonary vascular resistance decreases and pulmonary blood flow increases with the initiation of the neonatal respiration and resultant increase in partial pressure of oxygen ($Po_2$) and decrease in pulmonary arterial vasoconstriction. Pulmonary arterial pressure falls from a prenatal value of 70/45 torr to about 50/30 torr and 30/12 torr by 24 hours and 1 week after birth, respectively. Functional closure of the ductus arteriosus begins within 12 hours after birth as a result of an increase in partial pressure of arterial oxygen ($Pao_2$) and reflex neurogenic and vasoactive factors. In the majority of normal infants the ductus is physiologically closed by the second day of life.[22] Permanent anatomic closure normally occurs within the first 2 months of life, forming the ligamentum arteriosum.[5]

## PATHOPHYSIOLOGY

Only when the ductus remains patent as long as 3 months after full term birth is its presence considered abnormal. The patient with a persistent PDA has an abnormal communication between the aorta, with its relatively high pressure, and the pulmonary artery, with its low pressure. The amount and direction of blood flow vary with the size and shape of the communication and with the difference between the pulmonary and systemic vascular resistances. As the diameter of the PDA increases, the shunt volume also increases, resulting in volume overload of the left heart and pulmonary venous congestion. There is an absolute increase in the total circulating volume proportionate to the amount of left to right shunt. When PDA is large, aortic pressure can be transmitted directly into the pulmonary trunk, resulting in pulmonary hypertension and right heart failure. Because of the close anatomic relation of PDA to the left pulmonary artery, the effect on the left lung is greater than on the right lung. The direction of the blood flow or shunt through the PDA depends on the relationship between systemic and pulmonary vascular resistances. At birth the resistances in pulmonary and systemic vascular systems are identical. As pulmonary arterial pressure drops and a pressure gradient is created between the aorta and pulmonary artery, flow through the ductus can take place mainly during systole. Between 6 months and a year after birth, as maturation of pulmonary and systemic vessels takes place, a diastolic pressure gradient also develops and results in blood flow across the ductus both during systole and diastole. If the condition is untreated over several years, secondary changes—muscular hypertrophy, intimal fibrosis, increased pulmonary vascular resistance, and reversal of the flow of shunt (Eisenmenger's reaction)—occur in the small muscular pulmonary arteries and arterioles.

#### DUCTUS-DEPENDENT CARDIAC MALFORMATIONS

**Ductus-dependent lesions with restricted pulmonary blood flow**
- Pulmonary atresia or stenosis in association with ventricular septal defect (tetralogy of Fallot)
  - Atrial septal defect
  - Transposition of great arteries
- Tricuspid atresia in association with
  - atrial septal defect
  - Ventricular septal defect

**Ductus-dependent lesions with restricted systemic blood flow**
- Mitral atresia with atrial septal defect
- Aortic atresia with atrial and/or ventricular septal defects
- Preductal coarctation or complete interruption of aortic arch

## USUAL PRESENTATION

PDA may be an isolated form or associated with other cardiovascular malformations to compensate either for a decreased pulmonary blood flow or for proximal obstruction to aortic circulation (see the box).

In about 15% of patients with PDA there are associated extracardiac anomalies, which may include scoliosis, sternal deformities, clubfoot, eye defects, deafness, and mental retardation.

## CLINICAL PRESENTATION

The clinical picture of an infant with a persistent PDA depends very much on the size of the ductus, the pressures in the aorta and pulmonary artery, and the duration of shunt through the ductus. There is no characteristic history for a patient with persistent PDA. In the majority of patients a murmur is heard during a routine physical examination. A few patients may show signs of congestive heart failure including cough, dyspnea, tachypnea, tachycardia, and hepatosplenomegaly. Others may have a history of failure to thrive or diminished exercise tolerance.

A turbulent flow through the ductus mainly during systole under 6 months of age and during both systole and diastole after 6 moths of age can be heard as systolic and systolic-diastolic murmurs, respectively. The murmur can be best heard high on the left side of the sternum. The hallmark of the persistent PDA is the continuous or machinery murmur. If S2 can be heard, it may be single or paradoxically split. The other helpful diagnostic finding of PDA is wide pulse pressure leading to bounding pulses. A high-pitched diastolic decrescendo murmur of pulmonary vascular insufficiency (Graham Steell murmur) is heard in cases of the reversal of the flow of shunt (Eisenmenger's syndrome).

### Laboratory findings

A typical PDA can be diagnosed from the physical examination, chest x-ray film, and ECG, and usually confirmed with an echo-Doppler evaluation. In the case of an atypical PDA, the definitive diagnosis can be made by cardiac catheterization. The following lesions should be included in the differential diagnosis, as they may mimic the PDA:

1. Aortic pulmonary window
2. Truncus arteriosus
3. Venous hum
4. Ventricular septal defect with aortic regurgitation
5. Systemic arteriovenous fistula
6. Coronary arterial fistula
7. Pulmonary arteriovenous fistula
8. Ruptured sinus of valsalva fistula

***Chest x-ray films.*** Findings may range from normal to biventricular hypertrophy. Enlargement of the left atrium, left ventricle, ascending aorta, and aortic arch can be seen in the chest film. In addition, the pulmonary artery and its vasculature are enlarged (Fig. 14–3).

***Electrocardiogram.*** The ECG findings are equally variable, ranging from a normal tracing to either left ventricular or biventricular hypertrophy.

***Echocardiogram.*** Echo can document dilatation of the left heart structures. The left ventricular

A

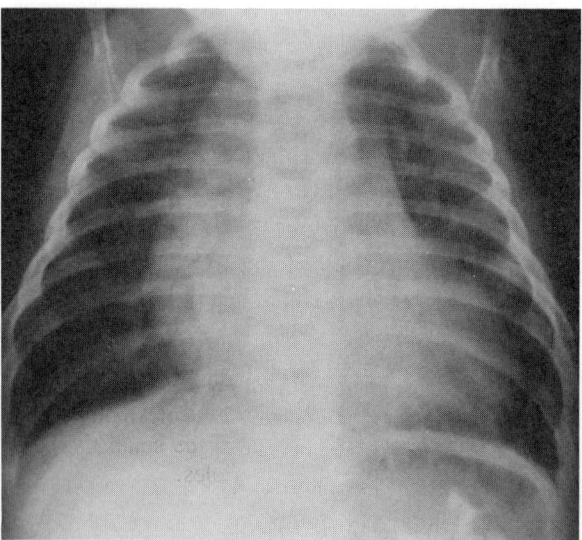

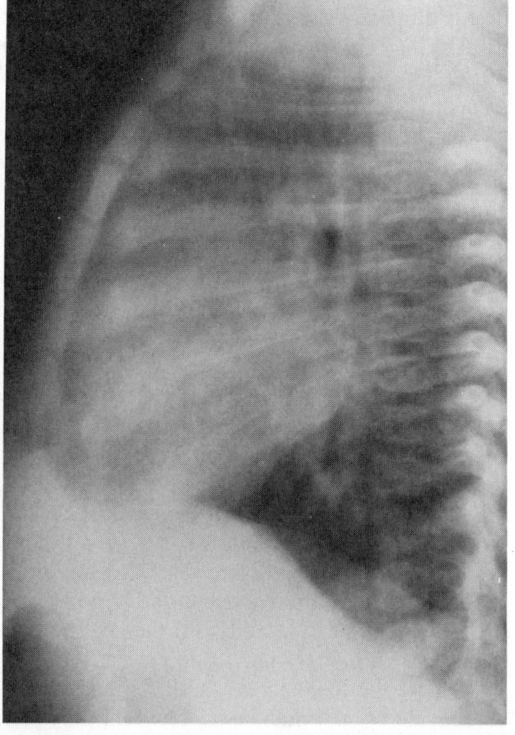

B

**Figure 14–3** Anteroposterior (**A**) and lateral (**B**) chest radiographs of a 2-month-old boy with a PDA. The heart is enlarged; left ventricular enlargement is suggested on the frontal view, and left atrial enlargement is noted on the lateral view. The pulmonary arterial flow is increased. (Courtesy of Sandra G. Kirchner, MD.)

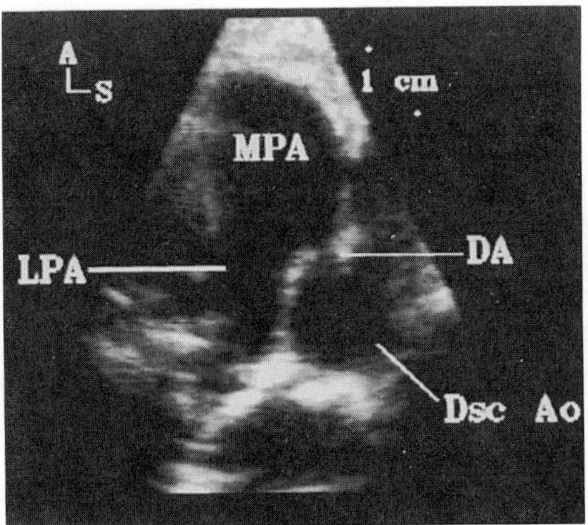


**Figure 14–4** Echocardiogram showing a PDA. *A,* anterior; *S,* superior; *MPA,* main pulmonary artery; *LPA,* left main pulmonary artery; *Dsc Ao,* descending aorta; *DA,* ductus arteriosus. (From Fyler DC, editor: *Nadas' pediatric cardiology,* Philadelphia, 1992, Hanley & Belfus.)

ejection fraction is often increased due to arteriovenous shunting. Doppler studies of flow in the pulmonary artery and aorta can document a PDA (Fig. 14–4).

***Catheterization data.*** The typical pressures and oxygen saturations are shown in Fig. 14–5.

## MEDICAL MANAGEMENT

Patients with PDA who have congestive heart failure are usually treated with fluid restriction, furosemide, digoxin, and occasionally dopamine. However, furosemide may actually promote patency of the ductus by its effects on prostaglandin metabolism.[11] Digoxin appears to have a little or no beneficial effect in infants weighing less than 1250 g.[16] Preterm infants treated with corticosteroids for more than 24 hours prior to birth may have a decreased incidence of PDA.[6]

### Indomethacin

Treatment with indomethacin has been shown to be effective in the closure of PDA.[3] Indomethacin is known to decrease the synthesis of prostaglandins by inhibiting cyclooxygenase enzymes.[18] A success rate of up to 80% has been reported with the use of indomethacin. Indomethacin (0.2 mg/kg) is usually given intravenously either three

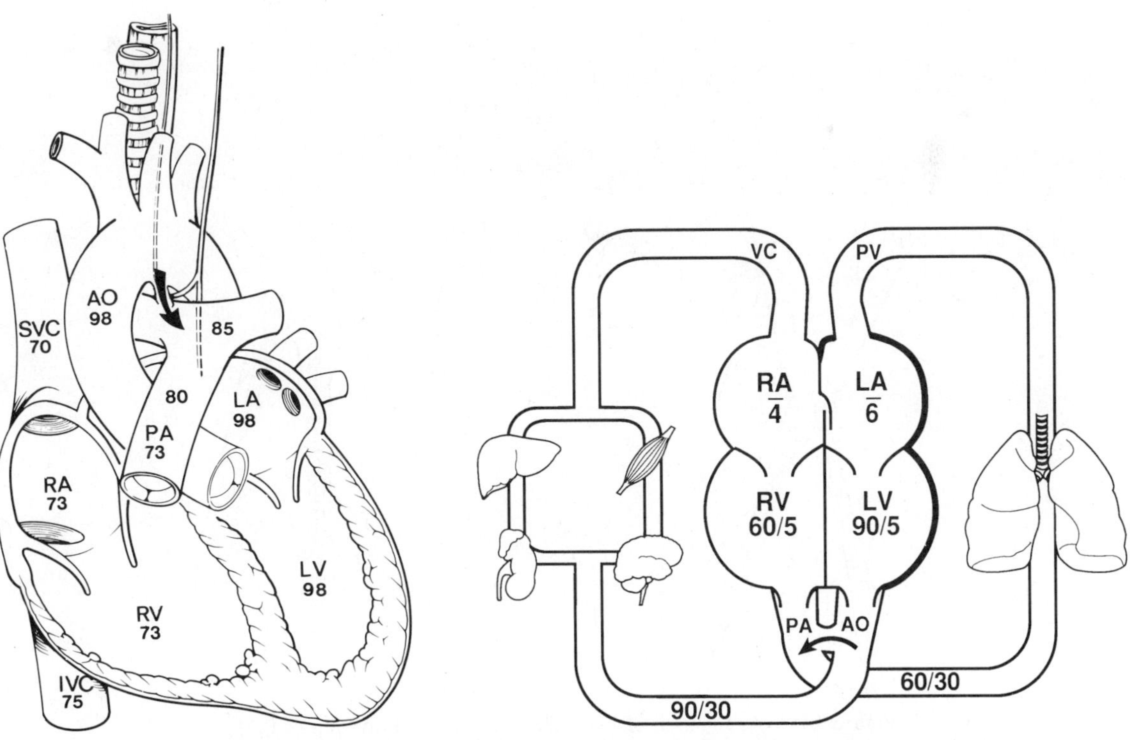


**Figure 14–5** Oxygen saturations and pressures in a patient with PDA.

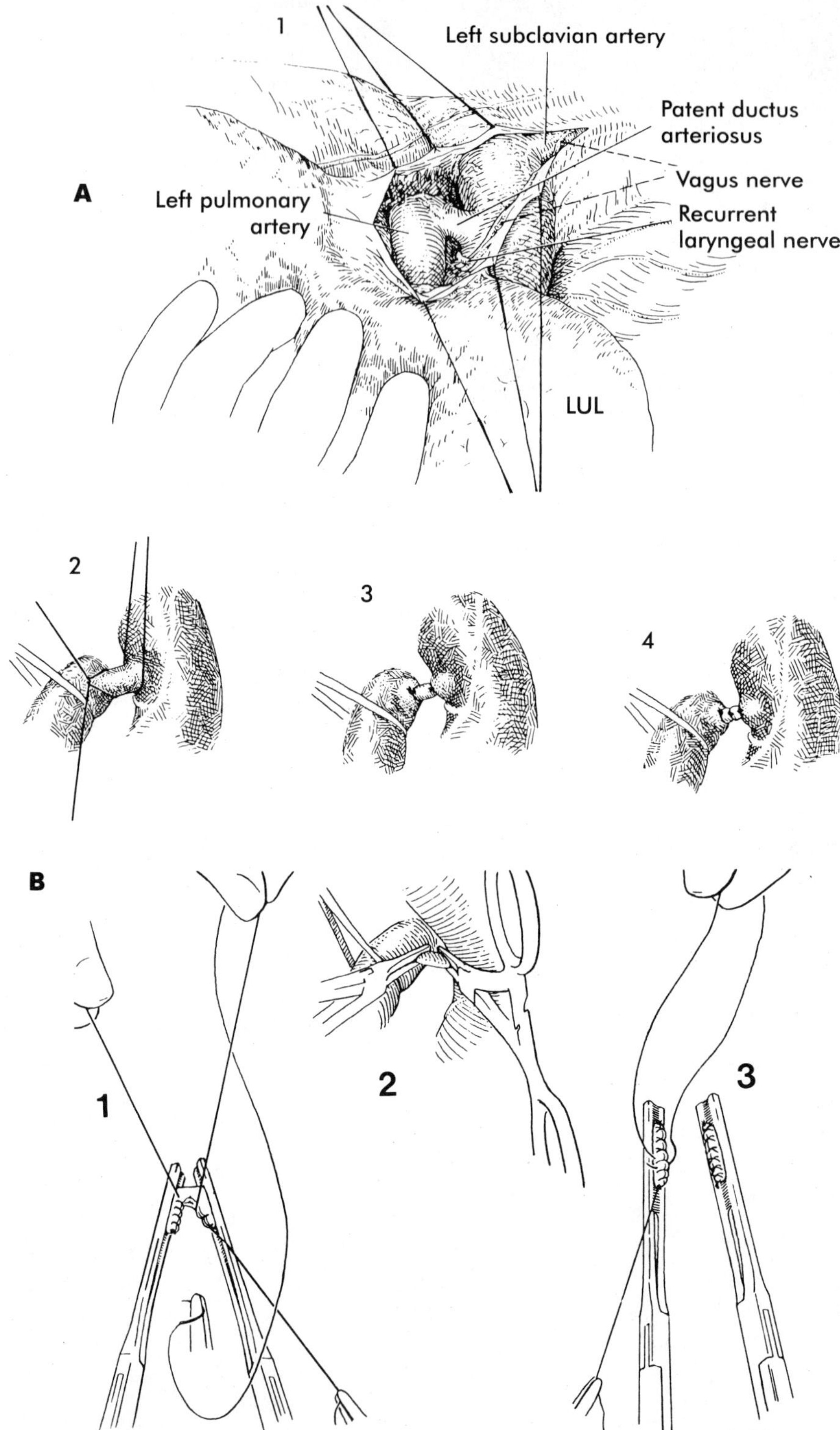


**Figure 14–6 A,** Ligation of PDA. **B,** Clamping and division of PDA.

times over 24 hours or daily for 72 hours. Indomethacin is frequently known to cause a transient diminution in renal function resulting in an increase in creatinine levels.[14] It is also known to prolong bleeding time.[9] Renal and hepatic insufficiency, sepsis, necrotizing enterocolitis, coagulation problems, and severe hyperbilirubinemia are some of the contraindications for use of indomethacin. Contrary to popular belief, it has been shown that indomethacin at the plasma concentrations achieved therapeutically does not displace bilirubin from the albumin.

### Prostaglandins

Prostaglandins $E_1$ and $E_2$ are used to keep the ductus patent in ductus-dependent lesions with little or no flow through the pulmonary valve until the time of surgical intervention to promote the flow through the pulmonary artery.[8] Likewise, prostaglandins are frequently essential to maintain the patency of ductus arteriosus until the time of surgery in ductus-dependent patients with limited systemic flow, as seen in coarctation or interrupted arch of the aorta.[15,17] Prostaglandin $E_1$ is infused intravenously in a starting dose of 50 to 100 ng/kg/min. Once the favorable effect is seen, this dose can be adjusted to 10 to 20 ng/kg/min. The following side effects of prostaglandins are reported: fever, bradycardia, apneic spells, hypotension, cutaneous flushing, and seizurelike activity. Apneic spells are more common in infants under 2 kg. Infants who receive prostaglandins should be monitored closely for apneic spells, and mechanical ventilation should be instituted when necessary.

## TRANSCATHETER CLOSURE

There are three types of transcatheter occlusion devices currently in use to close PDA nonsurgically.[20] These include Porstmann's Ivalon plug,[25,26] Rashkind's double disc,[28] and Sideris's button device.[27] A success rate close to 90% has been claimed for each device.[32]

## SURGICAL MANAGEMENT

In 1907 John Munro[23] was the first one to suggest surgical ligation as a treatment for PDA. In 1938 Graybiel and associates[10] performed the first surgical ligation of PDA. This 22-year-old patient died of complications postoperatively. In 1939 Robert Gross[13] performed the first successful surgical ligation of PDA.

Surgical intervention of PDA does not require cardiopulmonary bypass. Interruption of PDA is achieved by either division or ligation of the ductus (Fig. 14–6). Surgery is usually done with the patient in a right lateral decubitus position (left posterolateral thoracotomy). Perioperative surgical complications include the following:

1. Risk of tear, evulsion, and profuse bleeding
2. Residual shunt with ligation
3. Postoperative aneurysms
4. Systemic embolization from calcifications of the aorta (usually in older patients with pulmonary hypertension)
5. Transient or permanent left vocal cord palsy from recurrent laryngeal nerve injury
6. Trauma to the thoracic duct
7. Bacterial endocarditis
8. Left lung injury from pressure and retraction of the lung
9. Phrenic nerve injury

## ANESTHESIA MANAGEMENT

### Preoperative evaluation and preparation

In determining the appropriate anesthetic strategy it is important to understand the pathologic anatomy and physiology of the heart lesion. Other associated cardiac and extracardiac deformities also influence anesthetic management. Establishing systemic and pulmonary pressures and oxygen saturations is also helpful in choosing the appropriate drugs for patients with congenital heart disease with either intracardiac or extracardiac shunts. It is also important to know the effects of various drugs and conditions on the patency of the ductus arteriosus (see box below).

### Preoperative medications

Children under 6 months may not require any preoperative anesthesia. Older children, however, benefit from routine preoperative medication. Morphine sulfate 1 mg/kg IM can be given in the ward

**DUCTUS ARTERIOSUS: EFFECTS OF VARIOUS DRUGS AND OTHER FACTORS ON ITS PATENCY**

| Contraction of PDA | Relaxation of PDA |
|---|---|
| Increased $P_{O_2}$ | Prostaglandin $E_1$ |
| Prostaglandin $F_2a$ | Prostaglandin $E_2$ |
| Acetylcholine | High altitude |
| Norepinephrine | Hypoxemia |
| Histamine | Acidosis |
| Indomethacin | Hypothermia |
| Aspirin | |
| Nonsteroidal antiinflammatory drugs | |
| Succinylcholine (?) | |

before the child is brought to the holding room, and midazolam 0.5 to 0.6 mg/kg can be given orally about 30 minutes before the child comes to the operating room.

### Monitoring

Intraoperative monitoring of a patient with PDA necessitates an ECG and pulse oximeter (right hand), invasive or noninvasive blood pressure (preferably right hand), and body temperature.

### Precautions

It is absolutely necessary to have intravenous tubings bubble free and to take extreme care not to inject any air bubbles. These preventive measures are necessary because a left to right shunt can become a bidirectional shunt with anesthesia and operative manipulations.

Complications following surgery include left recurrent laryngeal nerve injury, phrenic nerve trauma, complications related to use of indomethacin or prostaglandin, systemic thromboembolism, necrotizing enterocolitis, and hypertension related to baroreceptor dysfunction.

### Induction

In patients with a functioning intravenous line anesthesia can be induced with IV ketamine (1 mg/kg), atropine (10 to 15 μg/kg), and a muscle relaxant to facilitate the endotracheal intubation. In a patient with no intravenous line anesthesia can be induced with halothane under mask; an IV line can then be started and tracheal intubation performed with the use of a muscle relaxant. Acetylcholine is known to contract the ductus and succinylcholine may also contract the ductus arteriosus. For this reason use of succinylcholine is not recommended if ductal patency must be maintained.

Pay a great deal of attention to ventilation and oxygenation of these patients. Hypoventilation and hypoxemia can acutely revert a left to right shunt to a right to left shunt in a neonate. Hyperventilation and hyperoxemia should be avoided, as they can reduce pulmonary vascular resistance, leading to an increase in left to right shunt. An increase in systemic vascular resistance can cause more shunting to the right side.

A left to right shunt theoretically does not change the uptake and induction time of any inhaled anesthetics; it slightly prolongs the onset of intravenous anesthetics. No clinical data support or contradict this theory. Many pediatric cardiac anesthesiologists believe a left to right shunt is of little practical concern with either type of anesthetic.

### Maintenance

In cases of uncomplicated PDA, usually in older children, either maintain anesthesia with halothane and a nondepolarizing muscle relaxant or a narcotic (fentanyl 10 to 15 μg/kg or sufentanil 1.5 to 2.5 μg/kg) with a low concentration of an inhalation anesthetic and a nondepolarizing muscle relaxant. An additional dose of atropine may be necessary at times to treat bradycardia, which may occur during the manipulation of the ductus. Maintaining hematocrit near normal is recommended, as hemodilution is known to be associated with an increase in left to right shunt.[21] With the interruption of the ductus there is usually an abrupt increase in diastolic and mean arterial blood pressure because of the elimination of low-resistance pulmonary circulation. Lung compliance has been shown to improve with the ligation of PDA.

### Postoperative care

The majority of patients with uncomplicated PDA can be extubated in the immediate postoperative period. Only the sick children need postoperative ventilation.

### Anesthetic management of a premature infant for ligation

In premature infants the physiologic closure of the ductus arteriosus may be delayed beyond the neonatal period. Most premature infants with PDA develop congestive heart failure early during postnatal life. They are also prone to develop respiratory distress syndrome because of an increased pulmonary blood flow and pulmonary hypertension. Because of a decreased systemic blood flow many of these patients develop renal dysfunction, gastrointestinal hypoperfusion, and necrotizing enterocolitis. Most of these patients come to the operating room with intravenous catheter and umbilical arterial catheter already in place. Often these patients require dopamine or dobutamine for maintenance of cardiac output and kidney perfusion. Anesthesia is usually maintained in these patients with a narcotic (fentanyl 10 to 15 μg/kg or sufentanil 1.5 to 2.5 μg/kg), a low concentration of an inhalational anesthetic, and a nondepolarizing muscle relaxant. Most of these patients require postoperative ventilatory support.

## REFERENCES

1. Alzamora-Castro V, Battilana G, Abugattas R et al: Patent ductus arteriosus and high altitude, *Am J Cardiol* 5:761, 1960.
2. Anderson RC: Causative factors underlying congenital heart malformations I: patent ductus arteriosus, *Pediatrics* 14:143, 1954.

3. Bhat R, Fisher E, Raju T et al: Patent ductus arteriosus: recent advances in diagnosis and management, *Ped Clin North Am* 29:1117, 1982.
4. Castiglioni A: *A history of medicine*, New York, 1947, Knopf.
5. Christie A: Normal closing time of the foramen ovale and ductus arteriosus. *Am J Dis Child* 40:323, 1930.
6. Clyman RI, Ballard PL, Sniderman S et al: Prenatal administration of β-methasone for prevention of patent ductus arteriosus, *J Pediatr* 98:123, 1981.
7. Daniolowicz D, Rudolph AM, Hoffman J: Delayed closure of the ductus arteriosus in premature infants, *Pediatrics* 37:74, 1966.
8. Freed MD, Heymann MA, Lewis AB et al: Prostaglandin $E_1$ infants with ductus arteriosus–dependent congenital heart disease, *Circulation* 64:899, 1981.
9. Friedman Z, Whitman V, Maisels MJ et al: Indomethacin disposition and indomethacin-induced platelet dysfunction in premature infants, *J Clin Pharmacol* 18:272, 1978.
10. Graybiel A, Strieder JW, Boyer NH: An attempt to obliterate the patent ductus arteriosus in a patient with bacterial endocarditis, *Am Heart J* 15:621, 1938.
11. Green TP, Thompson TR, Johnson DE et al: Furosemide promotes patent ductus arteriosus in premature infants with the respiratory distress syndrome, *N Engl J Med* 308:743, 1983.
12. Gregg NM: Congenital cataract following German measles in the mother, *Trans Ophthal Soc Australia* 3:35, 1941.
13. Gross RE, Hubbard JP: Surgical ligation of a patent ductus arteriosus: a report of first successful case, *JAMA* 112:729, 1939.
14. Halliday HL, Hirata T, Brady JP: Indomethacin therapy for large patent ductus arteriosus in the very low birth weight infants: results and complications, *Pediatrics* 64:154, 1979.
15. Hastreiter AR, van der Horst RL, Sepehri B et al: Prostaglandin $E_1$ infusion in newborns with hypoplastic left ventricle and aortic atresia, *Pediatr Cardiol* 2:95, 1982.
16. Heitz F, Fouron J-C, van Doesburg NH et al: Value of systolic time intervals in the diagnosis of large patent ductus arteriosus in fluid restricted and mechanically ventilated preterm infants, *Pediatrics* 74:1069, 1984.
17. Heymann MA, Berman W Jr, Rudolph AM et al: Dilatation of the ductus arteriosus by prostaglandin $E_1$ in aortic arch abnormalities, *Circulation* 59:169, 1979.
18. Heymann MA, Rudolph AM, Silverman NH: Closure of the ductus arteriosus in premature infants by inhibition of prostaglandin synthesis, *N Engl J Med* 295:530, 1976.
19. Heymann MA, Rudolph AM: Effects of congenital heart disease on fetal and neonatal circulations, *Prog Cardiovasc Dis* 15:115, 1972.
20. King TD, Thompson SL, Steiner C et al: Secundum atrial septal defect: nonoperative closure during cardiac catheterization, *JAMA* 235:2506, 1976.
21. Lister G, Hellenbrand WE, Kleinman CS et al: Physiologic effects of increasing hemoglobin concentration in left-to-right shunting in infants with ventricular septal defects, *N Engl J Med* 306:502, 1982.
22. Moss AJ, Emmanouilides GC, Duffie ER Jr: Closure of the ductus arteriosus in the newborn infant, *Pediatrics* 32:25, 1963.
23. Munro J: Ligation of the ductus arteriosus, *Ann Surg* 46:335, 1907.
24. Olley PM, Coceani F: Prostaglandins and the ductus arteriosus, *Ann Rev Med* 32:375, 1981.
25. Portsmann W, Wierny L, Warnke H: Der Verschluss des Ductus Arteriosus persistens ohne Thorakotomine (1, Mitfeilung), *Thoraxchirurgie* 15:199, 1967.
26. Porstmann W, Wierny L, Warnke H et al: Catheter closure of patent ductus arteriosus: 62 cases treated without thoracotomy, *Radiol Clin North Am* 9:203, 1971.
27. Rao PS, Wilson AD, Sideris EB et al: Transcatheter closure of patent ductus arteriosus with buttoned device: first successful clinical application in a child, *Am Heart J* 121:1799, 1991.
28. Rashkind WJ, Mullins CE, Hellenbrand WE et al: Nonsurgical closure of patent ductus arteriosus: clinical application of the Rashkind PDA occluder system, *Circulation* 75:583, 1987.
29. Rudolph AM, Heymann MA, Spitznas U: Hemodynamic considerations in the development of narrowing of the aorta, *Am J Cardiol* 30:514, 1972.
30. Samuelsson B, Goldyne M, Granstrom E et al: Prostaglandins and thromboxanes, *Ann Rev Biochem* 997, 1978.
31. Siassi B, Blanco C, Cabal LA et al: Incidence and clinical features of patent ductus arteriosus in low-birth-weight infants: a prospective analysis of 150 consecutively born infants, *Pediatrics* 57:347, 1976.
32. Wierny L, Plass R, Porstmann W: Transluminal closure of patent ductus arteriosus: long-term results of 208 cases treated without thoracotomy, *Cardiovasc Intervent Radiol* 9:279, 1986.
33. Zetterquist P: *A clinical and genetic study of congenital heart defects*, The Institute for Medical Genetics, University of Uppsala, Sweden, 1972.

# 15 Atrial Septal Defects

*Jay Kambam*



The types of atrial septal defects (ASD) vary from a slight perforation in the fossa ovalis to a complete absence of the interatrial septum. Complex defects involving the endocardial cushion will be presented in Chapter 17. Even though a patent foramen ovale is a type of interatrial communication, it is not generally considered an atrial septal defect. The incidence of probe patent foramen ovale in adults is about 25%.[1] Isolated secundum atrial septal defects account for approximately 7% to 11% of all congenital cardiac defects.[7,15] Girls are more frequently affected than boys, with a ratio of 2:1.[33] A familial incidence of ASD has also been reported. There is an increased incidence of ASD in populations living at high altitudes.[21] The average life span of a patient with an ASD, if not corrected surgically, is estimated to be about 40 years.[24]

## EMBRYOLOGY

The atrial portion of the heart tube is initially located outside the pericardial cavity in the transverse septum. A common atrium is formed through union of the right and left sides and becomes incorporated into the pericardial cavity. The common atrium grows transversely and appear as the right and left extremities on either side of the truncus. These two ventrolateral atrial extensions eventually become the right and left auricular appendages. As a result of expansion a depression is formed in the roof of the common atrium, and consequently a sickle-shaped crest appears in the lumen of the atrium. This is the first passively formed segment of the septum primum. Between the fourth and sixth weeks of gestational age, the single atrial chamber is divided into two. This begins with the extension of the septum primum toward the endocardial cushions formed in the atrioventricular canal (Fig. 15–1). The opening between the right and left primitive atria is the ostium primum. The endocardial thickening of the free margin of the septum primum fuses with both endocardial cushions of the atrioventricular canal, leading to the closure of the ostium primum. As the first septum continues to proliferate, fenestrations appear and eventually coalesce to form the ostium secundum in the cephalad portion of the septum primum. At about this time a thin septum called the septum secundum appears on the right of the septum primum. During this process the incorporation of the right sinus horn into the right atrium and that of the common pulmonary vein into the left atrium take place. The septum secundum covers the ostium secundum in an incomplete fashion, resulting in the formation of the foramen ovale. The concave free margin of the septum secundum persists as a thin flap, which balloons out into the left atrium, forming the valve of the foramen ovale. This valve overrides the or-

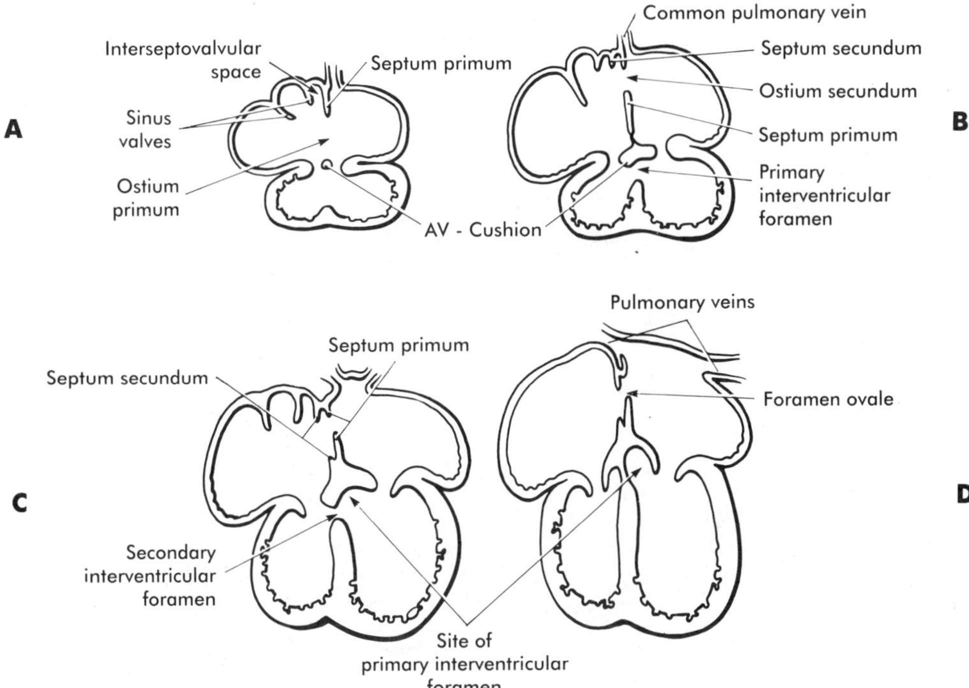


**Figure 15–1** Schematic representation of the atrial septa at successive stages of development. **A,** 30 days; **B,** 33 days; **C,** 37 days; **D,** newborn.

ifice of the inferior vena cava and effectively permits blood flow from the right atrium to the left atrium. The free margin of the septum secundum is sometimes called the crista dividens, as it separates the inferior vena caval stream into two; one passes directly through the foramen ovale into the left atrium, and the other spills into the right atrium. After birth, with the establishment of pulmonary circulation and increased pressure in the left atrium, the upper edge of the septum primum is pressed against the septum secundum, leading to the closure of the foramen ovale. However, in about 25% of the cases, this closure is incomplete.

## PATHOLOGIC ANATOMY

The single atrial chamber is divided into the right and left atria between the fourth and sixth weeks of gestation. The ultimate balance between proliferation and absorption of the septum primum and septum secundum leads to the formation of the atrial septum. ASD (an opening between the two atria) results when there is an error in the development of either septum. There should be no confusion, however, between an ASD and an open foramen ovale. Complete absence of the interatrial septum called cortriloculare biventriculare, or single atrium. There may be more than one type of defect in the interatrial septum in the same patient (Fig. 15–2).

### Sinus venosus defect

In the first variety the interatrial opening is high in the septum near the junction of the superior vena cava and the right atrium (Fig. 15–3). Such a defect is also called sinus venosus defect. This defect is frequently known to be associated with anomalous connections of the right pulmonary veins.

### Secundum defect

In the second variety the ASD is in the center of the septum at the site of the foramen ovale (Fig. 15–2). Secundum defects account for most instances of isolated ASD encountered in infancy.[8] When there are multiple fenestrations in the central portion of the septum, the defect is called a Chiari network. In approximately 15% of the cases there are associated extracardiac anomalies.[14] There is a significant familial incidence when the ASD is associated with certain skeletal abnormalities of the forearm and hand (Holt-Oram syndrome or cardiac-limb syndrome) or with prolongation of the P-R interval in the EKG.[7]

### Ostium primum defect

In the third variety the communication is at the ostium primum (the lower end of the septum) and is thus called ostium primum defect (Fig. 15–2). This defect is often associated with mitral valve incompetence due to a cleft in the anterior mitral

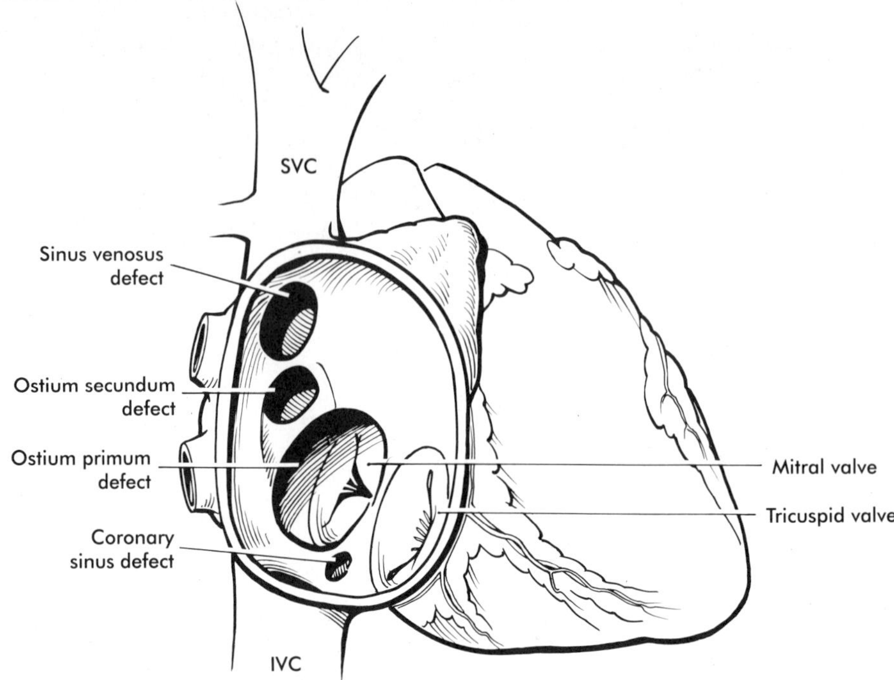


**Figure 15–2** Different types of atrial septal defects as viewed from the right atrium. *SVC,* superior vena cava; *IVC,* inferior vena cava.

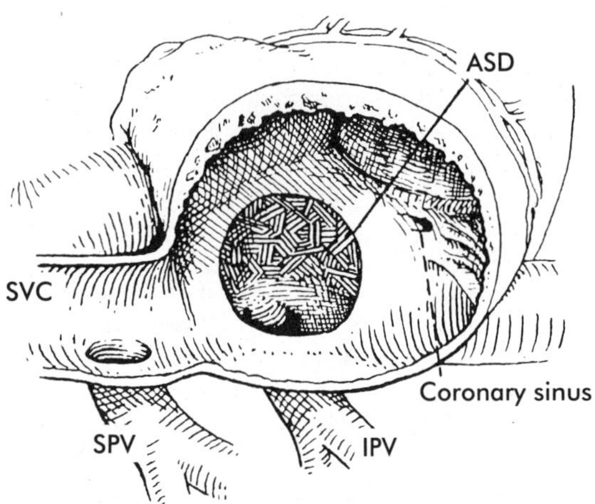


**Figure 15–3** Sinus venosus defect. Note the superior pulmonary vein *(SPV)* enter superior vena cava *(SVC).* (From Johnson J, editor: *Surgery of the chest,* St Louis, 1970, Mosby.)

leaflet. This defect is also classified as an incomplete atrioventricular canal or a partial endocardial cushion defect. Ostium primum defect is also frequently associated with tricuspid incompetence and/or VSD. The ostium primum defect is sometimes associated with Down's syndrome. The management of ostium primum defect is discussed in Chapter 17.

### Coronary sinus defect

The fourth category is the defect posterior to the fossa ovalis, a position normally occupied by the ostium of the coronary sinus (Fig. 15–2). Coronary sinus defect is frequently associated with anomalous connection of right pulmonary veins.

### Cor triloculare biventriculare (common atrium)

In this type of anomaly there are two atrial appendages, but one common atrial chamber is devoid of a septal partition. This anomaly is characterized by either total absence of the interatrial septum or the presence of only the vestigial elements of a poorly developed atrial septum (Fig. 15–4). The right-sided portion of the common atrium receives both venae cavae and the coronary sinus, and the left-sided portion receives the pulmonary veins. The hemodynamic findings seen in such an anomaly are very similar to those seen in large atrial septal defects. Common atrium is likely to be associated with asplenia.[28] Common atrium is often a part of the Ellis–Van Creveld syndrome of ectodermal dysplasia and polydactyly.[11] The other associated cardiac anomalies of common

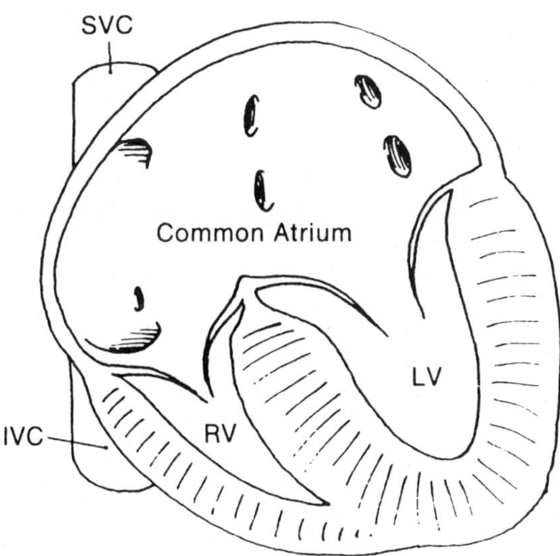


**Figure 15–4** Complete absence of the interatrial septum seen in single atrium (cor triloculare biventriculare). (From Gravanis MB, editor: *Cardiovascular pathophysiology*, New York, 1987, McGraw-Hill.)

atrium include systemic anomalous venous return (50%), partial or complete anomalous pulmonary venous return (25%), VSD (20%), and pulmonic valve stenosis (2%).

## PHYSIOLOGY AND PATHOPHYSIOLOGY

### Fetal circulation

There are two umbilical arteries and one umbilical vein. The two umbilical arteries carry relatively unoxygenated and hypoglycemic blood to the placenta, and the single umbilical vein carries relatively oxygenated blood with a higher glucose concentration from the placenta to the fetus. About 40% to 60% of this umbilical venous blood enters the portal vein to supply the liver. The remainder of the umbilical venous blood travels through the ductus venosus into the inferior vena cava. The ductus venosus connects the umbilical vein to the inferior vena cava near the junction of the hepatic veins. There may be a physiologic constrictor at the origin of the ductus venosus, which regulates the proportion of the umbilical and portal blood passing throught the liver. As it enters the right atrium, about one third of the blood from the inferior vena cave (mostly umbilical venous blood) is deflected across the foramen ovale into the left atrium by the crista dividens and eustachian valve, and the remainder enters the right ventricle via the tricuspid valve. Almost all of the blood from the superior vena cava enters the right ventricle and only about 3% of the blood enters the left atrium via the foramen ovale.

### Neonatal circulation

Once the umbilical cord is tied after birth, elimination of the low resistance placental circulation causes an increase in systemic vascular resistance. Pulmonary vascular resistance decreases and pulmonary blood flow increases with the initiation of neonatal respiration and the resultant increase in oxygen pressure and decrease in pulmonary arterial vasoconstriction. In addition there is a decrease in right atrial pressure as a result of elimination of large umbilical venous return. Thus, a decrease in right atrial pressure and an increase in left atrial pressure cause the foramen ovale to close and cease the right atrial to left atrial shunt. Physiologic closure of the foramen ovale occurs shortly after birth, but anatomic closure may be delayed as long as 1 year.

### Pathophysiology

The mean pressures in the left and right atria under normal conditions are about 7 and 4 mm Hg, respectively. In the presence of an ASD with a left to right shunt, there is equal pressure in both atria. The pressure changes are somewhat dependent on the right ventricular compliance. Because the compliance of the right ventricle at birth is low, the left to right shunt is minimal. As pulmonary vascular resistance decreases with time, the right ventricular compliance increases, resulting in an increase in the left to right shunt. In sinus venosus defect there may be an accompanying small right to left shunt due to the flow of a small portion of vena caval blood into the left atrium. In patients with a common atrium, instead of unidirectional shunt flow there are varying amounts of vena caval and pulmonary venous blood mixing inside the common atrium. The patient with an ASD has a burden on the right side of the heart as a result of an increase in volume flow through the septal defect from the left atrium to the right atrium. This results in the enlargement of both right atrium and right ventricle. A pressure gradient of about 20 mm Hg may be demonstrated across the pulmonic valve because of the increased right ventricular stroke volume. However, because of the reserved capacity of the pulmonary vascular system, it is only later in the natural history of the ASD that structural changes in the pulmonary arteries are observed. An increase in pulmonary vascular resistance adds pressure overload to the already volume-overloaded right ventricle. This will result in right ventricular hypertrophy leading to an increase in right atrial pressure. Rarely, when the right atrial pressure exceeds that of left atrium, a reversal of the shunt and cyanosis are seen (Eisenmenger's reaction).

Patients with ASD who acquire mitral stenosis

(usually of rheumatic origin) tend to develop pulmonary hypertension in an accelerated fashion. This anatomic association has been called Lutembacher's syndrome.[19] For reasons that are unclear, infective endocarditis is rare in patients with ASD.[14]

## CLINICAL PRESENTATION

The majority of patients with ASD lead a normal life without any symptoms during their childhood. Children symptomatic from ASD usually have congestive heart failure, failure to thrive, or recurrent respiratory infections. It is rare for an infant with an isolated ASD to show signs of congestive heart failure. Some children may have frequent respiratory infections because of increased pulmonary blood flow. Congestive heart failure and other symptoms become much more common in the fourth through sixth decades. Mild dyspnea and easy fatigue are the two most common early symptoms of a patient with an ASD. Patients with ASD may also have a variety of atrial arrhythmias including atrial flutter, atrial fibrillation, supraventricular tachycardia, and atrioventricular conduction abnormalities. Atrial arrhythmias are relatively uncommon in children but increasingly common in older children and adults with ASD.[2,3,4] Arrhythmias are usually the result of long-standing hypertrophy of the right atrium.

The general physical examination is usually normal in uncomplicated ASD. There may be associated skeletal deformities (Holt-Oram syndrome), notable facies (Down's syndrome), and visceral anomalies. Patients with a large ASD sometimes will have a prominent left costal cartilage as a result of cardiomegaly. The physical habitus of such a patient is often thin with long and narrow bones and poorly developed skeletal muscles (the gracile habitus). Cyanosis is usually not part of the clinical picture. The heart sounds are usually abnormal in patients with ASD. The first heart sound is usually accentuated because of a prominent tricuspid valve closure component. The hallmark of an ASD is the fixed splitting of a second heart sound that does not change with respirations. The murmurs associated with an ASD are typically soft and may not

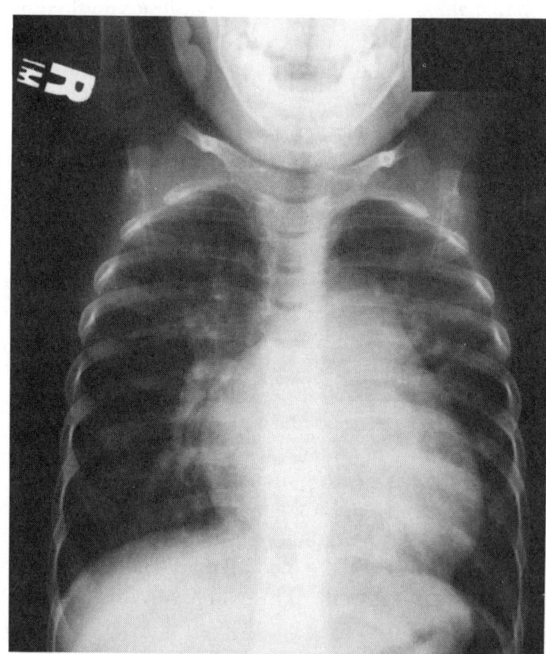


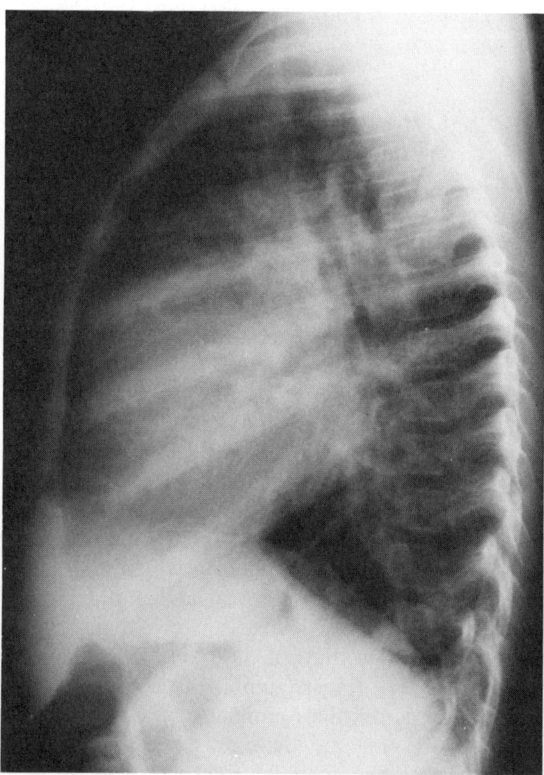


**Figure 15–5** Anteroposterior **(A)** and lateral **(B)** chest radiographs in a 2-year-old girl with a large atrial septal defect. Cardiomegaly is present, with evidence of right heart enlargement; the main pulmonary artery segment is also enlarged. The pulmonary arterial flow is increased. (Courtesy of Sandra G. Kirchner, MD.)

be audible in infancy and early childhood. Almost all patients with clinically recognizable ASD have a crescendo-decrescendo systolic murmur at the high left sternal border. This murmur is due to a rapid flow across the pulmonary valve. Respiration and position of the patient usually have no effect on the murmurs of ASD. With an increase in pulmonary vascular resistance and a resultant decrease in pulmonary blood flow, these murmurs tend to disappear.

### Laboratory findings

***Chest x-ray films.*** The heart usually appears distinctly large, with a marked enlargement of the right ventricle and right atrium (Fig. 15–5). Massive pulmonary artery enlargement with greatly engorged lung fields are also seen. The aortic knob is usually small and not apparent. In the majority of patients with SVD the radiologic findings are identical to those of a typical ostium secundum defect. In some patients, however, there may be a localized dilation of the superior vena cava at the entrance of the anomalous pulmonary veins. This gives rise to the appearance of higher than normal vascular pedicle in the right atrium.

***Electrocardiogram.*** In secundum defects ECG usually shows right axis deviation and right ventricular hypertrophy. Dilatation of the right ventricle as a result of the volume overload may stretch the right bundle branch, leading to incomplete right bundle branch block. In ostium primum ASD there is a left axis deviation and right ventricular hypertrophy.

***Echocardiogram.*** With echocardiography one can see a paradoxic anterior ventricular septal motion that contracts with the right ventricle rather than left ventricle. With two-dimensional echocardiography one can easily see enlargement of the right atrium and ventricle along with the location and size of the ASD (Fig. 15–6). Cardiac catheterization studies are not necessary, as the echocardiographic studies usually provide sufficient information, including an estimate of the left to right shunt.

***Catheterization data.*** On cardiac catheterization the diagnosis of ASD can be made by finding a rise in oxygen saturation between the superior vena cava and the right atrium (Fig. 15-7). A gradient of 20 to 40 mm Hg across a normal pulmonary valve can be demonstrated in patients with large shunts.

## MEDICAL MANAGEMENT

An isolated ASD is usually well tolerated without any symptoms for several years. Symptoms are rare in childhood. Only an occasional child with an ASD will have signs and symptoms of congestive heart failure. Medical management of such a patient usually consists of digitalis and diuretics. An occasional child may also require treatment for atrial arrhythmias, which may persist even after successful surgical correction of the ASD.

The usual dose of furosemide or ethacrynic acid is 1 mg/kg or 2 to 3 mg/kg body weight when given intravenously or orally, respectively. Diuretics are almost always used in combination with digitalis. Digoxin is the most commonly used digitalis preparation in neonates and infants with ASD. The usual recommended total oral digitalizing dose is 20 to 50 μg/kg (premature, 20 μg/kg; full term, 30 μg/kg; infants and children, 30 to 50 μg/kg) in three divided doses (½ + ¼ + ¼) at 6- to 8-hour intervals. The maintenance dose of digoxin (usually 25% of the total digitalizing dose) is 5 to

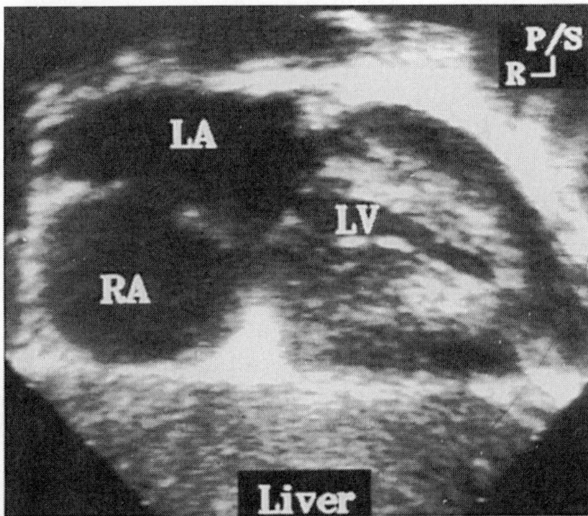


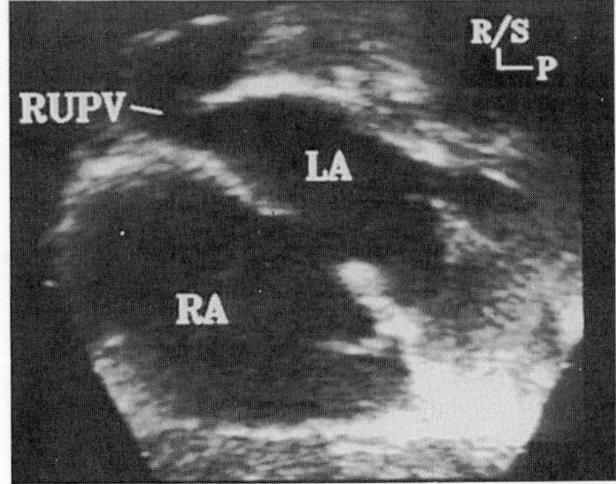


**Figure 15–6** Subxiphoid long-axis (**A**) and short-axis (**B**) views in a child with a typical secundum atrial septal defect. *LA*, left atrium; *LV*, left ventricle; *P*, posterior; *R*, right; *RA*, right atrium; *RUPV*, right upper pulmonary vein; *S*, superior. (From Fyler DC, editor: *Nadas' pediatric cardiology*, Philadelphia, 1992, Hanley & Belfus.)

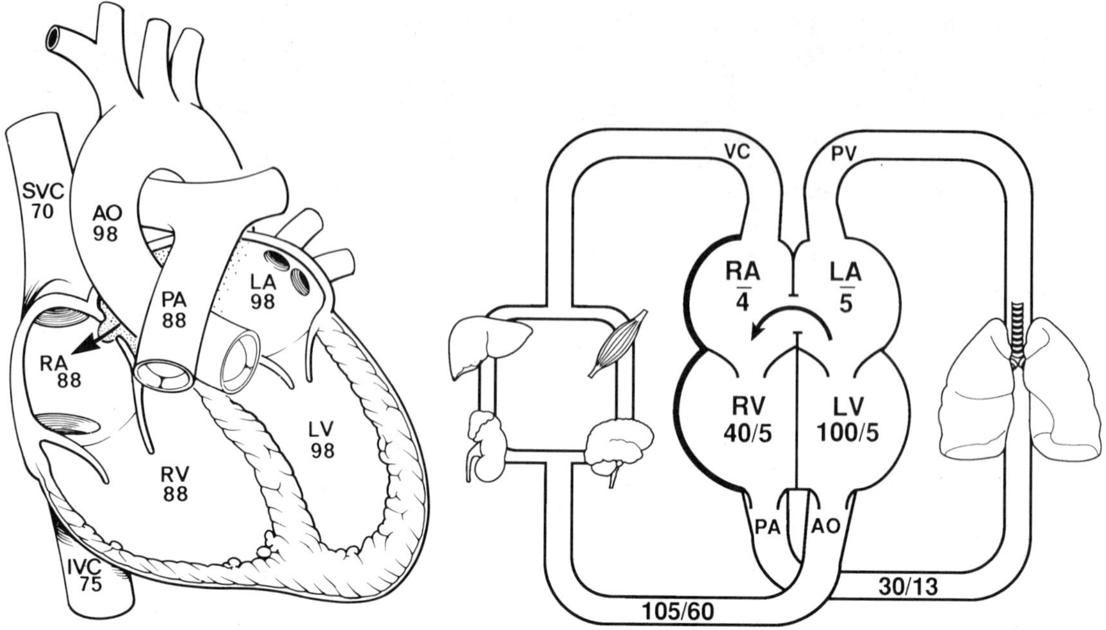


**Figure 15–7** Oxygen saturations and pressures in a patient with atrial septal defect.

10 μg/kg/day (premature, 5 μg/kg; full term, 8 μg/kg; infants and children, 8 to 10 μg/kg). These oral doses should be reduced to 75% when given by an intravenous route. For children with CHD who are in mild congestive heart failure, slow digitalization is usually chosen. Slow digitalization is usually accomplished by eliminating the initial digitalizing dose and just giving the maintenance dose once a day. The side effects of digoxin and diuretics are discussed in Chapter 6.

## SURGICAL MANAGEMENT

Surgery is frequently indicated on the basis of clinical and laboratory findings, laboratory determination of the size of the shunt, and the ratio of the pulmonary and systemic blood flow. Several studies indicate that spontaneous closure of ASD does occur in 25% to 50% of the cases during the first year of extrauterine life.[5,9,12,20,23]

The following are indications for surgery: (1) pulmonary to systemic blood flow ratio of more than 2:1, (2) marked cardiomegaly, (3) marked congestive heart failure, and (4) retarded growth and development. Otherwise surgery is usually undertaken when the patient is between 4 and 6 years of age, as the risks of cardiopulmonary bypass are low at this age. Between 1947 and 1953 multiple attempts were made to correct the ASD by closed techniques. In 1953 Lewis successfully closed an ASD by an open technique under hypothermia. Also in the same year Gibbon[10] employed the pump oxygenator successfully for the first time to suture an ASD.[11] A sternotomy is usually used, but a right thoracotomy in the fourth right intercostal space can also be used. Once cardiopulmonary bypass is initiated, the heart is arrested with a cardioplegia solution and the right atrium is opened. In the majority of cases closure of an ASD is done with a simple continuous suture. In only a few cases is either a pericardial patch or a prosthetic patch required (Fig. 15–8). Surgical repair of an ASD in an otherwise healthy patient has been associated with excellent results. The perioperative mortality rate is about 1%. Perioperative surgical complications include (1) postpericardiotomy syndrome (rare), (2) transient atrial arrhythmias (relatively common), (3) severe bradyarrhythmias and tachyarrhythmias (rare), (4) air embolism (rare), and (5) obstruction of the superior vena cava (rare, from sinus venosus defect closure). Cardiac dysrhythmias occasionally persist after surgical repair of ASD. These dysrhythmias are seen more often in patients with sinus venosus defects than in patients with secundum defects.[4]

## TRANSCATHETER CLOSURE

The pioneering work of Porstmann, King, and Rashkind has offered nonsurgical transcatheter closure of heart defects such as atrial and ventricular septal defects and patent ductus arteriosus as an alternative technique to surgery.[22,25,27]

King and his associates[16,17] used a catheter that

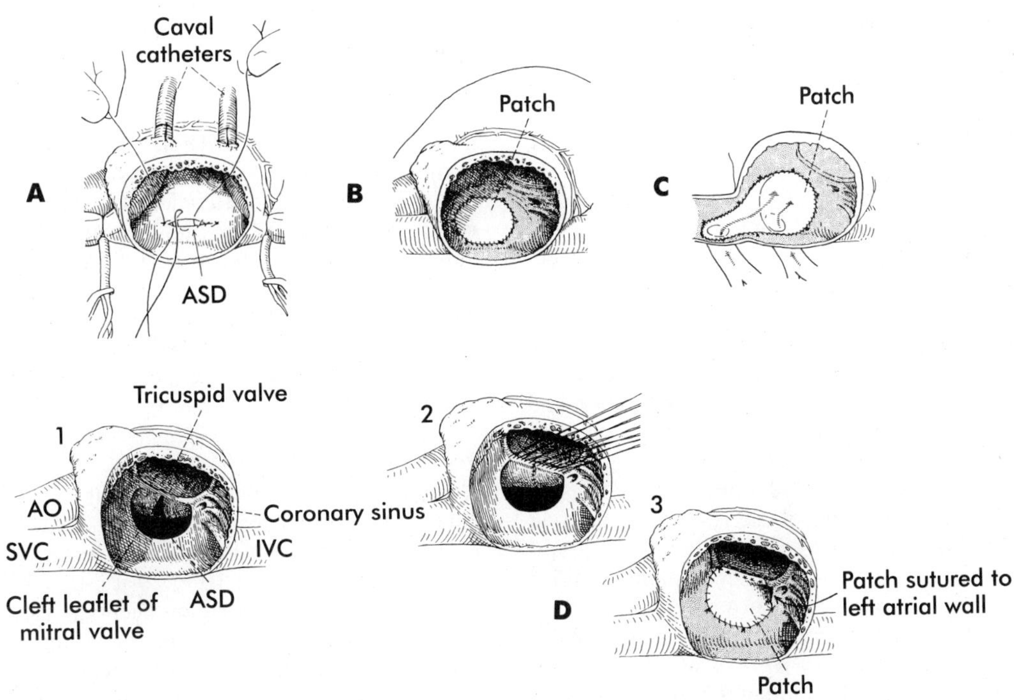


**Figure 15–8 A,** Closure of atrial septal defect with a simple running stitch. **B,** Closure of atrial septal defect with a patch. **C,** Closure of superior vena caval defect with a patch. **D,** Closure of septum primum. (From Johnson J, editor: *Surgery of the chest,* St Louis, 1970, Mosby.)

had paired opposed Dacron-covered stainless steel interlocking umbrellas, which collapse into a capsule at the tip of the catheter. Because of the complicated maneuvering required for implantation of this device and the bigger sheath required for the catheter (23 French), this technique has not been tried in humans.

Rashkind[26] designed a single foam umbrella with miniature hooks and an elaborate centering mechanism and tried it in both animal models and human subjects. This device is bulky and requires a 16-French sheath for insertion.

Because of the problems associated with implantation of the hooked single umbrella, Rashkind introduced a double-disc device. This device, also known as the clam shell device, was later modified by Lock and his associates.[18] It has no hooks and uses spring tension to allow the arms to fold back against each other. Recently the FDA suspended clinical trials with this device pending further study of breakage of its arms.

A buttoned double-disc device developed by Sideris and associates[2,9,30] is undergoing clinical trials. Initial trials have offered promise for application in human subjects. The advantage of this device is that it can be placed via an 8-French sheath and thus can be used in very young children.

Secundum ASD with a pulmonary to systemic flow ratio of more than 1.5:1 is generally considered an indication for surgical closure, and similar criteria are used for transcatheter closure. Defects larger than 25 mm, ostium primum defects, sinus venosus defects, and the defects that are associated with anomalous pulmonary venous connection and pulmonary vascular obstructive disease are considered contraindications for transcatheter techniques. Although transcatheter closure of ASD has been successfully accomplished in humans, it is not considered a best alternative to surgery because of the low morbidity and mortality and excellent postoperative results associated with open heart repair of ASD.

## ANESTHESIA MANAGEMENT

An understanding of pathologic anatomy and physiology and of pharmacology of various drugs that may alter the systemic and pulmonary blood flow is essential in managing patients with a functioning communication between the two sides of the heart. The anesthesia management of patients with ASD is very similar to that of VSD. Patients who come for surgery and anesthesia with ASD are usually older than those with VSD. The incidence of perioperative atrial arrhythmias, is higher in patients with ASD than with VSD.

### Premedication

Preoperative sedation in these patients depends on the age of the child and severity of the defect. Advantages of preoperative sedation include decrease or elimination of anxiety, reduction of oxygen demand, and avoidance of further hemodynamic deterioration. However, it is important not to oversedate these babies, as hypoventilation will have detrimental effects on oxygen saturation and pulmonary blood flow. Preoperative sedation should ideally be achieved in the holding room, where someone can watch for any undesirable side effects. Children with isolated ASD are usually in good health and do not pose a big challenge compared with children with other complex cardiac deformities. A narcotic and an anticholinergic drug combination (meperidine 2 mg/kg or morphine 0.1 mg/kg, and atropine 10 μg/kg) can be given intramuscularly 90 to 120 minutes before the scheduled time of operation. Oral midazolam (0.6 mg/kd) may also be given 30 minutes before the scheduled time of operation depending on the evaluation of the child in the holding room. For reasons that are not known, bacterial endocarditis is rare in patients with ASD. Because of the low incidence of bacterial endocarditis, prophylactic antibiotic administration is not used by all clinicians.[34]

### Monitoring

Monitoring during surgery includes an ECG, invasive arterial pressure, noninvasive blood pressure, pulse oximeter, capnogram, body temperature (esophageal and nasopharyngeal), central venous pressure, and urinometer. Pulmonary arterial or left atrial pressure monitoring is usually not necessary. Arterial blood gases, serum potassium, and hematocrit are monitored frequently throughout the operation.

### Induction of anesthesia

The majority of patients come to the operating room with no IV catheter. It is not difficult to start an IV line in a well sedated child before the induction of anesthesia. In these patients anesthesia can be induced with either 4 to 5 mg/kg of IV sodium thiopental or 1 to 2 mg/kg of ketamine depending on the underlying ventricular function. In children who are uncooperative and in small children who come to the operating suite without an IV line in place, anesthesia can be induced with either halothane by mask or ketamine by IM injection. I recommend using inspired concentrations of halothane under 2%, as complete heart block may result from concentrations in excess of 2%. A left to right shunt does not alter the speed of inhalational induction.[6,31] On the other hand, a left to right shunt is said to result in a slow intravenous induction.[32] But this difference is of theoretic interest only. Once the IV line is secured, tracheal intubation can be performed with either succinylcholine or a nondepolarizing muscle relaxant. Atropine 5 to 10 μg/kg should be given prior to the administration of succinylcholine (1 to 2 mg/kg, IV). An arterial cannula and a central venous catheter are usually inserted after the airway is secured.

### Maintenance

Anesthesia is maintained either with one of the inhaled anesthetic agents (halothane, enflurane, or isoflurane) or with an IV narcotic (fentanyl 50 to 100 μg/kg or sufetanil 10 to 20 μg/kg). If halothane or one of the inhalation agents is used as a sole anesthetic, one should either continue the inhaled agent or use a narcotic drug (fentanyl 15 μg/kg or sufentanil 2.5 μg/kg) and an amnestic agent (lorazepam, 25 μg/kg or midazalom, 50 μg/kg) at the time of extracorporeal circulation. Otherwise one will have a paralyzed patient without any anesthesia on board. Vecuronium or one of the newer nondepolarizing muscle relaxants (doxacurium or pipecuronium) can be used to maintain muscle paralysis throughout the operation.

If deep hypothermia and circulatory arrest are planned (usually in children under 10 kg body weight), I administer 10 ml/kg of dextran 40 in 5% dextrose solution before peripheral cooling is initiated. (See Chapter 4 for complete details of deep hypothermia.)

Patients with ASD and increased pulmonary blood flow may benefit by the addition of slight positive end expiratory pressure. Other conditions that increase left to right shunt should be avoided (see the box on next page).

Heparin is usually given into the right atrium by the surgeon just before the placement of cannulas. Protamine is administered by the anesthesiologist at the conclusion of extracorporeal circulation following the removal of cardiac cannulas. A few patients, especially the ones with pulmonary hypertension, require either isoproterenol (0.01 to 0.05 μg/kg/min) or dopamine (3 to 6 μg/kg/min) infusion after coming off bypass. Complete heart block is one of the well recognized complications of repair of an ostium primum defect. Unlike patients with ostium primum, patients with secundum type and sinus venosus type rarely require postoperative cardiac pacing. The routine patient fol-

**CONDITIONS THAT ARE KNOWN TO INCREASE LEFT TO RIGHT SHUNT**

1. Low hematocrit
2. Increased SVR
3. Decreased PVR
4. Hyperoxemia
5. Hyperventilation
6. Negative airway pressure

lowing a straightforward ASD repair presents little or no problem in postoperative care.

### Precautions

In all cases where there is a communication between right and left sides of the heart, it is absolutely necessary that all intravenous lines be free of air bubbles. In addition, one should use extra caution not to introduce any air bubbles when injecting drugs through an IV line. Even though the use of nitrous oxide is not contraindicated in patients with an ASD, many anesthesiologists avoid the use of it, especially once the chest is opened, for the fear of intravascular air bubble expansion.

### Postoperative ventilation

Even though the trachea can be extubated at the end of operation in most of the uncomplicated ASD patients, I routinely ventilate the patients mechanically for a few hours postoperatively, as the majority of my patients receive intravenous narcotic agents in high doses during surgery. In addition patients usually become somewhat hypothermic at the end of the surgery. Once a patient is awake, stable, and rewarmed to a normal body temperature, the trachea can be extubated safely in the cardiac recovery room.

### REFERENCES

1. Bedford E, Papp C, Parkinson J: Atrial septal defect, *Br Heart J* 3:37, 1941.
2. Bolens M, Friedli B: Sinus node function and conduction system before and after surgery for secundum atrial septal defect: an electrophysiologic study, *Am J Cardiol* 53:1415, 1984.
3. Campbell M: Natural history of atrial septal defect, *Br Heart J* 32:820, 1980.
4. Clark EB, Kugler JD: Preoperative secundum atrial septal defect with coexisting sinus node and atrioventricular node dysfunction, *Circulation* 65:976, 1982.
5. Cockerham JT, Martin TC, Gutierrez FR et al: Spontaneous closure of secundum atrial septal defect in infants and young children, *Am J Cardiol* 523:1267, 1983.
6. Eger EI: Uptake of inhaled anesthetics: the alveolar to inspired anesthetic difference: effect of ventilation/perfusion abnormalities. In: *Anesthetic uptake and action,* Baltimore, 1974, Williams & Wilkins.
7. Feldt RH, Avasthey P, Yoshimasu F et al: Incidence of congenital heart disease in children born to residents of Olmsted County, Minnesota, 1950-1969, *Mayo Clin Proc* 46:794, 1971.
8. Fyler DC, Buckley LP, Hellenbrand WE et al: Report of the New England Regional Infant Cardiac Program, *Pediatrics* 65(I):377, 1980.
9. Ghisla RP, Hannon DW, Meyer RA: Spontaneous closure of isolated secundum atrial septal defects: an echocardiographic study, *Am Heart J* 109:1327, 1985.
10. Gibbon JH: Application of a mechanical heart and lung apparatus to cardiac surgery, *Minn Med* 37:171, 1954.
11. Giknis FL: Single atrium and the Ellis-VanCreveld syndrome, *J Pediatr* 62:558, 1963.
12. Hoffman JIE, Rudolph AM, Danilowicz D: Left to right atrial shunts in infants, *Am J Cardiol* 30:868, 1972.
13. Holt M, Oram S: Familial heart disease with skeletal malformations, *Br Heart J* 22:236, 1960.
14. Kaplan EL, Anthony BF, Gijno A et al: American Heart Association report: prevention of bacterial endocarditis, *Circulation* 56:139A, 1977.
15. Keith JD: Atrial septal defect: ostium secundum, ostium primum and atrioventricularis communis (common AV canal). In Keith JD, Rowe RD, Vlad P, editors: *Heart disease in infancy and childhood,* ed 3, New York, 1978, MacMillan.
16. King TD, Thompson SL, Steiner C et al: Secundum atrial septal defect: nonoperative closure during cardiac catheterization, *JAMA* 235:2506, 1976.
17. King TD, Mills NL: Nonoperative closure of atrial septal defects, *Surgery* 75:383, 1974.
18. Lock JE, Rome JJ, Davis R et al: Transcatheter closure of atrial septal defects: experimental studies, *Circulation* 79:1091, 1989.
19. Lutembacher R: De la stenose mitrale avec communication intr'auriculaire, *Arch Mal Coeur* 9:237, 1916.
20. Mahoney LT, Truesdell SC, Krzmarzick TP et al: Atrial septal defects that present in infancy, *Am J Dis Child* 140:1115, 1986.
21. Miao C, Zuberbuhler JS, Zuberbuhler JR: Prevalence of congenital cardiac anomalies at high altitude, *J Am Coll Cardiol* 12:224, 1988.
22. Mills NL, King TD: Nonoperative closure of left-to-right shunts, *J Thorac Cardiovasc Surg* 72:371, 1976.
23. Mody MR: Serial hemodynamic observations in secundum atrial septal defects with special reference to spontaneous closure, *Am J Cardiol* 32:978, 1973.
24. Moss AJ, Siassi B: The small atrial septal defect: operate or procrastinate? *J Pediatr* 79:854, 1971.
25. Rao PS, Wilson AD, Levy JM et al: Role of buttoned double disc device in the management of atrial septal defects, *Am Heart J* 123:191, 1992.
26. Rashkind WJ: Transcatheter of congenital heart disease, *Circulation* 67:711, 1983.
27. Rome JJ, Keane JF, Perry SB et al: Double-umbrella closure of atrial defects: initial clinical applications, *Circulation* 82:751, 1990.
28. Ruttenberg HD, Neufeld RV, Lucas LS et al: Syndrome of congenital cardiac disease with asplenia, *Am J Cardiol* 13:387, 1964.
29. Sideris EB, Sideris SE, Fowlkes JP et al: Transvenous atrial septal occlusion in piglets using a buttoned double disc device, *Circulation* 81:312, 1990.
30. Sideris EB, Sideris SE, Thanopoulos BD et al: Transvenous atrial septal defect occlusion by the buttoned device, *Am J Cardiol* 66:1524, 1990.

31. Stoelting R, Longnecker DE: Effect of right-to-left shunt on rate of increase in arterial anesthetic concentration, *Anesthesiology* 365:352, 1972.
32. Tanner GE, Angers DG, Barash PG et al: Effect of left-to-right, mixed right-to-left, and right-to-left shunts on inhalational anesthetic induction in children: a computer model, *Anesth Analg* 64:101, 1985.
33. Weidman WH, Swan HJC, DuShane JW et al: A hemodynamic study of atrial septal defect and associated anomalies involving the atrial septum, *J Lab Clin Med* 50:165, 1957.
34. Zaver AG, Nadas AS: Atrial septal defect—secundum type, *Circulation* 31-32 (suppl 3):24, 1965.

# 16 Ventricular Septal Defects

*Jay Kambam*



If one excludes the patent ductus arteriosus associated with prematurity and bicuspid aortic valve, isolated ventricular septal defect is the most common cardiac abnormality found in children. Isolated ventricular septal defects (VSD) accounts for approximately 25% of all congenital heart defects. The incidence of VSD is higher in premature infants than in full term infants.[18] For some unknown reason the incidence of VSD in the United States has steadily increased in the past 2 decades. A male prevalence for VSD has been documented.

## EMBRYOLOGY

After cardiac looping between the fourth and fifth weeks of intrauterine life, the single ventricle is divided into two chambers. This is achieved by the union of the membranous portion of the ventricular septum, the bulbus cordis, and the endocardial cushions (Fig. 16–1). The primitive left ventricle is developed from the ventricular portion, and the primitive right ventricle is formed from the proximal portion of the truncus arteriosus (bulbus cordis). At this time the left and the right ventricles are connected by the primary interventricular foramen. Growth and trabeculation of the ventricles account for the formation of the major portion of the muscular septum. The muscular portion of the ventricular septum grows cephalad as each ventricular cavity enlarges to meet with the right and left ridges of the bulbus cordis. The left ridge unites with a ridge of the interventricular septum, and the right ridge fuses with the tricuspid valve and the endocardial cushion, thus separating the pulmonary valve from the tricuspid valve and leaving the aortic valve in continuity with the mitral valve.

The conus swellings appear at about the same time as the truncal swellings and the atrioventricular cushions. The conus and truncal swellings and the atrioventricular cushions eventually combine to form the conus septum, separating the conus cordis into the anterolateral and posteromedial portions. The endocardial cushion from the conus septum and the right superior endocardial cushion merge with the superior segment of the muscular septum, thus closing the interventricular foramen. The superior segment of the muscular septum thins to become the membranous segment of the interventricular septum. Deviations in the development of the membranous septum may result in perimembranous VSD. The failure of fusion of parts of the conus septum may give rise to defects in the outlet septum. The inlet defects are usually the result of failure of the proper fusion of the right superior endocardial cushion tissue with the muscular septum. VSD in the muscular septum is the result of either inadequate fusion of the medial walls of the left and right ventricles or excessive absorption of the septum during the growth of the ventricles.

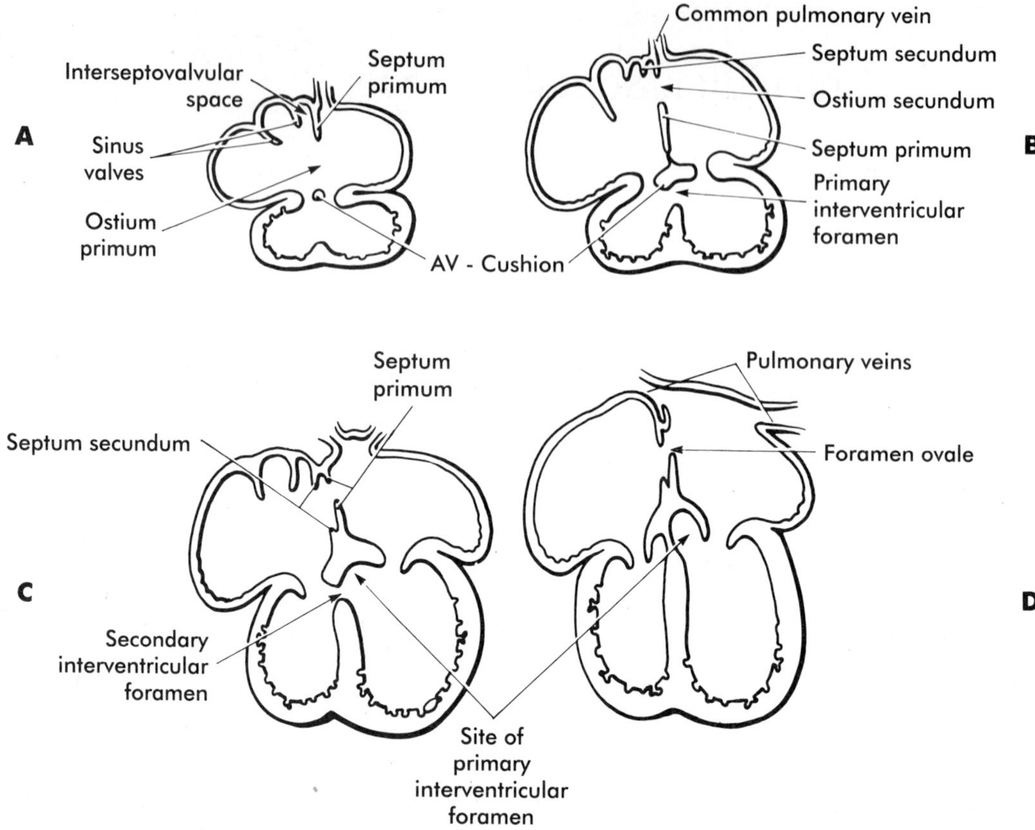


**Figure 16–1** Schematic representation of the atrial and ventricular septa at successive stages of development. **A,** 30 days. **B,** 33 days. **C,** 37 days. **D,** newborn.

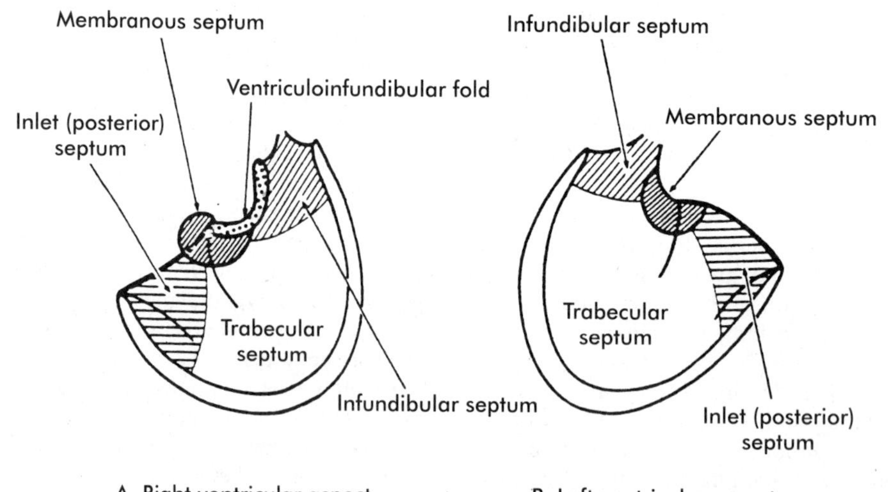


**Figure 16–2** Diagram illustrating the components of the ventricular septum (in the definitive heart the margins between muscular segments are indistinct). There are three muscular portions, inlet, trabecular, and infundibular. The fibrous membranous portion completes the septum. Note the ventriculoinfundibular fold in the right ventricle between the atrioventricular and arterial valves. (From Anderson RH, editor: Another look at cardiac embryology. In *Progress in cardiology,* Philadelphia, 1978, Lea & Febiger.)

## PATHOLOGIC ANATOMY

The ventricular septum is divided into a small membranous portion and a large muscular portion. The muscular septum is further subdivided into three parts, inlet, trabecular, and infundibular or outlet portions (Fig. 16–2).

## CLASSIFICATION

A VSD may be classified into one of three main varieties: perimembranous, muscular, and subarterial infundibular (see the box). VSD may be either supracristal or infracristal; the crista supraventricularis is the landmark. The muscular and membranous types of VSD are located below the crista supraventricularis and are thus infracristal, and the subarterial infundibular VSD is located above the supraventricularis and is supracristal. VSD may be small, medium, or large and are classified according to their size. VSDs may be single or multiple, and the shape varies.

**CLASSIFICATION AND RELATIVE INCIDENCE OF VENTRICULAR SEPTAL DEFECTS**

1. Perimembranous (70%)
    - Trabecular extension (typical type)
    - Inlet extension (AV canal type)
    - Outlet extension (Tetralogy of Fallot type)
2. Muscular (25%)
    - Trabecular
    - Inlet
    - Outlet
3. Subarterial infundibular (5%)

### Perimembranous defects

The membranous portion of the ventricular septum is a small area in close proximity to the segmental leaflet of the tricuspid valve and a small segment of the right atrium on the right side. The aortic valve is on the left side. As a consequence congenital or acquired abnormalities of the aortic and tricuspid valves may be associated with membranous VSD. The perimembranous type is by far the most common type, constituting about 70% of all VSD (Fig. 16–3). Isolated membranous VSD, however, is very rare. The membranous type of VSD usually extends into the adjacent muscular septum (box). Typically it extends into the trabecular portion of the muscular septum. In the AV canal type the defect extends into the inlet portion, and in the TOF type the defect extends into the outlet portion of the muscular septum.

### Muscular septum

The muscular septum is a large area of the ventricular septum, which is subdivided into trabecular, inlet, and outlet or infundibular portions.

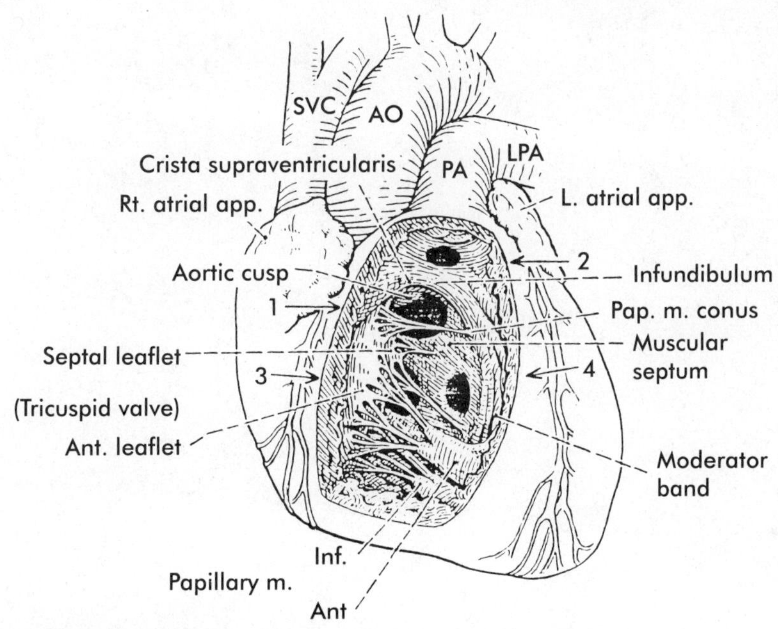


**Figure 16–3** Different types of ventricular septal defects as viewed from the right ventricle. *1,* infracristal membranous defect; *2,* supracristal defect; *3,* endocardial cushion defect; *4,* low muscular defect. *SVC,* superior vena cava; *AO,* aorta; *LPA,* left pulmonary artery; *PA,* pulmonary artery. (From Johnson J, editor: *Surgery of the chest,* St. Louis, 1970, Mosby.)

Muscular defects may be located in any of these areas and are often multiple. The muscular defects are the second most common type of VSD, accounting for about 25% (Fig. 16–3).

### Subarterial infundibular defects

These defects are located beneath the aortic valve when viewed from the left ventricle, and viewed from the right ventricle they are under the pulmonary valve (Fig. 16–3). Aortic insufficiency is frequently present in this type of defect because the adjacent aortic valve cusps often protrude into the infundibular VSD.

## PATHOPHYSIOLOGY

After birth, once the umbilical cord is tied, an increase in systemic vascular resistance results from elimination of the low-resistance placental circulation. Pulmonary vascular resistance (PVR) decreases and pulmonary blood flow increases with the initiation of neonatal respiration and the resultant increase in arterial oxygen pressure and decrease in pulmonary arterial vasoconstriction. Pulmonary arterial pressure falls from a prenatal value of 70/45 torr to about 50/30 torr and 30/12 torr by 24 hours and 1 week after birth, respectively. Since the decrease in PVR to a critical level does not occur until the age of 6 or 8 weeks, signs and symptoms of CHF from a VSD do not usually occur until that time.

In general the amount and direction of shunting depend on the difference between the systemic and pulmonary vascular resistances, pressure difference across the two sides, and the size (radius) of the defect. In cases of large VSD, pressure gradient essentially does not exist, and shunting across the defect is primarily governed by the ratio of pulmonary to systemic vascular resistance (SVR). This is usually called a nonrestrictive shunt. On the other hand, if the cardiac defect is small, the shunt across the defect is primarily influenced by the size of the lesion, and the ratio of PVR and SVR will have only a minor role. These are called restrictive shunts.

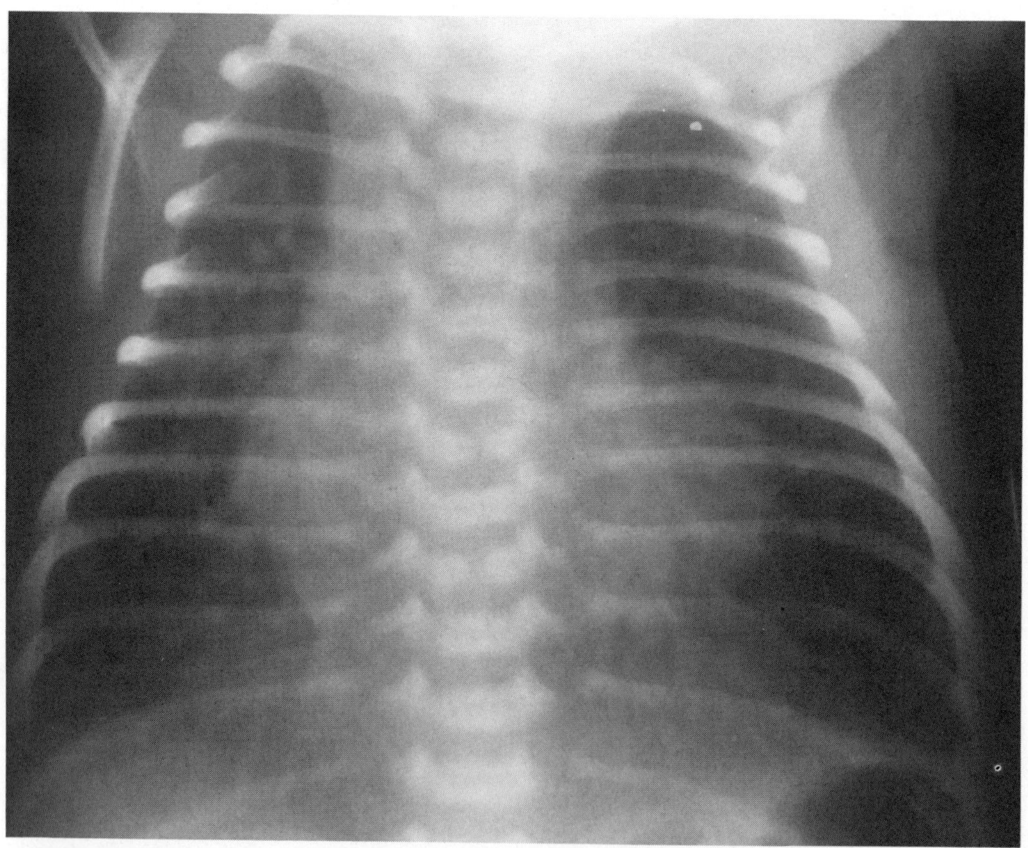

**Figure 16–4** Anteroposterior chest radiograph of a three-week-old baby boy with a ventricular septal defect. The heart is enlarged, but it is not possible to detect specific chamber enlargement, which is often the case in neonates. The pulmonary arterial flow is increased and the main pulmonary artery segment is prominent. (Courtesy of Sandra G. Kirchner.)

A left to right shunt is usually seen in children with acyanotic VSD. Since the shunt of VSD occurs mainly when both ventricles are contracting simultaneously, the blood is mainly shunted toward the pulmonary artery, resulting in increased pulmonary arterial flow and no significant increase in the right ventricular end systolic volume. This will result in enlargement of the main pulmonary artery and its vasculature, LA, and LV. Therefore, in VSD it is the left ventricle that is burdened, not the right ventricle, and there is no right ventricular enlargement. With a large VSD, however, there is a direct transmission of the LV pressure to the RV along with a large shunt resulting in biventricular hypertrophy. When a large VSD is left untreated, in years there will be gradual development of pulmonary vascular obstructive disease (PVOD) or Eisenmenger's syndrome.

## CLINICAL PRESENTATION

### History and physical findings

Children with small VSD usually have no problems and have normal growth and development. Children with moderate to large VSD, however, usually have decreased exercise tolerance, recurrent respiratory infections, impaired growth and development, and signs and symptoms of CHF. In longstanding cases where there is a significant PVOD, cyanosis may be present. Signs and symptoms of CHF are usually noticed by the end of 2 months, when PVR is significantly reduced. A regurgitant holosystolic murmur is usually audible at the left lower sternal border.

***Electrocardiogram.*** In small VSD the ECG findings may be totally normal. In moderate VSD both left atrial hypertrophy (LAH) and left ventricular hypertrophy (LVH) are noticeable, and in large VSD, in addition to LAH, there will be signs of biventricular hypertrophy. In patients with PVOD one may see right ventricular hypertrophy (RVH) without LAH or LVH.

***Chest x-ray film.*** Like ECG findings, chest x-ray findings may vary according to the size of the VSD and the duration of the shunt. An increase in the size of the PA and its vascular markings, along with an enlarged LA and LV, are usually seen in patients with VSD (Fig. 16–4). In large VSD, RV enlargement is seen in addition to enlargement of the other chambers.

***Echocardiography.*** Two-dimensional echocardiograms usually provide definitive and accurate diagnosis of the size and site of the VSD (Fig. 16–5). They also indicate the direction and magnitude of the shunt and estimated PA pressures and PVR.

***Cardiac catheterization.*** With the rapid progress of noninvasive assessment of VSD, diagnostic catheterization and angiography (Fig. 16–6) are performed less frequently than heretofore.

## MEDICAL MANAGEMENT

Spontaneous closure is believed to occur in 30% to 40% of all VSDs.[1,2,6,9,18,22] In the majority of cases closure occurs within the first year of life. Smaller VSDs are known to close spontaneously more often than larger defects. Subarterial (infundibular) and AV canal VSDs seldom close spontaneously. Patients with VSD usually develop signs and symptoms of CHF at the end of 2 months of age. Once the diagnosis is made, the medical man-

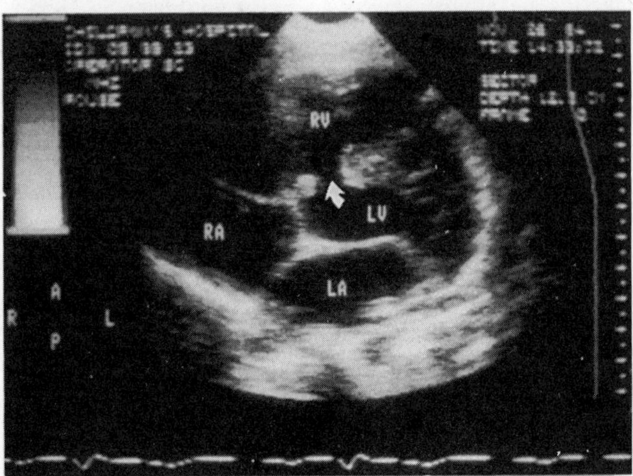


**Figure 16–5** An echocardiogram in parasternal short-axis view showing a membranous ventricular septal defect. Note the rightward and posterior location of the defect, behind the septal leaflet of the tricuspid valve and near the crux of the heart. *RV,* right ventricle; *LV,* left ventricle; *RA,* right atrium; *LA,* left atrium. (From Fyler DC, editor: *Nadas' pediatric cardiology,* 1992, Philadelphia, Hanley & Belfus.)

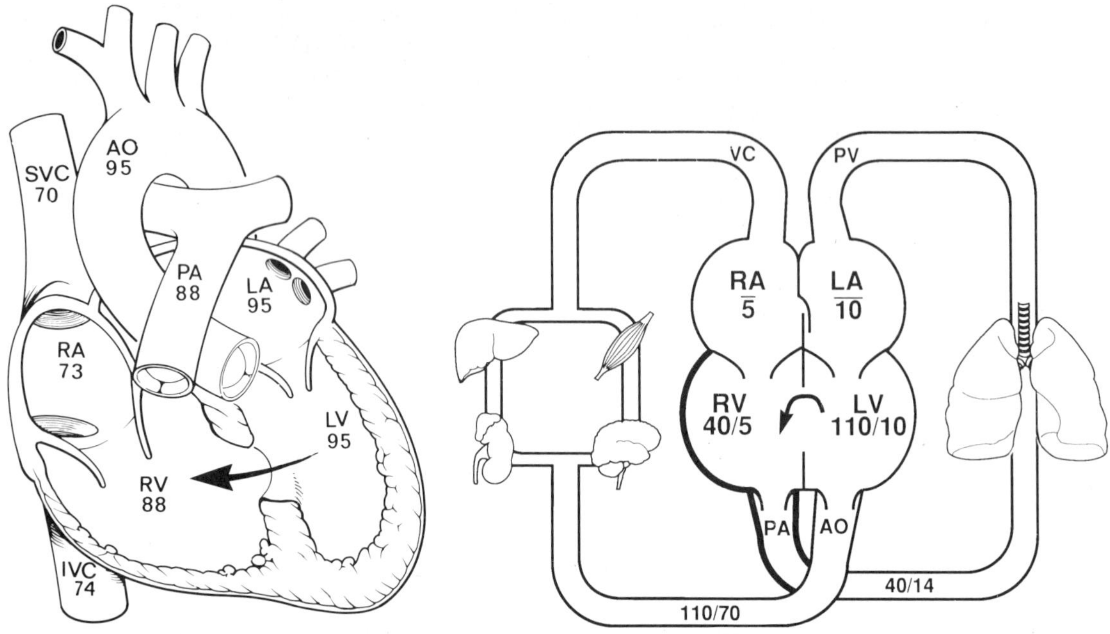


**Figure 16–6** Oxygen saturations and pressures in a patient with ventricular septal defect. *SVC*, superior vena cava; *AO*, aorta; *RA*, right atrium; *PA*, pulmonary artery; *LA*, left atrium; *RV*, right ventricle; *LV*, left ventricle; *IVC*, inferior vena cava.

agement consists of close follow-up of these patients and treatment with diuretics and digitalis preparations.[4,7] Maintenance of hematocrit is also important in these patients. As with anemia, left to right shunt increases, worsening CHF.[5,13] Patients with CHF may rapidly improve with the administration of a single dose of fast-acting diuretic such as furosemide or ethacrynic acid, usually dose 1 mg/kg and 2 to 3 mg/kg body weight IV and orally, respectively. Diuretics are almost always used with digitalis. Digoxin is the most commonly used digitalis preparation in neonates and infants with VSD. The usual recommended total oral digitalizing dose is 20 to 50 μg/kg (premature, 20 μg/kg; full term, 30 μg/kg; infants and children, 30 to 50 μg/kg) in three divided doses (½ + ¼ + ¼) at 6- to 8-hour intervals. The maintenance dose of digoxin (usually 25% of the total digitalizing dose) is 5 to 10 μg/kg/day (premature, 5μg/kg; full term, 8 μg/kg; infants and children, 8 to 10 μg/kg). Reduce these oral doses to 75% when given IV. For children with CHD who are in mild CHF, slow digitalization is usually chosen. Slow digitalization is usually accomplished by eliminating the initial digitalizing dose and just giving the maintenance dose once a day. The side effects of digoxin and diuretics are discussed in Chapter 6. The incidence of bacterial endocarditis is rare in patients with small VSDs. However, it is high in large VSDs.[26]

## SURGICAL MANAGEMENT

Children with VSD undergo either PA banding as a palliative procedure or surgical repair of the VSD. Palliative surgery in the form of pulmonary artery banding was recommended by Muller and Dammann[19] in 1952 as part of a two-stage repair for children with VSD. PA banding is infrequently performed as a palliative procedure unless additional heart defects warrant deferral of the complete repair until later. In 1955 Lillehei and associates[12] reported the first successful closure of VSD using the cross-circulation technique. For the majority of patients with simple VSD the present approach is primary intracardiac repair.[11,25] Surgical closure of VSD is accomplished by using extracorporeal circulation with or without deep hypothermia and circulatory arrest. An atrial or right ventricular approach is most frequently used, but a left ventricular approach is sometimes an option (multiple trabecular muscular defects).[3,17,23,27] Unless there is a technical problem, the majority of surgeons use the right atrial approach rather than the right ventriculotomy (Fig. 16–7). Distortion of tricuspid valve leaflets occurs frequently when the transatrial closure of VSD is performed, but this is rarely a problem.

The development of PVOD is rare before 1 year of age, but the incidence increases thereafter.[20,25] The incidence of PVOD is also higher with large VSDs, multiple VSDs, and with associated PDA.

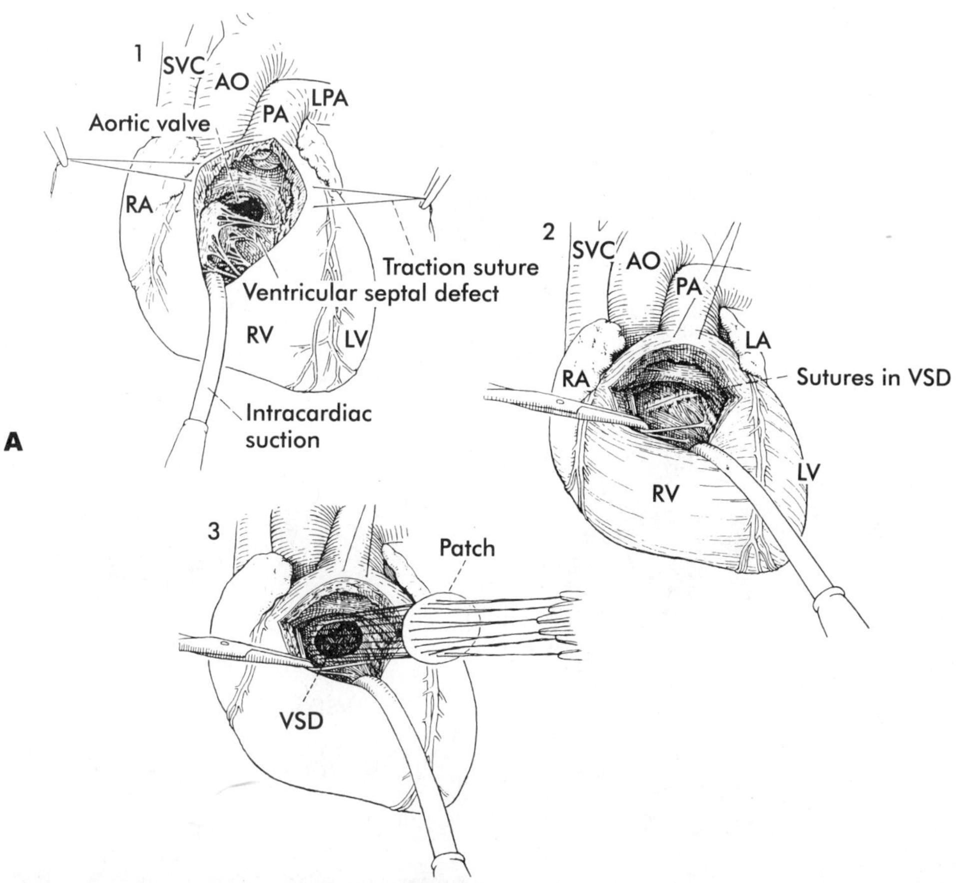


**Figure 16–7** Techniques for closing ventricular septal defects. **A,** Right ventricular approach. *Continued.*

The surgical mortality rate is high if the surgery is undertaken before the patient is 6 months of age (about 20%). But after the patient is 6 months of age, the mortality rate for such operations is much lower (about 2%).[3,17,23,27] For the reasons mentioned above the surgical correction of VSD is usually undertaken between 1 and 2 years of age. Indications for an earlier surgical correction include left to right shunt with Qp:Qs greater than 2; CHF unresponsive to medical therapy; significant growth retardation; and large VSD with signs of increasing PVR. Children with VSD and PDA will usually undergo closure of the PDA first, followed by correction of the VSD at a later time. Similarly, patients with VSD and coarctation of the aorta undergo repair of the coarctation first. Patients with endocardial cushion defect (AV canal type) and patients with subarterial infundibular VSD with aortic regurgitation require prompt surgery, even if their Qp:Qs is less than 2. Surgery is contraindicated in children with PVR:SVR of 0.75 or greater or PVOD with predominant right to left shunt. The surgical mortality rate for children with otherwise uncomplicated VSD is less than 2%. Perioperative complications include residual shunt, bacterial endocarditis, distortion of the tricuspid valve leaflets, isolated right bundle branch block (RBBB), RBBB with left anterior hemiblock, and complete heart block.

While the majority of patients who undergo closure of VSD become asymptomatic, their exercise tolerance and left ventricular performance remain abnormal for several years after the repair.[10,15,16,21]

## INTERVENTIONAL CATHETER CLOSURE

As in some other CHDs such as PDA and ASD, interventional catheter closure has become a reality for VSD. The clinical usefulness of interventional catheter closure for VSD remains to be seen.

## ANESTHESIA MANAGEMENT

An understanding of pathologic anatomy and physiology and of the pharmacology of various drugs that may alter the systemic and pulmonary blood flows is essential in managing patients with a functioning communication between the two sides of the heart. Special problems one encounters in a

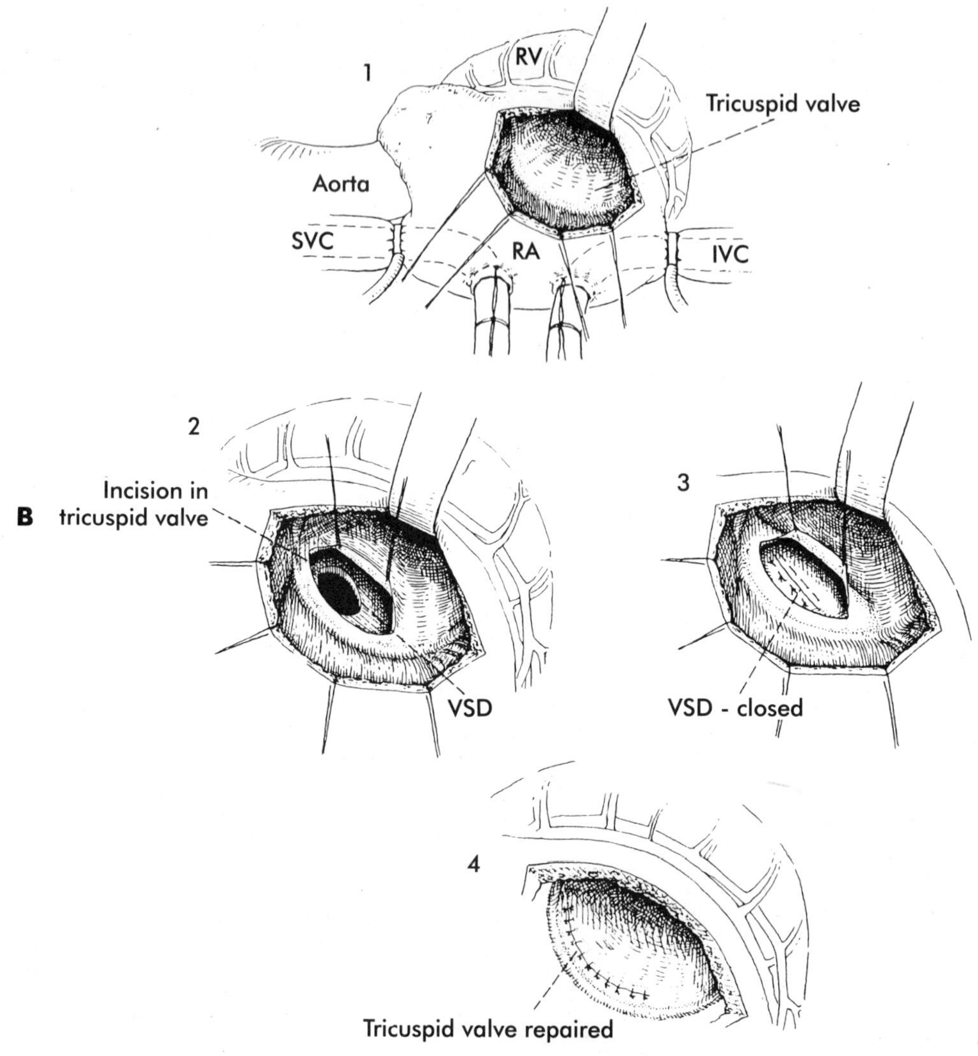


**Figure 16–7, cont'd B,** Right atrial approach. *SVC,* superior vena cava; *AO,* aorta; *RA,* right atrium; *PA,* pulmonary artery; *LA,* left atrium; *RV,* right ventricle; *LV,* left ventricle; *IVC,* inferior vena cava; *LPA,* left pulmonary artery; *VSD,* ventricular septal defect.

patient with VSD include increased pulmonary blood flow, CHF, and decreased ventricular function. In patients with supracristal VSD, aortic insufficiency is an additional problem. One should also remember that in smaller VSDs it is the left ventricle that is usually burdened, and in large VSD both ventricles are burdened.

### Preoperative assessment

Preoperative evaluation of a patient with VSD should include a thorough history, including past and present medications and physical examination; laboratory tests including chest x-ray film, EKG, echocardiogram, catheterization data, hemoglobin, glucose, and electrolytes; any history of palliative or corrective surgery (PDA or coarctation of aorta) or noncardiac surgery; and pediatric cardiologist's consult note. In addition, one should evaluate the status of both cardiac and pulmonary reserves.

Depending on the size of the defect, children with an isolated VSD may have various degrees of CHF and decreased lung compliance. Signs and symptoms of CHF may be absent in a patient with a mild defect and in patients who are being treated medically with digitalis and diuretic preparations.

### Premedication

Since left to right shunt increases in children with anxiety and apprehension, these children will benefit from preoperative medication. Premedication usually consists of an IM narcotic and anticholinergic drug combination (morphine 0.1 to 0.15 mg/

kg and atropine 10 μg/kg) in the ward and oral midazolam (0.5 to 0.6 mg/kg) in the holding room.

### Monitoring

Monitoring of children with VSD during surgery includes an ECG, invasive arterial pressure, non-invasive blood pressure, pulse oximeter, capnogram, body temperature (esophageal and nasopharyngeal), central venous pressure, and urinometer. The left upper extremity should not be used for the placement of a blood pressure cuff and arterial cannula in patients who previously underwent coarctation of the aorta. Pulmonary arterial or left atrial pressure monitoring is not necessary in the majority of cases. Arterial blood gases, serum potassium, and hematocrit are monitored frequently throughout the operation.

### Induction

The majority of patients come to the operating room with no intravenous catheter. However, it is not difficult to start an IV line in a well sedated child before the induction of anesthesia. In patients who arrive with a functioning IV line, anesthesia can be induced with either 4 to 5 mg/kg of sodium thiopental or 1 to 2 mg/kg of ketamine IV, depending on the underlying ventricular function. In children who are uncooperative and in small children who come to the operating suite without an IV line in place, anesthesia can be induced with either halothane by mask or ketamine by IM injection. I recommend inspired concentrations of halothane under 2%, as severe myocardial depression and/or complete heart block may result with concentrations in excess of 2%.

A left to right shunt does not alter the speed of inhalational induction.[8,25] On the other hand, a left to right shunt is said to result in a slow intravenous induction.[14] But this difference is of theoretical interest only. Once the IV line is secured, tracheal intubation can be performed with either succinylcholine or a nondepolarizing muscle relaxant. Atropine 5 to 10 μg/kg should be given prior to the administration of succinylcholine (1 to 2 mg/kg IV). An arterial cannula and a central venous catheter are usually inserted after the airway is secured.

### Maintenance

Anesthesia is maintained with either halothane (1% to 1.5%) in patients with normal ventricular function, or with an IV narcotic (fentanyl 50 to 100 μg/kg or sufentanil 15 to 30 μg/kg) in patients with decreased ventricular function. If halothane or one of the inhalation agents is used as a sole anesthetic, one should administer a narcotic drug (fentanyl 15 μg/kg or sufentanil 5 μg/kg) and an amnestic agent like lorazepam (30 μg/kg) at the time of rewarming during the extracorporeal circulation. Otherwise one will have a paralyzed patient without adequate anesthesia on board. Vecuronium or one of the newer nondepolarizing muscle relaxants (doxacurium or pipecuronium) can be used to maintain muscle paralysis throughout the operation.

One should closely watch the administration of intravenous fluids in these patients. Since the left ventricle is already burdened with signs of CHF in the majority of patients, minimal amounts of fluids should be used.

If deep hypothermia and circulatory arrest are planned (usually in children under 10 kg body weight), I administer 10 ml/kg of dextran 40 in 5% dextrose solution before peripheral cooling is initiated (see Chapter 4 for complete details of deep hypothermia).

Heparin is usually given into the right atrium by the surgeon just before the placement of cannulas. Protamine is administered by the anesthesiologist at the conclusion of extracorporeal circulation following the removal of cardiac cannulas. A few patients, especially the ones with pulmonary hypertension, require either isoproterenol (0.01 to 0.05 μg/kg/min) or dobutamine (3 to 6 μg/kg/min) infusion after coming off bypass.

Conditions that promote left to right shunt are listed in the accompanying box. Since patients with VSD will have increased pulmonary blood flow, they may benefit from the addition of slight positive end expiratory pressure (PEEP). Hyperventilation, high inspired oxygen concentrations, and low hematocrit are known to increase left to right shunt and pulmonary blood flow, so one should use low inspired concentrations, normal ventilation, and normal hematocrit to reduce the chances of increased pulmonary blood flow and CHF in patients with VSD. An increase in systemic vascular resistance and/or a decrease in pulmonary vascular resistance will promote a left to right shunt for reasons outlined in Chapter 10. Hypoventilation and hypoxemia should be avoided, as these can acutely

---

**CONDITIONS THAT ARE KNOW TO INCREASE LEFT TO RIGHT SHUNT**

1. Low hematocrit
2. Increased SVR
3. Decreased PVR
4. Hyperoxemia
5. Hyperventilation
6. Negative airway pressure

---

revert a left to right shunt into right to left shunt in a neonate.

## Precautions

In all cases where there is a communication between right and left sides of the heart, it is absolutely necessary that all intravenous lines be free of air bubbles. In addition, use extra caution not to push any air bubbles when injecting drugs through an IV line. Although the use of nitrous oxide is not contraindicated in patients with a VSD, many anesthesiologists avoid the use of it, especially once the chest is opened, for fear of intravascular air bubble expansion. Appropriate antibiotic prophylaxis therapy is also required for patients with VSD (please see Chapter 6).

## Postoperative ventilation

Patients with VSD are usually left intubated and mechanically ventilated postoperatively. Once a patient is awake, stable, and rewarmed to a normal body temperature, the trachea can be extubated safely in the cardiac recovery room.

## REFERENCES


1. Alpert BS, Cook DH, Varghese PJ et al: Spontaneous closure of small ventricular septal defects: 10-year follow-up, *Pediatrics* 63:204, 1979.
2. Anderson RH, Lenox CC, Zuberbuhler JR: Mechanisms of closure of perimembranous ventricular septal defect, *Am J Cardiol* 52:341, 1983.
3. Arciniegas E, Farooki ZQ, Hakimi M et al: Surgical closure of ventricular defect during the first 12 months of life, *J Thorac Cardiovasc Surg* 80:921, 1980.
4. Artman M, Graham TP: Congestive heart failure in infancy: recognition and management, *Am Heart J* 103:1040, 1982.
5. Beekman RH, Rocchini AP, Rosenthal A: Hemodynamic effects of hydralazine in infants with a large ventricular septal defect, *Circulation* 65:523, 1982.
6. Beerman LB, Park SC, Fischer DR et al: Vetricular septal defect associated with aneurysm of the membranous septum, *J Am Coll Cardiol* 5:118, 1985.
7. Berman W, Ybek SM, Dillon T et al: Effects of digoxin in infants with a congested circulatory state due to a ventricular septal defect, *N Engl J Med* 308:363, 1983.
8. Eger EI: Uptake of inhaled anesthetics: the alveolar to inspired anesthetic difference: effect of ventilation/perfusion abnormalities. In Eger EI, editor: *Anesthetic uptake and action,* Baltimore, 1974, Williams & Wilkins.
9. Freedom RM, White RD, Pieroni DR et al: The natural history of the so-called aneurysm of the membranous ventricular septum in childhood, *Circulation* 49:375, 1974.
10. Jarmakani JMM, Graham TP Jr, Canent RV Jr, et al: The effect of corrective surgery on left heart volume and mass in children with ventricular septal defect, *Am J Cardiol* 27:254, 1971.
11. Kirklin JW, Applebaum A, Bargeron LM Jr: Primary repair versus banding for ventricular septal defects in infants. In Langford-Kidd BS, Rowe RD, editors: *The child with congenital heart disease after surgery,* Mount Kisco, NY, 1976, Futura.
12. Lillehei CW et al: The results of direct vision closure of ventricular septal defects in eight patients by means of controlled cross circulation, *Surg Gynecol Obstet* 101:447, 1955.
13. Lister G, Hellenbrand WE, Kleinman CS et al: Physiologic effects of increasing hemoglobin concentration in left-to-right shunting in infants with ventricular septal defects, *N Engl J Med* 306:502, 1982.
14. Lucero V, Lerman J, Burrows F: Onset of neuromuscular blockade with pancuronium in children with congenital heart disease, *Anesth Analg* 66:788, 1987
15. Maron BJ, Redwood DR, Hirshfeld JW Jr et al: Postoperative assessment of patients with ventricular septal defect and pulmonary hypertension, *Circulation* 48:864, 1973.
16. McNamara DG, Latson LA: Long-term follow-up of patients with malformations for which definitive surgical repair has been available for 25 years or more, *Am J Cardiol* 50:560, 1982.
17. McNicholas K, DeLeval M, Stark J et al: Surgical treatment of ventricular septal defect in infancy, *Br Heart J* 41:133, 1979.
18. Moe DG, Guntheroth WG: Spontaneous closure of uncomplicated ventricular septal defect, *Am J Cardiol* 60:674, 1987.
19. Muller WH Jr, Dammann MF Jr: The treatment of certain congenital malformations of the heart by the creation of pulmonic stenosis to reduce pulmonary hypertension and excessive pulmonary blood flow, *Surg Gynecol Obstet* 95:213, 1952.
20. Nadas AS, Ellison RC, Weidman WH: Pulmonary stenosis, aortic stenosis, ventricular septal defect: clinical course and indirect assessment, *Circulation* 56:I-1, 1977.
21. Otterstad JE, Erikssen J, Froysaker T et al: Long-term results after operative treatment of isolated ventricular septal defect in adolescents and adults, *Acta Med Scand* (suppl)708:36, 1986.
22. Ramaciotti C, Keren A, Silverman NH: Importance of (perimembranous) ventricular septal aneurysm in the natural history of isolated perimembranous ventricular septal defect, *Am J Cardiol* 57:268, 1986.
23. Richardson JV, Schieken RM, Lauer RM et al: Repair of large ventricular septal defects in infants and small children, *Ann Surg* 195:318, 1982.
24. Tanner GE, Angers DG, Barash PG et al: Effect of left-to-right, mixed right-to-left, and right-to-left shunts on inhalational anesthetic induction in children: a computer model, *Anesth Analg* 64:101, 1985.
25. Van Hare GF, Soffer LJ, Sivakoff MC et al: Twenty-five-year experience with ventricular septal defect in infants and children, *Am Heart J* 114:606, 1987.
26. Weidman W: Second natural history study of congenital heart defects, *Circulation* 87:1-7, 1993.
27. Yeager SB, Freed MD, Keane JF et al: Primary surgical closure of ventricular septal defect in the first year of life: results in 128 infants, *J Am Coll Cardiol* 3:1269, 1984.

# 17 Endocardial Cushion Defects (Complete Atrioventricular Septal Defect)

*Jay Kamban, Frank Fish, and Walter Merrill*



The complete atrioventricular (AV) septal defect accounts for approximately 2% of all congenital heart defects in children. No sex prevalence for complete AV septal defect has been documented. The complete AV septal defect is the most common congenital cardiac anomaly seen in children with Down's syndrome.[5] Almost 70% of children with complete AV septal defect have Down's syndrome.

## EMBRYOLOGY

Between the fourth and sixth weeks of gestational age, the single atrial chamber divides into two parts. This separation begins with the extension of the septum primum toward the endocardial cushions formed in the AV canal (Fig. 17–1). The opening between the right and left primitive atria is the ostium primum. The endocardial thickening of the free margin of the septum primum fuses with both endocardial cushions of the atrioventricular canal, leading to the closure of the ostium primum. As the first septum continues to proliferate, fenestrations appear and eventually coalesce to form the ostium secundum in the cephalad portion of the septum primum. At about this time a thin septum called the septum secundum appears on the right of the septum primum. During this process the incorporation of the right sinus horn into the right atrium and that of the common pulmonary vein into the left atrium take place. The septum secundum covers the ostium secundum in an incomplete fashion, resulting in the formation of the foramen ovale. The concave free margin of the septum secundum persists as a thin flap, which balloons out into the left atrium forming the valve of the foramen ovale.

After cardiac looping occurs between the fourth and fifth weeks of intrauterine life, the single ventricle divides into two chambers. This is achieved by the union of the membranous portion of the ventricular septum, the bulbus cordis, and the endocardial cushions. The primitive left ventricle is developed from the ventricular portion, and the primitive right ventricle is formed from the proximal portion of the truncus arteriosus (bulbus cordis). At this time the left and the right ventricles are connected by the primary interventricular foramen. Growth and trabeculation of the ventricles account for the formation of the major portion of the muscular septum. The muscular portion of the ventricular septum grows cephalad as each ventricular cavity enlarges to meet with the right and left ridges of the bulbus cordis. The left ridge unites with a ridge of the interventricular septum, and the right ridge fuses with the tricuspid valve and the endocardial cushion, thus separating the pulmonary valve from the tricuspid valve and leaving the aortic valve in continuity with the mitral valve.

The conus swellings appear at about the same time as the truncal swellings and the atrioventricular cushions. The conus and truncal swellings and the AV cushions eventually combine to form the conus septum, separating the conus cordis into the anterolateral and posteromedial portions. The endocardial cushion from the conus septum and the

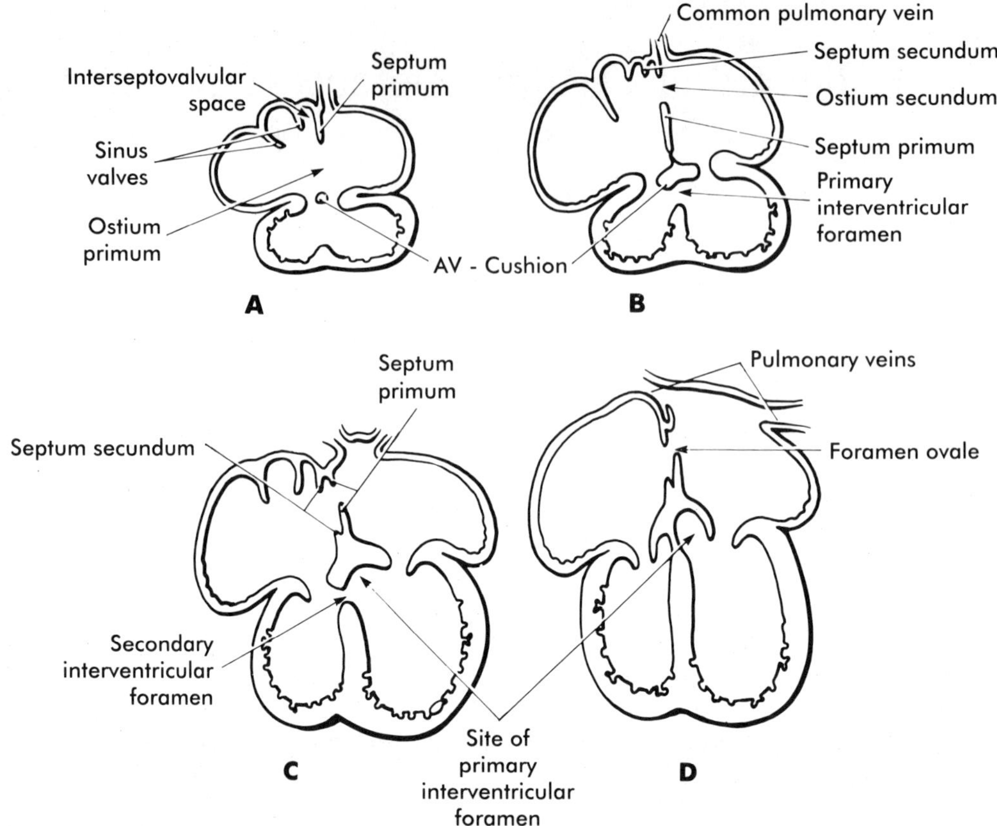


**Figure 17–1** Schematic representation of the atrial septa at successive stages of development. **A,** 30 days; **B,** 33 days; **C,** 37 days; **D,** newborn.

right superior endocardial cushion merge with the superior segment of the muscular septum, thus closing the interventricular foramen. The superior segment of the muscular septum thins to become the membranous segment of the interventricular septum.

In summary, the four essential components responsible for normal development of the heart are the septation of the atria, the septation of the ventricle, the proliferation of the endocardial cushions, and the development of the bulboconus area. Deviations in the development of these components can result in either partial or complete AV septal defect. The inlet defects are usually the result of failure of the proper fusion of the right superior endocardial cushion tissue with the muscular septum.

## PATHOLOGIC ANATOMY

The AV septal defects (endocardial cushion defects) are classified by many authors into various subtypes.[16,18] However, in this chapter these are classified into two main types: (1) complete atrioventricular septal defect, which is the most common congenital cardiac anomaly seen in children with Down's syndrome (Fig. 17–2), and (2) incomplete AV septal defect, or ostium primum defect, which is usually associated with a cleft in the anterior leaflet of the mitral valve. The principal components of the complete AV septal defect include an atrial septal defect; clefts of the anterior leaflet of the mitral valve and the septal leaflet of the tricuspid valve, which together form common anterior and posterior leaflets of the AV valve; and a membranous (inlet) type of VSD. In a normal patient the left ventricular outflow tract (LVOT) is wedged between the two AV valves. In patients with complete AV septal defect the LVOT is not wedged between the two AV valves. Instead it is displaced anteriorly in a narrow and elongated fashion that gives the characteristic gooseneck appearance in cineangiogram studies.[2,3] As a consequence abnormalities may involve virtually all intracardiac structures, and a wide array of complex cardiac lesions may be associated with complete AV septal defect. In such cases the associated lesions pri-

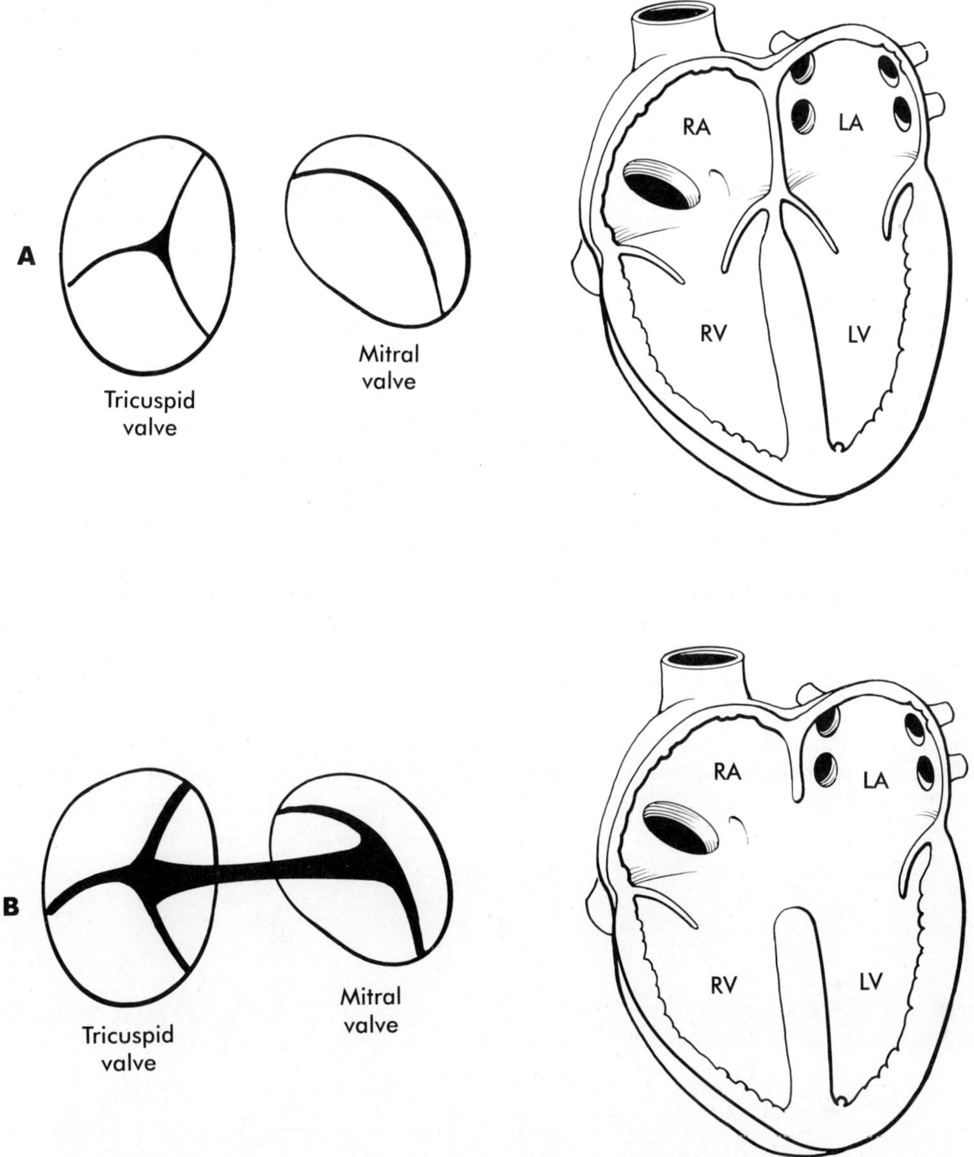


**Figure 17–2** Anatomy of a normal heart **(A)** and a heart with complete atrioventricular canal **(B).** Normal and cleft mitral and tricuspid valves with resulting common atrioventricular valve are also shown. *RA,* right atrium; *LA,* left atrium; *RV,* right ventricle; *LV,* left ventricle.

marily determine the medical and surgical therapy required, while the associated septal defect complicates or limits the options considered.

## PATHOPHYSIOLOGY

In complete AV septal defect, in addition to the abnormal development of both atrioventricular valves (mitral and tricuspid), the superior portion of the interventricular septum and inferior portion of the interatrial septum are defective. The combination of these defects usually results in variable shunting at the atrial or ventricular level, LV to right atrial shunting, interventricular shunts, and AV valve regurgitation. The paths of the blood flow through such a centrally located defect will be dependent on the relative pressures and compliance in all four heart chambers as well as the ratio of the pulmonary to systemic vascular resistance. The shunts are usually left to right (left atrium and/or left ventricle to the right atrium and/or the right ventricle). With the presence of a large ventricular septal defect and pulmonary hypertension from birth, the chance of developing pulmonary vascular obstructive disease is quite high in patients with complete AV septal defect at the age of 1 year and beyond, and patients with Down's syndrome may be at particular risk.[14]

## CLINICAL PRESENTATION

In the neonatal period AV septal defect may be manifest only as a murmur (due to AV valve regurgitation), possibly with mild hypoxemia due to intracardiac admixture. Older children symptomatic from AV septal defects usually have congestive heart failure, failure to thrive, poor feeding, or recurrent respiratory infections. CHF and other symptoms become much more common after 2 months of life as the left to right shunt increases with the gradual fall in pulmonary vascular resistance.

The general physical examination is usually normal in uncomplicated complete AV septal defect patients. The precordium is usually hyperactive. A systolic regurgitant murmur is audible, loudest at the areas of the left lower sternum and the apex of the heart. Additional murmurs due to increased pulmonary flow and a diastolic rumble may also be present. In addition to the signs of congestive heart failure, the pulmonary component of the second heart sound is accentuated, and systolic clicks may be heard. Cyanosis is usually not part of the clinical picture of patients with complete AV septal defect except when there are associated CHDs.

### Laboratory findings

***Chest x-ray films.*** In these patients the heart usually appears distinctly large, with a marked enlargement of the right ventricle, right atrium, and left ventricle (Fig. 17–3). Massive pulmonary artery enlargement with greatly engorged lung fields is also seen.

***Electrocardiogram.*** The characteristic ECG findings include superior QRS axis, right ventricular and left ventricular hypertrophy, RBBB, and variable degrees of AV block.

***Echocardiogram.*** With echocardiography and Doppler with color flow mapping, one can document the relative size and shape of the atrial and ventricular defects and evaluate the AV valve abnormalities. Critical features include the presence of crossing AV valve attachments, relative size of the right and left ventricles, extent of AV valve regurgitation and associated CHDs, particularly pulmonary stenosis or aortic coarctation.

***Catheterization data.*** Cardiac catheterization is usually indicated to evaluate the size of the intracardiac shunt, the status of the pulmonary vascular

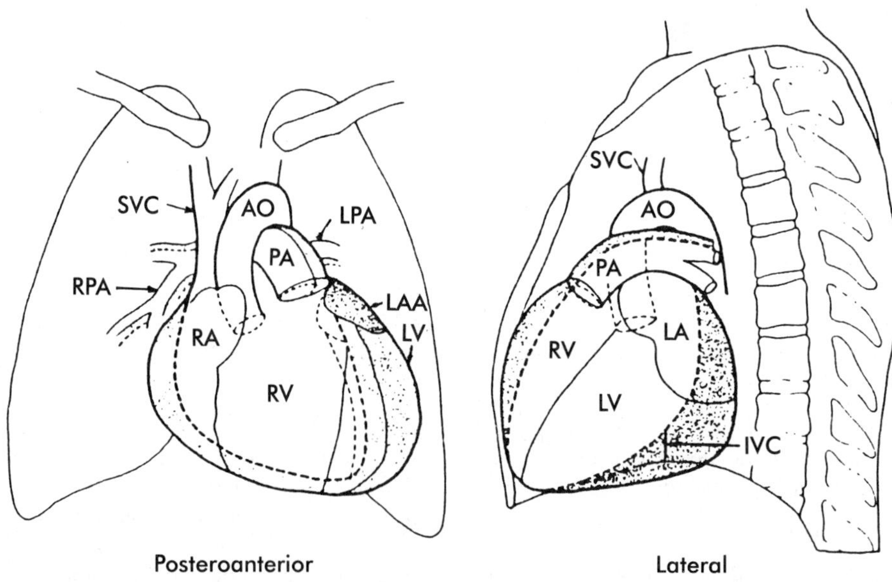


**Figure 17–3** Diagrammatic drawing of chest roentgenograms in the complete form of atrioventricular canal. All four cardiac chambers are enlarged with increased pulmonary vascular markings. *SVC,* Superior vena cava; *AO,* aorta; *LPA,* left pulmonary artery; *RPA,* right pulmonary artery; *RA,* right atrium; *PA,* pulmonary artery; *LAA,* left atrial appendage; *LV,* left ventricle; *RV,* right ventricle; *LA,* left atrium. (From Park MK, editor: *Pediatric cardiology for practitioners,* St Louis, 1988, Mosby.)

status, and the presence of associated abnormalities in the majority of patients with an echo diagnosis of complete AV septal defect.

## MEDICAL MANAGEMENT

Small infants who present with signs and symptoms of CHF are usually managed medically with digitalis, diuretics, and afterload reduction. The usual dose of furosemide is 0.5 to 1 mg/kg IV or 1 to 2 mg/kg body weight orally. Diuretics are almost always used in combination with digitalis. Digoxin is the most commonly used digitalis preparation in neonates and infants with CHF. The usual recommended total oral digitalizing dose is 20 to 50 μg/kg (premature, 20 μg/kg; full term, 30 μg/kg; infants and children; 30 to 50 μg/kg) in three divided doses (½ + ¼ + ¼) at 6- to 8-hour intervals. The maintenance dose of digoxin (usually 25% of the total digitalizing dose) is 5 to 10 μg/kg/day (premature, 5 μg/kg; full term, 8 μg/kg; infants and children, 8 to 10 μg/kg). In infants and young children the total dose is divided into twice daily doses. One should reduce these oral doses to 75% when given IV. For children with CHD who are in mild CHF, the initial digitalizing dose may be deleted and twice daily dose maintenance therapy initiated at the outset. Children who are refractory to medical therapy are referred for early surgical management.

## SURGICAL MANAGEMENT

The first successful surgical repair of an AV septal defect was performed by Lillehei and associates[12] in 1956, and the first successful repair of a partial AV septal defect was performd by Kirklin[9] in the same year. The majority of patients with complete AV septal defect currently undergo primary corrective operation at an earlier age than in the past.[1,4,6,7,13,15,17,19] Only selected patients who have defects not amenable to primary repair undergo palliative surgery (pulmonary artery banding procedure) followed later by corrective surgery (closure of ASD, VSD, and reconstruction of AV valves) when possible (Fig. 17–4). A large left to right shunt with pulmonary hypertension or increasing pulmonary vascular resistance, CHF refractory to medical therapy, recurrent respiratory infections, and failure to thrive are the usual indication for operation. Residual mitral regurgitation, residual ventricular septal defect, supraventricular dysrhythmias, and complete heart block are some of the complications of surgical repair. The perioperative mortality rate for corrective surgery is in the vicinity of 5 to 10%.

## ANESTHESIA MANAGEMENT

An understanding of pathologic anatomy and physiology and of the pharmacology of various drugs that may alter the systemic and pulmonary blood

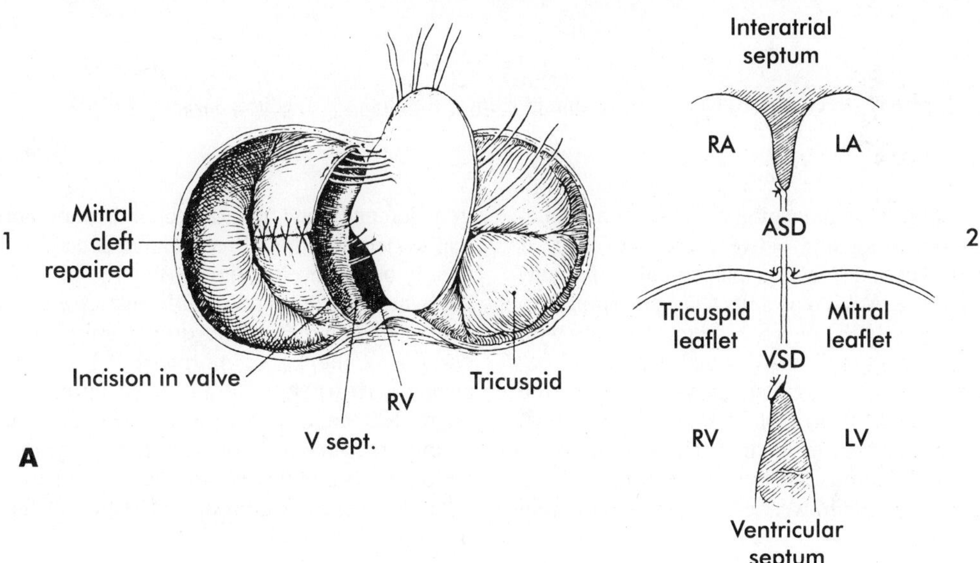


**Figure 17–4 A,** Repair of complete atrioventricular canal. *RV,* Right ventricle; *V sept,* ventricular septum; *RA,* right atrium; *LA,* left atrium; *ASD,* atrial septal defect; *VSD,* ventricular septal defect; *LV,* left ventricle; *RV,* right ventricle; *IVC,* inferior vena cava. (From Effler DB, editor: *Blades' surgical disease of the chest,* ed 4, St Louis, 1978, Mosby.)

*Continued.*

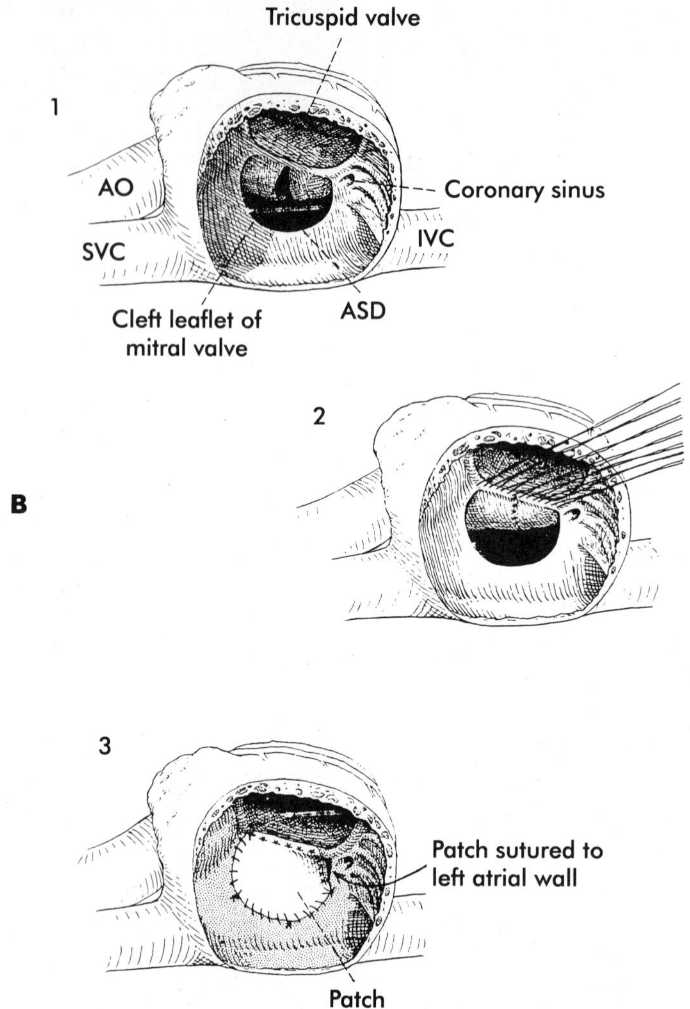


**Figure 17–4, cont'd B,** Closure of septum primum (From Johnson J, editor: *Surgery of the chest,* St Louis, 1970, Mosby.)

flows is essential in managing patients with a functioning communciation between the two sides of the heart. The anesthesia management of patients with complete AV septal defect is very similar to that for a large ASD or VSD. Many patients with uncomplicated complete AV septal defect will basically have a left to right shunt with an increased pulmonary blood flow. Conduction abnormalities, mitral regurgitation, residual VSD, and supraventricular dysrhythmias are frequently seen in these patients once they are weaned from extracorporeal circulation.

## Premedication

Preoperative sedation in these patients depends on the age of the child and severity of the defect. Advantages of preoperative sedation include a decrease or elimination of anxiety, reduction of oxygen demand, and avoidance of further hemodynamic deterioration. Preoperative sedation should ideally be achieved in the holding room, where one can watch for any undesirable side effects. A narcotic and anticholinergic drug combination (meperidine 2 mg/kg or morphine 0.1 mg/kg, and atropine 10 μg/kg) can be given intramuscularly 90 to 120 minutes before the scheduled time of operation. Oral midazolam (0.6 mg/kg) may also be given 30 minutes before the scheduled time of operation depending on the evaluation of the child in the holding room.

## Monitoring

Monitoring during surgery should include an ECG, invasive arterial pressure, noninvasive blood pressure, pulse oximeter, capnogram, body temperature (esophageal and nasopharyngeal), central venous pressure, and urinometer. Arterial blood gases, serum glucose and potassium, and hematocrit are monitored frequently throughout the operation.

### Induction

The majority of patients come to the operating room with no IV catheter. In patients who come to the operating room with a functioning IV line, anesthesia can be induced with 1 to 2 mg/kg of IV ketamine. In children who are uncooperative and in small children who come to the operating suite without an IV line in place, anesthesia can be induced with either halothane by mask or ketamine by IM injection, depending on the underlying ventricular function. We recommend using inspired concentrations of halothane under 2%, as complete heart block may result from concentrations in excess of 2%. A left to right shunt does not alter the speed of inhalational induction.[8,10] On the other hand, a left to right shunt is said to result in a slow intravenous induction.[11] This difference, however, is of theoretical interest only. Once the IV line is secured, trachal intubation can be performed with either succinylcholine or a nondepolarizing muscle relaxant. Atropine 5 to 10 μg/kg should be given prior to the administration of succinylcholine (1-2 mg/kg IV). An arterial cannula and a central venous catheter are usually inserted after the airway is secured.

### Maintenance

Anesthesia is maintained with an inhaled anesthetic agent (halothane or isoflurane) or an IV narcotic (fentanyl 50 to 100 μg/kg or sufentanil 10 to 20 μg/kg). If halothane or one of the inhalational agents is used as the sole anesthetic, one should either continue the inhaled agent or use a narcotic drug (fentanyl 15 μg/kg or sufentanil 2.5 μg/kg) and an amnestic agent (lorazepam 25 μg/kg or midazolam 50 μg/kg) at the time of extracorporeal circulation. Vecuronium or one of the newer nondepolarizing muscle relaxants (doxacurium or pipecuronium) can be used to maintain muscle paralysis throughout the operation.

If deep hypothermia and circulatory arrest are planned (usually in children under 10 kg body weight), we administer 10 ml/kg of dextran 40 in 5% dextrose solution before peripheral cooling is initiated (see Chapter 4 for complete details of deep hypothermia).

Patients with increased pulmonary blood flow may benefit by the addition of slight positive end expiratory pressure. Other conditions that increase left to right shunt should be avoided (box).

Heparin is usually injected into the right atrium by the surgeon just before the placement of cannulas. Protamine is administerd by the anesthesiologist at the conclusion of the extracorporeal circulation following the removal of cardiac cannulas. A few patients, especially the ones with pulmonary hypertension, require either isoproterenol (0.01 to 0.05 μg/kg/min) or dobutamine (3 to 6 μg/kg/min) infusion after coming off bypass. Complete heart block is one of the well recognized complications of repair of the complete AV defect. Unlike patients with secundum type and sinus venosus type ASD defects, patients with ostium primum and complete AV septal defects require more frequent postoperative cardiac pacing.

**CONDITIONS THAT ARE KNOWN TO INCREASE LEFT TO RIGHT SHUNT**

1. Low hematocrit
2. Increased SVR
3. Decreased PVR
4. Hyperoxemia
5. Hyperventilation
6. Negative airway pressure

### Precautions

In all cases where there is a communication between the right and left sides of the heart, it is absolutely necessary that all intravenous lines be free of air bubbles. In addition, one should use extra caution not to introduce any air bubbles when injecting drugs through an IV line.

### Postoperative ventilation

We routinely ventilate the patients with complete AV septal defect mechanically for a few days postoperatively.

### REFERENCES


1. Bender HW, Hammon JW, Hubbard SC et al: Repair of atrioventricular canan malformation in the first year of life, *J Thorac Cardiovasc Surg* 84:515, 1982.
2. Baron MG, Wolf BS, Steinfield L et al: Endocardial cushion defects: specific diagnosis by angiocardiography, *Am J Cardiol* 13:162, 1964.
3. Blieden LC et al: The gooseneck of the endocardial cushion defect: anatomical basis, *Chest* 65:13, 1974.
4. Bove EF, Sondhemier HM, Davey R-EW et al: Results with the two-patch technique for repair of complete atrioventricular septal defect, *Ann Thorac Surg* 38:157, 1984.
5. Bull C, Rigby ML, Shinebourne EA: Should management of complete atrioventricular canal defect be influenced by coexistent Down syndrome? *Lancet* 1:1147, 1985.
6. Castaneda AR, Mayer JE, Jonas RA: Repair of complete atrioventricular canal in infancy, *World J Surg* 9:590, 1985.
7. Clapp SK, Perry BL, Farooki ZQ et al: Surgical and medical results of complete atrioventricular canal: a 10-year review, *Am J Cardiol* 59:454, 1987.
8. Eger EI: Uptake of inhaled anesthetics: the alveolar to inspired anesthetic difference: effect of ventilation/perfu-

sion abnormalities. In Eger EI, editor: *Anesthetic uptake and action,* Baltimore, 1974, Williams & Wilkins.
9. Kirklin JW, Daugherty GW, Burchell HB et al: Repair of the partial form of persistent common atrioventricular canal: so-called ostium primum type of atrial septal defect with intraventricular communication, *Ann Surg* 142:858, 1955.
10. Kirkpatrick SE, Pitlick PT, Naliboff J et al: Frank-Starling relationship as an important determination of fetal cardiac output, *Am J Physiol* 231:495, 1976.
11. Komp DM, Sparrow AW: Polycythemia in cyanotic heart disease: a study of altered coagulation, *J Pediatr* 76:231, 1980.
12. Lillehei CW, Cohen M, Warden HE, et al: The direct-vision intracardiac correction of congenital anomalies by controlled cross circulation: results in 32 patients with ventricular septal defects, tetralogy of Fallot, and atrioventricularis communis defects, *Surgery* 38:11, 1956.
13. Mavroudis C, Weinstein G, Turley K et al: Surigcal management of complete atrioventricular canal, *J Thorac Cardiovasc Surg* 83:670, 1982.
14. Neufeld EA, Sher M, Paul MN et al: Pulmonary vascular disease in complete atrioventricular canal defect, *Am J Cardiol* 39:721, 1977.
15. Pan-Chih, Chen-Chun: Surgical treatment of atrioventricular canal malformations, *Ann Thorac Surg* 43:150, 1987.
16. Piccoli GP, Gerlis LM, Wilkinson JL et al: Morphology and classification of atrioventricular defects, *Br Heart J* 42:621, 1979.
17. Rastelli GC, Ongley PA, Kirklin JW et al: Surgical repair of complete form of persistent common atrioventricular canal, *J Thorac Cardiovasc Surg* 55:299, 1968.
18. Rastelli GC, Kirklin JW, Titus JL: Anatomic observations on the complete form of persistent common atrioventricular canal with special reference to atrioventricular valves, *Mayo Clinic Proc* 41:296, 1966.
19. Williams WH, Guyton RA, Michalik RF et al: Individualized surgical management of complete atrioventricular canal, *J Thorac Cardiovasc Surg* 83:670, 1982.

## Section B RIGHT-TO-LEFT SHUNTS

# 18 Truncus Arteriosus

*Thomas P. Graham Jr., Walter Merrill,* and *Jay Kambam*



Buchanan,[2] in 1864, published the first clinical and pathologic description of truncus arteriosus in a 6½-year-old child. Collett and Edwards[3] described the pathologic features of 80 cases in 1949 and provided the classification system frequently used. Rastelli and associates[11] indicated the feasibility of homograft repair of truncus in the modern era, and McGoon and associates in 1968[10] first reported the successful repair of this condition. Ebert and associates[4] subsequently reported the first series of infants undergoing correction of truncus arteriosus.

## EMBRYOLOGY AND PATHOLOGIC ANATOMY

There continues to be some disagreement regarding the morphogenesis of truncus arteriosus. The most widely accepted theory is failure of fusion of the conotruncal ridges. Recent embryologic studies have indicated that neural crest abnormalities in the developing chick embryo are associated with conotruncal anomalies,[7] and the possibility exists that abnormalities of neural crest cells in humans lead to failure of fusion of the conotruncal ridges with resultant truncus arteriosus.

The pathologic anatomy is one of a large truncal root overriding a large outlet ventricular septal defect with the pulmonary artery arising from the ascending aorta (Fig. 18–1). Pulmonary atresia with large ventricular septal defect and origin of multiple aorticopulmonary collateral arteries arising from the descending aorta is no longer considered a part of the truncus arteriosus complex.

In the so-called truncus type I there is a main pulmonary artery arising from the ascending aorta that branches into the right and left pulmonary arteries. In type II or type III truncus the pulmonary arteries appear to arise separately from the truncal root without a significant length of the main pulmonary artery (Fig. 18–1). The surgical distinction among these groups is minimal.

The truncal valve is usually tricuspid but can be bicuspid or quadracuspid. It is frequently thickened and can be regurgitant or stenotic.

Patients with truncus arteriosus usually have unobstructed pulmonary blood flow and show signs of progressive congestive heart failure beginning in the early postnatal period. When there is associated truncal valve incompetence, the patient can have severe congestive heart failure in the first few days of life. It has been postulated that in this condition the increased myocardial oxygen demand associated with cardiomegaly and tachycardia can be associated with an inadequate myocardial oxygen supply because of the low arterial diastolic pressure. This situation can cause myocardial ischemia, which can worsen the congestive heart failure. Frequently associated cardiovascular anomalies are listed in Table 18–1. Interrupted aortic arch occurs in a significant number of patients and presents a formidable surgical challenge.

In addition to cardiovascular abnormalities, the DiGeorge syndrome with immunologic abnormal-

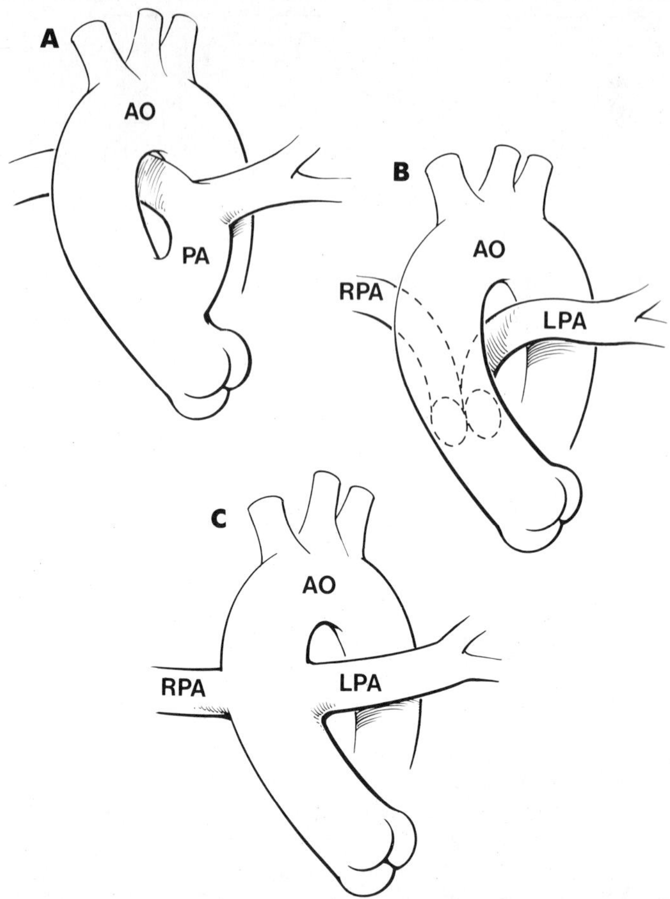


**Figure 18–1** Types of truncus arteriosus. **A,** Type 1, common trunk arising from the heart with a partial septation giving rise to the dominant aorta and main pulmonary artery. **B,** Type 2 has a common trunk and pulmonary arteries arising from the posterior surface of the common trunk. **C,** Type 3 has a common trunk and pulmonary arteries arising from the lateral walls of the common trunk. *AO,* aorta; *PA,* pulmonary artery; *LPA,* left pulmonary artery; *RPA,* right pulmonary artery.

**Table 18–1** Cardiovascular anomalies associated with truncus arteriosus

| | Prevalence (%) |
|---|---|
| Right aortic arch | 25-30 |
| Truncal insufficiency | 15-20 |
| Patent ductus arteriosus | 15-20 |
| Interrupted aortic arch | 10-20 |
| Secundum ASD | 10-20 |
| Pulmonary artery stenosis | 8-12 |
| Truncal stenosis | 5-12 |
| Unilateral absence of pulmonary artery | 5-10 |
| Left SVC to coronary sinus | 5-10 |

ities plus hypocalcemia should be considered in any patient with truncus arteriosus.

## CLINICAL PRESENTATION

The presentation usually involves an infant with early congestive heart failure associated with minimal or no cyanosis.[6] The physical signs include a very active precordium with increased right and left ventricular impulses. Usually there is an ejection click and a systolic murmur of increased outflow across the truncal valve. The diastolic murmur of truncal valve insufficiency can be present, and there is usually a diastolic apical rumble associated with increased pulmonary blood flow. The peripheral pulses are bounding and the aortic pulse pressure is wide.

The chest x-ray film shows an enlarged heart with a concave main pulmonary artery segment.

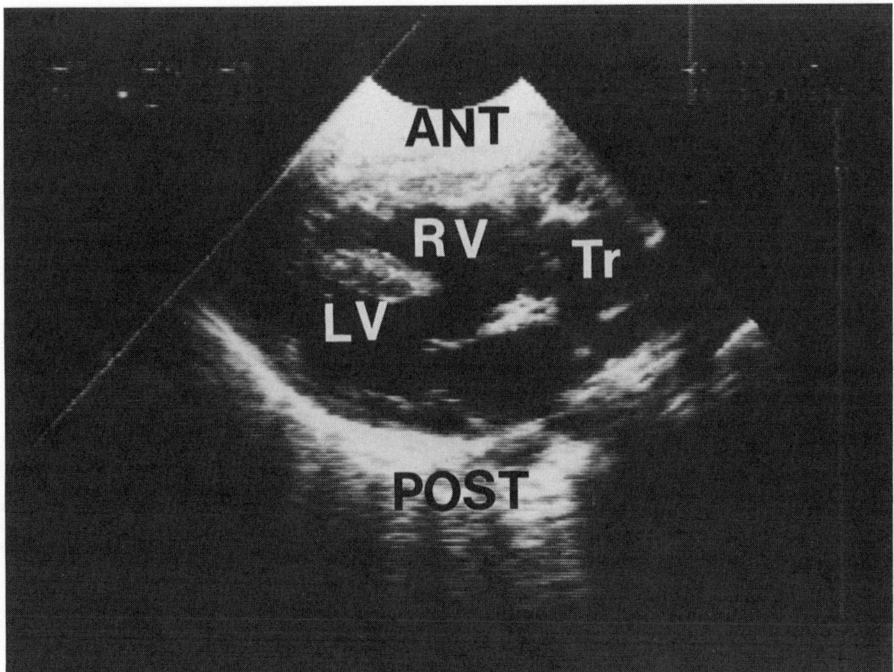


**Figure 18–2** Echocardiogram in a long axis view showing large ventricular septal defect with overriding of the septum by truncus arteriosus. *RV,* right ventricle, *LV,* left ventricle; *Tr,* truncus; *ANT,* anterior, *POST,* posterior. (From Graham TP, Gutgesell HP: Conotruncal abnormalities: In Long WA, editor: *Fetal and neonatal cardiology,* Philadelphia, 1990, Saunders.)

There is a right aortic arch in 25% to 30% of the patients, and the right pulmonary artery segment is somewhat higher in the chest than normal. Pulmonary vascularity is increased.

The ECG usually shows right atrial or biatrial enlargement, right axis deviation, and biventricular hypertrophy. There can be negative T waves in leads V5 and V6 consistent with a left ventricular strain pattern.

The echocardiogram is usually diagnostic, with aortic valve override and a large ventricular septal defect present. The pulmonary arteries can be seen to arise from the aorta (Fig. 18–2). This distinction is helped by color flow Doppler mapping.

Catheterization and angiocardiography are usually carried out. Typical features for oxygen saturation and pressure determinations are shown in Fig. 18–3. An aortic root angiogram is useful to determine the size and length of the main pulmonary artery and to determine if there is any associated pulmonary artery stenosis (Fig. 18–4). In addition aortic insufficiency, if present, is assessed as to severity, and any aortic arch abnormality is characterized. Interrupted aorta arch, which occurs in 10% to 20% of patients, greatly complicates the management.

## MEDICAL MANAGEMENT

Patients are treated initially with digoxin and diuretics. Prostaglandin $E_1$ is mandatory in cases with an associated interrupted arch. Medical management is rarely successful in providing anything but temporary alleviation of symptoms. Once the diagnosis is made, a plan should be made for early surgical repair. Patients with truncal stenosis or severe truncal insufficiency represent a most difficult surgical problem. Patients with truncus plus interrupted aortic arch have an extremely high morbidity and mortality. Only recently have reparative operations for these patients been reported to have any degree of success.

All patients with truncus arteriosus should be considered to have DiGeorge syndrome until proven otherwise. Because of the defective immune system only irradiated blood products should be used for transfusions and surgery to prevent graft versus host disease.

## SURGICAL MANAGEMENT

The overall experience with pulmonary artery banding for truncus arteriosus has been unsatisfactory. Operative mortality is high, and technical problems are frequently encountered in the placement of the band.[8,9,12] Improper band placement

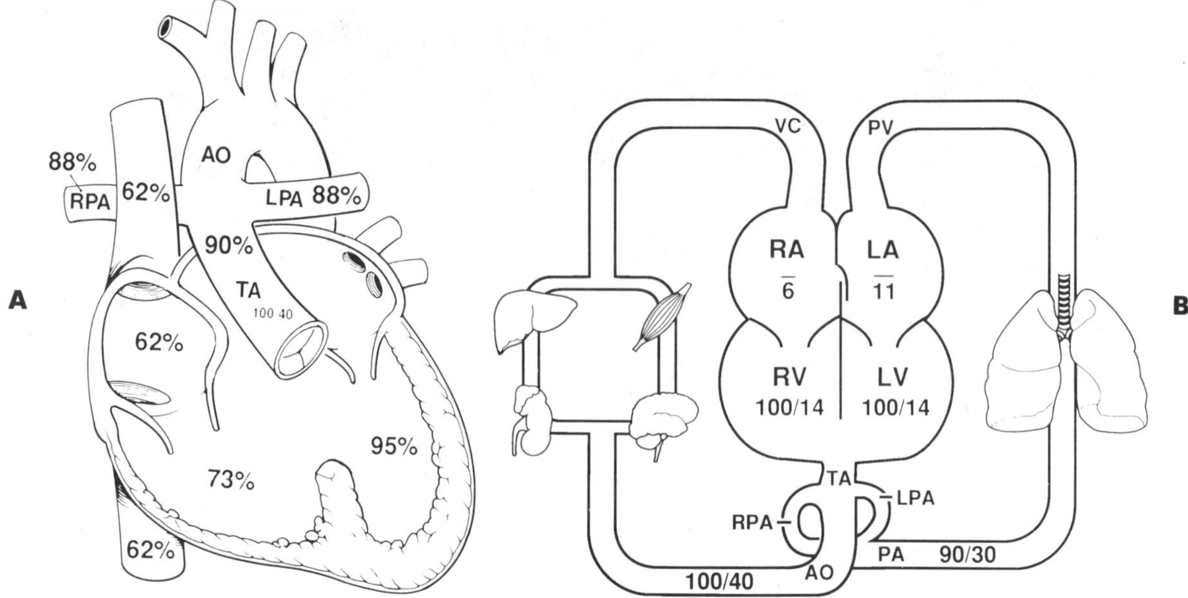


**Figure 18–3** Typical catheterization data from a young infant with truncus arteriosus. *AO*, aorta; *LPA*, left pulmonary artery; *RPA*, right pulmonary artery; *TA*, truncus arteriosus.

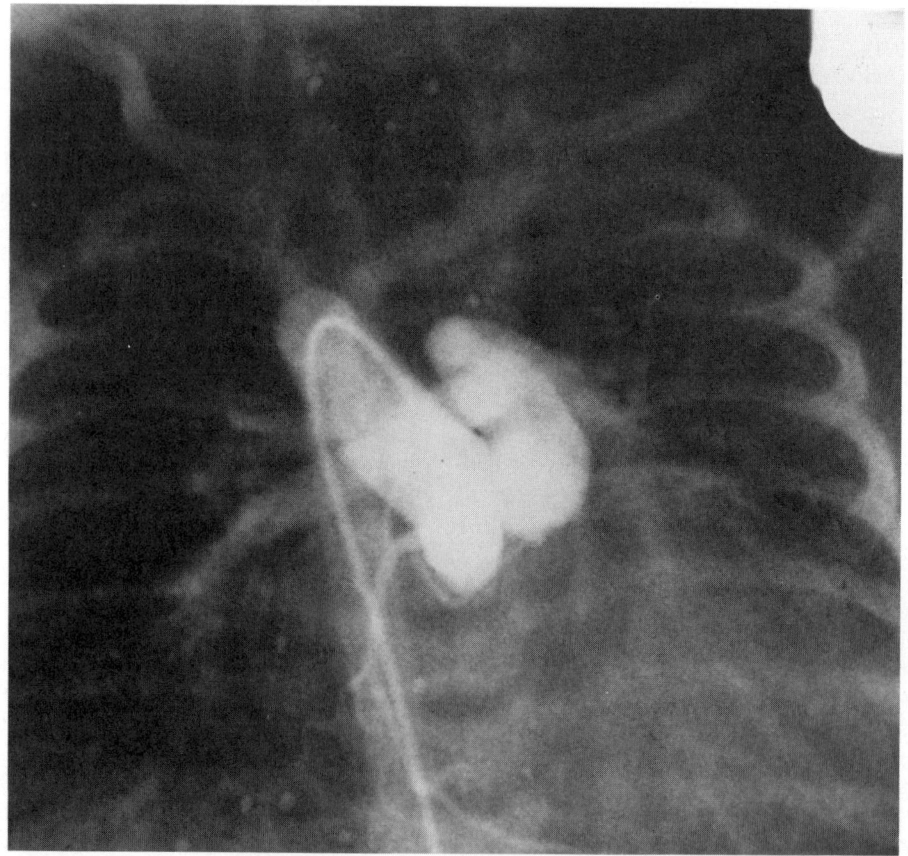

**Figure 18–4** Retrograde truncal root angiography showing truncus arteriosus type I, a right aortic arch, and no truncal valve insufficiency. (From Graham TP, Gutgesell HP: Conotruncal abnormalities. In Long WA, editor: *Fetal and neonatal cardiology*, Philadelphia, 1990, Saunders.)

may lead to excessive constriction of one branch pulmonary artery, resulting in poor growth, or inadequate constriction of another pulmonary artery, resulting in the development of pulmonary vascular obstructive disease in the ipsilateral lung. Distortion of one or both pulmonary arteries by banding may compromise subsequent operative options. In most centers pulmonary artery banding has been abandoned in favor of primary total correction.

Repair of truncus arteriosus involves the following primary steps (Fig. 18–5): detachment of the main pulmonary artery or the individual pulmonary arteries from the truncus, repair of the aorta with direct suture or a patch, closure of the ventricular septal defect, and connection of the right ventricle to the pulmonary artery or arteries with an extracardiac conduit.[4] Usually the extracardiac conduit of choice is an aortic homograft, but a Dacron tube graft with a porcine valve or a valveless prosthetic conduit can be used.

Mild to moderate truncal valve regurgitation is fairly common. Usually this is best handled by conservation of the truncal valve. Hemodynamically important truncal valve insufficiency or stenosis is an indication for valve replacement. This can be done with a mechanical prosthesis,[1] or alternatively two homografts may be inserted, one to connect the right ventricle to the pulmonary arteries and one to replace the truncal valve by connecting the left ventricle to the aorta.[5]

Operative mortality for repair of this lesion has ranged from 10% to 30%. Two of the major determinants of outcome are pulmonary vascular obstructive disease and poor preoperative condition.[13] If the pulmonary vascular resistance exceeds 10 units-m$^2$ the operative mortality is quite high.

Usually repair in an infant requires insertion of a small extracardiac conduit. Eventually this conduit will have to be replaced because of growth of the child or progressive conduit stenosis. In most instances conduit replacement is relatively safe, and the mortality rate is approximately 5%.

## ANESTHESIA MANAGEMENT

An understanding of pathologic anatomy and physiology and of the pharmacology of various drugs that may alter the systemic and pulmonary blood flows is essential in managing patients with a functioning communication between the two sides of the heart. Special problems one may encounter in a patient with truncus arteriosus include increased pulmonary blood flow (type I) with congestive heart failure, normal pulmonary flow (types II and III), and decreased ventricular function. As with other cyanotic cardiac lesions, the degree of systemic oxygen saturation is directly related to the patient's pulmonary blood flow. Thus, with a decreased pulmonary flow cyanosis is present, and with increased pulmonary flow the patient develops congestive heart failure. Myocardial ischemia secondary to cardiomegaly and low diastolic and high pulse pressures are common problems in these children. Hypocalcemia is frequently found in these children, especially when truncus arteriosus is associated with DiGeorge syndrome. As mentioned earlier, children with associated DiGeorge syndrome, because of the defective immune system, should receive only irradiated blood. Systemic hy-

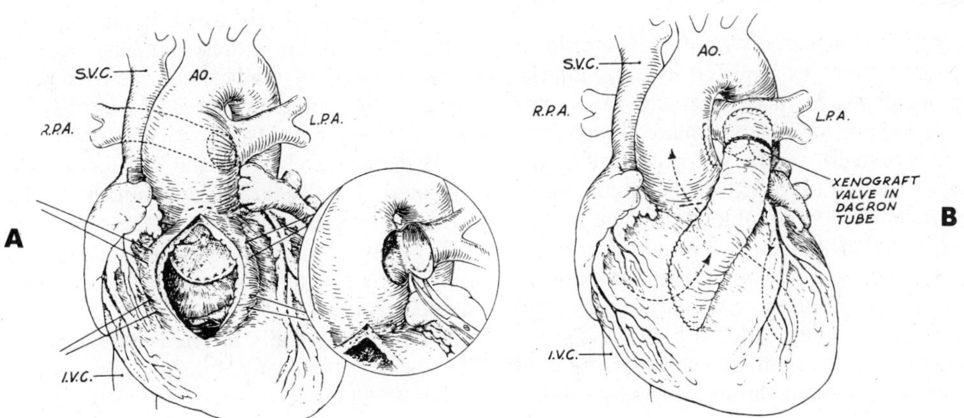


**Figure 18–5** Repair of truncus arteriosus. **A,** Ventricular septal defect has been closed with a patch, and the left ventricle is connected to the aorta. The only outlet for the right ventricle is the ventriculotomy. The inset shows the pulmonary artery has been disconnected from the truncus. **B,** completed repair has a valve in a Dacron graft connecting the ventriculotomy site and the pulmonary artery. (From Effler DB, editor: *Blades' Surgical Disease of the Chest,* ed 4, St Louis, 1978, Mosby.)

poperfusion and metabolic acidosis are also seen in children with associated interrupted aortic arch. Any prostaglandin infusion necessitates utmost attention. Accidental stoppage could lead to rapid deterioration of the child's condition.

### Preoperative assessment

Preoperative evaluation of a patient with truncus arteriosus should include a thorough history, including past and present medications and physical examination; laboratory tests including chest x-ray film, ECG, echocardiogram, catheterization data, hemoglobin, glucose and electrolyte levels; any history of palliative or corrective surgery (e.g., pulmonary artery banding or repair of coarctation of the aorta), or noncardiac surgery; and a pediatric cardiologist's consult note. Children with truncus arteriosus usually present with various degrees of congestive heart failure and decreased lung compliance.

### Premedication

Preoperative medication is given according to the age and severity of the cardiac lesion. In general preoperative sedation can be omitted in children under 6 months of age. However, since each child is different, one should make this decision during the preoperative visit. Because anxiety and apprehension can worsen congestive heart failure, some children will benefit from preoperative medication. Premedication usually consists of an intramuscular narcotic and an anticholinergic drug (morphine 0.1 to 0.15 mg/kg and atropine 10 μg/kg) in the ward and oral midazolam (0.5 to 0.6 mg/kg) in the holding room.

### Monitoring

Monitoring of the children with truncus arteriosus during surgery involves an ECG, invasive arterial pressure, noninvasive blood pressure, pulse oximeter, capnogram, body temperature (esophageal and nasopharyngeal), central venous pressure, and urinometer. The left upper extremity should not be used for the placement of a blood pressure cuff or arterial cannula in patients who have previously undergone repair of coarctation or interruption of the aorta. Left atrial pressure monitoring is useful in the majority of cases. Arterial blood gases, serum calcium and potassium, and hematocrit should be frequently monitored throughout the perioperative period.

### Induction

The majority of patients with truncus arteriosus come to the operating room with an intravenous catheter already in place. In patients who arrive with a functioning intravenous line, anesthesia can be induced with intravenous narcotic and/or 1 to 2 mg/kg of ketamine. In children who come to the operating suite without an IV line in place anesthesia can be induced with either halothane by mask or ketamine by intramuscular injection, depending on the underlying ventricular function. We recommend inspired concentrations of halothane under 2%, as severe myocardial depression and/or complete heart block may result with concentrations in excess of 2%.

Many pediatric cardiac anesthesiologists believe a right to left shunt slightly delays the induction time with commonly used inhaled anesthetics and is of little practical concern in the clinical setting. Theoretically a right to left shunt should slightly accelerate the onset of intravenous anesthetics. Again, there are really no clinical data to support or contradict this theory. Once the IV line is secured, tracheal intubation can be performed with either succinylcholine or a nondepolarizing muscle relaxant. We recommend avoiding succinylcholine in children with ductus dependent pulmonary to aortic shunt (see Chapter 14). Atropine 5 to 10 μg/kg should be given prior to the administration of succinylcholine (1 to 2 mg/kg IV). An arterial cannula and a central venous catheter are usually inserted after the airway is secured.

### Maintenance

Anesthesia is usually maintained with an IV narcotic (fentanyl 50 to 100 μg/kg or sufentanil 15 to 30 μg/kg) in these patients. Vecuronium or one of the newer nondepolarizing muscle relaxants (doxacurium or pipecuronium) can be used to maintain muscle paralysis throughout the operation.

One should closely watch the administration of intravenous fluids in these patients, and only minimal amounts of fluids should be used. Only irradiated blood products should be used for transfusions for the reasons already discussed.

If deep hypothermia and circulatory arrest are planned (usually in children under 10 kg body weight), we administer 10 ml/kg of dextran 40 in 5% dextrose solution before peripheral cooling is initiated (see Chapter 4 for complete details of deep hypothermia).

Heparin is usually injected into the right atrium by the surgeon just before the placement of cannulas. Protamine is administered by the anesthesiologist at the conclusion of extracorporeal circulation following the removal of cardiac cannulas. The majority of patients require either dopamine (3 to 6 μg/kg/min) or dobutamine (3 to 6 μg/kg/min) infusion during the perioperative period.

Since the majority of patients with truncus ar-

**CONDITIONS THAT ARE KNOWN TO INCREASE PULMONARY BLOOD FLOW**

1. Low hematocrit
2. Increased SVR
3. Decreased PVR
4. Hyperoxemia
5. Hyperventilation
6. Negative airway pressure

teriosus (type I) will have increased pulmonary blood flow, they may benefit from the addition of slight positive end expiratory pressure. Hyperventilation and low hematocrit are known to increase left to right shunt and pulmonary blood flow, so one should maintain normal ventilation and normal hematocrit to reduce the chances of increased pulmonary blood flow and congestive heart failure in patients with truncus arteriosus. An increase in systemic vascular resistance and/or a decrease in pulmonary vascular resistance will promote an increase in pulmonary blood flow (box above).

## Precautions

In all cases of communication between right and left sides of the heart it is absolutely necessary that all IV lines be free of air bubbles. In addition one should use extra caution not to push any air bubbles when injecting drugs through an IV line. Although the use of nitrous oxide is not contraindicated in patients with truncus arteriosus, many anesthesiologists avoid the use of it, especially once the chest is opened, for fear of intravascular air bubble expansion. Appropriate antibiotic prophylaxis is also required for patients with truncus arteriosus (see Chapter 9).

## Postoperative ventilation

Patients with truncus arteriosus are usually left intubated and mechanically ventilated postoperatively. Once the patient is awake, stable, and rewarmed to a normal body temperature, the trachea can be extubated in the cardiac recovery room.

## REFERENCES


1. Bove EL, Beekman RH, Snider AR et al: Repair of truncus arteriosus in the neonate and young infant, *Ann Thorac Surg* 47:499, 1989.
2. Buchanan A: Malformation of the heart: undivided truncus arteriosus: heart otherwise double, *Trans Path Soc Lond* 15:89, 1864.
3. Collett RW, Edwards JE: Persistent truncus arteriosus: a classification according to anatomic types, *Surg Clin North Am* 29:1245, 1949.
4. Ebert PA, Robinson SJ, Stanger P et al: Pulmonary artery conduit in infants younger than six months of age, *J Thorac Cardiovasc Surg* 72:351, 1976.
5. Elkins RC, Steinberg JB, Razook JD et al: Correction of truncus arteriosus with truncal valvar stenosis or insufficiency using two homografts, *Ann Thorac Surg* 50:728, 1990.
6. Graham TP Jr, Gutgesell HP: Conotruncal abnormalities. In WA Long, editor: *Fetal and neonatal cardiology,* Philadelphia 1990, Saunders.
7. Kirby ML: Cardiac morphogenesis: recent research advances, *Pediat Res* 21:219, 1987.
8. Mahle S, Nicoloff DM, Knight L et al: Pulmonary artery banding: long-term results in 63 patients, *Ann Thorac Surg* 27:216, 1979.
9. McFaul RC, Mair DD, Feldt RH et al: Truncus arteriosus and previous pulmonary arterial banding: clinical and hemodynamic assessment, *Am J Cardiol* 38:626, 1976.
10. McGoon DC, Rastelli GC, Ongley PA: An operation for the correction of truncus arteriosus, *JAMA* 205:69-73, 1968.
11. Rastelli GC, Titus JL, McGoon DC: Homograft of ascending aorta and aortic valve as a right ventricular outflow: an experimental approach to the repair of truncus arteriosus, *Arch Surg* 9S:698, 1967.
12. Singh AK, de Leval MR, Pincott JR et al: Pulmonary artery banding for truncus arteriosus in the first year of life, *Circ* 54(suppl 3):17, 1976.
13. Stark J, Gandhi D, de Leval M et al: Surgical treatment of persistent truncus arteriosus in the first year of life, *Br Heart J* 40:1280, 1978.

# 19 Tetralogy of Fallot

***Thomas P. Graham, Jr., Walter Merrill** and **Margaret Wood***



Tetralogy of Fallot is the cardiac condition in which there is a large subaortic outlet ventricular septal defect associated with right ventricular outflow tract obstruction. Additional features that make up the tetralogy include aortic override of the ventricular septum and right ventricular hypertrophy. The first anatomic description of tetralogy of Fallot is attributed to Nicholas Stenson in 1671.[28] A series of articles by Fallot[6] in 1888 describe the features of the lesion by distinguishing its characteristics from other causes of cyanosis, but the diagnosis of tetralogy during life was not made with any consistency until the 1930s and 1940s. In 1945 Blalock and Taussig[1] reported the first successful operation in a cyanotic child with heart disease in their classic paper describing the procedure in which the subclavian artery was anastomosed to the pulmonary artery to relieve hypoxemia. Open heart procedures for repair of tetralogy of Fallot were first applied by Lillehei and colleagues[23] in 1955. Although the surgical procedures were initially performed in older children, they were gradually adapted to younger infants. Tetralogy of Fallot is estimated to occur approximately twice per 10,000 live births and is one of the three most common cardiac lesions necessitating cardiac catheterization or surgery during the first year of life.

## EMBRYOLOGY AND PATHOLOGIC ANATOMY

The basic embryologic abnormality in tetralogy of Fallot is anterior displacement of the conal septum, which results in a large ventricular septal defect, right ventricular outflow tract obstruction, and aortic override of the ventricular septum. Since normally the conal septum contributes to the formation of the anterior leaflet of the tricuspid valve, minor abnormalities of this leaflet are almost always present in tetralogy of Fallot, and the medial or conus papillary muscle is usually small or absent. Extreme degrees of displacement of the conal septum may lead to atresia of the pulmonary valve.

In all patients with tetralogy of Fallot the ventricular septal defect is large and unrestrictive and the pulmonary stenosis sufficiently severe to result in normal or decreased pulmonary artery pressure. The ventricular septal defect is a perimembranous, outlet malalignment deficit, and infundibular pulmonary stenosis is frequently associated with a bicuspid pulmonary valve that can be stenotic (Fig. 19–1). In addition, varying degrees of annular hypoplasia as well as main pulmonary artery hypoplasia frequently are present. Additional important features that can occur with tetralogy of Fallot include diffuse hypoplasia of the pulmonary artery and stenosis of the right or left pulmonary arteries. Rarely, one pulmonary artery may lack a connection with the main pulmonary artery; this phenomenon more often involves the left pulmonary artery, which is supplied by a patent ductus arteriosus. Important associated abnormalities and their relative frequencies are listed in Table 19–1.

The basic pathophysiology in tetralogy of Fallot is related to the degree of right ventricular outflow tract obstruction. When this obstruction is only moderately severe, the predominant shunt will be left to right and the patient will not be cyanotic at rest. With increasing severity of stenosis, right to left shunting becomes significant and cyanosis more apparent. Acute increases in right to left shunting can be associated with a decrease in systemic vascular resistance or an increase in right

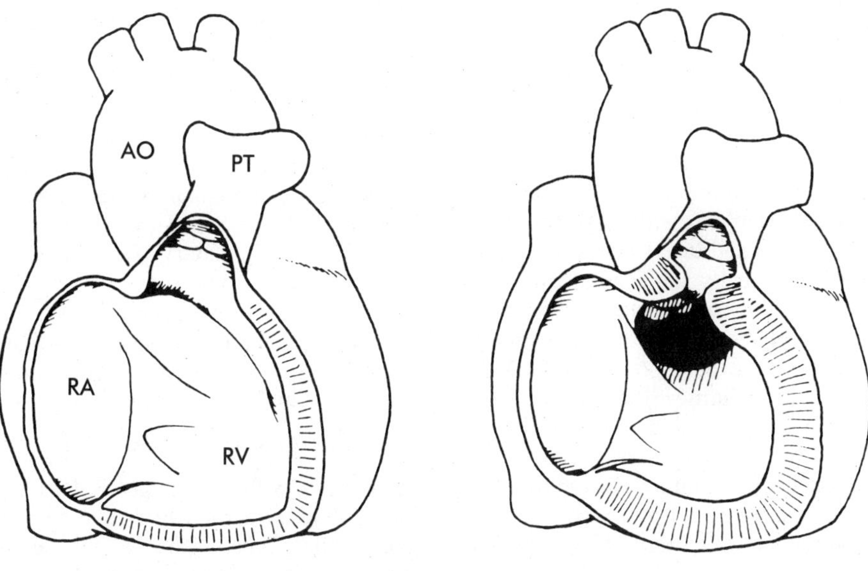


**Figure 19–1** Tetralogy of Fallot, right ventricular view. Note the high ventricular septal defect, infundibular stenosis, overriding of the aorta, and right ventricular hypertrophy. *AO*, aorta; *RA*, right atrium; *RV*, right ventricle; *PT*, pulmonary trunk. (From Gravanis MB, editor: *Cardiovascular pathophysiology*, New York, 1987, McGraw-Hill.)

**Table 19–1** Cardiovascular anomalies associated with tetralogy of Fallot

| Anomalies | Prevalence (percent) |
|---|---|
| Right aortic arch | 20-25 |
| Left anterior descending coronary artery assessing from right coronary or single coronary artery with major branch crossing right ventricular outflow tract | 3-8 |
| Second muscular ventral septal defect | 5-8 |
| Pulmonary artery stenosis | 15-30 |
| Absent connection of main to left or right pulmonary artery | 1-3 (left more common than right) |
| Secundum atrial septal defect | 5-15 |
| Patent foramen ovale | 50-60 |
| Left superior vena cava to coronary sinus | 10-15 |
| Supravalvular mitral stenosis | <1 |
| Patent ductus arteriosus | 5-10 |

ventricular outflow obstruction. These conditions can occur during increases in heart rate and/or increase in myocardial contractility associated with cardiac sympathetic stimulation at times of excitement or stress.

## CLINICAL PRESENTATION

Patients with severe tetralogy of Fallot as characterized by severe right ventricular outflow tract obstruction have cyanosis as young infants. A more typical presentation is a loud systolic murmur that can be mistaken for a small ventricular septal defect. These patients frequently are acyanotic or show only mild cyanosis at rest in early infancy. Hypercyanotic spells can occur but commonly do not begin until after 6 months of age. These spells are most common in patients who are acyanotic or only mildly cyanotic at rest. Spells occur most commonly in the morning and begin with irritability and crying. Progression to increasing cyanosis is usual and if untreated can result in seizures and a semicomatose condition.

### Physical signs

Patients with tetralogy of Fallot exhibit right ventricular hypertrophy and demonstrate a right ventricular parasternal lift on palpation. There is usually a prominent systolic murmur along the mid to upper left sternal border that can vary from pansystolic in patients who are pink to a softer short systolic murmurs in patients with more severe outflow tract obstruction and increased cyanosis. The second sound is classically single and helps to differentiate this condition from simple ventricular septal defect or isolated pulmonary stenosis. It is extremely rare to have an ejection click. When present, it is usually an aortic click in patients with a large right to left shunt and increased aortic outflow. Patients with pulmonary atresia and ventricular septal defect have no outflow tract murmur but have continuous murmurs typical of a patent ductus arteriosus at the upper left sternal border or murmurs due to aorticopulmonary collateral circulation over the anterior or posterior chest bilaterally. Older patients with long-standing tetralogy have aortic root dilatation and may exhibit a diastolic decrescendo murmur of aortic regurgitation. An uncommon variant of tetralogy of Fallot is the so-called absent pulmonary valve syndrome. This condition is characterized by a small pulmonary annulus and rudimentary pulmonary valve leaflets. Patients have a typical to and fro murmur of pulmonary stenosis and insufficiency. The pulmonary arteries frequently are markedly dilated and may cause severe respiratory distress due to the tracheobronchial compression.

## ANCILLARY STUDIES

In patients with tetralogy of Fallot the typical electrocardiogram exhibits right axis deviation and right ventricular hypertrophy. In the newborn after 3

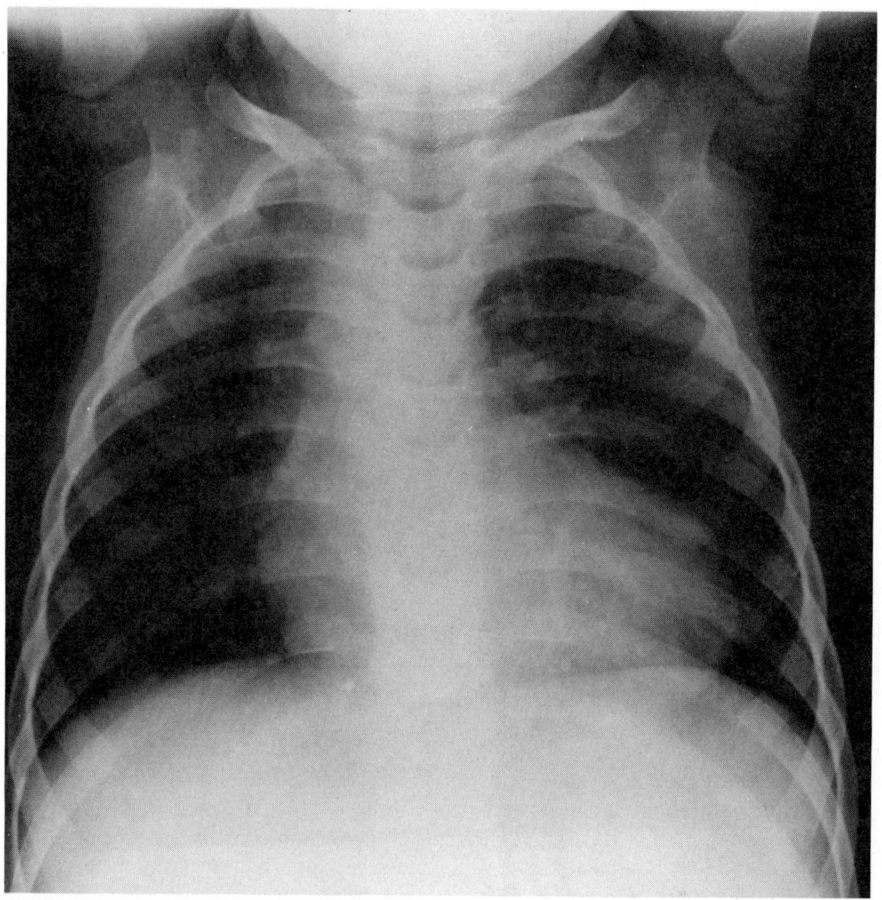

**Figure 19–2** Frontal chest film in an infant with tetralogy of Fallot and pulmonary atresia showing a right aortic arch, large aorta, concave main pulmonary artery segment, decreased pulmonary vascularity, and tilted up cardiac apex. (From Graham TP Jr, Gutgesell HP: Conotruncal abnormalities in fetal and neonatal cardiology. In Long WA, editor: *Fetal and neonatal cardiology,* Philadelpha, 1990, Saunders.)

days of age, the only feature for right ventricular hypertrophy can be an upright T-wave in leads $V_1$ and $V_4R$. In patients with the so-called pink tetralogy with prominent left to right shunting, biventricular hypertrophy can be present. If a superior axis is present in the frontal plant, complete atrioventricular septal defect with right ventricular outflow tract obstruction should be considered.

Although the chest x-ray film may be normal, most patients will show subtle or more significant features of tetralogy. These include a concave segment in the main pulmonary artery area with a tilted up cardiac apex and normal to decreased pulmonary vascularity. In addition a right aortic arch can be present. The features are shown in Fig. 19–2.

Echocardiography is usually diagnostic. On the parasternal long axis view a large perimembranous outlet ventricular septal defect is present with aortic override. In addition, on short axis and subcostal views a narrowed right ventricular outflow tract area, frequently a bicuspid pulmonary valve, and a small pulmonary annulus can be shown. The four-chamber view is also useful to delineate the ventricular septal defect, aortic override, atrioventricular valve anatomy, and ventricular sizes (Fig. 19–3). It is important to use the echocardiogram to attempt to determine whether there is continuity between the main pulmonary artery and right and left pulmonary arteries. Doppler echocardiography is used to estimate the gradient between right ventricle and pulmonary artery and also to attempt to determine if there is a patent ductus arteriosus or other associated features such as a left superior cava. In some patients the origin of the left anterior descending coronary artery from the right coronary artery can be demonstrated.

Catheterization and angiography can be carried out on most patients prior to surgical intervention. Typical pressures and oxygen saturations for a patient with tetralogy of Fallot are shown in Fig. 19–4.

Angiocardiography is an important part of the catheterization study, with right ventricular imaging in a shallow left anterior oblique and 30-40° cranial orientation demonstrating the characteristic outflow tract obstruction as well as determining the degree of narrowing of the pulmonary annulus, main pulmonary artery, and any obstructions in the right or left pulmonary artery (Fig. 19–5). In addition, left ventricular angiography is used to determine whether there is a separate muscular ventricular septal defect from the usual per-

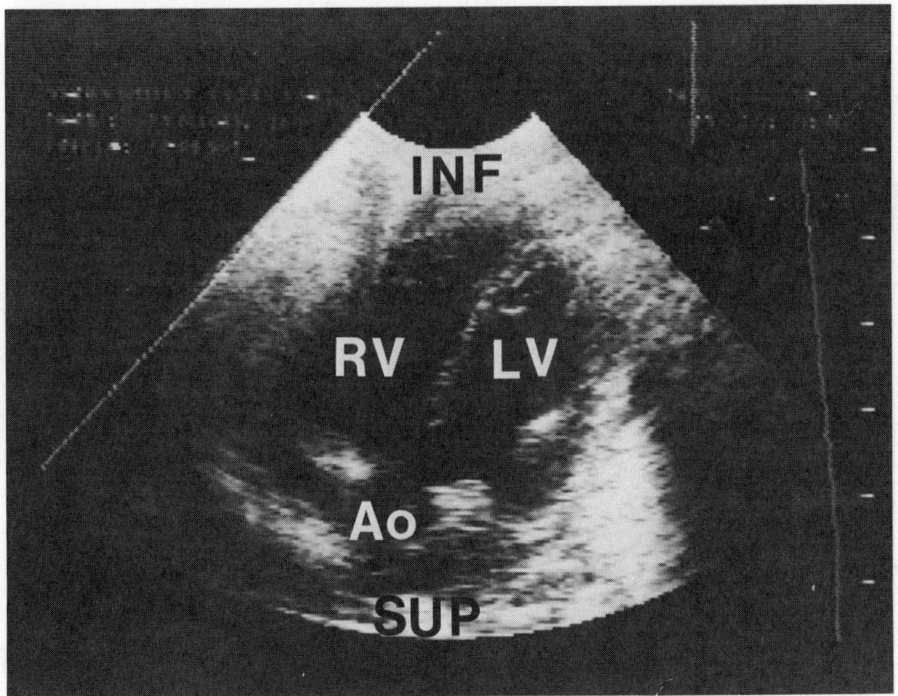


**Figure 19–3** Echocardiogram in a four-chamber view demonstrating relatively equal ventricular sizes, large outlet, malalignment ventricular septal defect and aortic override. *RV*, right ventricle; *LV*, left ventricle; *Ao*, aorta; *INF*, inferior; *SUP*, superior. (From Graham TP Jr, Gutgesell HP: Conotruncal abnormalities in fetal and neonatal cardiology. In Long WA, editor: *Fetal and neonatal cardiology*, Philadelphia, 1990, Saunders.)

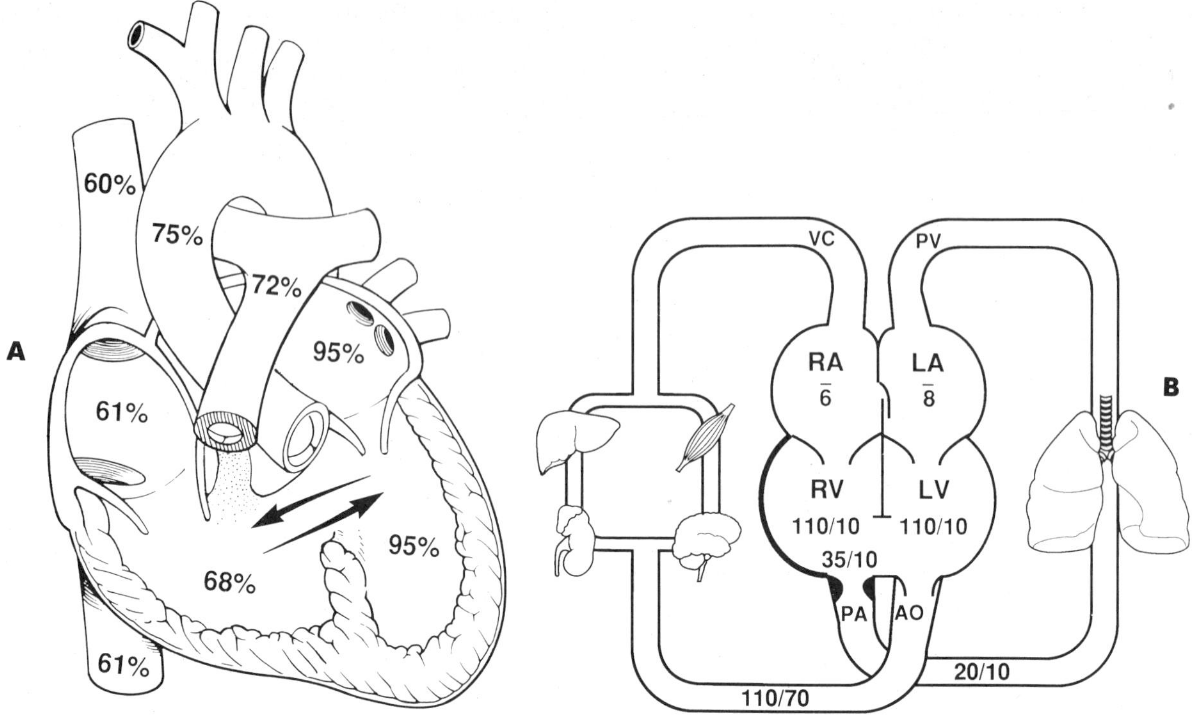


**Figure 19–4** Typical findings in tetralogy of Fallot. **A,** Oxygen saturations. **B,** pressures. VC, vena cava; *PV,* pulmonary vein; *RA,* right atrium; *LA,* left atrium; *LV,* left ventricle; *RV,* right ventricle.

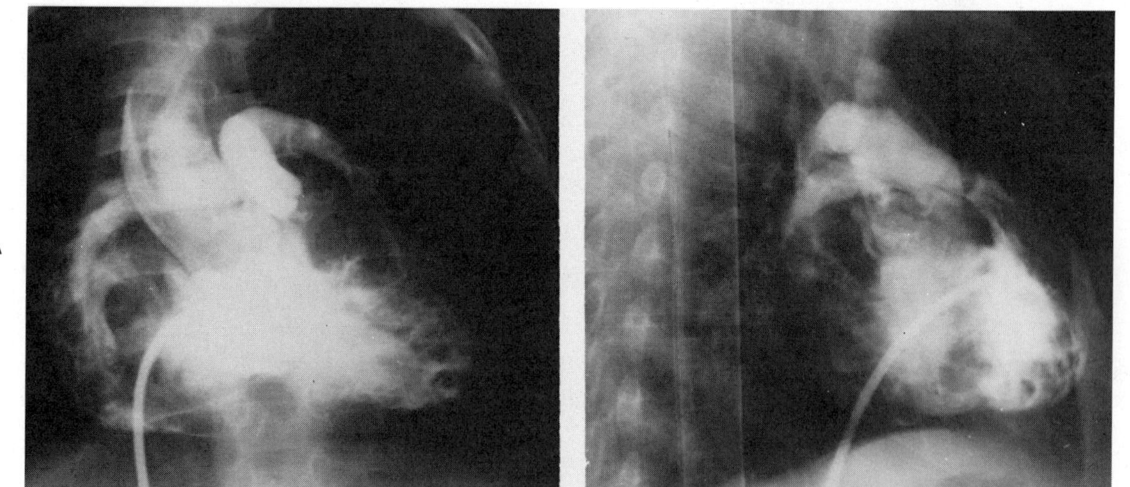


**Figure 19–5** **A,** Cranial and shallow left anterior oblique right ventricular angiogram showing severe infundibular pulmonary stenosis and good-sized right and left pulmonary arteries. The right to left shunt is demonstrated with aortic opacification. **B,** Lateral view of the same angiogram. The pulmonary annulus is approximately a third of the size of the aortic annulus.

imembranous outlet defect. Finally, left ventricular or aortic angiography is important in demonstrating coronary artery anatomy and in ruling out anomalous origin of the left anterior descending coronary artery or single coronary artery with a major branch crossing the right ventricular outflow tract.

## MEDICAL MANAGEMENT

Patients with questionable hypercyanotic spells should be treated prophylactically with propranolol as a preventive measure. The dosages usually used are 0.5 to 1 mg/kg given orally three times a day. Side effects such as excess bradycardia and central nervous system depression should be looked for as well as the rare case of hypoglycemia in patients who have decreased oral intake vomiting or diarrhea.

Treatment of the acute hypercyanotic spell includes immediate placement of the child in the knee-to-chest position to increase systemic afterload and decrease right to left shunting, 100% oxygen administration by mask or nasal cannula, again to increase systemic resistance and be certain that the infant is fully oxygenated. Morphine 0.1 mg/kg is also used; it probably serves to decrease irritability and excitement, resulting in decreased heart rate and cardiac sympathetic stimulation, which in turn decreases right ventricular infundibular narrowing and diminishes right to left shunting. Blood gases should be checked and any metabolic acidosis treated with sodium bicarbonate. Phenylephrine as a bolus (0.25 to 0.5 μg/kg) and/or continuous infusion (0.025 to 0.05 μg/kg/min) can be used to increase systemic resistance and decrease right to left shunting. Finally, intravenous propranolol in a dose of 0.05 mg/kg IV can be used to decrease heart rate and decrease systolic infundibular narrowing. Occasionally patients are unresponsive to all these interventions and require tracheal intubation and emergency surgery. It is critically important to try to prevent hypercyanotic spells by avoiding prolonged examinations or venipunctures in an irritable child.

In most patients there is no need for prolonged medical management, and surgical repair should be carried out in infants beyond 2 to 3 months of age who exhibit progressive cyanosis or hypercyanotic spells. Elective operations generally are performed on patients between 6 and 18 months of age who continue to do well clinically but have typical features of tetralogy of Fallot. The two-stage repair with preliminary shunting operation is generally reserved for patients who have severe cyanosis in early infancy or severely hypoplastic pulmonary arteries.

## SURGICAL MANAGEMENT

Palliative systemic to pulmonary artery shunts are no longer commonly performed in patients with tetralogy of Fallot. However, very small young babies with severe cyanosis and patients who have quite small pulmonary arteries usually undergo a preliminary shunt because primary total correction can be associated with increased risk in these situations (Fig. 19–6). A preliminary shunt procedure will allow an opportunity for the pulmonary arteries to enlarge piror to total repair, and a shunt will alleviate severe hypoxemia and polycythemia.

Complete repair most commonly involves a right ventriculotomy, closure of the ventricular septal defect with a patch, excision of obstructing right ventricular outflow tract muscle bundles, and closure of the right ventricular outflow tract (Fig. 19–7). Some authors have advocated closure of the ventricular septal defect from the right atrial approach accompanied by resection of obstructing musculature through a combined approach from the right atrium and the pulmonary artery.

Hospital mortality for total repair in good risk patients is 5% or less.[3,13] Postoperative complications include excessive bleeding, low cardiac output, residual ventricular septal defect, and heart block. Many patients experience transient early postoperative heart failure, especially if the repair has included a transannular outflow tract patch, which results in pulmonary valvar insufficiency. Late reoperation is required in approximately 2% of patients for recurrent or residual ventricular septal defect or right ventricular outflow obstruction.

## ANESTHESIA MANAGEMENT

The most important goal of the anesthesiologist in the management of tetralogy of Fallot is avoiding factors that can lead to a decrease in systemic vascular resistance, an increase in pulmonary vascular resistance, or right ventricular outflow obstruction. The anesthesia management, therefore, is predicated on (1) manipulation of factors that affect right ventricular outflow obstruction and cause increased pulmonary vascular resistance, (2) knowledge of the effect of anesthetic agents on pulmonary and systemic vascular resistance, and (3) maintenance of cardiac output.

### Preoperative assessment

Although it is expected that patients with tetralogy of Fallot will have undergone an extensive investigation of their cardiac defect as outlined in the previous section, it is important that the anesthesiologist also undertake a preoperative assessment. The history and physical examination should be reviewed and particular attention paid to previous

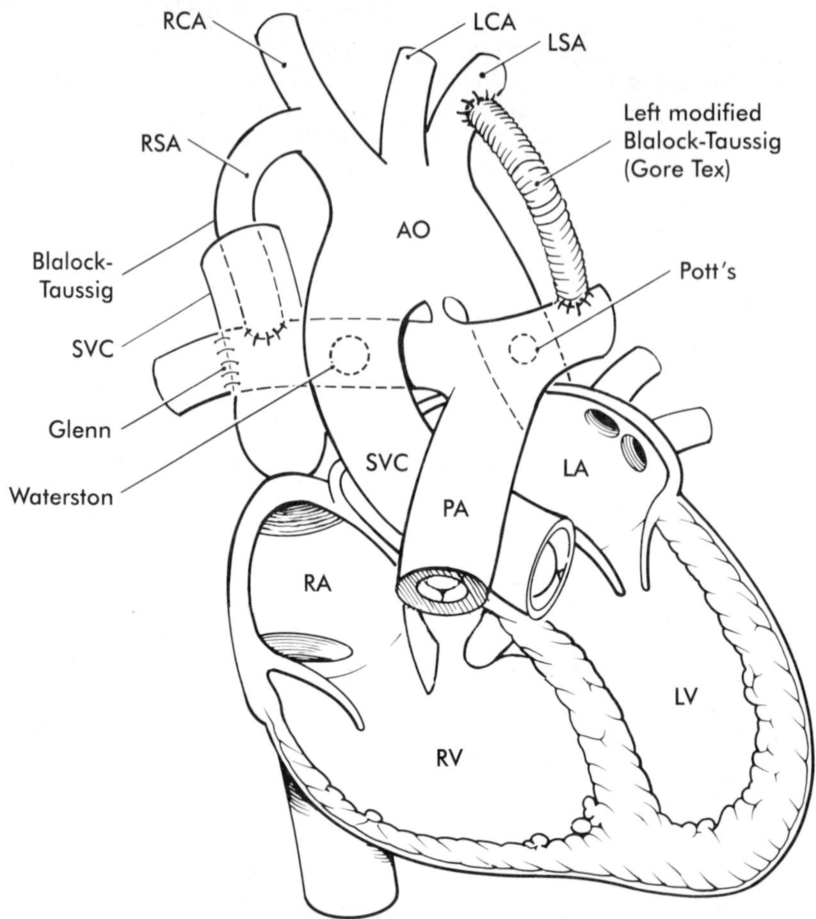


**Figure 19–6** Various palliative surgical procedures to increase the pulmonary blood flow. (1) Blalock-Taussig shunt (classic BT shunt), right subclavian artery to right pulmonary artery. (2) Modified Blalock-Taussig shunt, left subclavian artery to left pulmonary artery with a Gore-Tex material. (3) Glenn shunt, superior vena cava to right pulmonary artery. (4) Pott's shunt, descending aorta to left pulmonary artery. (5) Waterston's shunt, ascending aorta to right pulmonary artery. *RCA,* right coronary artery; *LCA,* left coronary artery; *LSA,* left subclavian artery; *AO,* aorta; SVC, superior vena cava; PA, pulmonary artery; *LA,* left atrium; *LV,* left ventricle; *RV,* right ventricle; *LA,* left atrium.

surgical procedures. The laboratory data should be examined; serum electrolytes, hematocrit, and a coagulation profile should be noted. In addition a serum calcium, blood glucose, and the patient's acid-base status should be measured and any abnormalities corrected before surgery. The cardiologist's assessment of the degree of right ventricular outflow obstruction should also be considered, since this will give an indication of problems that might be encountered during anesthesia.

## Premedication

It is important to choose a premedication that results in a calm child and thus avoids cardiac sympathetic stimulation that might increase right to left shunting and result in a hypercyanotic spell either preoperatively or during anesthesia induction. On the other hand, it is essential to avoid respiratory depression because hypoxia and hypercarbia can also lead to increased pulmonary vascular resistance and cyanosis. In general, generous premedication that allays anxiety and aids in anesthesia induction is usually given. However, in neonates and infants under 6 months of age, usually no premedication, or atropine alone, is required. Older children are usually given a classic premedication consisting of an opioid and anticholinergic agent; for example morphine 0.05 to 0.2 mg/kg and atrophine 0.02 mg/kg or glycopyrrolate 0.01 mg/kg. Oral medication is well tolerated by children, and an oral benzodiazepine may be added to the regimen.[10] Bradycardia is a common complication of

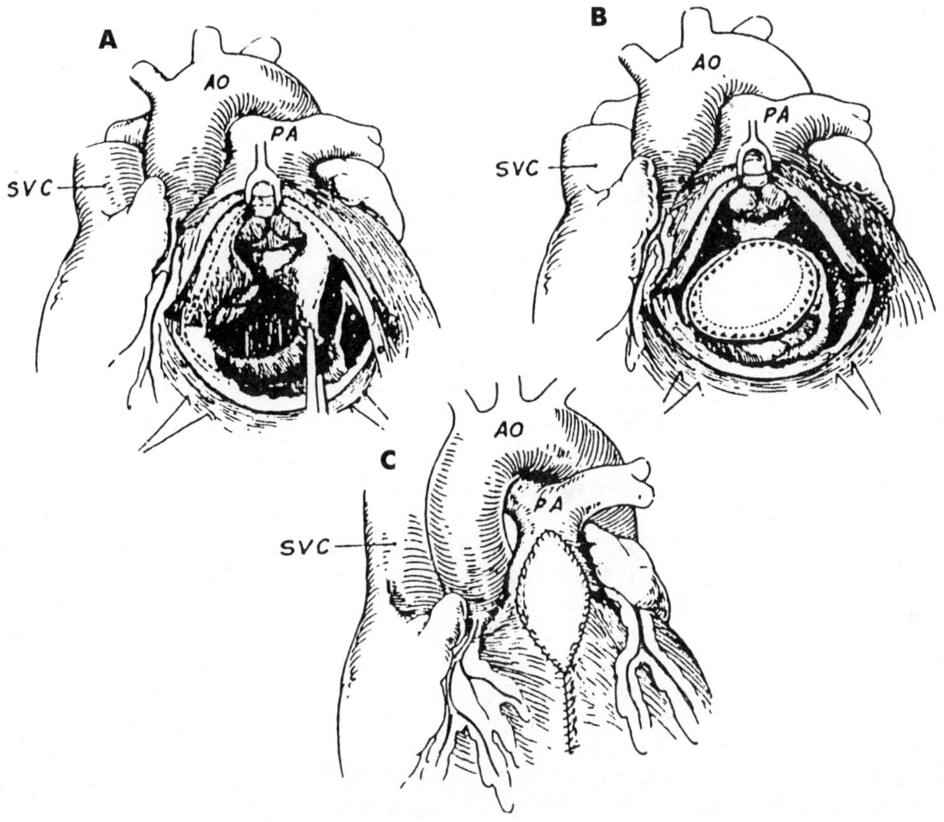


**Figure 19–7** Operation for correction of the tetralogy of Fallot. **A,** Infundibulectomy, or removal of the outflow tract obstruction to the right ventricle by sharp dissection. **B,** Closure of the ventricular septal defect. **C,** If the pulmonary annulus is too narrow or if the infundibulectomy does not open the outflow obstruction adequately, a patch in the outflow tract may be necessary. *AO,* aorta; *SVC,* superior vena cava; *PA,* pulmonary artery. (From Effler DB, editor: *Blades' surgical diseases of the chest,* ed 4, St. Louis, 1978, Mosby.)

anesthesia induction, and an anticholinergic agent should be routinely added to the premedication, especially if the child is concurrently receiving a β-adrenergic blocking agent.[20,25] Recently esmolol, an ultra–short-acting cardioselective β-adrenergic blocking agent, has been suggested to aid in the management of hypercyanotic spells.[25]

### Induction

Factors that increase pulmonary vascular resistance should be avoided. These include hypoxia, acidosis, excitement, and agitation. Anesthesia induction, which may be either inhalational or intravenous, is usually determined by the clinical condition and age of the patient.[12,14,21] Neonates and small infants are usually anesthetized with a combination of fentanyl (with midazolam or diazepam in some instances) followed by succinylcholine or a nondepolarizing muscle relaxant such as vecuronium. Although older children usually receive an inhalational anesthetic in many pediatric centers, intravenous administration is a satisfactory alternative for cooperative children. Factors affecting induction (cardiac output, ventilation, right to left shunt) are discussed in Chapter 10. An inhalational induction in a patient with tetralogy of Fallot with a right to left shunt may be prolonged.[27] In cyanotic patients either 100% oxygen or 50% nitrous oxide in oxygen (with an inhalational agent) is usually administered during induction. The patient should be observed during induction for peripheral systemic vasodilation and for hypotension.

If the patient becomes hypotensive and tissue perfusion is decreased, metabolic acidosis may occur. It is important to recognize that these patients may have a small preoperative baseline metabolic acidosis, and thus a worsening of acid-base status may lead to increased pulmonary vascular resistance, hypoxia, and cyanosis. In addition a decreased in systemic vascular resistance may increase right to left shunting in patients with tetralogy of Fallot. A previously performed palliative systemic pulmonary artery shunt may exist, and if arterial blood pressure is decreased, then flow through the shunt is decreased, which leads to decreased pulmonary perfusion. This situation then leads to hypercarbia, acidosis, and further hypoxia. Therefore, intravenous and inhalational anesthetic agents that decrease myocardial contractility and systemic vascular resistance should be used with caution.

The effect of intravenous and inhalational anesthetic agents on pulmonary vascular resistance has been carefully studied both in vivo and in vitro.[8,16-19] High-dose thiopental (10 mg/kg) has been shown to decrease pulmonary vascular resistance. Thiopental can also decrease cardiac output and systemic vascular resistance due to its well recognized hemodynamic effects. Narcotics in general do not have marked effects on pulmonary vascular resistance. Hickey and co-workers[17,18] have shown that fentanyl (25 μg/kg) has minimal effect on pulmonary and systemic hemodynamics in small infants after repair of congenital heart defects. Thus, induction of anesthesia with fentanyl is becoming widespread. The effect of ketamine on pulmonary vascular resistance is controversial. Ketamine has been shown to increase pulmonary vascular resistance in adult humans.[9] However, in some studies under controlled conditions pulmonary vascular resistance responses appear to be minimally affected in infants.[4,5,15,22] Although it is important to maintain cardiac output, if myocardial contractility increases, right ventricular outflow obstruction (dynamic infundibular stenosis) increases, ventricular filling decreases, and pulmonary blood flow is limited. Therefore, a right to left shunt develops with ensuing cyanosis and acidosis. Thus, a balance must be maintained between systemic vascular resistance and infundibular right ventricular outflow obstruction.

Management of an increased right to left shunt during anesthesia includes discontinuation of the precipitating agent, correction of a metabolic acidosis, and the administration of an inotrope such as phenylephrine to increase systemic vascular resistance. Isoproterenol should be avoided because of $\beta_2$-adrenergic induced vasodilation.

The initiation of ventilation and possibly increased airway pressure should be approached cautiously, since a raised mean intrathoracic pressure may reduce stroke volume and cardiac output. It is important to exercise great care in patients with tetralogy of Fallot with a right to left shunt to avoid introducing air emboli into the circulation because of the risk of paradoxical embolism.

The effect of a right to left cardiac shunt on drug pharmacokinetics is an area that has not been extensively investigated. In an animal model the influence of a right to left shunt on lidocaine pharmacokinetics has shown that lidocaine peak concentrations were higher and clearance reduced.[2] In the normal circulation the lungs absorb 60% to 80% of a lidocaine bolus on the first passage. Thus, although it is difficult to extrapolate laboratory experimental findings to the clinical setting, it is important to recognize that a large right to left shunt has the potential to affect pharmacokinetics, especially of drugs administered through a central venous catheter.

### Maintenance

Anesthesia is usually maintained with an IV narcotic (fentanyl 50 to 100 μg/kg or sufentanil 15 to 25 μg/kg) in these patients. Vecuronium or one of the newer nondepolarizing muscle relaxants (doxacurium or pipecuronium) can be used to maintain muscle paralysis throughout the operation.

In contrast with adult patients, in children with CHD pulmonary arterial pressure and pulmonary vascular resistance were not significantly changed by administration of 50% nitrous oxide in either the group with normal PVR or the group with elevated PVR.[24,26]

If deep hypothermia and circulatory arrest are planned (usually in children under 10 kg body weight), we administer 10 ml/kg of dextran 40 in 5% dextrose solution before peripheral cooling is initiated (see chapter 4 for complete details of deep hypothermia).

Heparin is usually injected into the right atrium by the surgeon just before the placement of cannulas. Protamine is administered by the anesthesiologist at the conclusion of extracorporeal circulation following the removal of cardiac cannulas. The majority of patients require isoproterenol (0.01 to 0.05 μg/kg/min) infusion during the perioperative period.

Since patients with tetralogy of Fallot have decreased pulmonary blood flow, one should avoid using excessive positive airway pressure or positive end expiratory pressure during ventilation.

Patients with tetralogy of Fallot are usually left intubated and mechanically ventilated postoperatively. Once the patient is awake and stable, and rewarmed to a normal body temperature, the trachea can be extubated in the cardiac recovery room, usually after 24 to 72 hours.

### Surgery without bypass: systemic to pulmonary artery shunt

The principles of anesthesia outlined in the previous section also apply to anesthesia for nonbypass operations. Anesthesia usually includes an intravenous induction with fentanyl, a nondepolarizing muscle relaxant, and ventilation with oxygen and in some instances nitrous oxide. It is important postoperatively to assess carefully the adequacy of the shunt and degree of oxygenation before the decision is made to wean the patient from the ventilator. In addition any metabolic acidosis can be corrected during this period. Since these patients routinely require postoperative ventilation, maintenance of anesthesia is often accomplished by fentanyl administration.

At induction cross-matched blood should be available and excellent intravenous access obtained. A radial artery cannula should be placed in the area opposite the side of operation, since the radial pulse on the side of surgery will be obliterated during the operation due to clamping of the subclavian artery. Some patients will arrive in the operating room receiving an infusion of prostaglandin $E_1$ to maintain pulmonary blood flow if ductal flow is important.[7] This should be continued until the shunt is completed.

The position of the patient is either lateral or supine, depending on the type of pulmonary-systemic shunt being performed and whether a thoracotomy is required. Arterial oxygen saturation may decrease with the onset of one-lung ventilation and further decrease on clamping of the pulmonary artery to allow graft anastomosis. Therefore, 100% inspired oxygen is usually administered, and it is important to correct bradycardia and metabolic acidosis quickly. Heart rate and blood pressure may decrease. If hemodynamic stability does not resolve, then the administration of an inotrope such as dopamine should be contemplated. Dopamine (5 to 10 $\mu g/kg/min$) administration also results in increased flow through the new shunt. Some surgeons administer heparin to help maintain graft patency. Once the shunt has been completed and the surgeon has removed the clamp, the systemic pressure may decrease because of runoff into the pulmonary artery. Inotrope support may be required at this time. These infants usually have a high preoperative hematocrit and should volume replacement be required, whole or packed cells should be avoided.

## REFERENCES


1. Blalock A, Taussig HB: The surgical treatment of malformations of the heart in which there is pulmonary stenosis or pulmonary atresia, *JAMA* 128:189, 1945.
2. Bokesch PM, Castaneda AR, Ziemer G et al: The influence of a right-to-left cardiac shunt on lidocaine pharmacokinetics, *Anesthesiology* 67:739, 1987.
3. Castaneda AR, Freed MD, Williams RG et al: Repair of tetralogy of Fallot in infancy: early and late results, *J Thorac Cardiovasc Surg* 74:372, 1977.
4. Coppel DL, Dundee JW. Ketamine anesthesia for cardiac catheterization, *Anesthesia* 27:25, 1972.
5. Faithfull NS, Haider R: Ketamine for cardiac catheterization: an evaluation of its use in children, *Anesthesia* 26:318, 1971.
6. Fallot A: Contribution a l'anatomie pathologique de la maladie bleu (cyanose cardiaque), *Marseille Medicine* 25:77, 138, 207, 270, 341, 402, 1988.
7. Freed MA, Heymann MA, Lewis AB et al: Prostaglandin $E_1$ in infants with ductus arteriosus–dependent congenital heart disease, *Circulation* 64:889, 1981.
8. Friesen RH, Henry DB: Cardiovascular changes in preterm neonates receiving isoflurane, halothane, fentanyl, and ketamine, *Anesthesiology* 54:238, 1986.
9. Gassner S, Cohen M, Aygen M et al: The effect of ketamine on pulmonary artery pressure: an experimental and clinical study, *Anesthesia* 29:141, 1974.
10. Goldstein-Dresner MC, Davis PJ, Kretchman E et al: Double-blind comparison of oral transmucosal fentanyl citrate with oral meperidine, diazepam, and atrophine as preanesthetic medication in children with congenital heart disease, *Anesthesiology* 74:28, 1991.
11. Graham TP Jr., Gutgesell HP: Conotruncal abnormalities in fetal and neonatal cardiology. In Long WA, editor: *Fetal and Neonatal Cardiology,* Philadelphia, 1990, Saunders.
12. Greeley WJ, Bushman GA, Davis DP et al: Comparative effects of halothane and ketamine on systemic arterial oxygen saturation in children with cyanotic congenital heart disease, *Anesthesiology* 65:666, 1986.
13. Gustafson RA, Murray GF, Warden HE et al: Early primary repair of tetralogy of Fallot, *Ann Thorac Surg* 45:235, 1988.
14. Hensley FA, Larach DR, Stauffer RA et al: The effect of halothane/nitrous oxide/oxygen mask induction on arterial hemoglobin saturation in cyanotic congenital heart disease, *J Cardiothorac Anesth* 1:289, 1987.
15. Hickey PR, Hansen DD, Cramolini GM et al: Pulmonary and systemic hemodynamic responses to ketamine in infants with normal and elevated pulmonary vascular resistance, *Anesthesiology* 62:287, 1985.
16. Hickey PR, Hansen DD, Strafford M et al: Pulmonary and systemic hemodynamic effects of nitrous oxide in infants with normal and elevated pulmonary vascular resistance, *Anesthesiology* 65:374, 1986.
17. Hickey PR, Hansen DD, Wessel DL et al: Blunting of stress responses in the pulmonary circulation of infants by fentanyl, *Anesth Analg* 64:1137, 1985.
18. Hickey PR, Hansen DD, Wessel DL et al: Pulmonary and systemic hemodynamic responses to fentanyl in infants, *Anesth Analg* 64:483, 1985.
19. Hilgenberg JC, McCammon RL, Stoelting RK: Pulmonary and systemic vascular responses to nitrous oxide in patients with nitrous oxide and pulmonary hypertension, *Anesth Analg* 59:323, 1980.
20. Honey M, Chamberlain DA, Howard J: The effect of β-sympathetic blockade on arterial oxygen saturation in Fallot's tetralogy, *Circulation* 30:501, 1964.
21. Laishley RS, Burrows FA, Lerman J et al: Effect of anesthetic induction regimens on oxygen saturation in cyanotic congenital heart disease, *Anesthesiology* 65:673, 1986.
22. Levin RM, Seleny FL, Streczyn MV: Keamine-pancuronium-narcotic technique for cardiovascular surgery in infants: a comparative study. *Anesth Analg* 54:800, 1975.
23. Lillehei CW, Cohen M, Warden HE, et al: Direct vision intracardiac surgical corrections of the tetralogy of Fallot and pulmonary atresia defects, *Ann Surg* 142:418, 1955.
24. Murray D, Forbes R, Murphy K et al: Nitrous oxide: cardiovascular effects in infants and small children during halothane and isoflurane anesthesia, *Anesth Analg* 67:1059, 1988.
25. Nussbaum J, Zane EA, Thys DM: Esmolol for the treatment

of hypercyanotic spells in infants with tetralogy of Fallot, *J Cardothorac Anesth* 3:200, 1989.
26. Schulte-Sasse U, Hess W, Tarnow J: Pulmonary vascular responses to nitrous oxide in patients with normal and high pulmonary vascular resistance, *Anesthesiology* 57:9, 1982.
27. Tanner GE, Angers DG, Barash PG et al: Effect of left-to-right, mixed left-to-right, and right-to-left shunts on inhalational anesthetic induction in children: a computer model, *Anesth Analg* 64:101, 1985.
28. Willius FA: Cardiac clinics 124: an unusually early description of the so-called tetralogy of Fallot, *Proc Staff Mayo Clin* 23:316, 1948.

# 20 Transposition of the Great Arteries

*Jay Kambam*



D-transposition of the great arteries (TGA) is one of the most frequently seen congenital heart defects producing cyanosis in the newborn. The incidence of TGA among infants born with congenital heart defects (CHD) is about 5%.[3,11,18] TGA is the second most common CHD encountered in early infancy (the most common type of CHD is ventricular septal defect). The etiologic factors of TGA are unknown. TGA is not associated with any genetic component. Males are more affected than females by a ratio of about 3:1. The incidence of TGA is higher in infants born to mothers of advanced age and those with diabetes mellitus.

## EMBRYOLOGY

A number of important events that take place during intrauterine cardiac development result in a normal relationship of the aorta and the pulmonary artery. Between the third and fourth weeks of gestation the aorticopulmonary trunk divides into the aorta and the pulmonary artery. This is accomplished by the development of the truncoconal ridges, which grow caudad in a spiral fashion, placing the aorta in a posterolateral position and the pulmonary artery in an anteromedial position (Fig. 20–1).

There are at least two theories that attempt to explain transposition of the great arteries. One has to do with differential conal absorption. The second theory posits abnormal formation of the aorticopulmonary septum.

### Differential conal absorption theory

In normal embryologic development a bilateral conus develops beneath the aorta and the pulmonary artery. At this stage the developing aortic valve assumes the rightward position, and the pulmonary valve assumes the leftward position. According to this hypothesis there is further growth

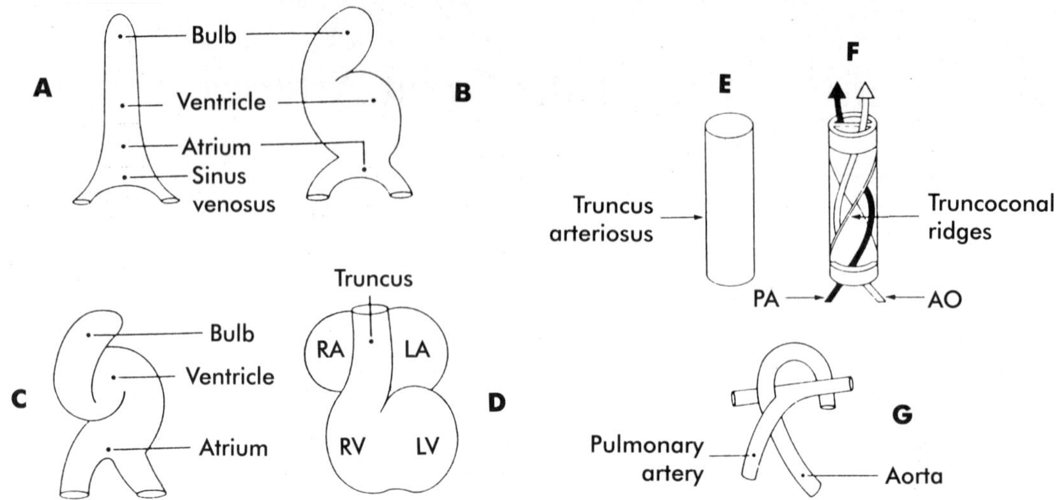


**Figure 20–1** Schematic representation of the development of the primitive cardiac tube into the definitive four-chambered heart. **A,** 18 days; **B,** 21 days; **C,** 23 days; **D,** 28 days. Note the initial rightward convex bending of the tube in **B. E, G,** The division of the truncus arteriosus into the aorta and the pulmonary artery. **F,** septation and the spiral direction of the pulmonary artery and the aorta. *RA,* Right atrium; *LA,* left atrium; *RV,* right ventricle; *LV,* left ventricle; *PA,* pulmonary artery; *AO,* aorta. (From Fink BW, ed: *Congenital heart disease: a deductive approach to its diagnosis,* ed 3, St Louis, 1991, Mosby.)

of the subpulmonic conus and absorption of the subaortic conus. This differential growth and absorption result in the normal pulmonary valve and aortic valve relationships with their corresponding ventricular outflow tracts. However, according to this theory, in transposition of the great arteries the reverse occurs. There is further growth of the subaortic conus and absorption of the subpulmonic conus. This is thought to result in the left ventricle emptying its blood into a vessel that becomes the pulmonary artery and the right ventricle emptying its blood into a vessel that becomes the aorta.

### Theory of abnormal formation of the aorticopulmonary septum

The aorticopulmonary system normally develops in a spiral fashion to separate the truncus arteriosus. According to this theory transposition of the great arteries occurs as a result of the abnormal formation of the aorticopulmonary septum. It is hypothesized that abnormal fusion of the truncal ridges results in septation of the truncus arteriosus in a straight fashion, resulting in an anterior aorta and a posterior pulmonary artery.

## PATHOLOGIC ANATOMY

Normal development of the heart and great vessels results in the left ventricle emptying its oxygenated blood into the aorta and the right ventricle emptying its poorly oxygenated blood into the pulmonary artery. In transposition of the great arteries the aorta arises from the right ventricle, and its route is anterior and rightward. The pulmonary artery originates from the left ventricle, and its route is posterior and leftward (Fig. 20–2). In a heart with TGA the two great vessels appear to sit side by side. The salient pathoanatomic features of a patient with TGA are summarized in Table 20–1.

## PATHOPHYSIOLOGY

In the normal heart the circulation is connected in series, but in TGA there are two separate parallel circulations (Fig. 20–2). In the normal heart the deoxygenated systemic blood returns to the right heart and is pumped into the pulmonary circulation by the right ventricle via the pulmonary artery. Once oxygenated, the blood returns to the left heart and is pumped into the systemic arterial circulation by the left ventricle via the aorta. In the heart with TGA the deoxygenated blood returns to the right heart and is pumped into the systemic arterial circulation by the right ventricle via the aorta, while the oxygenated blood returns to the left heart and is pumped by the left ventricle back into the pulmonary circulation via the pulmonary artery. The result is complete isolation of the two circuits, with hypoxemic blood circulating in the body and oxygenated blood circulating in the pulmonary circuit. Survival is not possible in a patient with TGA unless there is adequate mixing between the two circulations. Some of the ways by which mixing of blood between the pulmonary and systemic circulations can occur are (1) at the atrial level, as in open foramen ovale or an atrial septal defect

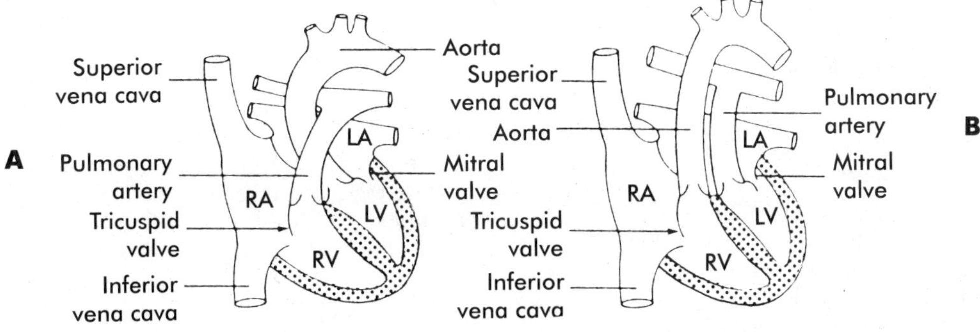


**Figure 20–2** Diagram of the great arteries. **A,** Normal. **B,** transposed. *RA,* Right atrium; *LA,* left atrium; *RV,* right ventricle; *LV,* left ventricle; *PA,* pulmonary artery. (From Fink BW, ed: *Congenital heart disease: a deductive approach to its diagnosis,* ed 3, St Louis, 1991, Mosby.)

**Table 20–1** Pathologic anatomy of transposition of the great arteries

| | Normal heart | Heart with TGA |
|---|---|---|
| Right atrium | Normal | Normal |
| Tricuspid valve | Normal | Normal |
| Pulmonary valve | | |
| Subpulmonary infundibulum | Present | Absent |
| Fibrous continuity | Absent | Present |
| Right ventricle | Coarsely trabeculated | Coarsely trabeculated |
| Left atrium | Normal | Normal |
| Left ventricle | Finely trabeculated | Finely trabeculated |
| Mitral valve | Normal | Normal |
| Aortic valve | | |
| Subaortic infundibulum | Absent | Present |
| Fibrous continuity | Present | Absent |
| Atrioventricular connection | Concordant | Concordant |
| Ventriculoarterial connection | Concordant | Discordant |
| Great arteries | Spiral fashion | Parallel fashion |
| Pulmonary artery arises from | Right ventricle | Left ventricle |
| Aorta arises from | Left ventricle | Right ventricle |
| Conduction system | Normal | Normal |
| Coronary arteries | | |
| Right coronary origin | Above right sinus | Above posterior sinus |
| Left coronary origin | Above left sinus | Above left sinus |
| Coronary sinuses | Faces pulmonary artery | Faces pulmonary artery* |
| Noncoronary sinuses | Faces posterior and right | Faces anterior and right |

*Facilitates transplantation of the coronary arteries from the aorta to the pulmonary artery.

(ASD), (2) at the ventricular level as a ventricular septal defect (VSD), and (3) at the great arterial level as a patent ductus arteriosus (PDA). The mixing between the two circulations must be equal; otherwise the total blood volume ends up either in the systemic or the pulmonary circulation. Bidirectional shunt is not possible at the level of PDA, as it usually allows blood to flow from the aorta to the PA in patients wtih simple TGA. Thus the presence of PDA without ASD or VSD is not compatible with life. Systemic oxygenation is mainly dependent on the left to right shunt (remember, the aorta arises from the right ventricle), and return of deoxygenated blood to the pulmonary circulation depends on the right to left shunt.

### Atrial and ventricular septal defects

The presence of an ASD or a VSD in a patient with TGA gives an entirely different picture. Even though there is a bidirectional shunting of blood via an ASD or VSD, shunting is predominantly from right to left at the ventricular level and left to right at the atrial level. Because of the sufficient mixing of blood both at the atrial and ventricular levels, only mild cyanosis is seen in these patients in the neonatal period. As pulmonary vascular resistance gradually decreases in the first few weeks after birth, these patients develop congestive heart failure from excessive pulmonary blood flow.

### Ventricular septal defect and pulmonary stenosis

The presence of VSD and mild to moderate pulmonary stenosis (PS) is associated with diminished pulmonary blood flow. There is usually a bidirectional shunt present at the ventricular level. Cyanosis is absent in neonates with mild PS and may be present in patients with moderate PS. However, patients with severe PS or pulmonary atresia are very cyanotic and require a palliative operation to restore adequate pulmonary blood flow for survival.

### L-transposition of the great arteries (corrected transposition)

The frequency of this defect is less than 1% of all CHDs. In patients with L-TGA there is abnormal looping of the great arteries and truncoconal septation. In this malformation twisting of the loop to the left results in the arterial ventricle (anatomic right ventricle) displaced leftward and posteriorly and the venous ventricle (anatomic left ventricle) displaced rightward and anteriorly. Abnormalities of septation and rotation also result in the origin of the pulmonary artery rightward and posteriorly and the origin of the aorta leftward and anteriorly. As a result the pulmonary artery originates from the venous ventricle and the aorta originates from the arterial ventricle (Fig. 20–3). The right atrium (RA) empties blood into the anatomic left ventricle (LV) through the mitral valve (MV), and the left atrium (LA) empties into the anatomic right ventricle (RV) via the tricuspid valve (TV). The sites of origin of the coronary arteries are also usually reversed in this malformation. The right coronary artery arises from the left posterior aortic sinus and the anterior descending and circumflex arteries arise from a vessel that originates from the right posterior aortic sinus. Patients with L-TGA lead normal lives provided there are no other cardiac defects. However, in the majority of patients with L-TGA there are other cardiac defects including VSD (80%), PS (50%), TV deformity (30%), and congenital heart block. The cardiac apex is in the right chest (dextrocardia) in about 50% of the patients with L-TGA.

### Transposition of the aorta and overriding of pulmonary artery (Taussig-Bing syndrome)

In this malformation the aorta arises from the RV, and the PA overrides the ventricular septum. A VSD is always present. Pulmonary hypertension usually dominates the clinical picture in these patients.

## CLINICAL PRESENTATION

Infants with TGA usually have normal or above average birth weights. In the majority of patients with D-TGA, hypoxemia and cyanosis are present at birth. However, the degree of cyanosis can be altered by the presence of other associated cardiac defects. These patients may also present with signs of CHF and with breathing and feeding difficulties in the newborn period. On auscultation of the chest no heart murmur is audible in most patients with an intact ventricular septum. When there is a VSD, a pansystolic murmur is audible. A soft systolic ejection murmur is present in the presence of pulmonary stenosis.

### Laboratory findings

***Electrocardiography.*** In the majority of newborns with TGA, the ECG is within normal limits. But rightward QRS axis deviation and right ventricular hypertrophy are present in the ECG in some

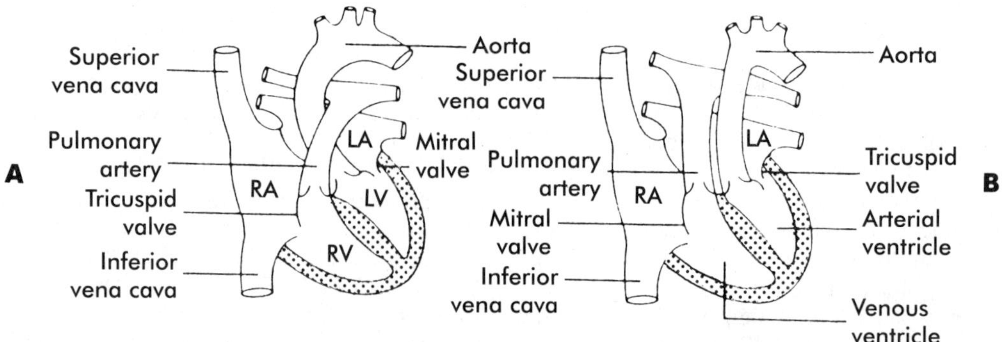


**Figure 20–3** Diagram of corrected transposition of the great arteries. **A,** Normal. **B,** Corrected. *RA,* right atrium; *LA,* left atrium; *LV,* left ventricle; *RV,* right ventricle.

patients with TGA. In the presence of a large VSD and/or PS, signs of biventricular hypertrophy are seen in the ECG. Occasionally right atrial hypertrophy (RAH) is seen, but left atrial hypertrophy (LAH) in a patient with TGA is a very rare finding. Cardiac arrhythmias are also uncommon in patients with D-TGA.

***Chest x-ray film.*** In almost half of the neonates with TGA there may be a normal chest roentgenogram. In about one third of the patients with an intact ventricular septum, because of the altered course of the great vessels, the mediastinum is narrow. Radiographically, one can also see increased pulmonary vascular markings, especially on the right lung. The heart appearance in the chest x-ray film shows an ovoid shape (a shape of an egg on a string) (Fig. 20–4).

***Echocardiogram.*** One can readily make the diagnosis of TGA with the help of an echocardiogram. The salient echocardiographic features of a patient with TGA are (1) an anterior aorta arising from the right ventricle, (2) a posterior pulmonary artery arising from the left ventricle, which divides into a right and a left pulmonary artery, and (3) absence of a usual circle and sausage view of the normal great arteries; instead, two circular structures are seen (Fig. 20–5). Other associated cardiac abnormalities including PDA, PS, ASD, VSD, and coronary and valve deformities can also be seen in the echo.

***Cardiac catheterization data.*** The typical oxygen saturations and pressures in the various heart chambers and great arteries are shown in Fig. 20–6.

## MEDICAL MANAGEMENT

Without proper medical and surgical management, the prognosis of these patients is exceedingly poor. The availability of prostaglandins since the mid-1970s has dramatically changed the survival rate and preoperative course of many neonates with certain CHDs including TGA.[10,23,30,31]

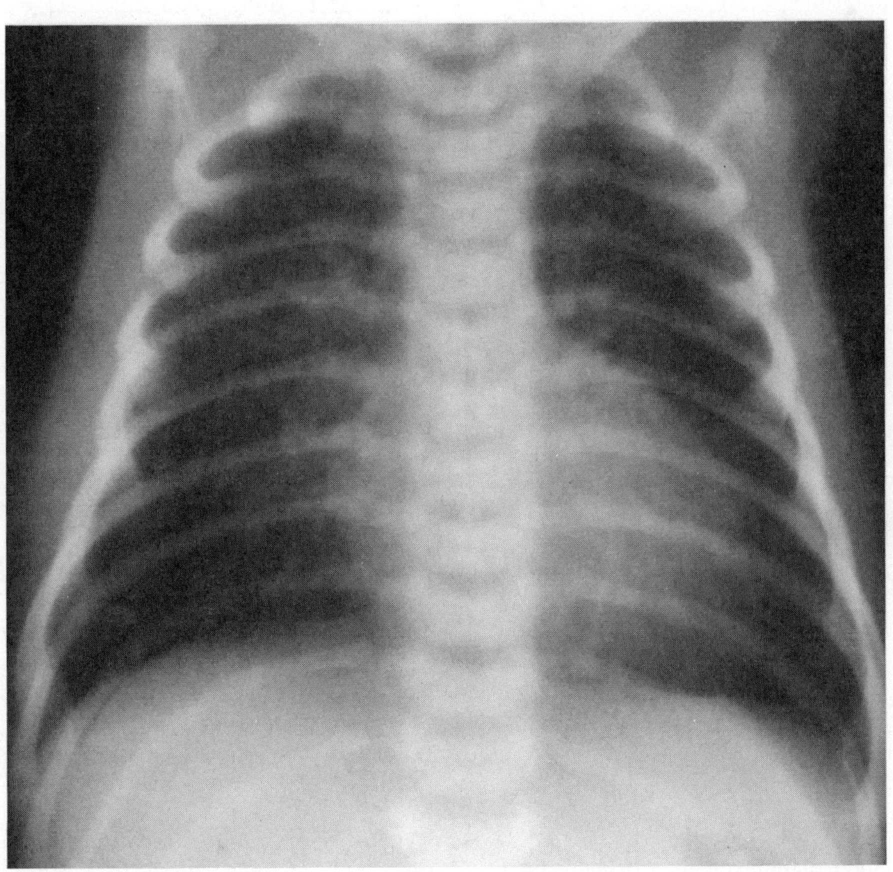

**Figure 20–4** Anteroposterior chest radiograph in an infant with complete transposition of the great arteries: Salient radiographic features are cardiomegaly (the heart has egg-on-a-string configuration), a concave main pulmonary artery segment, and increased pulmonary arterial flow. (Courtesy of Sandra G. Kirchner, MD.)

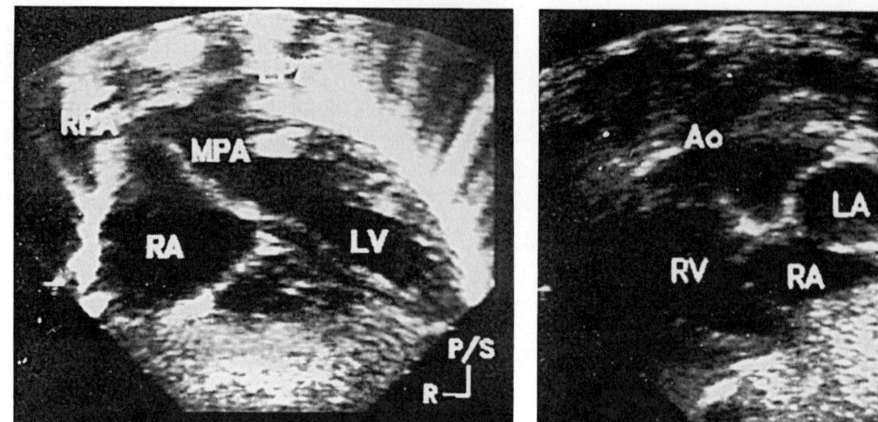


**Figure 20–5** D-transposition of the great arteries. **A,** Subxiphoid long axis view showing the bifurcating pulmonary artery aligned with the left ventricle. **B,** subxiphoid short axis view demonstrating the aorta, including the arch and brachiocephalic vessels, aligned with the right ventricle. *RPA,* right pulmonary artery; *MPA,* main pulmonary artery; *RA,* right atrium; *LV,* left ventricle; *AO,* aorta. (From Fyler DC, ed: *Nadas' pediatric cardiology,* Philadelphia, 1992, Hanley & Belfus.)

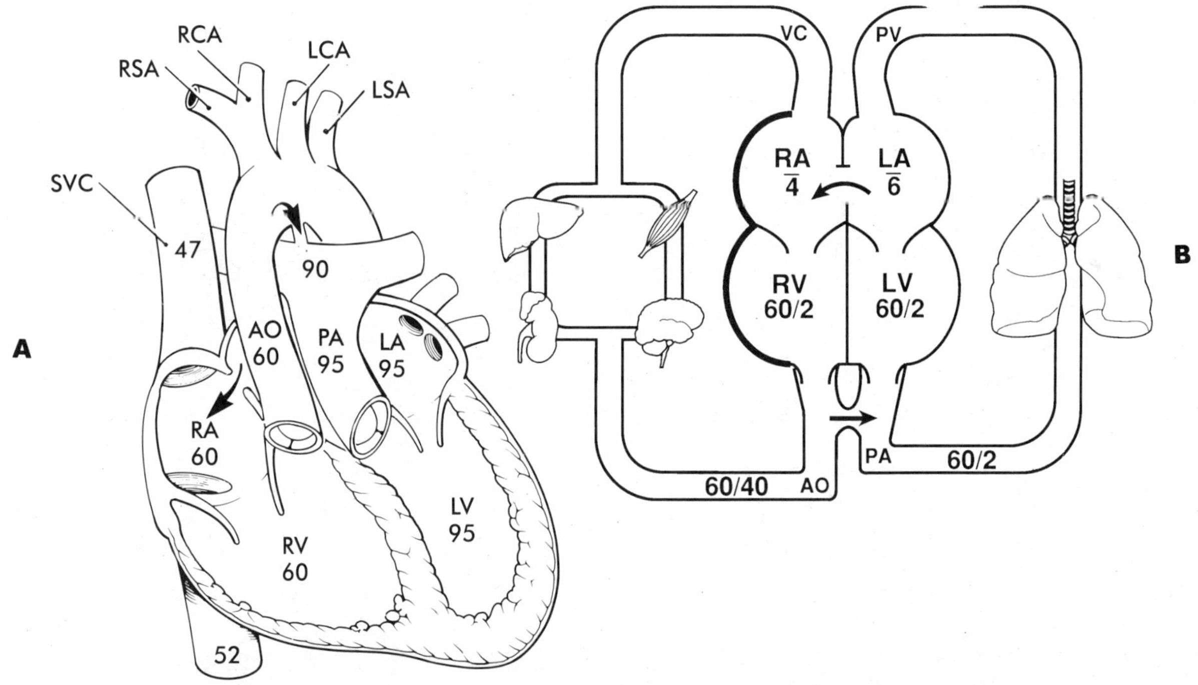


**Figure 20–6** Oxygen saturations and pressures in a patient with transposition of great arteries. *RCA,* right coronary artery; *LCA,* left coronary artery; *LSA,* left subclavian artery; *SVC,* superior vena cava; *AO,* aorta; *PA,* pulmonary artery; *LA,* left atrium; *LV,* left ventricle; *RV,* right ventricle.

### Prostaglandin therapy

The introduction of intravenous prostaglandin $E_1$ provides a pharmacologic means of dramatically improving oxygenation of newborns with TGA until palliative or definitive procedures can be performed. Prostaglandin $E_1$ infusion improves arterial oxygen pressure either by reopening or maintaining patency of the ductus arteriosus.

### Hematocrit

Because of the extreme hypoxemia in cases where the defect is uncorrected at birth or immediately thereafter, these patients quite often gradually develop polycythemia in an attempt to provide adequate systemic oxygen delivery. However, if the hematocrit exceeds 60%, then phlebotomy and an exchange transfusion with a plasma substitute are advised to improve the cardiovascular status, to reduce peripheral sledging, and to improve the coagulation status of the patient perioperatively.[9,14,15,17,28,35] On the other hand, patients with a low hematocrit develop signs of congestive heart failure as well as worsening of hypoxemia and acidosis.[5,22,25] Patients with either a high hematocrit (above 60%) or a low hematocrit (below 40%) are also frequently prone to certain neurologic complications ranging from minor headaches to major cerebrovascular accidents.[5,22,25]

### Other therapy

Correction of metabolic acidosis and treatment of hypoglycemia and hypocalcemia are frequently necessary, especially in patients with severe hypoxemia. Oxygen therapy usually helps lower the PVR and increases the oxygen saturation to a certain extent in some seriously ill patients.

### Treatment of congestive heart failure

Patients with TGA and a VSD or a large PDA usually develop CHF in the first few weeks of life. These patients are usually treated with a diuretic or a combination of diuretic and digitalis.

## SURGICAL MANAGEMENT[1,2,13,16,19,24,26,27,29]

The landmark events in the management of TGA are listed in Table 20–2. Since the introduction of the Rashkind procedure (balloon atrial septostomy) in the mid-1960s and the availability of the prostaglandin $E_1$ infusion in mid-1970s the perioperative survival rate of infants with D-TGA has been markedly improved. The surgical treatment of patients with TGA can be divided into (1) palliative procedures (Blalock-Hanlon operation, and pulmonary artery banding), and (2) definitive procedures. These include switching the right and left side structures at the atrial level (Senning's and Mustard's procedures), the ventricular level (Rastelli procedure), or the great arterial level (Jatene operation). Timing and selection of procedures and the resultant mortality rate vary widely from one medical center to another. Since the mid 1980s the arterial switch operation (Jatene operation) has gained popularity.

### Palliative procedures

***Blalock-Hanlon operation.*** If the prostaglandin $E_1$ infusion and Rashkind procedure (balloon or blade atrial septostomy) fail to produce satisfactory results, then an emergency palliative Blalock-Hanlon operation or definitive surgery is usually performed, depending upon the underlying pathology (Fig. 20–7). The Blalock-Hanlon operation consists of a right thoracotomy and excision of the posterior aspect of the atrial septum. This operation does not require cardiopulmonary bypass. The perioperative mortality rate is 10% to 25%.

**Table 20–2** Surgical milestones of TGA

| Procedure | Year |
|---|---|
| Blalock-Hanlon atrial septectomy | 1950 |
| Pulmonary artery banding | 1952 |
| Senning's repair | 1959 |
| Mustard operation | 1964 |
| Rashkind balloon septostomy | 1966 |
| Rastelli operation | 1969 |
| Park blade septostomy | 1975 |
| Jatene operation (arterial switch) | 1976 |
| Senning's activated operation | 1977 |

***Pulmonary artery banding.*** A thoracotomy for PA banding may be necessary to limit the pulmonary blood flow, to control CHF,and to minimize pulmonary vascular obstructive disease.

### Definitive procedures

***Atrial level operations***

*Mustard's operation.* This is the oldest of the definitive surgical procedures for TGA.[21] It redirects the pulmonary and systemic venous return to the right ventricle and left ventricle respectively at the atrial level by the use of either a pericardial or prosthetic baffle (Fig. 20–8, *A*).

*Senning's operation.* This is a modification of Mustard's operation. In this operation a patient's own atrial septal flap and right atrial free wall are used to redirect the systemic and pulmonary venous return to the right and left ventricles respectively (Fig. 20–8, *B*).

Complications following intraarterial surgery are more frequently seen with Mustard's operation. Complications include obstruction to either pulmonary venous return (less than 5%) or systemic venous return (less than 5%); residual atrial shunt; arrhythmias (mostly atrial in nature: tachyarrhythmias, bradyarrhythmias, sick sinus syndrome, and atrioventricular conduction abnormality); sudden death, usually from arrhythmias (3%); pulmonary vascular obstructive disease; and right ventricular dysfunction, especially with exercise.

***Ventricular level operation***

*Rastelli's operation.* This operation is usually indicated for patients with VSD and severe PS. In this operation the left ventricle is directed to the aorta by creating an intraventricular tunnel between

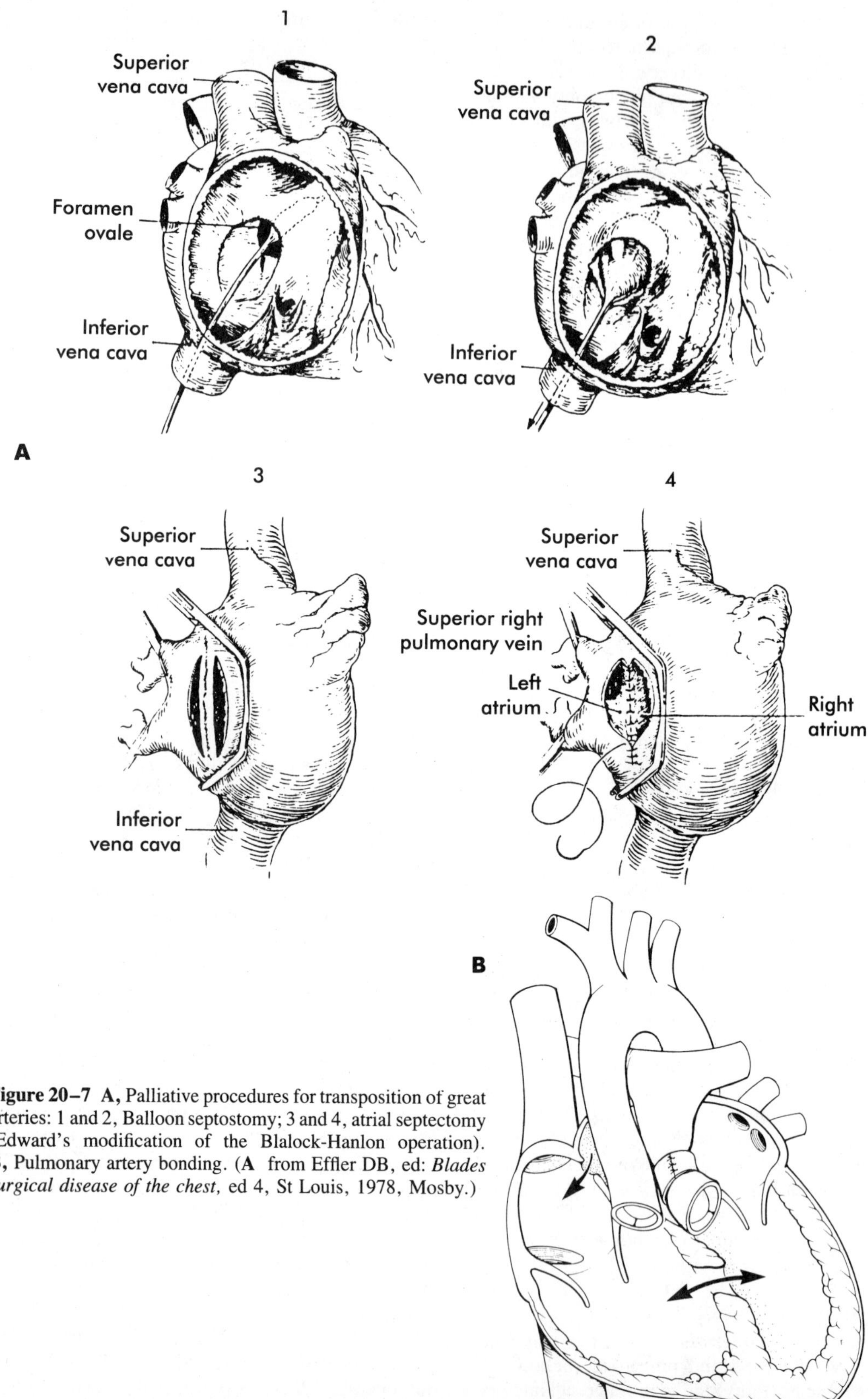


**Figure 20–7** **A,** Palliative procedures for transposition of great arteries: 1 and 2, Balloon septostomy; 3 and 4, atrial septectomy (Edward's modification of the Blalock-Hanlon operation). **B,** Pulmonary artery bonding. (**A** from Effler DB, ed: *Blades surgical disease of the chest,* ed 4, St Louis, 1978, Mosby.)

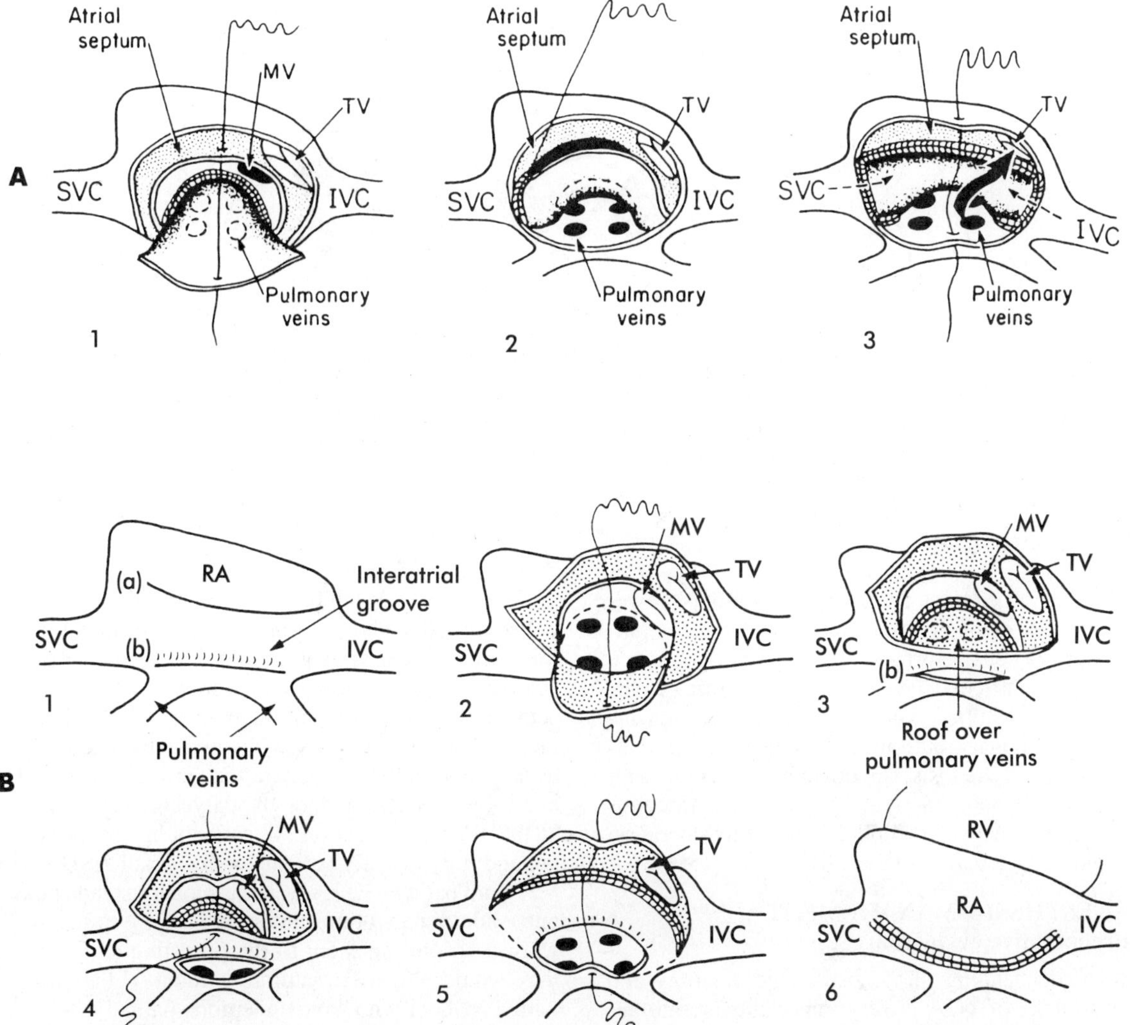


**Figure 20–8** Repair of transposition of great arteries at the atrial level. **A,** Mustard procedure. **B,** Senning's procedure. *SVC,* Superior vena cava; *MV,* mitral valve; *TV,* tricuspid valve; *IVC,* inferior vena cava; *RA,* right atrium; *RV,* right ventricle.

the VSD and the aortic valve. A prosthetic conduit or an aortic homograft is connected between the PA and RV (Fig. 20–9). Postoperative complications of the Rastelli operation are conduit narrowing and obstruction (frequent) and complete heart block (infrequent).

***Great arterial level operation***

*Jatene operation*. The anatomic correction of TGA by switching the great arteries and retransplanting the coronary arteries (Fig. 20–10) was proposed by Jatene in 1975.[13] This is the newest of the definitive procedures for TGA. In 1982 Jatene reported the successful use of this operation in infants and young children with TGA and a large VSD with high LV and PA pressures.[12] Successful anatomic repair of TGA in neonatal patients with intact ventricular septa has also been reported by other investigators.[4,20] In these patients, if the Jatene operation is delayed into the later part of infancy, one can expect postoperative LV failure with poor results. This is the result of an unprepared LV, as the LV pressures decrease in accordance with PVR during infancy. In view of this some surgeons perform the PA banding procedure in the neonatal period to prepare the LV for future anatomic repair. The growth of the heart and LV prepared to withstand high systemic pressures make this anatomic repair technically easier and excellent results more likely.

The advantages of this operation compared with

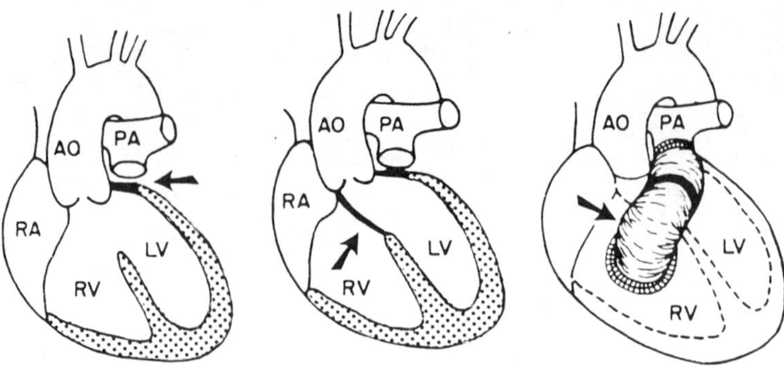


**Figure 20–9** Repair of transposition of great arteries at the ventricular level. External valved conduit reconstruction for transposition of the great vessels (Rastelli's procedure). *AO*, Aorta; *PA*, pulmonary artery; *RA*, right atrium; *RV*, right ventricle; *LV*, left ventricle. (From Park MK, ed: *Pediatric cardiology for practitioners*, St Louis, 1988, Mosby.)

the other procedures are fewer arrhythmias, fewer incidences of obstruction to the systemic or pulmonary venous return, and infrequent occurrence of right ventricular (systemic) dysfunction. Complications resulting from the Jatene operation include pulmonary outflow tract stenosis, supravalvular aortic stenosis, myocardial ischemia with ventricular dysfunction, and myocardial infarction. The most frequent complication of this operation is pulmonary outflow tract obstruction (15%).

## ANESTHESIA MANAGEMENT

### Preoperative evaluation

An understanding of the pathologic anatomy and physiology of TGA is very important for safe anesthetic management of these patients, as it is for any other CHD patient. In patients with most types of CHD, hypoxemia and cyanosis usually result from a right to left shunting of blood, and this may or may not be associated with an inadequate pulmonary blood flow. But in the majority of patients with TGA, hypoxemia and cyanosis are due to inadequate mixing of blood between right and left circulations. As a matter of fact, creation of a shunt between the two sides of the heart is absolutely necessary for survival and usually improves the oxygenation of the blood in children with TGA. Temporary improvement can usually be achieved by using prostaglandin $E_1$ infusion and creation of an ASD by balloon septostomy (Rashkind procedure). If this therapy fails to improve oxygenation, then patients come to the operating room either for an emergency Blalock-Hanlon atrial septectomy operation (palliative) or for a definitive operation at the atrial, ventricular, or great arterial level, depending on the underlying pathology.

The majority of the babies born with TGA have either normal or above normal weight at birth. Children with severe hypoxemia are prone to metabolic acidosis, hypoglycemia, and hypocalcemia. A recent analysis of arterial blood gases and electrolyte measurement in patients with severe hypoxemia, usually just before the operation, are essential to avoid hypotensive and/or hypoglycemic episodes at the time of induction. If patients are on prostaglandin $E_1$ (usually patients with a small ASD or VSD and patients with severe pulmonary stenosis), one should pay utmost attention to $E_1$ infusion while transporting them to the operating suite, as they would quickly desaturate without it. Patients with a VSD or who have undergone palliative surgery previously are usually not that hypoxemic when they return to undergo definitive surgery. However, children in this latter category may have a different problem. Their hematocrit may be in the 60% range. If the hematocrit is more than 65%, an exchange hemodilution may be necessary to avoid renal, hematologic, neurologic, and other complications.[9,14,15,17,28,35] Children with a big VSD may be in CHF and may come to the operating suite for a PA banding operation. Since these patients are usually treated with digoxin and a diuretic, checking electrolytes preoperatively is recommended. These children may not do well with a hematocrit less than 40%. Patients with a low hematocrit frequently develop signs of congestive heart failure as well as worsening of hypoxemia and acidosis.[5,22,25]

### Preoperative medication

Preoperative sedation in these patients depends on the age of the child and severity of the defect.

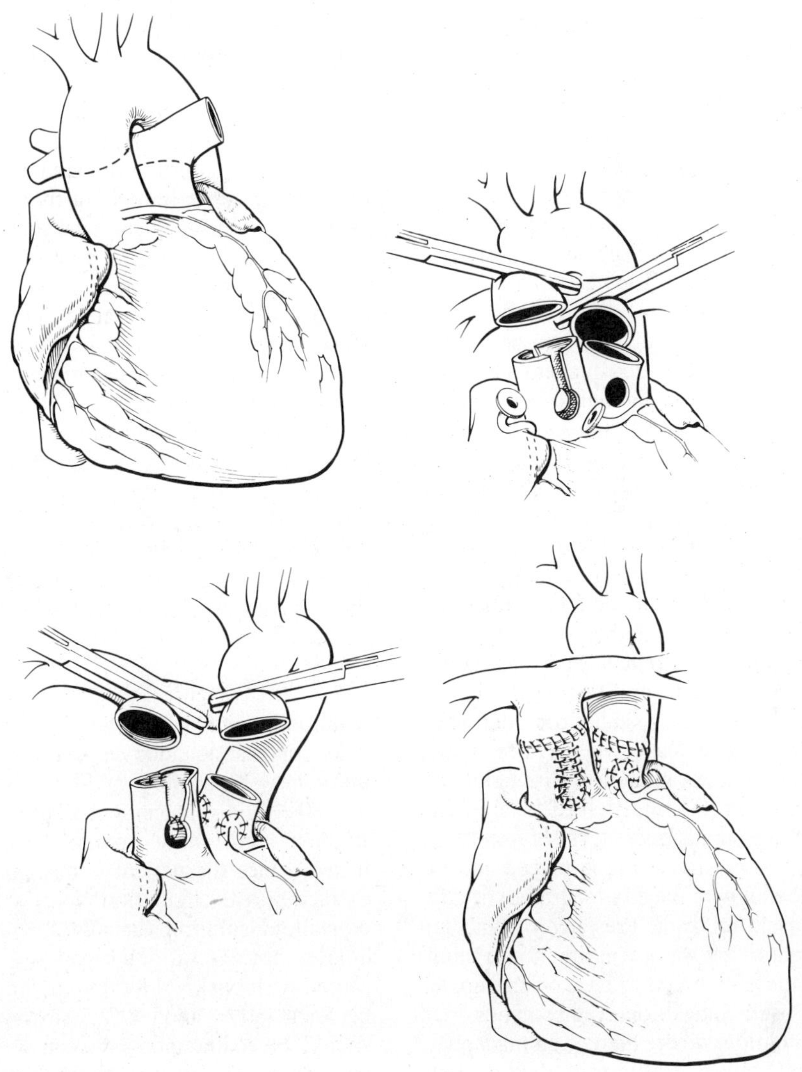

**Figure 20–10** Jatene operation: repair of transposition of great arteries at the level of great arteries (arterial switch).

Advantages of preoperative sedation include decrease or elimination of anxiety, reduction of oxygen demand, and avoidance of further hemodynamic deterioration. However, one should not oversedate these children, as hypoventilation will have detrimental effects on oxygen saturation and pulmonary blood flow.[6,7,33] Preoperative sedation should ideally be achieved in the holding room, where someone can watch for any undesirable side effects. A small dose of narcotic and a paralyzing dose of a neuromuscular blocker may be given to some, especially the ones on a ventilator and prostaglandin $E_1$, to facilitate a smooth transport from the ICU. Babies who later return for definitive surgery usually receive either oral benzodiazepine (midazolam 0.5 to 0.6 mg/kg) or an IM dose of morphine sulphate (0.1 to 0.15 mg/kg) or both preoperatively.

### Intraoperative monitoring

Monitoring of the children with TGA during surgery should include an ECG, invasive arterial pressure, noninvasive blood pressure, pulse oximeter, capnogram, temperature (esophageal and nasopharyngeal), central venous pressure, and urinometer. Arterial blood gases, serum glucose, calcium, potassium, and hematocrit are monitored frequently throughout the operation. Myocardial ischemia, ventricular dysfunction, and even frank myocardial infarction are sometimes associated with Jatene operation. One should therefore monitor for and treat these perioperative complications appropriately.

### Induction of anesthesia

Critically ill children usually arrive in the operating room with an IV line in place. In these children anesthesia can be induced either with small incremental doses of a narcotic (fentanyl 15 to 25 μg/kg or sufentanil 5 to 10 μg/kg) or an IV dose of ketamine (1 to 2 mg/kg) followed by a narcotic. Either a depolarizing (succinylcholine 2 mg/kg) or a nondepolarizing muscle relaxant can be used to facilitate the endotracheal tube placement. However, since acetylcholine is known to constrict the ductus, the use of succinylcholine is not recommended in ductus-dependent lesions. Since these patients' oxygen status is marginal to start with, it is absolutely necessary to make sure that the tracheal tube is not advanced too far down into one of the bronchi. Also, I routinely reintubate the trachea if the trachea has been intubated for more than 12 hours, as I have seen a number of endotracheal tubes gradually develop a mucus plug obstruction during the operation. If the child comes to the operating room without an IV (usually for a definitive operation), there are at least two ways to induce anesthesia, by slow mask induction with halothane (my choice) or by an IM injection of ketamine (4 to 6 mg/kg). Once an adequate level of anesthesia is achieved, an intravenous line is placed and the trachea is intubated with the administration of atropine and a muscle relaxant. Presence of both left to right and right to left shunts (bidirectional shunt) usually does not have much impact on the uptake of currently used inhalational anesthetics.[8,32,34] However, in situations where there is an inadequate mixing of blood between the two circulations, both the uptake and elimination of inhalational anesthetics will be much slower. Fortunately, the patients in this group usually come to the operating room with an IV line and with a prostaglandin $E_1$ infusion, and therefore their anesthesia can be induced with an intravenous agent.

### Maintenance

In view of the poor mixing of the blood between the two sides of the heart, it not only takes a long time to increase the blood concentration of an inhaled anesthetic, but it is also difficult to get the concentration decreased rapidly when desired. I recommend turning off the inhaled anesthetic once the trachea is intubated and an IV line is established. The desired level of anesthesia can be achieved by using additional doses of either fentanyl (up to a total dose of 100 μg/kg) or sufentanil (up to a total dose of 30 μg/kg) and a nondepolarizing muscle relaxant. If the operation is palliative (Blalock-Hanlon atrial septectomy, for example), the narcotic dose should be reduced (fentanyl 25 μg/kg or sufentanil 10 to 15 μg/kg). Vecuronium, pancuronium, atracurium, or one of the newer nondepolarizing muscle relaxants (doxacurium or pipecuronium) can be used to maintain muscle paralysis throughout the operation. In patients in whom deep hypothermia and circulatory arrest are used, I routinely give 10 ml/kg of dextran 40 in dextrose 5% solution intravenously before the initiation of peripheral cooling (see chapter 4). Heparin is usually given into the right atrium by the surgeon just before the placement of cannulas. Protamine is administered by the anesthesiologist at the conclusion of extracorporeal circulation following the removal of cannulas. The majority of patients require either an isoproterenol (0.01 to 0.05 μg/kg/min) or dopamine (3 to 6 μg/kg/min) infusion after coming off bypass. If there are signs of myocardial ischemia and ventricular dysfunction, use of nitroglycerin may be helpful for certain patients.

### Fluid and blood management

Minimal amount of crystalloid solutions should be used for maintenance in patients with increased pulmonary blood flow and CHF. For children not in CHF, fluid replacement should be about 5 ml/kg/hour until extracorporeal circulation is established. Once the patient is disconnected from the extracorporeal circulation along with maintenance crystalloid solution (usually 5% dextrose in one quarter normal saline) blood loss should be replaced with banked blood to maintain a hematocrit between 30% and 40%. However, hematocrit should be maintained between 45% and 55% in patients undergoing palliative surgery. Children who undergo a Jatene operation commonly require fresh blood and blood products (fresh frozen plasma and platelets) to control the suture line bleeding from the great arteries as well as the coronary arteries (abnormal coagulation related bleeding).

### Ventilation

Patients are mechanically ventilated to maintain a nearly normal carbon dioxide pressure. Addition of low levels of PEEP may be beneficial in patients with excessive pulmonary blood flow and CHF.

### General precautions

In all cases where there is a communication between the right and left sides of the heart, it is absolutely necessary that all intravenous lines be free of air bubbles. In addition, one should use extra caution not to introduce any air bubbles when injecting drugs through an IV line. Even though the use of nitrous oxide is not contraindicated in patients with TGA, many anesthesiologists avoid the use of it, especially once the chest is opened, for fear of intravascular air bubble expansion.

### Postoperative ventilation

Patients who undergo palliative surgery usually require short-term ventilatory support postoperatively. Patients who undergo definitive surgery are ventilated postoperatively for 1 or 2 days along with adequate narcotic administration for pain relief.

## REFERENCES


1. Benson LN, Olley PM, Patel RG et al: Role of prostaglandin $E_1$ infusion in the management of transposition of the great arteries, *Am J Cardiol* 44:691, 1979.
2. Blalock A, Hanlon CR: The surgical treatment of complete transposition of the aorta and the pulmonary artery, *Surg Gynecol Obstet* 90:1, 1950.
3. Campbell M: Incidence of cardiac malformations at birth and later, and neonatal mortality, *Br Heart J* 35:189, 1973.
4. Castenada AR, Norwood WI, Jonas RA et al: Transposition of the great arteries and intact ventricular septum: anatomic repair in the neonate, *Ann Thorac Surg* 38:438, 1984.
5. Cottrill CM, Kaplan S: Cerebral vascular accidents in cyanotic congenital heart disease, *Am J Dis Child* 125:484, 1973.
6. DeBock TL, Petrilli RL, Davis PJ et al: Effect of premedication on preoperative arterial oxygen saturation in children with congenital heart disease, *Anesthesiology* 67:A492, 1987 (abstract).
7. Edelman NH, Lahiri S, Braudo L et al: The blunted ventilatory response to hypoxia in cyanotic congenital heart disease, *N Engl J Med* 282:405, 1980.
8. Eiger EI: Uptake of inhaled anesthetics: the alveolar to inspired anesthetic difference: effect of ventilation/perfusion abnormalities. In Eiger EI, editor: *Anesthetic uptake and action,* Baltimore, 1974, Williams & Wilkins.
9. Gross S, Keffer V, Leibman J: The platelets in cyanotic congenital heart disease, *Pediatrics,* 42:651, 1968.
10. Heymann MA, Rudolph AM, Silverman NH: Closure of the ductus arteriosus in premature infants by inhibition of prostaglandin synthesis, *N Engl J Med* 295:530, 1976.
11. Hoffman JIE, Christianson R: Congenital heart disease in a cohort of 19,502 births with long-term follow-up, *Am J Cardiol* 42:641, 1978.
12. Jatene AD, Fontes VF, Souza LCB et al: Anatomic correction of transposition of the great arteries, *J Thorac Cardiovasc Surg* 83:20, 1982.
13. Jatene AD, Fontes VF, Paulista PP et al: Anatomic correction of transposition of the great vessels, *J Thorac Cardiovasc Surg* 72:364, 1976.
14. Komp DM, Sparrow AW: Polycythemia in cyanotic heart disease: a study of altered coagulation, *J Pediatr* 76:231, 1980.
15. Kontras SB, Bodenbender JG, Cranen J et al: Hyperviscosity in congenital heart disease, *J Pediatr* 76:214, 1970.
16. Lang P, Freed MD, Bierman FZ et al: Use of prostaglandin $E_1$ in infants with d-transposition of the great arteries and intact ventricular septum, *Am J Cardiol* 44:76, 1979.
17. Maurer HM, McCue CM, Robertson LW et al: Correction of platelet dysfunction and bleeding in cyanotic congenital heart disease by simple red cell volume reduction, *Am J Cardiol* 35:831, 1975.
18. Mitchell SC, Korones SB, Berendes HW: Congenital heart disease in 56,109 births: incidence and natural history, *Circulation* 43:323, 1971.
19. Muller WH, Dammann JR Jr: The treatment of certain congenital malformations of the heart by the creation of pulmonic stenosis to reduce pulmonary hypertension and excessive pulmonary blood flow: a preliminary report, *Surg Gynecol Obstet* 95:213, 1952.
20. Murphy ME, Aglira BA, Chin AJ et al: Two-dimensional and Doppler echocardiographic assessment of transposition of the great arteries following neonatal anatomic correction (Jatene operation), *Circulation* 72:345, 1985.
21. Mustard WT: Successful two-stage correction of transposition of the great vessels, *Surgery* 55:469, 1964.
22. Newburger JW, Sibert AR, Buckley LP et al: Cognitive function and age at repair of transposition of the great arteries in children, *N Engl J Med* 310:1495, 1984.
23. Olley PM, Coceani F, Bodach E: E-type prostaglandins: a new emergency therapy for certain cyanotic heart malformations, *Circulation* 53:728, 1976.
24. Park SC, Zuberbuhler JR, Neeches WH et al: A new atrial septostomy technique, *Cathet Cardiovasc Diagn* 1:195, 1975.
25. Phornphutkul C, Rosenthal A, Nadas AS et al: Cerebrovascular accidents in infants and children with cyanotic congenital heart disease, *Am J Cardiol* 32:329, 1973.
26. Quaegebeur JM, Rohmer J, Brom AG et al: Revival of the Senning operation in the treatment of transposition of the great arteries, *Thorax* 32:517, 1977.
27. Rashkind WJ, Miller WW: Creation of an atrial septal defect without thoractomy: a palliative approach to complete transposition of the great arteries, *JAMA* 196:991, 1966.
28. Rosenthal A, Nathan DG, Marty AT et al: Acute hemodynamic effects or red cell volume reduction in polycythemia of cyanotic congenital heart disease, *Circulation* 42:297, 1970.
29. Senning A: Surgical correction of transposition of the great vessels, *Surgery* 45:966, 1959.
30. Sharpe GL, Larsson KS: Studies on closure of the ductus arteriosus X; in vivo effects of prostaglandins, *Prostaglandins* 9:703-709, 1975.
31. Starling MB, Elliott RB: The effects of prostaglandins, prostaglandin inhibitors, and oxygen on the closure of the ductus arteriosus, pulmonary arteries, and umbilical vessels in vitro, *Prostaglandins* 8:187, 1974.
32. Stoelting R, Longnecker DE: Effect of right-to-left shunt on rate of increase in arterial anesthetic concentration, *Anesthesiology* 365:352, 1972.
33. Stow PJ, Burrows FA, Lerman J et al: Arterial oxygen saturation following premedication in children with cyanotic congenital heart disease, *Can J Anaesth* 35:63, 1988.
34. Tanner GE, Angers DG, Barash PG et al: Effect of left-to-right, mixed right-to-left, and right-to-left shunts on inhalational anesthetic induction in children: a computer model, *Anesth Analg* 64:101-107, 1985.
35. Wells R: Syndrome of hyperviscosity, *N Engl J Med* 283:183, 1980.

# 21 Anomalous Pulmonary Venous Connection

*James Johns, Walter Merrill, and Jay Kambam*



Total anomalous pulmonary venous connection (TAPVC) is a congenital abnormality in which all the pulmonary veins drain to the right atrium, either directly or via systemic veins, and there is no direct connection between the pulmonary veins and the left atrium. In partial anomalous pulmonary venous connection one or more pulmonary veins drain to the right atrium and some pulmonary veins drain normally to the left atrium. Despite the similarity of the names of these lesions, their clinical presentation and management are quite different. Partial anomalous pulmonary venous connection is usually but not always associated with an atrial septal defect, and its hemodynamic effects are virtually indistinguishable from those of an atrial septal defect. Anesthetic management of patients with partial anomalous venous connection is nearly the same as that for patients with atrial septal defects, and thus only total anomalous pulmonary venous connection will be considered in this chapter.

TAPVC is a relatively uncommon form of congenital heart disease, accounting for approximately 2% to 3% of congenital heart disease presenting in infancy. Overall TAPVC occurs in about 1 of 15,000 live births.[2] TAPVC is generally an isolated abnormality, but it may be part of one of the heterotaxy syndromes (abnormal sidedness, or situs ambiguus), usually asplenia[1] (bilateral right-sidedness). Without treatment TAPVC is generally fatal in the first year of life. Muller[6] successfully repaired TAPVC in 1951, but it was not until the 1970s that successful repair in infancy became common.

## EMBRYOLOGY

In normal development the pulmonary veins develop as part of a vascular plexus from the developing lungs, and the veins form a confluence posterior to what will become the left atrium.[1,5] Eventually the pulmonary venous confluence will join the left atrium, becoming the posterior wall of the left atrium. Prior to the joining of the pulmonary venous confluence with the left atrium, the blood leaving the lungs returns to the heart via the connections between the pulmonary venous system and the umbilicovitelline and cardinal veins. After the pulmonary venous confluence joins the left atrium, the pulmonary to systemic venous connections normally involute.

In a total anomalous pulmonary venous connection the pulmonary venous confluence fails to join the posterior portion of the left atrium. Instead, the normal embryologic connections between the pulmonary venous system and the systemic venous system persist. Indeed, the "anomalous" connections in TAPVC are not in fact anomalous but rather are normal connections that abnormally persist throughout fetal development.[1] The primary defect in TAPVC is the failure of the confluence of pulmonary veins to join the left atrium.[5]

In some cases the connection between the pulmonary venous confluence and the true left atrium may be stenotic, resulting in a proximal and a distal portion of the left atrium separated by a membrane with a restrictive opening. Because this phenomenon gives the appearance of three atria, this abnormality is known as cor triatriatum. In cor triatriatum as well as in TAPVC there may be persistence of some of the pulmonary to systemic venous connections, resulting in mixed types of pulmonary venous drainage.[14]

## ANATOMY

There are several types of TAPVC, depending largely on the sites of connections between the pulmonary venous confluence and the systemic venous system.[1,2,5] In approximately a third to half of patients with TAPVC, the persistent connection is between the pulmonary venous confluence and a left-sided vertical vein that joins the left innominate vein. The vertical vein is the remnant of the left anterior cardinal vein. Since the flow of blood in this instance is up the vertical vein to the innominate vein to the superior vena cava, these patients are said to have supracardiac TAPVC. In a quarter to a third of patients the persistent connection drains to the right atrium directly or through the coronary sinus (cardiac TAPVC). In the remaining quarter to a third of patients the connection is through the remnant of the umbilicovitelline system, with pulmonary venous blood going below the diaphragm to the portal or hepatic venous system and returning to the right atrium via the inferior vena cava (infradiaphragmatic TAPVC). In all these types of TAPVC there is generally a confluence of pulmonary veins into which all the pulmonary veins drain. Less commonly there may be several sites of connection between the pulmonary and systemic venous systems, and in these patients there may not be a well-developed confluence of pulmonary veins (Fig. 21–1).

In many patients with TAPVC there is obstruction to the pulmonary venous return to the heart. In supracardiac TAPVC obstruction is seen in about half of patients, most commonly at the junction of the vertical and innominate veins, where the vertical vein passes between the left pulmonary artery and the left main stem bronchus, or at the junction of the pulmonary venous confluence and the vertical vein. The pulmonary venous return in cardiac TAPVC is generally not obstructed. Virtually all patients with infracardiac TAPVC have obstruction at the level of the diaphragm, within the liver, or at the ductus venosus as it closes. In any of the types of TAPVC there may be obstruction at the level of the atrial septum.

In utero the fetal lungs normally receive approximately 5% to 10% of the combined ventricular output, and thus pulmonary venous return accounts for approximately 5% to 10% of the total venous return to the heart.[9] In TAPVC, since the left atrium and left ventricle do not receive the pulmonary venous return, they are often somewhat smaller than normal.

## PATHOPHYSIOLOGY

TAPVC is a complete mixing lesion: all the systemic and pulmonary venous blood must traverse the right atrium before entering the right or left ventricle. As in all patients with complete mixing lesions (TAPVC, tricuspid atresia, mitral atresia, pulmonary atresia, aortic atresia, single ventricle, truncus arteriosus, etc.), there is some degree of desaturation. Even a small amount of systemic venous blood going out the aorta will result in a

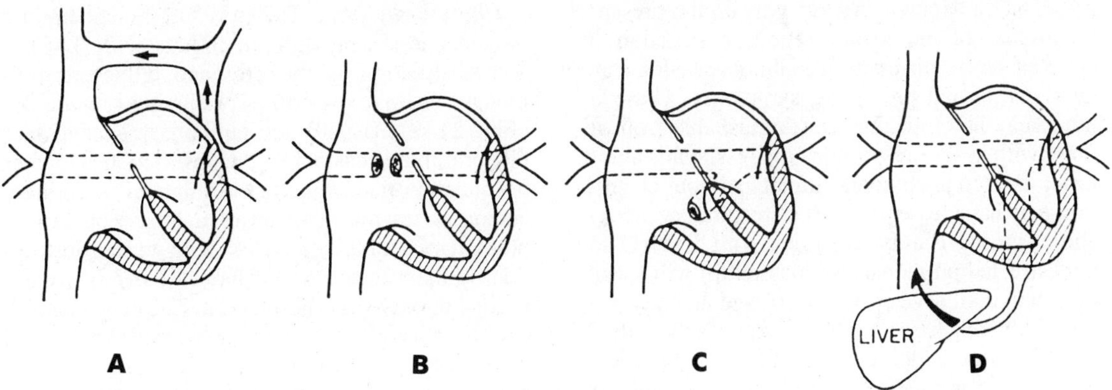


**Figure 21–1** Four types of TAPVC. **A,** Common pulmonary vein → vertical vein → innominate vein → superior vena cava → right atrium. **B,** Pulmonary veins → right atrium. **C,** Common pulmonary vein → coronary sinus → right atrium. **D,** Common pulmonary vein → portal vein → ductus venosus → inferior vena cava → right atrium.

decrease in the arterial $Po_2$. The degree of cyanosis with any complete mixing lesion depends on the relative amounts of pulmonary and systemic flow. If there is unrestricted pulmonary flow (such as in truncus arteriosus or single ventricle without pulmonic stenosis), a large amount of pulmonary venous blood with a high oxygen saturation will mix with a smaller amount of systemic venous blood with a low oxygen saturation, resulting in only mild cyanosis. In contrast, in lesions with decreased pulmonary flow (such as pulmonary atresia), there will be only a small amount of oxygenated blood mixing with the systemic venous blood, and the resulting mixture will have a very low oxygen saturation.

In patients with TAPVC the degree of cyanosis depends on whether there is obstruction to the pulmonary venous flow. Obstruction of the pulmonary venous return will result in limitation of pulmonary flow and therefore increased cyanosis. Furthermore, if there is obstruction the pulmonary capillary pressure will be increased, resulting in severe pulmonary edema. If there is no obstruction of the pulmonary venous return, there may be excessive pulmonary flow, which increases as pulmonary vascular resistance falls in the postnatal period, sometimes to several times the systemic flow.

Since the pulmonary veins do not enter the left atrium in TAPVC, all the blood entering the left ventricle must cross the atrial septum from the right atrium to the left atrium, usually across a patent foramen ovale. If the foramen ovale is restrictive, there will be limitation of flow into the left ventricle and therefore decreased left ventricular output. In such cases there may be decreased systemic perfusion, hypotension, shock, or acidosis.

## CLINICAL PRESENTATION

Patients with TAPVC usually become symptomatic within the first few hours or days of life. Their presentation depends in large part on the presence or absence of pulmonary venous obstruction. In cases of severe obstruction, pulmonary edema and cyanosis are the presenting symptoms. These infants may be clinically indistinguishable from infants with severe respiratory distress syndrome or group B strep pneumonia. Infants without obstruction may have lesser degrees of respiratory distress and cyanosis. Rarely, an infant with TAPVC and unobstructed pulmonary venous return will escape detection until several months of age and then present with congestive heart failure. Infants with restrictive atrial septal defects and a closing ductus will present with shock, poor perfusion, and acidosis. Fyler[2] and Lucas and Krabill[5] discuss clinical findings in TAPVC in more detail.

### Laboratory findings

***Physical examination.*** The physical signs of TAPVC are nonspecific. The general examination is usually remarkable for respiratory distress with grunting, retracting, and cyanosis. On cardiac examination the right ventricular impulse may be increased, and the intensity of the pulmonary component may be increased as well. However, these findings are often present in sick neonates without cardiac disease. There may be increased splitting of the second heart sound as a result of the increased right ventricular stroke volume as compared with the left. There often is no murmur; if a murmur is present, it is usually systolic. Patients with unobstructed pulmonary venous flow may additionally have a diastolic rumble from the increased flow across the tricuspid valve. Hepatomegaly is common. Since the clinical signs of TAPVC are generally nonspecific, it is essential that physicians caring for neonates consider TAPVC in the differential diagnosis of cyanotic infants with severe pulmonary edema.

***Arterial blood gases.*** Arterial blood gases on 100% inspired oxygen can be helpful in distinguishing pulmonary disease from cyanotic congenital heart disease, including TAPVC. If the arterial $Po_2$ on 100% oxygen is greater than 200 torr, then it is very unlikely that there is an intracardiac right to left shunt. Occasionally it may be possible to obtain an arterial $Po_2$ of 100 to 150 torr in patients with TAPVC because of streaming of oxygenated blood, but in general the $Po_2$ is less than 100 torr even on 100% oxygen in any patient with intracardiac right to left shunting.

***Electrocardiogram.*** As with the physical findings, the ECG findings of TAPVC are nonspecific. Right ventricular hypertrophy is almost always present, and right atrial enlargement is commonly seen.

***Chest x-ray film.*** The most prominent finding on the chest x-ray film in infants with TAPVC and obstruction is the presence of severe pulmonary edema, sometimes producing a white-out (Fig. 21–2). Usually the pulmonary changes are bilateral, but occasionally the obstruction is greater on one side than the other. Unilateral pulmonary edema raises the question of a mixed pattern of pulmonary venous connection with greater obstruction on the affected side. The heart size is usually normal or only slightly enlarged. The classic snowman heart (with the head representing the vertical vein, innominate vein, and SVC, and the body representing the rest of the heart) is seen only in patients with supracardiac TAPVC, and even then is not seen in infancy. The presence of bilateral

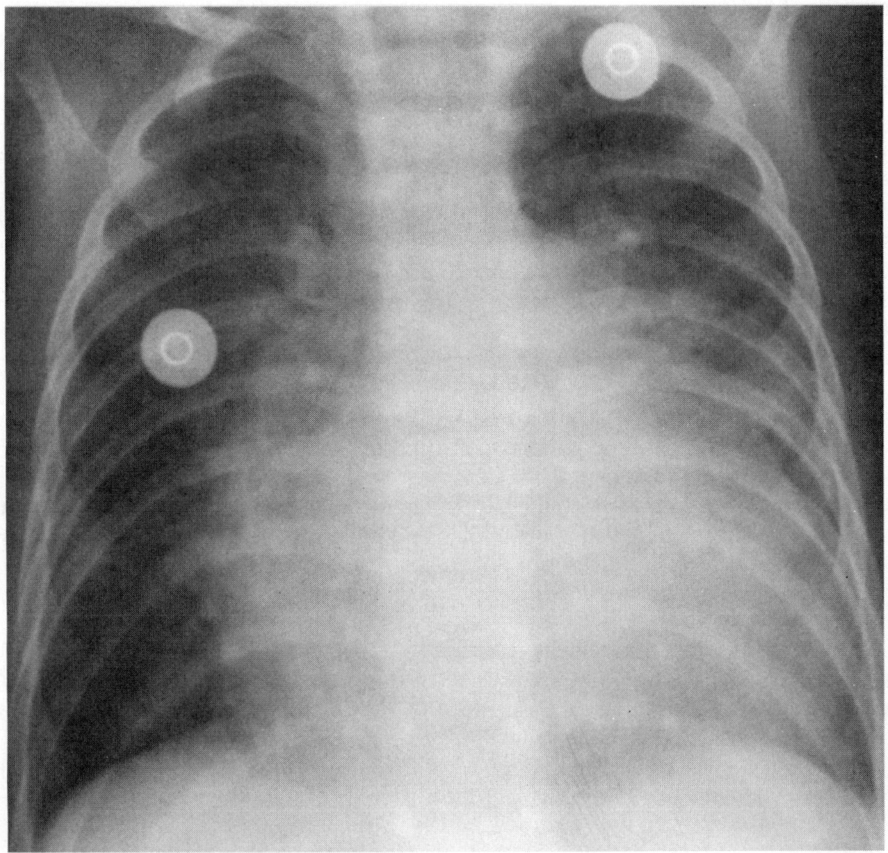

**Figure 21–2** Anteroposterior chest radiograph of a 2-month-old cyanotic infant with total anomalous pulmonary venous connection. Severe cardiomegaly, congestive failure, and a large main pulmonary artery segment are the important features. (Courtesy of Sandra G. Kirchner, MD.)

right bronchial morphology (eparterial bronchi) should raise the question of asplenia, in which TAPVC is often associated with pulmonary atresia.

***Echocardiography.*** Echocardiography is the mainstay of diagnosing TAPVC.[12,13] In patients with TAPVC the pulmonary venous confluence can usually be seen behind the left atrium, and the pulmonary veins are not seen entering the left atrium directly. Color Doppler flow mapping can be very helpful in tracing the connection of the pulmonary venous confluence up to the innominate vein, down below the diaphragm, or to the right atrium via the coronary sinus. Sites of obstruction can sometimes be detected by the increase in flow velocity downstream of the obstruction. It is important to try to visualize all the pulmonary veins entering the pulmonary venous confluence to exclude the possibility of mixed pulmonary venous drainage. In TAPVC the left atrium and left ventricle are commonly smaller than normal because of the decreased venous return to the left side of the heart. There should be right to left flow across the atrial septal defect or patent foramen ovale in patients with TAPVC. A net left to right flow across the atrial septum precludes the possibility of TAPVC, although one must be careful not to mistake SVC flow for a left to right atrial shunt.

With echocardiography it is often possible to obtain all the required preoperative data in a patient with TAPVC, thus avoiding the need for preoperative cardiac catheterization.

***Cardiac catheterization.*** If there is uncertainty about the diagnosis of TAPVC, the site of pulmonary venous drainage, or associated lesions, cardiac catheterization may be indicated. Although the infants in question are often very sick, with appropriate attention to acid-base status, ventilation, hemodynamics and temperature stability, they can be catheterized with a low risk of morbidity or mortality. It should be recognized, however, that many infants with TAPVC do not require catheterization prior to repair.

Oximetry provides very useful data in patients with TAPVC. The characteristic finding of TAPVC is the presence of a high oxygen saturation in the right atrium (Fig. 21–3). In the case of supracardiac TAPVC the SVC saturation is usually high, and in infradiaphragmatic TAPVC the IVC saturation is usually high. In patients with obstructed TAPVC there may be sufficient pulmonary edema to decrease the pulmonary venous saturation, so that oximetry may not help find the abnormal pulmonary venous connection. If an umbilical venous catheter is present, right atrial saturations may be obtained without a trip to the catheterization laboratory. High saturations suggest either an anomalous pulmonary venous connection or that the tip of the catheter has passed across the foramen ovale to the left atrium. Typically in TAPVC the saturations in all four chambers of the heart are approximately equal, owing to the complete mixing in the right atrium.

Catheterization pressure measurements are often not very helpful in patients with TAPVC. Right ventricular and pulmonary artery pressures are usually elevated, especially in patients with obstructed pulmonary venous connection. Occasionally in patients without obstruction the pulmonary artery pressures are only slightly elevated. Right atrial pressure may be elevated, and in the presence of a restrictive atrial communication there will be a pressure gradient from the right atrium to the left atrium. It may be possible to measure the pressure in the pulmonary venous confluence directly and by performing a pull-back pressure measurement from the pulmonary vein to the right atrium to determine the site of obstruction, if present.

Angiography can help delineate the anatomy of the abnormal pulmonary venous connection in patients with TAPVC. A pulmonary arteriogram with a balloon catheter occluding the ductus arteriosus allows visualization of the pulmonary venous flow and connections. In patients with supracardiac or cardiac TAPVC it is sometimes possible to pass an angiographic catheter from the right atrium or SVC into the pulmonary venous confluence and to perform a pulmonary venogram showing the anomalous pulmonary venous connections.

## MEDICAL MANAGEMENT

The initial step in the management of infants with TAPVC is stabilization. Infants with obstructed pulmonary veins often require intubation and ventilation with high airway pressures and high ventilatory rates because of severe pulmonary edema.

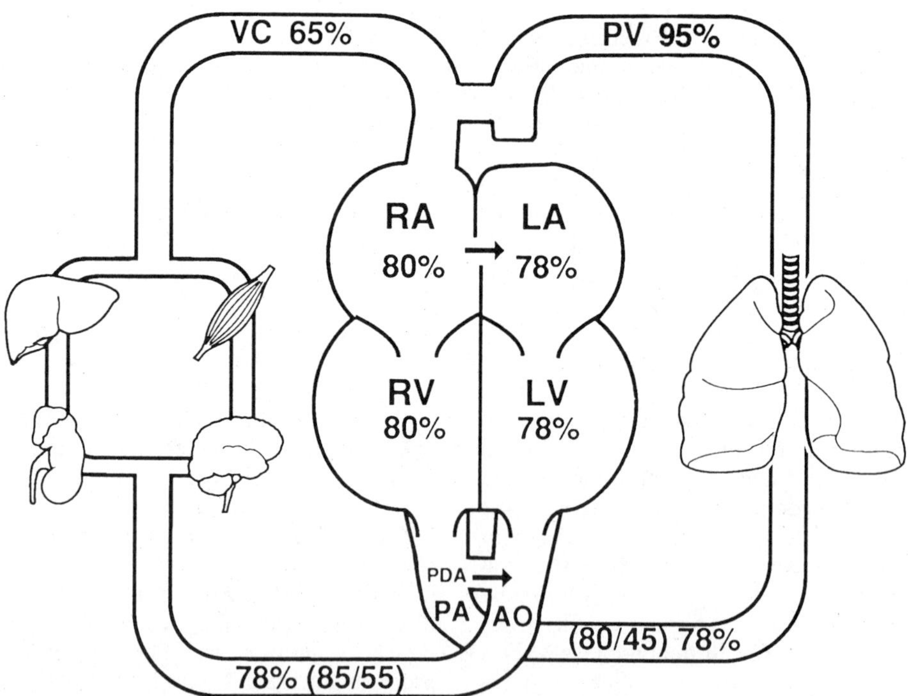


**Figure 21–3** Typical oxygen saturation findings in a case of TAPVC. *VC*, Vena cava; *PV*, pulmonary vein; *RA*, right atrium; *LA*, left artery; *RV*, right ventricle; *LV*, left ventricle; *PDA*, patent ductus arteriosus; *PA*, pulmonary artery; *AO*, aorta.

Once the diagnosis is made, the definitive therapy is surgical repair. There is little role for medical management in infants with TAPVC, except as needed to stabilize the infant while the diagnosis is made by echocardiography and/or catheterization and while preparations are made for surgical repair.

Prostaglandin $E_1$ infusion may have several beneficial effects in patients with TAPVC. In patients with restrictive atrial communications and decreased left ventricular output, the presence of a patent ductus arteriosus will allow the right ventricle to pump blood to the systemic circulation. Since there is complete mixing, the oxygen saturation of the blood pumped by the right ventricle is very similar to that pumped by the left ventricle. In patients with infradiaphragmatic TAPVC prostaglandin $E_1$ may also help maintain patency of the ductus venosus,[7] thus reducing obstruction of the pulmonary venous flow to the IVC and right atrium. Finally, prostaglandin $E_1$ may have beneficial effects on pulmonary vascular resistance. The usual starting dose of prostaglandin $E_1$ is 0.05 μg/kg/min.

Patients with TAPVC are at risk for pulmonary hypertensive crises preoperatively and postoperatively.[4,8] If pulmonary vascular resistance rises, the pulmonary flow will decrease, resulting in increasing cyanosis and acidosis, which may cause a further increase in pulmonary vascular resistance. Hyperventilation, sedation, and the use of pulmonary vasodilators such as oxygen and prostaglandin may help avoid or abort this vicious cycle.

## SURGICAL MANAGEMENT

Repair of TAPVC in infancy is generally performed with deep hypothermia and circulatory arrest,[3,8,10] although some surgeons prefer to use continuous low-flow perfusion.[4,11,15] In patients with cardiac TAPVC via the coronary sinus, the repair is accomplished by enlarging the os of the coronary sinus by cutting back into the atrial septal defect and by placing a pericardial baffle directing all the coronary sinus flow across the ASD to the left atrium. In patients with supracardiac or infradiaphragmatic TAPVC, the surgical approach is to perform as large an incision as possible in the pulmonary venous confluence, to create a corresponding incision in the back of the left atrium, and to create as large an anastomosis as possible. Sometimes enlargement of the left atrium by enlarging the atrial septal defect and repositioning the atrial septum to the right with a pericardial patch is necessary. The ascending vertical vein is always ligated above the orifice of the left superior pulmonary vein. The descending vertical vein may be ligated or left alone (Fig. 21–4). Early mortality is in the range of 3% to 20%, with much of the mortality occurring because of low cardiac output or pulmonary hypertensive crises.[3,4,8,10,11,15] Late surgical results are generally good, although there have been reports of subsequent pulmonary venous obstruction and arrhythmias.[3,10,11,15]

## ANESTHESIA MANAGEMENT

An understanding of pathologic anatomy and physiology and of the pharmacology of various drugs that may alter the systemic and pulmonary blood flows is essential in managing patients with a functioning communication between the two sides of the heart. TAPVC is a complete mixing congenital cardiac lesion. Special problems one may encounter in a patient with TAPVC include increased pulmonary blood flow with pulmonary edema (unobstructed type), increased pulmonary capillary pressure and pulmonary edema (obstructed type), and systemic hypoperfusion with hypoxemia and acidosis. As with other cyanotic cardiac lesions,

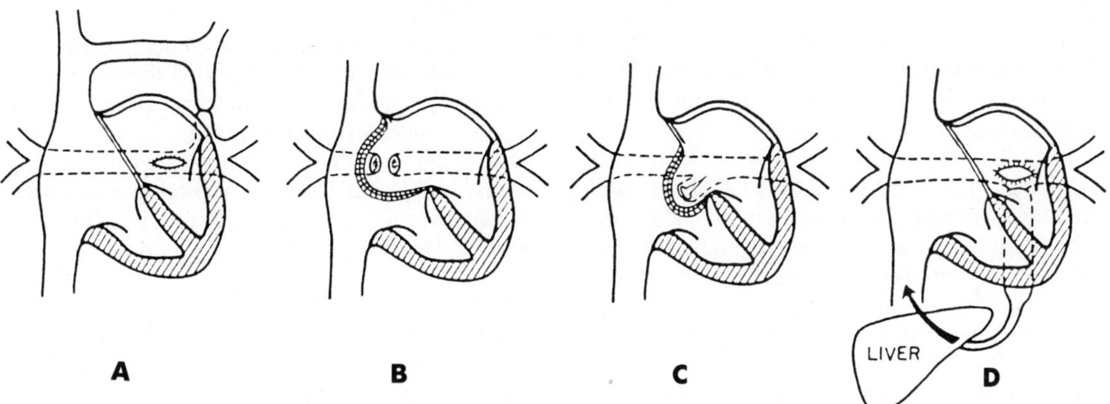


**Figure 21–4** Surgical correction of TAPVC: **A-D,** refer to Fig. 21–1.

the degree of systemic oxygen saturation is directly related to the patient's pulmonary blood flow. Thus, with decreased pulmonary flow cyanosis is present, and with increased pulmonary flow the patient develops congestive heart failure. If patient is receiving prostaglandin $E_1$ infusion to maintain the patency of ductus arteriosus and/or ductus venosus, one should pay utmost attention to this infusion. Accidental stoppage could lead to rapid deterioration of the child's condition.

### Preoperative assessment

Preoperative evaluation of a patient with TAPVC should include a thorough history, including present medications and physical examination; laboratory tests including chest x-ray film, ECG, echocardiogram and/or catheterization data, hemoglobin, glucose, and electrolyte levels; and a pediatric cardiologist's consult note. Children with TAPVC usually have various degrees of pulmonary edema and decreased lung compliance.

### Premedication

Preoperative medication is given according to the age of the patient and severity of the cardiac lesion. In general, preoperative sedation can be omitted in children undergoing correction of TAPVC who are under 6 months of age.

### Monitoring

Monitoring of a child with TAPVC during surgery involves an ECG, invasive arterial pressure, noninvasive blood pressure, pulse oximeter, capnogram, body temperature (esophageal and nasopharyngeal), central venous pressure, and urinometer. Left atrial pressure monitoring is useful in the majority of cases. Arterial blood gases, serum calcium and potassium, and hematocrit levels should be frequently monitored throughout the perioperative period.

### Induction

Almost all patients with TAPVC come to the operating room with an intravenous catheter in place. In these patients anesthesia can be induced with intravenous narcotic (fentanyl 10 to 20 μg/kg, sufentanil 2 to 3 μg/kg), and/or 1 to 2 mg/kg of ketamine. Theoretically a right to left shunt should slightly accelerate the onset of intravenous anesthetics. However, in mixed shunts there may be a diminished overall effect of right to left shunt on the onset of anesthetic action. There are really no clinical data to support or contradict this theory. Tracheal intubation can be performed with either succinylcholine or a nondepolarizing muscle relaxant. However, we recommend avoiding succinylcholine in children if patency of ductus arteriosus and/or ductus venosus is essential for hemodynamic stability (see Chapter 14). Atropine 5 to 10 μg/kg should be given prior to succinylcholine (1 to 2 mg/kg IV). An arterial cannula and a central venous catheter are usually inserted after the airway is secured.

### Maintenance

Anesthesia is usually maintained with an IV narcotic (fentanyl 50 to 100 μg/kg or sufentanil 15 to 20 μg/kg) in these patients. Vecuronium or one of the newer nondepolarizing muscle relaxants (doxacurium or pipecuronium) can be used to maintain muscle paralysis throughout the operation.

One should closely watch the administration of intravenous fluids in these patients, and only minimal amounts of fluids should be used.

If deep hypothermia and circulatory arrest are planned, we administer 10 ml/kg of dextran 40 in 5% dextrose solution before peripheral cooling is initiated (see Chapter 4 for complete details of deep hypothermia).

Heparin is usually injected into the right atrium by the surgeon just before the placement of cannulas. Protamine is administered by the anesthesiologist at the conclusion of extracorporeal circulation following the removal of cardiac cannulas. The majority of patients require infusion of either dopamine (3 to 6 μg/kg/min) or dobutamine (3 to 6 μg/kg/min) during the perioperative period.

Since the majority of patients with TAPVC have decreased lung compliance with pulmonary congestion, they may benefit from mechanical ventilation with high airway pressures and from hyperventilation. Since systemic perfusion and oxygenation are compromised in these patients, one should keep systemic vascular resistance on the normal to low side.

### Precautions

In all cases where there is a communication between the right and left sides of the heart, it is absolutely necessary that all intravenous lines be free of air bubbles. In addition one should use extra caution not to push any air bubbles when injecting drugs through an IV line. Appropriate antibiotic prophylaxis is also required for patients with TAPVC (see Chapter 6).

### Postoperative ventilation

Patients with TAPVC are usually left intubated and mechanically ventilated postoperatively. Once the patient is awake, stable, and rewarmed to a normal body temperature, the trachea can be extubated in the cardiac recovery room.

## REFERENCES


1. Delisle G, Ando M, Calder AL et al: Total anomalous pulmonary venous connection: report of 93 autopsied cases with emphasis on diagnostic and surgical considerations, *Am Heart J* 91:99, 1976.
2. Fyler DC: Total anomalous pulmonary venous return. In Fyler DC, editor: *Nadas' pediatric cardiology,* Philadelphia, 1992, Hanley & Belfus.
3. Lamb RK, Qureshi SA, Wilkinson JL et al: Total anomalous pulmonary venous drainage: 17-year surgical experience, *J Thorac Cardiovasc Surg* 96:368, 1988.
4. Lincoln CR, Rigby ML, Mercanti C et al: Surgical risk factors in total anomalous pulmonary venous connection, *Am J Cardiol* 61:608, 1988.
5. Lucas RV, Krabill KA: Anomalous venous connections, pulmonary and systemic. In Adams GA, Emmanouilides GC, Riemenschneider TA, editors: *Moss' heart disease in infants, children and adolescents,* Baltimore, 1989, Williams & Wilkins.
6. Muller WH: The surgical treatment of transposition of the pulmonary veins, *Ann Surg* 134:683, 1951.
7. Morin FC: Prostaglandin $E_1$ opens the ductus venosus in the newborn lamb, *Pediatr Res* 21:225, 1987.
8. Raisher BD, Grant JW, Martin TC et al: Complete repair of total anomalous pulmonary venous connection in infancy, *J Thorac Cardiovasc Surg* 104:443, 1992.
9. Rudolph AM: *Congenital diseases of the heart,* Chicago, 1974, Mosby.
10. Sano S, Brawn WJ, Mee RBB: Total anomalous pulmonary venous drainage, *J Thorac Cardiovasc Surg* 97:886, 1989.
11. Serraf A, Bruniaux J, Lacour-Gayet F et al: Obstructed total anomalous pulmonary venous return, *J Thorac Cardiovasc Surg* 101:601, 1991.
12. Snider AR, Serwer GA: *Echocardiography in pediatric heart disease,* Chicago, 1990, Mosby.
13. Van der Velde ME, Parness IA, Colan SD et al: Two-dimensional echocardiography in the pre- and postoperative management of totally anomalous pulmonary venous connection, *J Am Coll Cardiol* 18:1746, 1991.
14. Van Praagh R, Corsini I: Cor triatriatum: pathologic anatomy and a consideration of morphogenesis based on 13 postmortem cases and a study of normal development of the pulmonary vein and atrial septum in 83 human embryos, *Am Heart J* 78:379, 1969.
15. Wilson WR, Ilbawi MN, DeLeon SY et al: Technical modifications for improved results in total anomalous pulmonary venous drainage, *J Thorac Cardiovasc Surg* 103:861, 1992.

# 22 Pulmonary Atresia with Intact Ventricular Septum

*Volker Striepe*



Pulmonary atresia with an intact ventricular septum is an uncommon congenital abnormality, affecting about 1% to 3% of patients with congenital heart disease. This abnormality was first reported in 1783 by Hunter. It affects 30% of patients with cyanotic heart disease and is a frequent cause of cyanosis and death in the neonatal period.[14,23]

In the patient with this abnormality, pulmonary blood flow is dependent upon patency of the ductus arteriosus, and death commonly follows functional ductal closure. Therefore, early intervention is required. Despite surgery only one in four patients survive their first year of life. As with other types of congenital heart disease, this disorder is thought to be familial and multifactorially determined, although a recent report suggests an autosomal recessive inheritance.[5,11]

## EMBRYOLOGY

The semilunar valves form from small tubercles found on the main truncus swellings. They are visible when the truncus partitioning is nearly complete (16 mm embryo). Two pairs of these tubercles form the pulmonary and aortic valves, respectively. These tubercles gradually hollow out on their upper surfaces, thereby forming the semilunar valves by the time the embryo has reached the 40 mm stage.

In pulmonary atresia the valve remains fused and may form a dome-shaped structure without an opening or a horizontal fibrous plate.[23] The pulmonary trunk may be narrow or atretic, and the only outlet from the right heart will then be a patent foramen ovale. A patent ductus arteriosus forms the path of blood to the pulmonary circulation.

In the most common type of this disorder the right ventricle is hypoplastic with a muscular right ventricle and a stenotic or atretic pulmonary valve (type I of the Greenwold classification). A rarer type has a thin and flabby right ventricular wall (type II). The development of sinusoidal ventriculocoronary communications is discussed in the next section.

## PATHOLOGIC ANATOMY

The pulmonary valve is atretic; an atrial septal defect and a patent ductus arteriosus are usually present (Fig. 22–1). Variable degrees of right ventricular and pulmonary artery hypoplasia as well as tricuspid abnormalities are seen.

Despite its name this condition is largely a disorder dictated in its prognosis by the accompanying abnormalities of the right ventricular structures rather than the pulmonary valve itself.

There is usually moderate cardiomegaly, predominantly due to right atrial enlargement. With extreme enlargement the right atrium may almost fill the right hemithorax, compressing the right lung. The great vessels are usually normally related.

### Atrial septum

An atrial septal defect, which is common, is of the secundum type in 20% of patients.[15] The atrial septal defect may be severely restrictive in 5% to 10% of cases. An intact atrial septum has been reported and was associated with a rare coronary sinus atrial fenestration.[14,33]

### Tricuspid valve

The most common tricuspid abnormality is stenosis, with some degree of dysplasia usually evident. A parachute deformity has been described.[14] Some present with combined stenosis and regurgitation. Free regurgitation only is rarely present. In rare instances the right ventricle and the tricuspid valve are normal.

### Right ventricle

The right ventricle also presents a broad range in the degree of its deformity.[34] Greenwold and associates[19] classified the condition into two broad groups:

1. Those with small right ventricular cavities
2. Those with normal size or dilated right ventricular cavities

Approximately 75% fall into type 1. It is now generally considered that this classification is a gross simplification in that ventricular cavity sizes present a broad spectrum and may actually grow.[18,33,34]

Goor and Lillehei[17] described the tripartite concept of ventricular organization. They described a

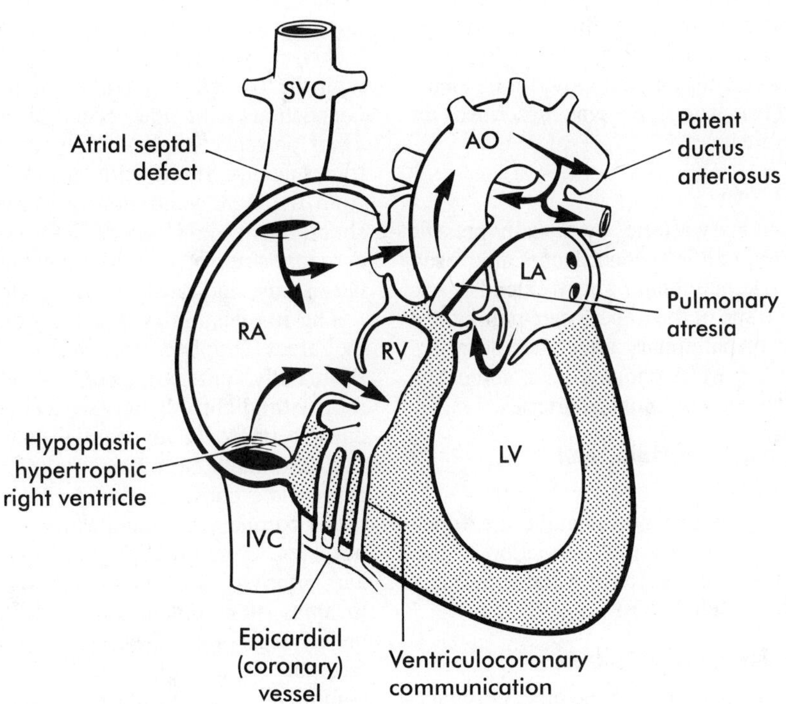


**Figure 22–1** Pathologic anatomy of pulmonary atresia with intact ventricular septum. Arrows indicate direction of blood flow. Note the sinusoidal ventriculocoronary artery communications. These may communicate with the left or right coronary arteries or their branches. *SVC,* Superior vena cava; *AO,* aorta; *RA,* right atrium; *LA,* left atrium; *RV,* right ventricle; *LV,* left ventricle; *IVC,* inferior vena cava.

sinus (inlet zone), trabecular portion, and a conus (outlet zone). Bull and colleagues[4] subdivided the hearts into three categories based on this morphologic organization:

1. Hearts with all three zones present
2. Those without the trabecular portion
3. Those with an inlet zone only

It appears that those with an inlet zone only are the most severely affected. However, Freedom and co-workers[14] point out that a deficient inlet zone may be an acquired phenomenon, and the most severely affected patients often have all three portions present at autopsy.

On the one end of the spectrum are those with diminutive right ventricular cavities and significant free wall hypertrophy. On the other are those with enlarged ventricular cavities. The latter usually exhibit regurgitant tricuspid valves that are dysplastic, displaced (Ebstein's anomaly), or both. Both extremes may have all three zones (inlet, trabecular, infundibular) present. The hearts with marked right ventricular enlargement show wall thinning of the right ventricle, which may occasionally even be devoid of myocardium (Uhl's anomaly).

### Pulmonary valve

Two major types of appearances have been described. In one, prominent commissural ridges converge at the center of the valve. In the second type the ridges are present only at the periphery, with the center composed of a smooth imperforate membrane. An intermediate type was described by Braunlin and colleagues.[3]

### Pulmonary arteries

Mediastinal pulmonary arteries are usually present and are connected to a left-sided ductus arteriosus in most cases. The pulmonary artery extends back to the heart to the site of the imperforate pulmonary valve. Absence of pulmonary artery has been described but is rare. Most patients have some hypoplasia of the branch pulmonary arteries.

### Pulmonary veins, left atrium, and mitral valve

The pulmonary veins and mitral valve are functionally normal, but aneurysmal herniation of the septum primum with a restrictive atrial septal defect may distort the left atrium.

### Coronary arteries and aortic arch

Proximal discontinuity of one or the other coronary arteries (but not both) have been described.[14,25] This occurs more commonly in patients with small right ventricles. The aortic arch is almost always left-sided.

Fistulous communication between right ventricular myocardial sinusoids and the coronary arterial tree may be present (Fig. 22–1).[8,14,20,24,26,30] Their incidence ranges between 10% and 57%. They most commonly connect the hypertensive right ventricle to the left anterior descending coronary artery, but connections to either or both coronary vessels may occur. Some of these communications may dilate with the high right ventricular pressures they are exposed to, or (but rarely) they may become attenuated with progressive endocardial sclerosis.

These fistulous communications originate from the abnormal development of the pulmonary valve. The heart muscle forms from a trabecular network of spongelike musculature supplied with blood from the intertrabecular spaces and sinusoids connecting to the heart chambers. The myocardium thus receives its blood supply mostly from the ventricular cavity at the time of valve formation. Since the pulmonary valve primordia fuse in this abnormality, the blood will exit the right ventricle along the path of least resistance, which will be through the sinusoidal connections to the developing coronary veins and arteries.

The higher the right ventricular pressure, the more frequent the communications. With free tricuspid regurgitation, however, these communications are absent. Their morphology varies considerably, ranging from long thin hairline connections with the coronary system to multiple aneurysmal connections with either or both coronary arteries.[24] Their presence implies that portions of both ventricles are perfused with blood at high pressure from the right ventricle. This leads to a circular shunt, from right ventricle through sinusoids to coronary arteries, coronary venous system, coronary sinus, and back to the right ventricle.

The implication is that myocardial viability in the areas supplied may become compromised. Postnatally, antegrade perfusion from the aortic root with slightly better oxygenated blood during diastole improves myocardial viability.

Additionally, significant intimal hyperplasia occurs in the coronary vessels linked to these ventriculocoronary communications, leading to what has been termed coronary fibroelastosis[12] or coronary arteritis.[36] Epicardial nodules may correspond to areas of complete luminal obliteration of the underlying coronary arteries.[36] Subendocardial infarction of the right or left ventricle is a common complication of pulmonary atresia.[15] Sinusoids are abnormal intramural vascular spaces and thus distinct from the ventriculocoronary communications.[18] Coronary anatomy may be a critical consideration with regard to surgery.[2,25]

### Ductus arteriosus

Survival, even in the short term, depends on a patent ductus arteriosus and/or an atrial septal defect.

## PATHOPHYSIOLOGY

The fusion of the pulmonary valve cusps into a membrane that does not allow blood to exit from the right ventricle in the normal manner is the basic abnormality. The venous return is shunted from the right to the left atrium through an atrial septal defect. The blood that enters the right ventricle has no way to exit except by regurgitation to the right atrium or through the ventriculocoronary artery communications.

A patent foramen ovale allows some blood to flow through the pulmonary vascular bed (Fig. 22–1). This is the most frequent type of disorder and is associated with a small hypertrophied right ventricular chamber (often with ventricular-coronary communications as described above) oligemic lung fields, and severe cyanosis.

Survival will depend on the patency of the ductus arteriosus and the presence of an atrial septal defect. Abnormalities of the tricuspid valve may change the presentation considerably. A regurgitant tricuspid valve will lead to marked right atrial dilatation and severe cardiomegaly, with large right ventricular cavities and thin ventricular walls. Ebstein's anomaly may be present.

## CLINICAL PRESENTATION

These infants show early severe cyanosis and tachypnea. On physical examination of the cardiovascular system a quiet precordium is noted. Cardiomegaly may be noted. There is a single second heart sound.

On auscultation of the heart there may be no murmur, or there may be a holosystolic murmur of tricuspid regurgitation at the lower sternal border. A machinery murmur of the patent ductus arteriosus may be auscultated. With progressive right ventricular failure, hepatomegaly and a prominent a wave in the jugular venous pulse may be observed.

### Laboratory findings

***Chest x-ray film.*** Heart size may be normal or enlarged. The right atrium is usually dilated, particularly in the presence of tricuspid regurgitation. The lung fields are oligemic.

***Electrocardiogram.*** Some 75% of cases have hypoplastic right ventricles and a QRS axis that is normal or slightly leftward shifted for age. The normal right ventricular dominance is absent. With right ventricular enlargement there may be right axis deviation. Right ventricular hypertrophy may be seen on occasion.

***Echocardiogram.*** The atretic pulmonary valve is demonstrated. The decreased size of the right ventricle, diminished tricuspid valve excursion, and normal or small left ventricle are demonstrated. The presence of Ebstein's anomaly or other tricuspid valve abnormality may be visualized.

Valve dimensions correlate well with angiographically derived values.[32] The condition can be diagnosed by echocardiography during fetal life, although two scans (one at 20 weeks and one at 30 weeks gestation) are required.[35] In some instances the decision to operate is based on echocardiographic findings alone.[25]

***Catheterization and ventriculogram.*** The findings of a typical catheterization report are shown in Fig. 22–2. Right ventricular angiography allows demonstration of cavity size, shape of infundibulum, and the degree of tricuspid regurgitation. Right atrial pressures are elevated and the atrial level fixed right to left shunt is demonstrated.

Right ventricular pressures are often very high and may exceed systemic pressures. Coronary artery anatomy is an important consideration in the surgical management of this condition. Sinusoids and fistulous communications with the coronary arteries may be illustrated in 10% to 57% of patients. Proximal coronary artery obstruction may be present.

There is a close correlation between the angiocardiographic appearance of the pulmonary valve and the state of the valve when examined directly as well as with right ventricular morphology.[3]

Right ventricular volume studies can be done, although the bizarre shape of the abnormal ventricle may make the calculated volumes inaccurate.[31] Double catheter techniques may help define the length of the atretic segment.[14]

## MEDICAL MANAGEMENT

Infants with pulmonary atresia and intact ventricular septum develop severe cyanosis and tachypnea soon after birth. Most die in the first month of life as the ductus arteriosus closes, although some may survive longer if the ductus remains open long enough for collateral circulation to develop.

Prostaglandin $E_1$ therapy is essential to improve oxygenation and acidosis. The infusion of prostaglandins is continued into the postoperative period. The introduction of this drug has had a highly significant effect on the survival statistics for this condition. Without surgery all such infants die in their first year of life. Even with surgery the risk of death is high for the first 2 postoperative years (only 47% survive to 2 years).[28]

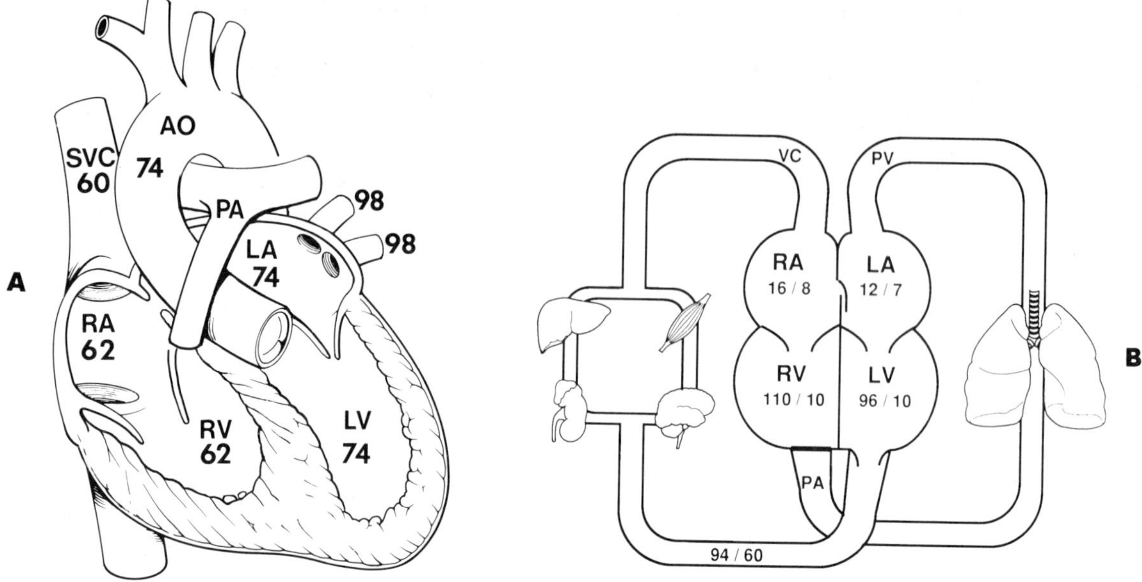


**Figure 22–2** Catheterization findings in pulmonary atresia with an intact ventricular septum. *SVC*, Superior vena cava; *AO, aorta; PA,* pulmonary artery; *RA,* right atrium; *LA,* left atrium; *RV,* right ventricle; *LV,* left ventricle; *PV,* pulmonary vein; *VC,* vena cava.

## SURGICAL MANAGEMENT

Early surgical results have improved considerably over the past few years.[14,20] Survival at 5 and 10 years with surgery remains somewhat disappointing and is reported to be 45% to 50% and 20% to 25% respectively.[6,7,9] The aim of surgical management is the decompression of the right ventricle, allowing growth of the ventricular cavity, and the improvement of pulmonary blood flow. Surgical management for this heterogeneous condition continues to evolve. The type of surgical procedure required is individualized according to the type of abnormality present.

Very few of these cases present the possibility of a single-stage repair. Many require an initial palliative procedure followed by another type of operation later, although the use of prostaglandin $E_1$ has allowed more adventurous surgery on healthier patients and has virtually eliminated the need for emergency surgery.[13] Greenwold's classification of right ventricular pathology, in its modified form has been used to help classify surgical management for this condition (see Pathologic Anatomy).[4] More quantitative approaches such as ventricular volume indices have been developed in an attempt to predict the value of different surgical procedures in the individual. These approaches also attempt to assess the degree of right ventricular growth. A discussion of possible surgical procedures follows.

### Balloon septostomy

Patients with severely restrictive atrial septal defects and a small ventricle may require a balloon septostomy under echocardiographic control as the initial procedure.[14,24]

### Palliative shunt

If the right ventricle is severely hypoplastic or there is infundibular hypoplasia, a systemic-pulmonary shunt such as a Blalock-Taussig may be performed to sustain pulmonary blood flow. These are used in patients deemed unsuitable for a pulmonary valvotomy. A Pott's anastomosis is no longer favored by some because the anatomical distortion may make a subsequent Fontan procedure difficult.[14]

Prostaglandin $E_1$ infusions are started immediately after birth and only gradually weaned postoperatively. Sudden discontinuation may be associated with increased mortality even after surgical corrective procedures.[14] It is important to realize that a shunt will improve hypoxemia but will not relieve right ventricular hypertension and the deleterious effects on coronary blood flow.

### Right ventricular outflow tract reconstruction

In patients with significant right ventricular hypertension or retrograde coronary filling, right ventricular outflow tract reconstruction using pericardium or polytetrafluoroethylene (PTFE) is advisable.[13,14] This can be placed in virtually all cases, even those with a narrow infundibulum, and will relieve right ventricular hypertension and allow right ventricular growth. This is a definitive repair.[6]

A contraindication may be the presence of sinusoidal ventriculocoronary communications, although some surgeons still consider a right ventricular outflow tract patch provided the left coronary artery is not interrupted.[13] Decompression of the right ventricle in the presence of these communications potentiates a steal phenomenon in the coronary circulation,[24] leading to ischemic events involving both ventricles, decreased ventricular function, and increased mortality.[14,27]

### Transventricular valvotomy and central shunt.

Patients with a patent infundibulum (i.e., outlet portion of the right ventricle) may undergo a transventricular valvotomy with or without a central aorta–pulmonary artery shunt; this provides low initial mortality and good palliation.[20] However, this procedure does not decrease right ventricular pressures immediately and all children require an outflow patch eventually.[13] Lewis and associates[26] and de Leval and coauthors[9] have described angiographic measurements of the dimensions of the right ventricle to predict which patients require a shunt in addition to a valvotomy.

The rare patients with almost normal-size right ventricles can undergo a transventricular valvotomy without a shunt.[9,10,29] However, some reports show a 100% reoperation rate after this procedure by 6 years of age.[6] This type of procedure is usually followed by an outflow patch operation for definitive repair. Failure after this procedure occurs in a subset of patients whose right ventricles fail to increase in size. The Fontan procedure or one of its modifications as well as cardiac transplantation are options in these patients.[13,28]

### Tricuspid valve closure

In the presence of ventriculocoronary artery fistulae but unobstructed coronary arteries a systemic pulmonary shunt has been suggested as the initial procedure, since right ventricular decompression could lead to coronary ischemia.[25] Right ventricular decompression can be considered later if the communications close. Otherwise closure of the tricuspid valve at a second stage is possible, thus preventing retrograde perfusion of the coronary arteries. It is difficult to identify the subset of patients in whom the ventriculocoronary communications close spontaneously.

### Fontan procedure

A modified Fontan procedure is performed in patients with inadequate right ventricular growth and/or persistent major ventriculocoronary artery communications.

## ANESTHESIA MANAGEMENT

The newborn arriving for a palliative shunt or any of the procedures detailed above will be cyanosed, tachycardiac, and frequently totally dependent on the patent ductus arteriosus for survival. All require endocarditis prophylaxis. The following management priorities should be considered:

1. Appropriate premedication
2. Open ductus arteriosus
3. No rise in pulmonary vascular resistance
4. Meticulous purging of all air from intravenous lines
5. Ventriculocoronary communications

### Premedication

Infants under 6 months of age are usually not premedicated. These infants only require continuation of the prostaglandin infusion and endocarditis prophylaxis. For older infants I prefer oral premedication, often oral midazolam in doses of 0.5 to 0.75 mg/kg. Diazepam in oral doses of 0.1 to 0.5 mg/kg may also be used.

Oral combinations of meperidine 3 mg/kg and pentobarbital 2 to 4 mg/kg have been suggested as alternatives. If the oral route is not available, intramuscular midazolam 0.08 mg/kg or morphine 0.1 to 0.2 mg/kg is considered. Crying and agitation induced by the pain of an intramuscular injection will aggravate shunting, hypoxemia, and acidosis, and that route is therefore best avoided. No premedication is given if the child is severely compromised or in cardiac failure.

It is possible to obtain adequate sedation with oral midazolam in 60% to 70% of patients when used in the given dose, and the incidences of respiratory and cardiovascular side effects increase with the dose.[1] All sedated patients require monitoring and the presence of a care giver with airway expertise.

### Maintaining an open ductus arteriosus

On review of the pathophysiology it is apparent that closure of the patent ductus arteriosus would lead to demise of the patient. Continuation of the prostaglandin E infusion at rates of 0.03 to 0.1 μg/kg/min until the repair has been accomplished and in most centers even into the postoperative period is strongly advised. Since acetylcholine constricts the ductus arteriosus, succinylcholine is best avoided.

### Pulmonary vascular resistance

The pulmonary vascular resistance is a crucial consideration in this condition. The pulmonary vas-

**Table 22–1** Pulmonary vascular resistance

| Decrease | Increase |
|---|---|
| Oxygen | Hypoxia |
| Hypocarbia | Hypercarbia |
| Anemia | Hypovolemia |
| Alkalosis | Hyperacidemia |
| Normal lung volume (FRC) | Hyperinflation (PEEP) |
| | Hypothermia |
| Sympathetic block | Sympathetic stimulation |
| Drugs (e.g., vasodilators) | Atelectasis |
| | High hematocrit |
| | Surgical constriction |
| | Drugs |

culature is highly reactive and any rise may cause significant falls in pulmonary perfusion and therefore hypoxemia. Consider the following relationship:

$Q = P/R$

Q, flow; P, pressure gradient; R, resistance

A rise in pulmonary vascular resistance will require a higher pressure to maintain the same flow. In pulmonary atresia the pressure is generated by the left ventricle, and since perfusion depends on the ductus arteriosus (nonrestrictive), the flow will be dependent on the ratio of pulmonary to systemic vascular resistance. Any increase in pulmonary vascular resistance leads to a fall in pulmonary blood flow unless there is a greater rise in systemic vascular resistance.

The factors used to manipulate the pulmonary vascular resistance are given in Table 22–1. It is important to avoid hypothermia, hypoxia, hypovolemia, and hypercarbia during the anesthetic management of these cases. Ventilation management is the least hazardous way of manipulating pulmonary vascular resistance. Frequently infants diagnosed with this condition are emergently intubated and ventilated prior to surgical intervention.[24]

Studies of ketamine and nitrous oxide in infants with normal or elevated pulmonary vascular resistance have shown no increase in resistance provided ventilation is controlled.[21,22]

### Purging air from intravenous lines

Any patient with an anatomical shunt is considered to be at risk of a paradoxical embolus. This is an embolus that has traversed a right to left shunt and therefore threatens to cause a cerebral event. It is imperative that all lines be free of air. Remember, the solubility coefficient of a gas in a liquid is temperature dependent: with the warming of fluids bubbles may form as gas escapes from the fluid.

### Ventriculocoronary communications

Awareness of the presence of communications is vital both in selecting the type of operation and in deciding on the anesthetic management. Decompression of the right ventricle (e.g., pulmonary valvotomy) or systemic hypotension will lead to decreased coronary perfusion and perioperative subendocardial infarction.

The presence of these communications is associated with an increased risk of death and decreased systolic and diastolic ventricular function.[27] Up to 50% of patients have additional coronary abnormalities including intimal thickening, tortuosity, or luminal obstruction.[25]

### Monitoring

Prior to induction of anesthesia routine monitors include ECG, pulse oximetry, and noninvasive blood pressure measurement. Placement of arterial and central venous pressure lines is performed after the patient's trachea is successfully intubated.

### Induction and maintenance

Since all patients require prostaglandin infusions, they will have intravenous access. An intravenous induction after adequate preoxygenation is performed using an opioid (fentanyl 10 to 50 μg/kg, sufentanil 1.5 to 2.5 μg/kg), or ketamine (1 mg/kg) and is tolerated with little hemodynamic compromise if the drugs are carefully titrated and the patient is relatively isovolemic. Endotracheal intubation is facilitated using a nondepolarizing muscle relaxant (vecuronium 0.1 to 0.2 mg/kg or pancuronium 0.1 mg/kg).

Maintenance is usually with an opioid unless a short shunt procedure is planned and the patient is not required to be on ventilatory support postoperatively. Pulmonary valvotomies may be performed through the main pulmonary artery under direct vision without bypass. Surgical exposure is gained via a left thoracotomy when this is the sole procedure being performed.[24]

Anesthetic considerations for the Fontan procedure are discussed in Chapter 23 and are the same as for patients with ventricular outflow tract reconstruction. Pulmonary vascular resistance is again extremely important; venous pressure will be the only driving force for pulmonary perfusion after a Fontan procedure.[15] Right ventricular failure may be fatal after outflow tract reconstructions.

Complications of the Fontan procedure include myocardial infarction (patients who have ventriculocoronary communications), mechanical obstruction at any level, dysrhythmias, rise in right atrial pressure, residual right to left shunt, venous hypertension, and the superior vena caval syndrome.

Pleural and pericardial effusions, hepatic dysfunction, and enteropathy have been described following modified Fontan procedures.

## REFERENCES


1. Berry FA: *Anesthetic management of difficult and routine pediatric patients,* ed 2, New York, 1990, Churchill-Livingstone.
2. Billingsley AM, Laks H, Boyce SW et al: Definitive repair in patients with pulmonary atresia and intact ventricular septum, *J Thorac Cardiovasc Surg* 97:746, 1989.
3. Braunlin EA, Formanek AG, Moller JH et al: Angiopathological appearance of pulmonary atresia with intact ventricular septum: interpretation of nature of right ventricle from pulmonary angiography, *Br Heart J* 47:281, 1982.
4. Bull C, de Leval MR, Mercanti C et al: Pulmonary atresia and intact ventricular septum: a revised classification, *Circulation,* 66(2):266, 1982.
5. Chitayat D, McIntosh N, Fouron J: Pulmonary atresia with intact ventricular septum and hypoplastic right heart in sibs: a single gene disorder? *Am J Med Genet* 42:304, 1992.
6. Cobanoglu A, Metzdorff MT, Pinson CW et al: Valvotomy for pulmonary atresia with intact ventricular septum: a disciplined approach to achieve a functioning right ventricle, *J Thorac Cardiovasc Surg* 89:482, 1985.
7. Coles JG, Freedom RM, Lightfoot NE et al: Long term results in neonates with pulmonary atresia and intact ventricular septum, *Ann Thorac Surg* 47:213, 1989.
8. Cornell SH: Myocardial sinusoids in pulmonary valvular atresia, *Radiology* 86:421, 1966.
9. De Leval M, Bull C, Hopkins R et al: Decision making in the definitive repair of the heart with a small right ventricle, *Circulation* 72(part 2):II52, 1985.
10. Dobell ARC, Grignon A: Early and late results in pulmonary atresia, *Ann Thorac Surg* 24:264, 1977.
11. Erikson NL, Buttino L, Juberg R: Congenital pulmonary atresia with intact ventricular septum, tricuspid insufficiency, and patent ductus arteriosus in two sibs, *Am J Med Genet* 32:187, 1989.
12. Essed CE, Klein HW, Krediet P et al: Coronary and endocardial fibroelastosis of the ventricles in the hypoplastic left and right heart syndromes, *Virchows Arch (A)* 368:87, 1975.
13. Foker JE, Braunlin EA, St. Cyr JA et al: Management of pulmonary atresia with intact ventricular septum, *J Thorac Cardiovasc Surg* 92:706, 1989.
14. Freedom RM, Wilson G, Trusler GA et al: Pulmonary atresia and intact ventricular septum: a review of the anatomy, myocardium, and factors influencing right ventricular growth and guidelines for surgical intervention, *Scand J Thorac Cardiovasc Surg* 17:1, 1983.
15. Gale AW, Danielson GK, McGoon DW et al: Modified Fontan operation for univentricular heart and complicated congenital lesions, *J Thorac Cardiovasc Surg* 78:831, 1979.
16. Gittenberger-de Groot AC, Sauer U, Bindl L et al: Competition of coronary arteries and ventriculocoronary arterial communications in pulmonary atresia with intact ventricular septum, *Int J Cardiol* 18:243, 1988.
17. Goor DA, Lilleihei CW: *Congenital malformations of the heart,* New York, 1975, Grune and Stratton.
18. Graham TP, Bender HW, Atwood GF et al: Increase in right ventricular volume following valvulotomy for pulmonary atresia or stenosis with intact ventricular septum, *Circulation* 49(suppl 2):69, 1974.
19. Greenwold WE, DuShane JW, Burchell HB et al: Congenital pulmonary atresia with intact ventricular septum: two anatomic types, *Circulation* 14:945, 1956 (abstract).
20. Hawkins JA, Kent Thorne J, Boucek MM et al: Early and late results in pulmonary atresia and intact ventricular septum, *J Thorac Cardiovasc Surg* 100:492, 1990.
21. Hickey PR, Hanson DD, Cramolini GM et al: Pulmonary and systemic responses to ketamine in infants with normal and elevated pulmonary vascular resistance, *Anesthesiology* 62:287, 1985.
22. Hickey PR, Hanson DD, Strafford M et al: Pulmonary and systemic effects of nitrous oxide in infants with normal and elevated pulmonary vascular resistance, *Anesthesiology* 65:374, 1986.
23. Hurst JW, Schlant RC: *The heart,* vol 1, ed 7, New York, 1990, McGraw-Hill.
24. Joshi SV, Brawn WJ, Mee RBB et al: Pulmonary atresia with intact ventricular septum, *J Thorac Cardiovasc Surg* 91:192, 1986.
25. Kasznica J, Ursell PC, Blanc WA et al: Abnormalities of the coronary circulation in pulmonary atresia and intact ventricular septum, *Am Heart J* 114(6):1415, 1987.
26. Lewis AB, Wells W, Lindesmith GC: Evaluation and surgical treatment of pulmonary atresia and intact ventricular septum in infancy, *Circulation* 67:1318, 1983.
27. Lightfoot NE, Coles JG, Dasmahapatra HK et al: Analysis of survival in patients with pulmonary atresia and intact ventricular septum treated surgically, *Int J Cardiol* 24:159, 1989.
28. Merrill WM, Frist WH, Stewart JR et al: Heart transplantation in children, *Ann Surg* 213(5):393, 1991.
29. Moulton AL, Bowman FO, Edie RN et al: Pulmonary atresia with intact ventricular septum: 16-year experience, *J Thorac Cardiovasc Surg* 78:527, 1979.
30. O'Connor WN, Cottrill CM, Johnson GL et al: Pulmonary atresia with intact ventricular septum and ventriculocoronary communications: surgical significance, *Circulation* 65:805, 1982.
31. Patel RM, Freedom RM, Moes CAF et al: Right ventricular volume determinations in 18 patients with pulmonary atresia and intact ventricular septum: analysis of factors influencing right ventricular growth, *Circulation* 61:428, 1980.
32. Rao PS, Liebman J, Borkat G: Right ventricular growth in case of pulmonic stenosis with intact ventricular septum and hypoplastic right ventricle, *Circulation* 53:389, 1976.
33. Rose AG, Beckman CB, Edwards JE: Communications between coronary sinus and left atrium, *Br Heart J* 36:182, 1974.
34. Scognamiglio R, Daliento L, Razzolini R et al: Pulmonary atresia with intact ventricular septum: a quantitative cineventriculographic study of the right and left ventricular function, *Pediatr Cardiol* 7:183, 1986.
35. Todros T, Gaglioti P, Demarie D: Pulmonary stenosis with intact ventricular septum: documentation of development of the lesion echocardiographically during fetal life, *Int J Cardiol* 19:355, 1988.
36. Vigorita V: Epicardial nodules: a possible sign of coronary endarteritis with hypoplastic right heart syndrome, *Johns Hopkins Medical Journal* 142:215, 1978.
37. Waldman JD, Lamberti JJ, Mathewson JW et al: Surgical closure of the tricuspid valve for pulmonary atresia, intact ventricular septum, and right ventricle to coronary artery communications, *Pediatr Cardiol* 5:221, 1984.

# 23 Tricuspid Atresia

*Volker Striepe*



The congenital agenesis, or absence, of the tricuspid valve is known as tricuspid atresia.[5,29] The first documented case of tricuspid atresia was described by Keysig in 1817. The condition is now known to be the third most common cause of cyanotic congenital heart disease, comprising between 1.4% and 2.9% of congenital heart defects.[31] The condition has a 50% mortality by 6 months of age without surgical intervention, but 50% survive past the second decade of life with palliative surgery.[18]

The initial surgery is usually a shunt procedure aimed at improving pulmonary blood flow so that a later physiologic correction by means of a Fontan-Kreutzer procedure (or a modification thereof) may be carried out. This procedure still carries considerable risk of morbidity and mortality: as of February 1992 documented survival after a modified Fontan was 79% at 30 days, 74% at 6 months, 73% at 1 year, 69% at 5 years, and 63% at 10 years.[8] The anesthetic management of these ill patients is greatly aided by an understanding of the pathophysiology of the condition as well as the surgical procedure.

## EMBRYOLOGY

Between the twenty-seventh and thirty-seventh days of development the embryo grows from 5 mm to a length of 16 or 17 mm. The major septa of the heart form during this stage, thus dividing the cardiac loop into four chambers. Simultaneous with atrial expansion and septum formation, two mesenchymal cushions, the superior and inferior atrioventricular endocardial cushions, appear in the atrioventricular canal (Fig. 23–1). These gradually grow toward each other until they fuse at the 10-mm stage, thereby dividing the atrioventricular canal into left and right atrioventricular orifices. Two lateral endocardial cushions develop at the same stage. The mesenchymal tissue that surrounds the atrioventricular canals gradually hollows out from the ventricular side, and the resulting atrioventricular valves are initially attached to the ventricular walls by muscular cords. The muscle tissue in the cords degenerates and is replaced by dense connective tissue. The valves eventually consist of connective tissue covered by endocardium and connected to papillary muscle by chordae tendineae. The tricuspid valve consists of a medial, an anterior, and a posterior cusp, and the mitral valve has an anterior and posterior cusp (Fig. 23–2). In addition to the division of the atrioventricular canal, the endocardial cushions are also responsible for the formation of the membranous portion of the interventricular septum as well as the closure of the ostium primum. If the endocardial cushions fail to fuse, a persistent atrioventricular canal combined with a defect in the cardiac septum will occur.

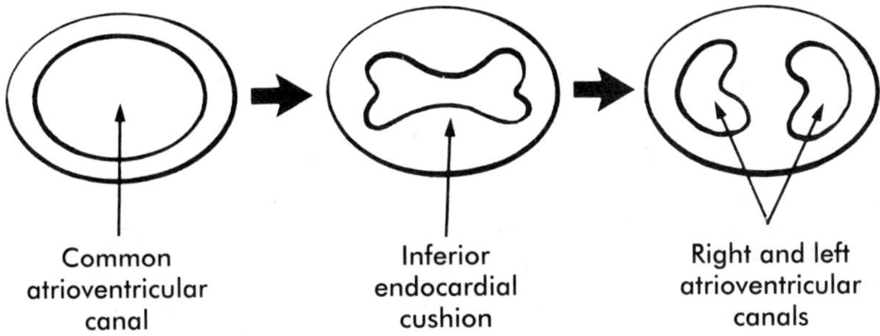


**Figure 23–1** Embryology of normal atrial and tricuspid valves. Note the formation of endocardial cushions. Their fusion divides the atrioventricular canal into right and left orifices. This precedes the development of the tricuspid and mitral valves from the surrounding mesenchymal tissue.

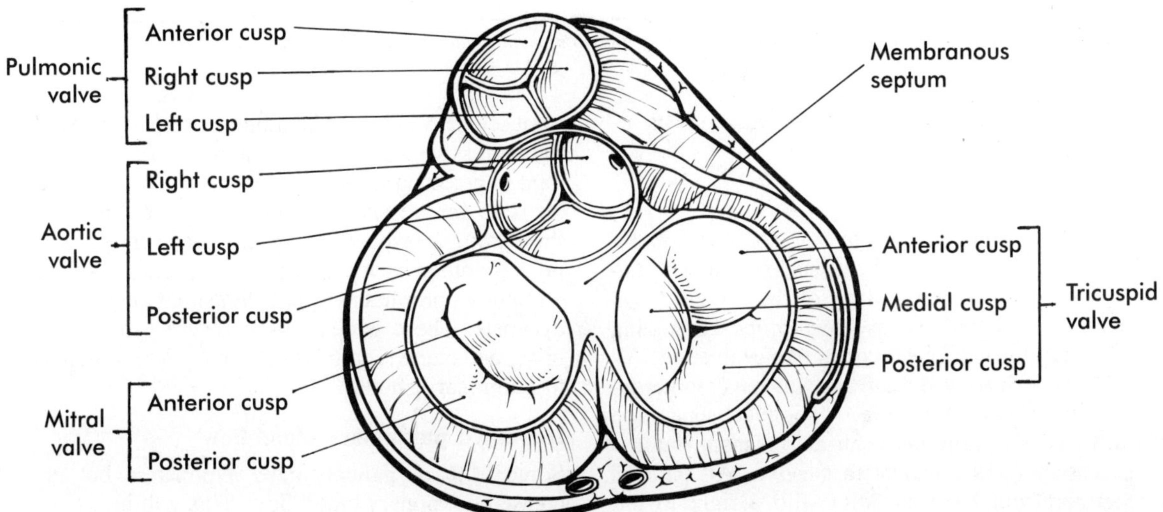


**Figure 23–2** Normal anatomy of the mitral and tricuspid valves.

Tricuspid atresia results if there is obliteration of the right atrioventricular orifice. This will be associated with a patent foramen ovale, a ventricular septal defect (VSD), underdevelopment of the right ventricle, and hypertrophy of the left ventricle.[24]

## PATHOLOGIC ANATOMY

Morphologic heterogeneity has led to considerable controversy in the literature and a variety of classifications.[1,30,32] The classifications were based on morphology of the valve,[33] x-ray appearance of pulmonary lung markings,[2] or associated anatomic defects. The most common classifications of the different types of tricuspid atresia are based on associated anatomic defects. Kühne classified tricuspid atresia as those with and those without associated transposition of the great arteries. The most common morphology consists of a dimple or a localized fibrous thickening in the floor of the right atrium in place of the tricuspid valve. No valvular material can be identified on macroscopic or microscopic examination. A practical classification based on Rao's modification is summarized in Table 23–1. Approximately 70% of cases involve tricuspid atresia without transposition of the great arteries (type I). Types Ia and Ib are both associated with decreased pulmonary blood flow (oligemic lung fields), with the associated anesthetic implications. Type Ic is distinguished by the presence of a large unrestrictive VSD without pulmonary atresia or stenosis with possibly increased pulmonary blood flow. Type II is associated with D-transposition, and type III, which is extremely rare, consists of L-transposiion with tricuspid atresia. Type III, unlike the first two groups, is not divided on the basis of pulmonary artery anatomy. This inconsistency was changed in a revision of the classification by P.S. Rao.[30] In the revised classification type II encompasses all types of transposition, and type III in-

**Table 23–1** Tricuspid atresia

| Type | | Pulmonary blood flow | Frequency (%) |
|---|---|---|---|
| Type I | Normally related great vessels | | 70 |
| | a. Pulmonary atresia | ↓ | 10 |
| | b. Ventricular septal defect and pulmonary atresia | ↓ | 50 |
| | c. Ventricular septal defect without pulmonary atresia | ↔ ↑ | 10 |
| Type II | D-transposition of the great vessels | | 30 |
| | a. Pulmonary atresia with ventricular septal defect | ↓ | 2 |
| | b. Pulmonary stenosis with ventricular septal defect | ↔ ↓ | 8 |
| | c. Normal or large pulmonary artery with ventricular septal defect | ↑ ↑ | 20 |
| Type III | L-transposition of the great vessels | | very rare |
| | a. Pulmonary or subpulmonary stenosis | ↓ | |
| | b. Subaortic stenosis | ↑ | |

Adapted from Rao PS: A unified classification for tricuspid atresia, *Am Heart J* 99:6, 1980.

cludes tricuspid atresia associated with truncus arteriosus.

## PATHOPHYSIOLOGY

A careful preoperative evaluation demands an elucidation of the associated cardiac anomalies to understand the pathophysiology of the lesion. A variety of classifications have been proposed, adding some confusion to the preoperative evaluation. All patients with tricuspid atresia will have some degree of arterial hypoxemia. A complete separation of the right atrium and ventricle means a shunt is necessary for the patient to survive. All patients therefore will have an ASD with a right to left shunt. If the ASD or patent foramen ovale is restrictive, a large pressure gradient may exist between the right and left atria, and right atrial emptying will be impeded, leading to venous congestion. The venous return has to be shunted to the left atrium, where complete or incomplete mixing (due to streaming) with pulmonary venous blood occurs. The left atrium is therefore usually large and muscular. The mitral valve leaflets are thick, and mitral insufficiency may develop in the young adult as left ventricular volume loading progressively increases. Left and right ventricular, pulmonary, and systemic arterial saturations will be equal unless mixing is incomplete.

### Decreased pulmonary blood flow

Most patients (over 70%) have pulmonary atresia or pulmonary or subpulmonary stenosis. This implies decreased pulmonary blood flow and cyanosis as the predominant presenting feature. In the presence of pulmonary atresia, an additional downstream shunt (PDA, bronchial collaterals) will exist. Cyanotic spells not unlike those of patients with tetralogy of Fallot may occur. Gradual closure of a muscular VSD or infundibular narrowing leads to progressive worsening of cyanosis. The concomitant hypoxic pulmonary vasoconstrictive response leads to progressive pulmonary hypertension. In these complex shunts the degree of cyanosis will be determined by the $Q_p$:$Q_s$ ratio. A ratio less than 1 implies a prominent right to left shunt and greater cyanosis. These patients have severe cyanosis at birth, and many require an early palliative systemic to pulmonary shunt.

### Increased pulmonary blood flow

Some 30% of patients have hypoxemia but increased pulmonary blood flow. This will be due to either a large VSD without pulmonary stenosis (type Ic, type IIc) or very rarely, subaortic stenosis (type III b). Since tricuspid atresia already imposes a volume load on the left ventricle, the large VSD will accentuate this, usually leading to congestive heart failure as part of the presentation. Muscular VSDs and infundibular stenotic areas tend to shrink gradually,[23] which will increase pulmonary blood flow while decreasing systemic flow in patients with transposition (type IIc). Conversely, patients with normally related arteries and a large VSD and those with IIIb lesions may benefit from a more balanced pulmonary to systemic flow caused by the gradual narrowing.

## CLINICAL PRESENTATION

The presentation will depend on the type of associated cardiac abnormalities and therefore the specific pathophysiology of the complex shunt. The correct diagnosis depends on history, physical examination findings, radiologic examination, and catheterization data. The patient will usually have a history of cyanosis from an early age; indeed, patients often show cyanosis on the first day of life.

The majority (70%) of patients with tricuspid atresia have diminished pulmonary blood flow and are profoundly cyanotic (type Ia,b; type IIa,b; type IIIa). Approximately 50% have type Ib abnormalities: normally related vessels, tricuspid atresia, and a small VSD. The less cyanotic patients with increased pulmonary blood flow often have some degree of congestive heart failure (type Ic, type IIc, type IIIb). These patients may go on to develop pulmonary obstructive disease in the first year of life.[9] The parents may report that the child is frequently short of breath, and they may recall cyanotic spells. Squatting may be reported if the child is older. Physical examination will reveal cyanosis as well as clubbing of fingers and toes in children older than 1 year.[9] A prominent a wave in the jugular venous pressure may be noted. Pulses are normal unless there is accompanying coarctation. Examination of the precordium reveals the absence of a right ventricular impulse and a prominent left apical impulse. A systolic thrill may be palpable. There is a single first heart sound and either a loud single or a closely split second sound. The loud second sound is due to aortic valve closure and is prominent with transposition, due to its anterior position in this condition.

Continuous bruits due to thoracic collateral circulation may be auscultated. A loud systolic murmur radiates along the sternal border if a VSD is present. A gradual decrease of this murmur in older patients may be an ominous sign of VSD closure or right ventricular infundibular narrowing.[9] A systolic murmur of pulmonary stenosis may be heard as well as a machinery murmur of a patent ductus arteriosus. Symptoms and signs of congestive heart failure (hepatomegaly, pedal edema, distended neck veins) will be dominant in patients with increased pulmonary blood flow. Chronic left ventricular volume overload leads eventually to cardiomyopathy with a low ejection fraction, which would persist after surgery. This will appear on history as progressive exertional dyspnea with frequent episodes of tachycardia, progressing to symptoms of cardiac failure.

### Laboratory findings

Clinical investigations aid in the diagnosis as well as in deciding which surgical procedure will be most beneficial to the patient.

***Electrocardiogram.*** ECG findings include left ventricular hypertrophy and ST and T wave changes of left ventricular strain. The latter are present in nearly 50% of patients.[9] Biatrial hypertrophy is common. The QRS axis is between 0 and -90 degrees in 75% of cases. Patients with transposition have an axis between 0 and +90.

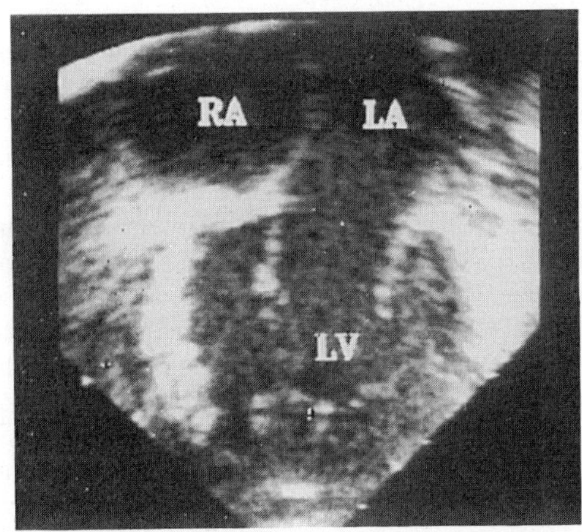


**Figure 23–3** Echocardiogram in a patient with tricuspid atresia, apical view. Note the absence of the right atrioventricular valve and the bowing of the atrial septum into the left atrium. *RA*, right atrium; *LA*, left atrium; *LV*, left ventricle. (From Fyler DC, ed: *Nadas' pediatric cardiology*, Philadelphia, 1992, Hanley & Belfus.)

***Hematocrit.*** These patients usually have polycythemia with a hematocrit greater than 65%.

***Arterial blood gas.*** Patients demonstrate arterial hypoxemia on arterial blood gas analysis.

***Chest x-ray film.*** Radiographic findings depend on volume of pulmonary blood flow and the size of the shunt. The heart is not enlarged, but the right heart border is straight and the apex is elevated and blunt as in a tetralogy of Fallot. A lateral view shows the absence of the right ventricular silhouette and shows left atrial enlargement. Numerous collateral vessels may lead to a reticulated, nodular, or honeycombed appearance in lung fields in older patients.[9] Rib notching due to collaterals may be seen. The pulmonary vascular markings may be increased, normal, or decreased, depending on pulmonary blood flow. Those with a small ASD tend to have a large right atrium and a small pulmonary artery with oligemic lung fields.

***Echocardiogram.*** This will confirm the diagnosis of tricuspid atresia (Fig. 23-3). It will allow the estimation of chamber size and the demonstration of flow velocities across the septal defects, using color flow Doppler and spectral analysis. An enlarged right atrium and a hypertrophied left venricle are visualized. This can be used to assess the mitral valve, which usually has a dilated annulus and may be regurgitant in advanced cases. Transposition can be diagnosed, as can the presence and degree of pulmonary stenosis and pulmonary hypertension. The ejection fraction can be estimated and will give an estimate of ventricular function.

***Catheterization data.*** An example of catheterization data is shown in Fig. 23–4. This investigation confirms the diagnosis and allows the detection of complications. Right atrial pressures are elevated and the a waves are usually accentuated. Right ventricular hypoplasia is common to all types, and inability to pass the catheter into this chamber will suggest but does not prove the diagnosis.[9] The usual approach is from the groin. The venous catheter can be passed through the atrial defect into the left atrium, and if pulmonary flow is high enough, on into the hypoplastic right ventricle.[16] Two thirds of patients show a patent foramen ovale (as opposed to an ASD).[19] Saturations will be low in the superior vena cava and the right atrium. Saturations in the left atrium, left ventricle, right ventricle, aorta, and pulmonary artery will all be the same. Arterial hypoxemia is invariably present. Right atrial pressures are high, often with a waves, particularly if the ASD is restrictive. Pulmonary artery, left ventricular, and systemic pressures are mostly normal.

***Angiography.*** This investigation gives the diagnosis. An injection of dye into the inferior vena cava will show the dilated right atrial chamber, and all the contrast will cross over to the left atrium through the atrial septal defect. A left ventriculogram is essential to determine the number and size of ventricular septal defects (Fig. 23–5).

## MEDICAL MANAGEMENT

Medical treatment is used primarily in the treatment of cyanosis, congestive heart failure and complications associated with tricuspid atresia. Cyanosis is frequently the first sign of this condition and will become progressively more severe due to shunt closure (VSD or PDA) or infundibular narrowing. Prostaglandins $E_1$ and $E_2$ are useful to maintain ductal patency.[28] Prostaglandin $E_1$ can be infused intravenously at an initial rate of 50 to 100 ng/kg/min, followed by a drop in rate to 10 to 20 ng/kg/min once clinical improvement is noted.[12] Cyanotic spells similar to those found in tetralogy of Fallot may occur and should be treated as they would for that condition. Intercurrent infections should be treated vigorously, and antibiotic prophylaxis for endocarditis is important. Congestive heart failure may be initially managed by conventional therapy with digoxin, fluid restriction, and diuretics. When catheterization shows a large pressure gradient between the two atria and signs of congestive heart failure intervene, a balloon atrial septostomy or atrial septectomy may be urgently

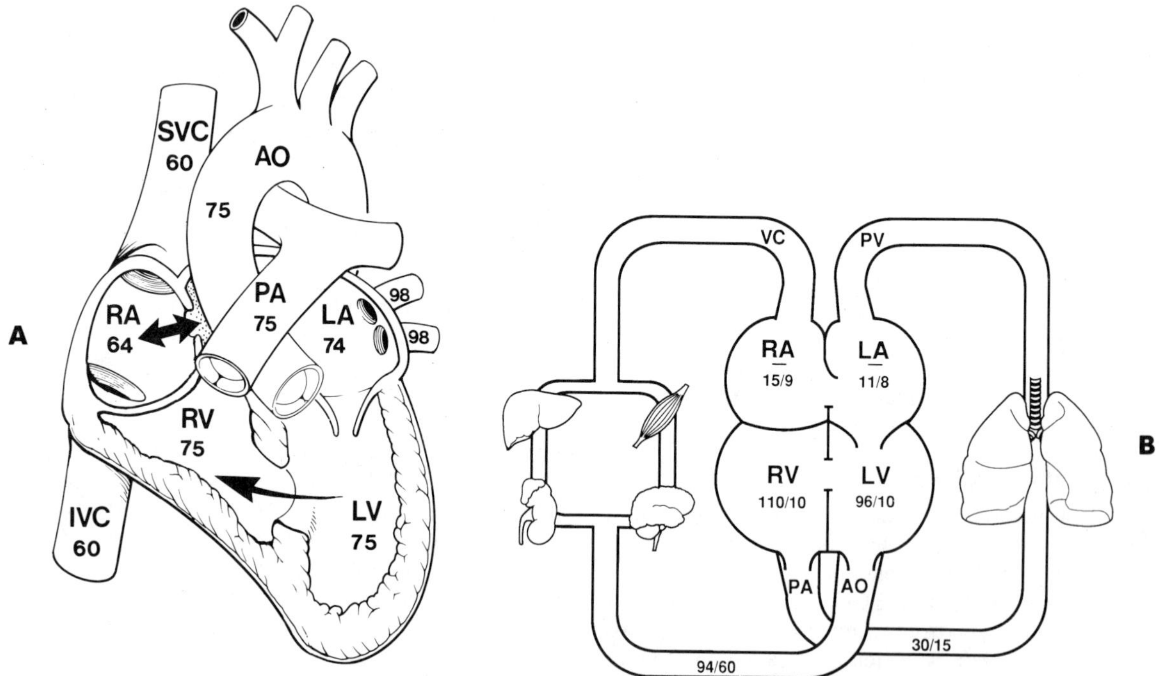


**Figure 23–4** Typical catheterization findings in a case of tricuspid atresia. **A,** Oxygen saturations in a patient with tricuspid atresia. **B,** Pressures in a patient with tricuspid atresia. *SVC,* Superior vena cava; *AO,* aorta; *PA,* pulmonary artery; *RA,* right atrium; *LA,* left atrium; *RV,* right ventricle; *LV,* left ventricle; *PV,* pulmonary vein; *IVC,* inferior vena cava.

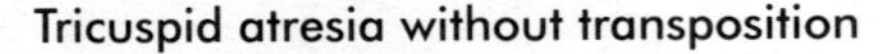


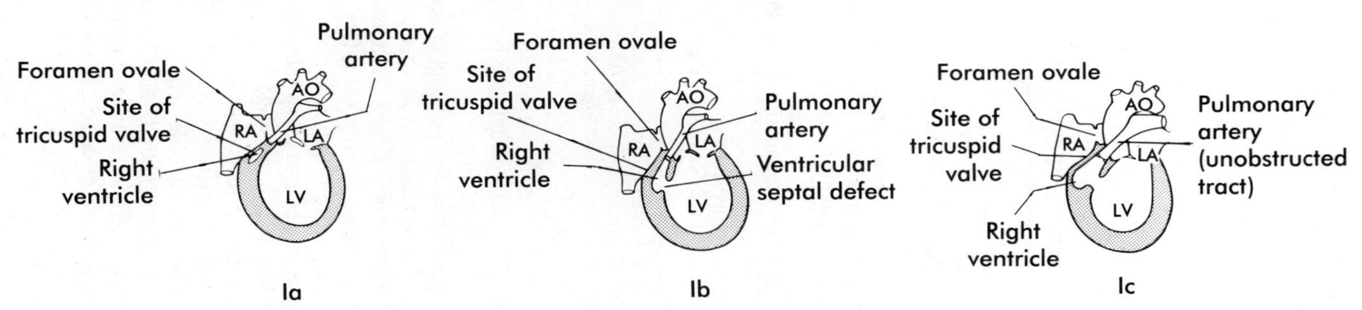


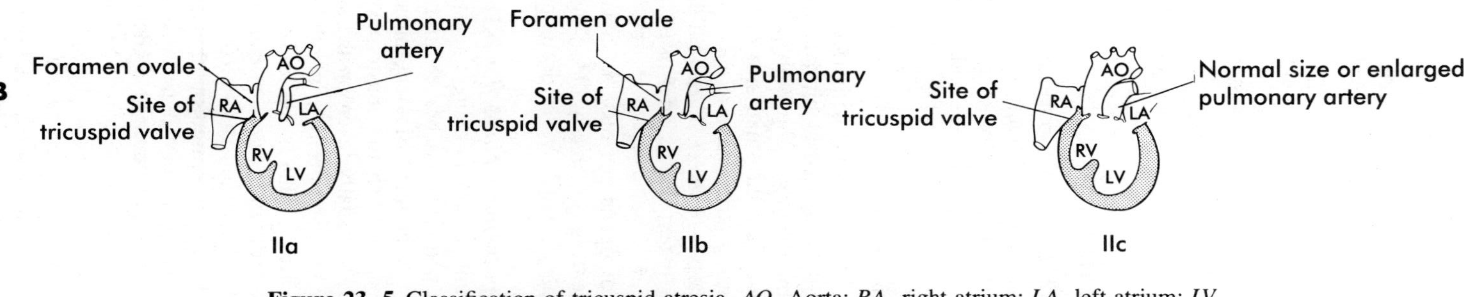


**Figure 23–5** Classification of tricuspid atresia. *AO*, Aorta; *RA*, right atrium; *LA*, left atrium; *LV*, left ventricle; *RV*, right ventricle; *PA*, pulmonary artery. (From Rao PS: A unified classification for tricuspid atresia, *Am Heart J*, 99:6, 1980.)

*Continued.*

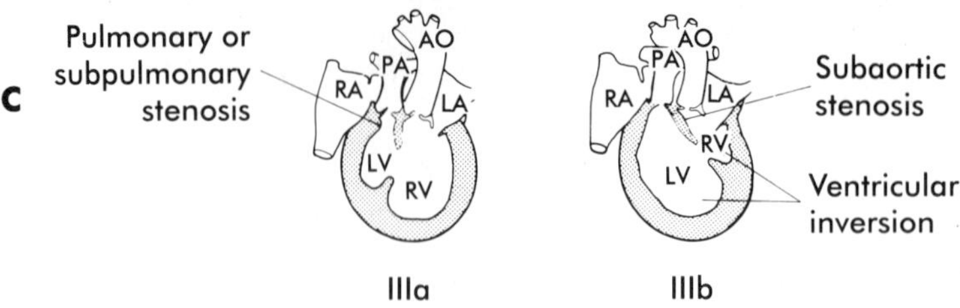


**Figure 23–5, cont'd**

needed. Ultimately, surgery best improves life expectancy.

## SURGICAL MANAGEMENT

Surgical procedures in tricuspid atresia can be grouped into palliative operations (e.g., palliative shunts) and those aimed at physiologic correction (Fontan-Kreutzer type procedures and heart transplantation).

### Palliative procedures

Approximately 70% of patients with tricuspid atresia are profoundly cyanosed at birth and require early surgical intervention. The high pulmonary vascular resistance and the small size of the pulmonary arteries and atria preclude a Fontan procedure at this early age (box). These children are dependent on a patent ductus arteriosus for survival.

Three types of operations may be considered: procedures increasing pulmonary blood flow, decreasing pulmonary blood flow, and decompressing the right atrium.

***Increase of pulmonary blood flow.*** The Blalock-Taussig shunt consists of a direct anastomosis of the subclavian artery to a branch of the pulmonary artery.[17] A modified Blalock-Taussig uses a tube graft to accomplish the anastomosis. The subclavian artery is usually taken on the side opposite the aortic arch and inserted into the ipsilateral pulmonary artery. This is the most common shunt performed early in tricuspid atresia. Central shunts such as the Waterston and Potts are not favored, as they lead to increased pulmonary pressures and possibly to pulmonary hypertension. This would make a Fontan procedure or a Glenn shunt unfeasible. Glenn demonstrated in 1958 that adequate pulmonary perfusion could be achieved by anastomosing the superior vena cava end to end to the distal end of the divided right pulmonary artery.[15] This improves pulmonary flow without concomitant left ventricular volume overload. A variation of the Glenn shunt, the bidirectional cavopulmonary anastomosis, has been employed as an interim procedure for patients at increased risk for the Fontan procedure.[5] In this procedure the upper end of the divided SVC is anastomosed end to side to the right pulmonary artery without dividing this artery from the main pulmonary artery. Both of these procedures allow adaptation to a Fontan correction at a later stage but require a low pulmonary vascular resistance to allow the low venous pressures to perfuse the lungs. Their role is therefore primarily in older children not suitable for Fontan-Kreutzer procedures. Complications of these procedures may be either immediate (in the operating room) or delayed. Immediate complications include hypoxemia due to inadequate pulmonary blood flow (e.g., shunting, kinked or obstructed graft, sudden rise in pulmonary vascular resistance). When the shunt is not restrictive enough, excessive pulmonary blood flow leading to pulmonary edema may occur. A low diastolic

**SELECTION CRITERIA FOR THE FONTAN PROCEDURE**

1. Age over 4 years
2. Sinus rhythm
3. Normal vena caval drainage
4. Right atrium of normal volume
5. Mean pulmonary artery pressure up to 15 mm Hg
6. Pulmonary resistance below 4 units/$m^2$
7. Diameter of pulmonary artery at least 75% of diameter of aorta
8. Normal function of primitive ventricle (ejection fraction at least 0.60)
9. No mitral incompetence
10. No impairment due to previous shunt

From Choussat A, Fontan F, Besse P et al: Selection criteria for Fontan's procedure. In Anderson RH, Shinebourne EA (eds): *Pediatric Cardiology,* Edinburgh, 1978, Churchill Livingstone.

pressure and a wide pulse pressure with good arterial saturations may be noted. Postoperatively the patient will be tachypneic with a hyperdynamic precordium and may exhibit rales on auscultation of the lung fields. A postoperative chest x-ray film may occasionally show unilateral pulmonary edema. Late complications include a dilated, chronically volume-overloaded ventricle and pulmonary vascular obstructive disease.

***Decrease of pulmonary blood flow.*** Patients with unobstructed pulmonary blood flow may have congestive heart failure and are usually not profoundly cyanosed. Here, the danger is that of developing pulmonary venous obstructive disease or progressive congestive failure. Pulmonary artery banding reduces pulmonary blood flow and protects its vasculature from high pressures so that a more definitive procedure can be attempted later. The procedure is performed through a left thoracotomy or a median sternotomy, without bypass. A band placed around the pulmonary artery is most effective if the pressure distal to the band drops to 30% to 50% of systemic pressure. Other than measuring the pressure drop, the adequacy of banding is assessed by monitoring a rise in systemic pressure and a concomitant acceptable fall in arterial saturation. The hemodynamic results are difficult to predict. A band that is too tight gives the ventricle a high afterload, and arterial desaturation followed by systemic hypotension and bradycardia may occur. The band may eventually migrate to a more distal branch and may distort the anatomy sufficiently to complicate a future repair.[20]

***Decompression of the right atrium.*** An atrial defect is common to all subtypes of tricuspid atresia. Even a small pressure gradient between the two atria (2 to 5 mm Hg) may lead to gradual right atrial enlargement and systemic venous congestion. A Rashkind-Miller balloon septostomy can be performed in the catheterization laboratory to enlarge the atrial defect or foramen ovale and thereby lower right atrial pressures. In an extremely ill neonate a balloon septostomy may be performed under transesophageal echocardiographic control at the bedside immediately after the diagnosis is established.[20] If either of these techniques is unsuccessful, a blade atrial septostomy performed at the time of catheterization and the Blalock-Hanlon procedure are useful alternatives. The Blalock-Hanlon procedure is an atrial septectomy performed through a right lateral thoracotomy incision without cardiopulmonary bypass.

### Physiologic correction

Fontan and Baudet[11] described their operation for the physiologic pulmonary blood flow restoration in tricuspid atresia in 1971. It is based upon the realization that venous (or atrial) pressure alone is adequate to drive blood through the pulmonary circulation. The original operation completely separated the pulmonary and systemic circulations.

The operation consisted of the following:

1. Classic cava-pulmonary anastomosis (end to side) between distal end of right pulmonary artery and right posterolateral aspect of the superior vena cava (Glenn).
2. Proximal end of right pulmonary artery is anastomosed to right atrium by means of an aortic valve homograft.
3. ASD is closed under cardiopulmonary bypass.
4. Pulmonary valve homograft is inserted into inferior vena cava.
5. Main pulmonary artery is ligated or transected.
6. SVC is ligated where it enters the right atrium.

Fig. 23–6 illustrates that the blood returning from the superior vena cava now perfuses the right pulmonary artery, and blood from the inferior vena cava passes though the right atrium and then into the left pulmonary artery. The atrial septal defect is closed, and the pulmonary and systemic circulations are thus completely separated. A low pulmonary vascular resistance is imperative for the procedure to succeed. Choussat and associates[6] described the ideal selection criteria for the Fontan procedure (box). The criteria are not absolute. Pulmonary hypertension, for instance, may not be an absolute contraindication provided the pulmonary vascular resistance is low.[14,26] Waterston and Potts shunts are no longer favored if a Fontan procedure is contemplated for the future. A Glenn shunt, by contrast, protects patients from postoperative hemodynamic instability and has been suggested to decrease morbidity from the Fontan procedure.[7] A 5- to 15-year follow-up after Fontan operations has shown that the Choussat criteria are still appropriate and that alternatives should be considered in high-risk patients.[8] Although the procedure could be termed a physiologic correction, it was concluded that it really is palliative in that considerable long-term morbidity and mortality are associated with it. Early complications include ascites and pleural effusion due to high venous pressures, arrhythmias, chylothorax, renal failure, low cardiac output, and deterioration of valves and conduits. Mid- to long-term complications include cirrhosis, subaortic obstruction, protein-losing enteropathy, atrioventricular valve insufficiency, cardiomyopathy and death.[8] Many variations of the Fontan procedure have been described. Kreutzer described an

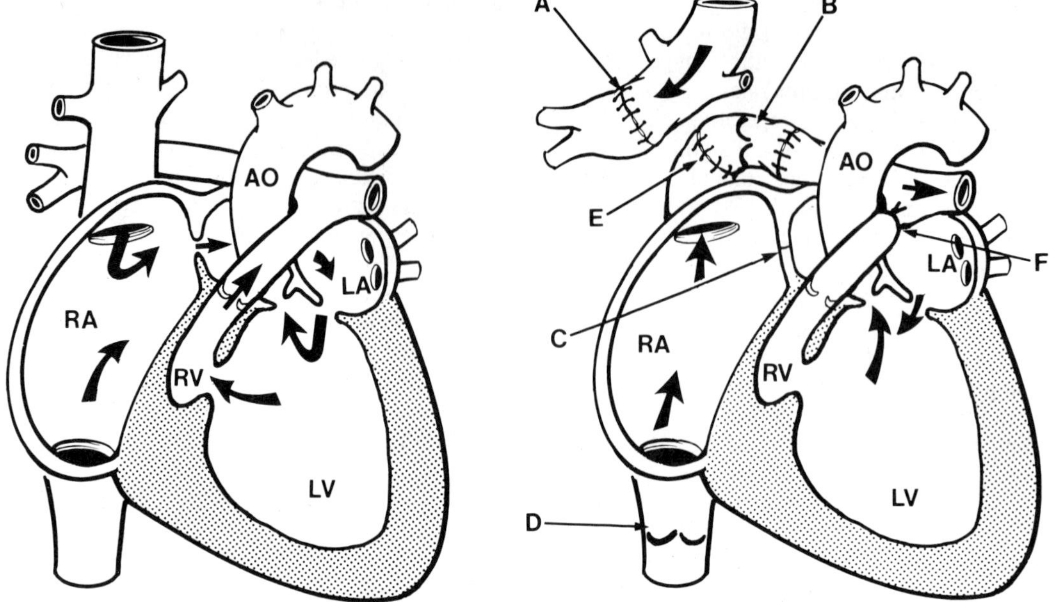


**Figure 23–6** The original Fontan procedure. **A,** Anastomosis between distal end of the right pulmonary artery and the right posterolateral aspect of the superior vena cava. **B,** Proximal end of the right pulmonary artery anastomosed to right atrium by an aortic valve homograft. **C,** Atrial septal defect closure. **D,** Pulmonary valve homograft inserted into inferior vena cava. **E,** Superior vena cava ligation. **F,** Main pulmonary artery ligation. *AO,* Aorta; *RA,* right atrium; *LA,* left atrium; *RV,* right ventricle; *LV,* left ventricle.

end to end anastomosis between the right atrial appendage and the pulmonary artery.[21] The ASD was closed, but neither a prosthetic valve nor a Glenn procedure was used. He commented that a direct connection was the preferred technique because it avoided the complications of conduits. The underlying rationale for the operation was the thought that the atrium was not acting as a pump at all and that the system relied on the left ventricle as a suction pump.[22]

Complications of valved and nonvalved conduits include fibrous peel formation, thrombotic occlusion, calcification and obstruction of the valve, and abnormal valve function (with possible reoperation to relieve obstruction).[3,5] Conduits to the pulmonary artery are preferable to those to a ventricle.[10] The aim is the formation of a wide-open, nonobstructive direct atriopulmonary communication. A patient who is not yet suitable for a modified Fontan procedure may be a candidate for a bidirectional cavopulmonary anastomosis.[4,22] This is a modification of the Glenn procedure. The upper end of the divided superior vena cava is anastomosed end to side to the right pulmonary artery, which diverts its flow to both right and left pulmonary arteries. A decrease in cyanosis and improvement in hemodynamics during future Fontan procedures have been the promising result.[4]

## ANESTHESIA MANAGEMENT

### Palliative shunt operations

These are often performed on severely cyanotic newborns. The overriding consideration in their management is whether pulmonary blood flow is restricted or excessive. The common scenario is limited pulmonary blood flow. These patients survive by virtue of their open ductus arteriosus and their often small ASD. Pulmonary blood flow must be maintained: remember to avoid all causes of PDA contraction (Table 23–1, box), continue prostaglandin therapy, and maintain a warm, humidified, and oxygenated environment. Small infants under 6 months of age may not require premedication. I frequently premedicate infants older than this with oral midazolam 0.5 to 0.6 mg/kg approximately 30 minutes before surgery under direct supervision of the anesthesiologist. Such infants may be prone to cyanotic spells not unlike those of infants with tetralogy of Fallot. Stimulation or distress during the induction phase may precipitate these spells. Airway stimulation should be avoided until the surgical plane of anesthesia is reached and intravenous access is obtained. It is of vital importance that all intravenous and arterial lines be carefully purged of all air bubbles during the preparation for surgery and that this maneuver be repeated just prior to their use. Paradoxical air embolism is a real risk.

Monitoring prior to induction of anesthesia consists of ECG, noninvasive blood pressure measurements, and pulse oximetry.

Induction of anesthesia is preferably intravenous, with fentanyl in doses of 20 to 50 μg/kg along with a nondepolarizing muscle relaxant such as vecuronium 0.1 to 0.2 mg/kg and atropine 10 μg/kg or pancuronium 0.1 mg/kg. Succinylcholine is preferably avoided because of its potential effects on the ductus arteriosus (see Chapter 14). Ketamine has the theoretic potential to increase pulmonary vascular resistance and has a negatively inotropic effect in adults, usually offset by its vagolytic side effect. In children the effect on pulmonary vascular resistance does not occur, and I use ketamine when the child is inadequately sedated and no intravenous access is available. When no intravenous access is available, an inhalational induction with nitrous oxide 50% and incremental halothane is acceptable. Once the patient has reached an acceptable plane of anesthesia, an intravenous line is established and intravenous anesthesia using a narcotic (fentanyl 10 to 20 μg/kg or sufentanil 1.5 to 2.5 μg/kg) is substituted. The inspired oxygen tension can then be elevated to 100%. Retrolental fibroplasia is not a concern in these types of congenital heart disease because a high arterial oxygen pressure cannot be attained in the presence of such large shunts. Halothane is a negative inotrope and is therefore best discontinued, as low cardiac output states and CHF are frequent complications in these patients.

The Blalock Hanlon procedure deserves special attention: After right lateral thoracotomy, a portion of each atrium is isolated from the circulation using a vascular clamp. After two atrial incisions the atrial septum is pulled into the surgical field and excised. Significant reductions in pulmonary and systemic return may occur during the few minutes of partial occlusion, leading to a reduction of cardiac output and worsening hypoxia. A 2-minute period of hyperventilation on 100% oxygen and the administration of bicarbonate 1 mEq/kg and atropine 0.15 mg/kg may be useful prior to clamp application. This will help compensate for the anticipated period of hypotension and acidosis. Packed red cells should be checked and ready for rapid administration when the clamp is removed, and pH correction of the transfused blood should be considered.

### Fontan procedure

***Premedication.*** The patients for this procedure or one of its modifications are usually older than 4 years (selection criteria for the Fontan procedure). These children are old enough to experience considerable anxiety prior to surgery. Adequate premedication and communication are very important. Premedication may be in the form of oral benzodiazepines (e.g., midazolam 0.5 mg/kg or diazepam 0.1 mg/kg) or in combination with intramuscular opiates (meperidine 1 mg/kg or morphine 0.1 mg/kg).[13] The premedication is usually given about 90 minutes prior to transfer to the operating room, except for midazolam, which is given orally 20 minutes prior to transfer, under direct supervision, to patients who have no intravascular access.

***Induction and prebypass period.*** Adults usually have radial arterial lines and intravenous access placed under local anesthesia while receiving 100% oxygen. All patients are monitored with an automated blood pressure measuring device (in the absence of an arterial line), ECG, and pulse oximetry from the time of induction of anesthesia. In the period before bypass the management goals can be divided into those for patients with decreased pulmonary blood flow (pulmonary atresia) and those with increased pulmonary flow. In those with decreased pulmonary blood flow, goals are aimed at optimizing arterial saturations by maintaining a low pulmonary vascular resistance and a good cardiac output. Airway stimulation during light anesthesia, bucking, coughing, acidosis, hypoxia, hypothermia, and a screaming unpremedicated child are incompatible with this goal. Ventilation to normocarbia or slight hypocarbia to reduce PVR is suggested. Prostaglandin infusions must be continued.

Patients with high pulmonary blood flow (frequently in cardiac failure) require a normal to high pulmonary vascular resistance. Positive pressure ventilation to normocarbia is recommended. If the patient is in congestive heart failure, inhalational agents for anesthetic induction are best avoided. Intramuscular ketamine with atropine allows the establishment of intravenous access and the use of an opioid anesthetic for maintenance. A careful titration of fentanyl increments of 1 μg/kg and diazepam 0.1 mg/kg up to a total of 1 mg/kg diazepam and 100 μg/kg fentanyl is a useful technique. Ventilation is gently controlled manually and neuromuscular paralysis obtained using pancuronium 0.1 mg/kg once the patient has lost consciousness. Patients who are not in failure at the time of surgery will usually tolerate an inhalational induction with halothane.[13,25] Many infants require inotropic support in the prebypass period. Hypovolemia secondary to fluid deficit and the hyperviscosity due to a high hematocrit lead to a high systemic and pulmonary vascular resistance and the danger of sludging. Patients who had no prior intravenous access and who have low pulmonary blood flow states benefit from a rapid intravenous infusion of 5 ml/kg of a crystalloid solution after the induction of anesthesia.

***Post-CPB phase.*** The Glenn shunt and the various modifications of the Fontan procedure have in common the reliance on venous or atrial pressures to perfuse the pulmonary vasculature. This means a relatively high right atrial or central venous pressure (15 mm Hg) and a low pulmonary vascular resistance are required. During rewarming from hypothermic bypass an infusion of isoproterenol 0.1 μg/kg/min or a combination of dopamine (up to 10 μg/kg/min) and sodium nitroprusside 1 to 2 μg/kg/min are begun.[27,34] The infusions are continued for 24 to 48 hours postoperatively. A central venous pressure of 15 mm Hg and an atrial pressure of about 10 mm Hg often optimize hemodynamic parameters. PEEP and other causes of raised intrathoracic pressure are avoided. Large tidal volumes, a short inspiratory phase, and ventilation to normocapnea as well as the avoidance of hypothermia and acidosis are again the goals of management. Although early return to spontaneous ventilation has the benefit of improving pulmonary blood flow, in my experience early hemodynamic instability often makes a 24-hour period of sedation, relaxation, and ventilatory support the preferred approach.

## REFERENCES


1. Anderson RH, Rigby ML: The morphologic heterogeneity of tricuspid atresia, *Int J Cardiol* 16:67, 1987.
2. Astley R, Oldham JS, Parson C: Congenital tricuspid atresia, *Br Heart J* 15:287, 1953.
3. Ben-Shachar G, Nicoloff DM, Edwards JE: Separation of neointima from Dacron graft causing obstruction, *J Thorac Cardiovasc Surg* 82:268, 1981.
4. Bridges N, Jonas RA, Mayer JE et al: Bidirectional cavopulmonary anastomosis as interim palliation for high-risk Fontan candidates, *Circulation* 82:170 (suppl 4), 1990.
5. Chopra PS, Rao PS: Corrective surgery for tricuspid atresia: which modification of Fontan-Kreutzer should be used? a review, *Am Heart J* 123(3):758, 1992.
6. Choussat A, Fontan F, Besse P et al: Selection criteria for Fontan's procedure. In Anderson RH, Shinebourne EA (eds): *Pediatric cardiology,* Edinburgh, 1978, Churchill Livingstone.
7. De Leon SY, Ilbawi MN, Idriss FS et al: Fontan operation for complex lesions: surgical considerations to improve survival, *Cardiovasc Surg* 92:1029-1037, 1986.
8. Driscoll D, Offord KP, Feldt RH et al: Five- to 15-year follow-up after Fontan operation, *Circulation* 85(2):469 February 1992.
9. Eagle KA, Habor E, DeSanctis RW et al: *The practice of cardiology,* ed 2, Boston, 1989, Little Brown.
10. Fernandez G, Costa F, Fontan F et al: Prevalence of reoperation for pathway obstruction after Fontan operation, *Ann Thorac Surg* 48:654-9, 1989.
11. Fontan F, Baudet E: Surgical repair of tricuspid atresia, *Thorax* 26:240, 1971.
12. Freed MD, Heymann MA, Lewis AB et al: Prostaglandin $E_1$ in infants with ductus arteriosus–dependent congenital heart disease, *Circulation* 64:899, 1981.
13. Fyman PN, Goodman K, Casthely PA et al: Anesthetic management of patients undergoing Fontan procedure, *Anesth Analg* 65:516, 1986.
14. Gildein HP, Ahmadi A, Fontan F et al: Special problems in Fontan-type operations for complex cardiac lesions, *Int J Cardiology* 29:21-28, 1990.
15. Glenn WWL: Circulatory bypass of the right side of the heart IV: shunt between superior vena cava and distal right pulmonary artery, *N Engl J Med* 259:117-24, 1958.
16. Grossman W: *Cardiac catheterization and angiography,* ed 3, Philadelphia, 1986, Lea & Febiger.
17. Kaplan JA: *Cardiac anesthesia,* ed 1, vol 2, Philadelphia, 1987, Saunders.
18. Katz J, Steward DJ: *Anesthesia and uncommon pediatric diseases,* Philadelphia, 1987, Saunders.
19. Keith JD, Rowe RD, Vlad P: *Heart disease in infancy and childhood,* ed 3, Macmillan, New York, 1978.
20. Kipel G, Arnon R, Ritter SB: Transesophageal echocardiographic guidance of balloon atrial septostomy, *J Am Soc Echocardiogr* 4(6):631, 1991.
21. Kreutzer G, Galindez E, Bono H et al: An operation for the correction of tricuspid atresia, *J Thorac Cardiovasc Surg* 66: 1973.
22. Kreutzer G, Vargas FJ, Schlichter AJ et al: Atriopulmonary anastomosis, *J Thorac Cardiovasc Surg* 83:427, 1982.
23. Lake C, editor: *Pediatric cardiac anesthesia,* East Norwalk, Conn, 1988, Appleton & Lange.
24. Langman J: *Medical embryology,* ed 3, Baltimore, 1975, Williams & Wilkins.
25. Lowe DA: Abormalities of the atrioventricular valves. In Lake C, editor: *Pediatric cardiac anesthesia,* East Norwalk, Conn, 1988, Appleton & Lange.
26. Mayer JE, Helgason H, Jonas RA et al: Extending the limits for the modified Fontan procedures, *J Thorac Cardiovasc Surg* 92:1021, 1986.
27. Mentzer RM, Alegre CA, Nolan SP: The effects of dopamine and isoproterenol on the pulmonary circulation, *J Thorac Cardiovasc Surg* 71:807, 1976.
28. Olley PM: Nonsurgical palliation of congenital heart malformations, *N Engl J Med* 297:951, 1972.
29. Rao PS: Terminology: tricuspid atresia or univentricular heart. In Rao PS, editor: *Tricuspid atresia,* Mt Kisco, NY, 1982, Futura.
30. Rao PS: A unified classification for tricuspid atresia, *Am Heart J* 99:799, 1980.
31. Rashkind WJ: Tricuspid atresia: a historical review, *Pediatr Cardiol* 2:85, 1982.
32. Tandon R, Edwards JE: Tricuspid atresia: a reevaluation and classification, *J Thorac Cardiovasc Surg* 67:530, 1974.
33. Van Praagh R, Ando M: Anatomic types of tricuspid atresia: clinical and developmental implications, *Circulation* 44(suppl 2):115, 1971 (abstract).
34. Williams DB, Kiernan PD, Schaff HV et al: The hemodynamic response to dopamine and nitroprusside following right atrium–pulmonary artery bypass (Fontan procedure), *Ann Thorac Surg* 34:51, 1982.

## Section C OBSTRUCTIVE LESIONS

# 24 Coarctation of the Aorta

*Wesley W. Kinney*



First described in 1750, coarctation of the aorta affects approximately 7% to 9% of patients with congenital heart disease. It is associated with both Marfan's and Turner's syndromes. It most commonly occurs near the ductus arteriosus but also occurs in the lower thoracic and abdominal aorta. Although the incidence of abdominal coarctation is equal in the two sexes, males are two to five times as often affected by thoracic coarctation.

## EMBRYOLOGY

The aortic arch normally arises predominantly from the left fourth arch of the primitive arches of the truncus arteriosus between the fifth and seventh weeks of gestation (Fig. 24–1). The cause of coarctation is uncertain. For whatever reason—intrusion of ductal arteriosus closure into adjacent normal aorta, extension of ductal muscle into aortal wall, or primary aortic malformation or hypoplasia—the aorta proximal to the site of ductal insertion, arising from the embryologic left fourth arch, is the most frequent site of clinically significant coarctation (Fig. 24–2). This produces the common preductal coarctation. When anomalous development occurs from the regions of the sixth primitive aortic arch to the point of fusion of the two dorsal aortae, postductal coarctation results. Juxtaductal coarctation results from an intraluminal tissue shelf—hemodynamically insignificant with fetal circulation—arising from the aortic wall directly opposite aortic insertion of the ductus arteriosus (Fig. 24–2). Upon transition from fetal to neonatal circulation, with both ductal constriction and increased aortic arch flow, this abnormal tissue shelf becomes manifest as the clinical consequence of reduced aortic flow. The typical coarctation results in reduction of aortic luminal diameter to as little as 1 to 3 mm. In an extreme form there is complete interruption of the aortic arch *(vide infra)*.

## PATHOPHYSIOLOGY

Infants with preductal coarctation have little or no collateral circulation because intrauterine perfusion of the lower body occurs via the ductus arteriosus. Systemic pressures in the right ventricle ensure profusion of the ascending aorta and the lower body of the neonate with preductal coarctation so long as the ductus remains patent. As a result no pressure gradient, upon which development of collateral circulation depends, ever occurs. When the ductus arteriosus closes, these neonates promptly develop congestive heart failure, shock, oliguria, and renal

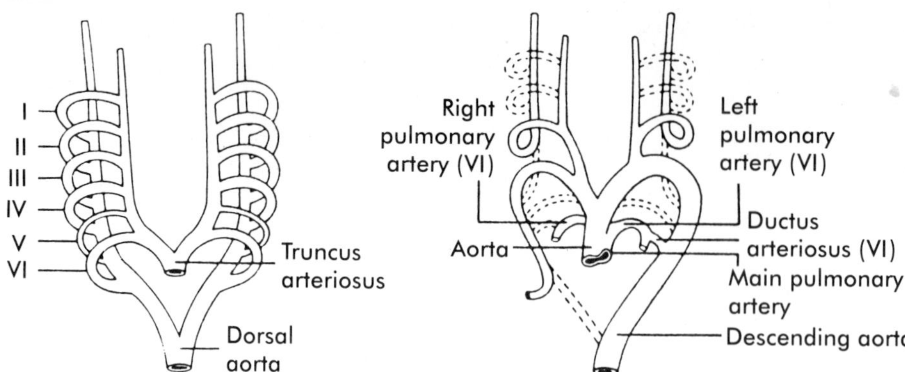


**Figure 24–1** Diagram of the development of the aortic arch system as it relates to the ductus arteriosus. (From Fink BW, editor: *Congenital heart disease: a deductive approach to its diagnosis,* ed 3, St. Louis, 1991, Mosby.

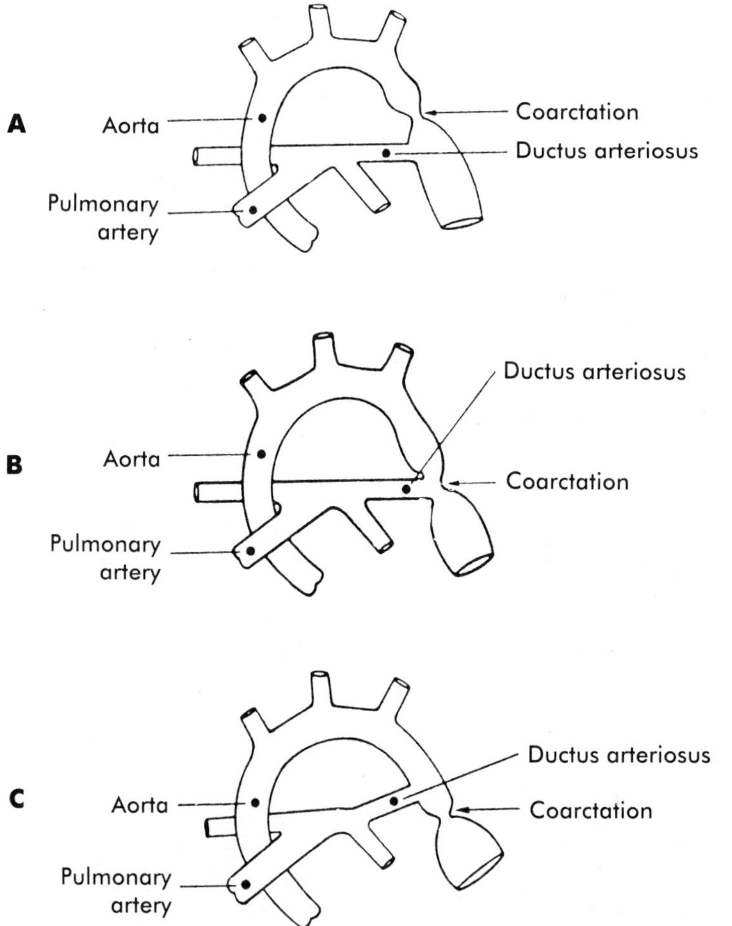


**Figure 24–2** Diagram of the anatomic variations of coarctation of the aorta as it relates to the location of the ductus arteriosus. **A,** preductal type. **B,** Ductal type. **C,** Postductal type. (From Fink BW, editor: *Congenital heart disease: a deductive approach to its diagnosis,* ed 3, St. Louis, 1991, Mosby.

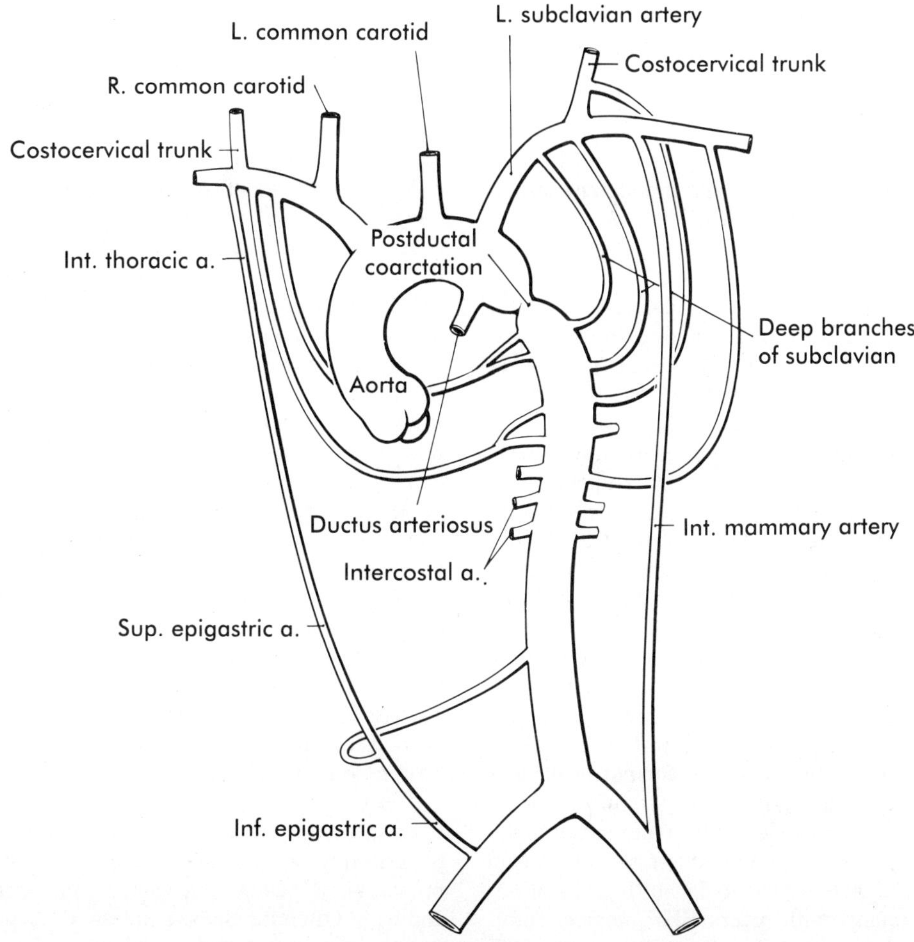


**Figure 24–3** Collateral circulation in coarctation of the aorta. Note that branches of the subclavian arteries are completely responsible for the collaterals proximal to the coarctation, but distal to the block, blood reaches the descending aorta through the intercostal arteries and the anastomoses between the superior and inferior epigastric vessels.

shutdown. Prostaglandin $E_1$ infusion, in the hope of maintaining ductal patency, is essential treatment for this group of patients. These neonates are likely to have the many congenital heart defects to which patients with coarctation are prone, further aggravating their circulatory decompensation when the ductus does close.[7,8,14,15,17]

Patients with postductal coarctation develop pressure gradients, typically 30 to 40 mm Hg, that stimulate collateral circulation development involving intercostal, internal mammary, and internal thoracic arteries, among others (Fig. 24–3). Thus closure of the ductus arteriosus has far less effect upon patients with postductal coarctation than on those with preductal coarctation. Patients in this group often remain asymptomatic into their teens or later, in contradistinction to those with preductal coarctation, who typically become chronically quite ill within the first couple of weeks of life.

## CLINICAL PRESENTATION

The majority of neonatal and infant patients with preductal coarctation manifest tachypnea, dyspnea, poor feeding, weight gain, and signs of congestive heart failure within the initial 3 months of life. In fact, coarctation is the most common cause of CHF diagnosed at the age of 1 to 3 weeks. Bicuspid aortic valve is present in up to 75% of patients with coarctation, most often without symptoms in neonates and infants. VSD, PDA, or transposition of the great arteries is associated in approximately 40% of patients with coarctation, and these associated lesions will have a major impact on the presence and severity of signs and symptoms, which typically develop early in the neonatal period. With associated VSD, left ventricular peak systolic pressure and the degree of left to right shunting are determined by the degree of coarctation. Mitral stenosis, mitral insufficiency, ASD, or endocardial fibroelastosis may also coexist. When CHF develops, mitral regurgitation secondary to papillary muscle necrosis often follows. Almost all congenital heart defects have been associated with coarctation except tetralogy of Fallot and pulmonary atresia and stenosis. All these associated cardiac defects are more common with preductal coarctation.

### Laboratory findings

***Physical examination.*** The classic findings in coarctation are pulses in the lower extremities that are delayed and diminished or absent, in association with reduced blood pressure readings in the lower extremities and abnormally elevated blood pressure readings in the upper extremities; these may exceed those in the lower extremities by 20 mm Hg or more. The pattern of pulse abnormality sometimes may suggest the location of the coarctation. When pulses are present in the right arm, right carotid artery, and left arm but absent on the left side, coarctation is at the aortic isthmus. If the pulse is palpable in the right arm but absent in the left arms and legs, or if the right arm blood pressure is greater than the left arm blood pressure, coarctation is proximal to or adjacent to left subclavian artery takeoff. If the pulse is palpable in the left arm but not in the right upper extremity or legs, coarctation is distal to left subclavian artery in association with a rare anomalous right subclavian artery that originates distal to the aortic coarctation. In sicker infants with severe CHF medical stabilization and significant improvement of the CHF may be required before the differential pulse and blood pressure findings are manifest. Prostaglandin $E_1$ infusion can maintain ductal patency, and sodium bicarbonate is used to correct acidemia. It is apparent that blood pressure measurements must be made in both arms and the lower extremities.

Patients who develop normally and remain asymptomatic, predominantly those with localized postductal coarctation, may only be detected on screening physical exam with detection of a systolic ejection murmur, usually grade 2/6 to 3/6 radiating over the upper right sternal border, left sternal border, apical area, or occasionally posteriorly in the interscapular area left of the midline. Because up to half of patients with coarctation have associated bicuspid aortic valve, an ejection click is often heard, and occasionally the diastolic murmur of aortic insufficiency is also found. A systolic thrill may be palpable in the suprasternal notch area.

Infants with preductal coarctation are usually in variable degrees of respiratory distress, often with accompanying metabolic acidemia and oliguria or anuria reflecting the degree of CHF. Frequently there is a prominent $S_3$ gallop and a diffuse systolic ejection murmur. With greater degrees of CHF there may be only a faint murmur or even none at all. With effective medical therapy and improvement in the CHF the murmur may become more prominent.

When a right to left shunt via the PDA is present, the lower half of the body may be differentially cyanotic. In that case the upper half of the body receives well oxygenated blood via the vessels originating from the aortic arch above the level of the coarctation, but the lower half of the body is poorly perfused with lower-saturation blood from the right ventricle via the pulmonary artery and PDA, from which tissue oxygen extraction is high relative to local tissue perfusion and blood oxygen content, resulting in the cyanosis. Metabolic acidemia, and eventually renal failure, will develop when systemic hypoperfusion persists long enough.

***Electrocardiogram.*** In individuals with postductal coarctation whose condition is detected during asymptomatic later life, ECG usually shows ventricular hypertrophy, often with leftward axis deviation of the QRS complex. A significant proportion of these older patients with postductal coarctation will have a normal ECG.

The hallmark on ECG of the asymptomatic patients presenting early in life is right ventricular hypertrophy, often with strain or right bundle branch block pattern, associated with dominant $R_I$ and $S_{AVF}$. Often the S wave in lead $V_1$ is quite deep and the R wave in the lateral precordial leads is very tall.

***Chest x-ray film.*** In individuals presenting asymptomatically in later life, heart size may be entirely normal or occasionally slightly enlarged, with or without dilatation of the ascending aorta. When chest film is taken so as to result in overpenetration, a 3 sign representing prestenotic and poststenotic dilatation may be seen (Fig. 24–4). The reverse 3 sign, or E sign, especially on the left anterior oblique projection of the barium swallow, will show displacement of the barium-filled esophagus anterially where the poststenotic aortic dilatation causes an indentation leading to a configuration that looks somewhat like an E. Rarely seen in infancy and infrequent in patients under 5 years of age, rib notching involving ribs 4, 5, 6, 7, 8 or 9 in some combination is the classic pathognomonic hallmark of increased collateral circulation resulting from thoracic coarctation of the aorta.

In patients presenting symptomatically younger in life, findings are those typical of but nonspecific for CHF, that is, any combination of marked cardiomegaly, pulmonary edema, and pulmonary venous congestion.

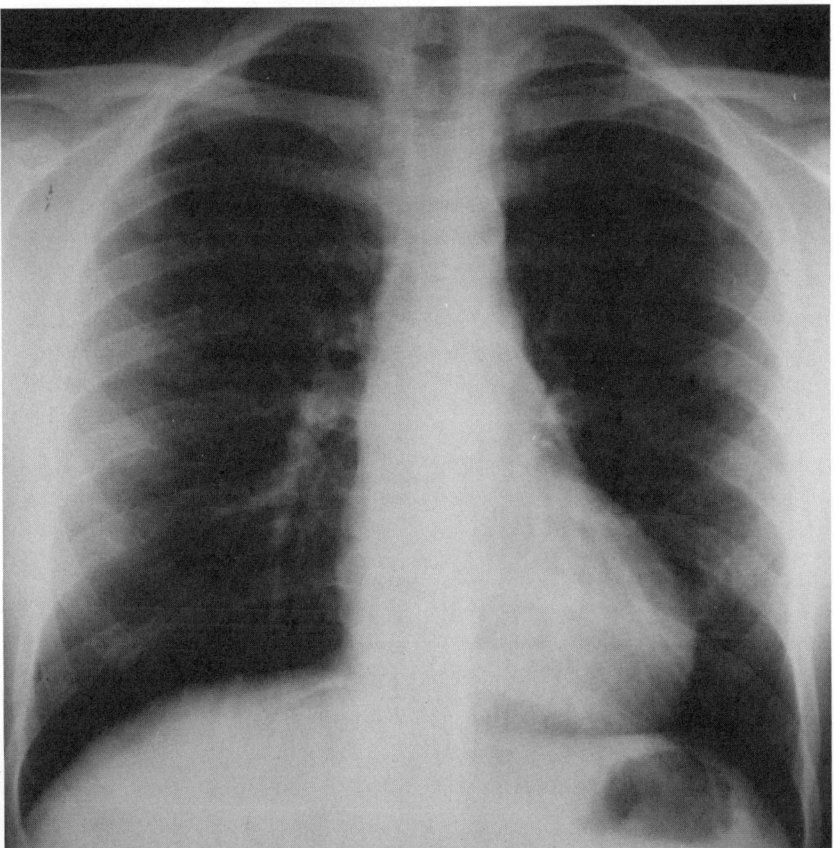

**Figure 24–4** Posteroanterior chest radiograph of a 16-year-old girl with coarctation of aorta. Note the rib notching, particularly that involving the left fourth rib. In addition there is a 3 sign abnormality of the aortic arch. Although the heart is not enlarged, the configuration is consistent with left ventricular hypertrophy. (Courtesy of Sandra G. Kirchner, MD.)

***Echocardiogram.*** In patients presenting asymptomatically later in life, a shelflike membrane is often visualized posteriorly and laterally in the descending aorta, especially from the suprasternal notch view, with two-dimensional echocardiography. Associated anomalies such as bicuspid aortic valve or a VSD can often be demonstrated with echo, rendering cardiac catheterization unnecessary for diagnosis in many instances. However, certain critical views required for successful demonstration of the usual location of coarctation, such as suprasternal notch imaging, demand cervical hyperextension and somewhat elevated shoulder support, difficult to achieve and maintain in children. The certainty with which diagnosis can be made by echocardiogram varies from one center to another, depending on the skill and experience of the echocardiographer and the quality of the images obtained.

***Cardiac catheterization.*** Cardiac catheterization, when necessary, will show a clear pressure differential between ascending and descending aorta with a significant pressure drop distal to the site of coarctation. It also can definitively identify any associated lesion such as bicuspid aortal valve with or without stenosis, VSD, transposition of the arteries, and so on. Indications for cardiac catheterization include incomplete information from echocardiogram, concern over collateral flow that may affect the planning of the operative repair, and complex associated congenital heart disease that needs to be better delineated. Usual collateral circulation includes dilated subdivisions and branches of subclavian arteries, internal mammary arteries, superior intercostal arteries except the first two pairs, internal thoracic arteries, intercostal arteries (which over years cause rib notching), superior epigastric arteries, and perhaps anterior spinal ar-

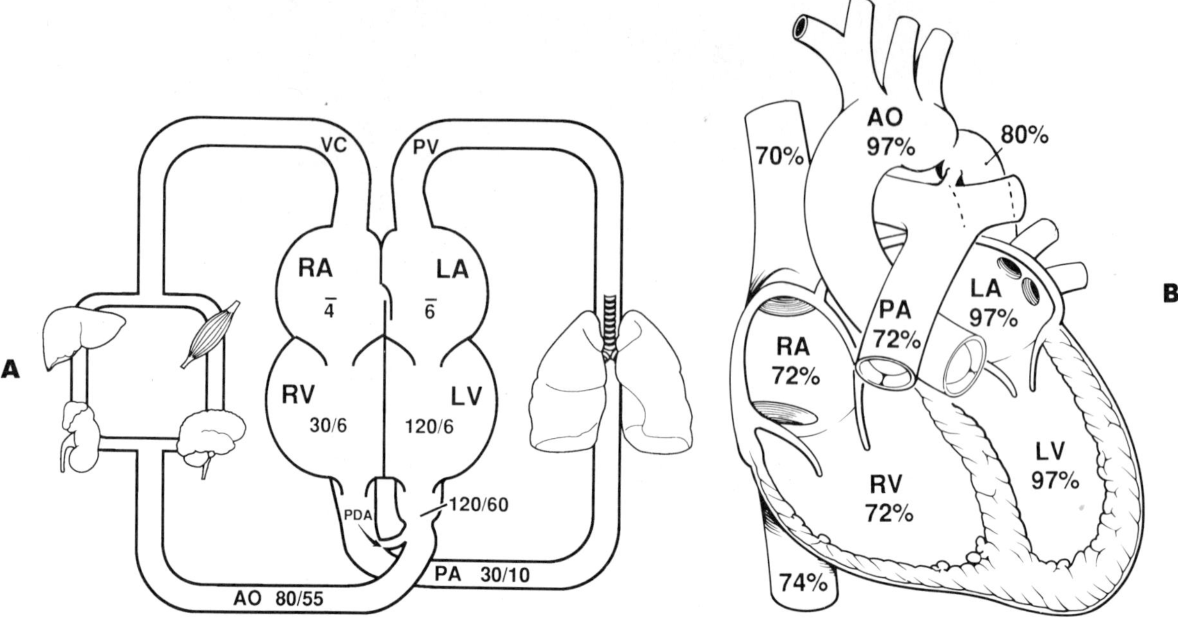


**Figure 24–5** Typical pressures (mm Hg) and oxygen saturations in a patient with preductal type of coarctation of the aorta. *VC,* Vena cava; *PV,* pulmonary vein; *RA,* right artery; *LA,* left artery; *RV,* right ventricle; *LV,* left ventricle; *PDA,* patent ductus arteriosus; *PA,* pulmonary artery; *AO,* aorta.

tery and vertebral arteries. Patients who have adequate collateral circulation are less likely to develop paraplegia as a result of aortic cross-clamping intraoperatively.[9,10,16,18] Patients with poorly developed collateral flow may benefit from information gained at the time of preoperative catheterization to allow for consideration of possible intraoperative shunting procedures and selection of location of any cross-clamp applications. Fig. 24–5 shows typical pressures and oxygen saturations of a patient with preductal coarctation of the aorta.

## MEDICAL MANAGEMENT

Patients with coarctation of the aorta who pass through infancy undiagnosed are apt to develop significant hypertension that becomes evident in childhood. The hypertension should be detected on screening examination such as a school physical. Coupled with recognition of pulse discrepancies and pressure gradients between upper and lower extremities, the diagnosis of coarctation should be made promptly. Surgical therapy is usually planned for ages 4 to 8 years, depending on the aortic size, and is often scheduled for the surgeon's and family's preferences.[17]

For the sick neonate or infant with CHF, digitalization, diuresis, oxygen therapy, and inotropic support will be employed. Prostaglandin $E_1$ may be given to maintain the patency of the ductus arteriosus in patients whose systemic perfusion depends on the right to left shunt. All these medications must be continued until the patient arrives for anesthesia in surgery.

Prognosis with medical treatment alone is poor for preductal coarctation: about 50% mortality in the first month of life, more than 80% in the first 3 months. With surgical correction the mortality rate decreases to less than 5%.

For postductal coarctation the average prognosis for survival is to about age 35 years, with a fatality rate by age 40 increasing to 60% to 70%, usually due to rupture of the aorta, CHF, bacterial endocarditis, or an intercerebral bleed. In adults and asymptomatic children operative mortality is less than 1%.

## SURGICAL MANAGEMENT

A variety of surgical techniques are employed for coarctation repair (Fig. 24–6).[1-6,9-11,16,18] When feasible, the procedure of choice is resection of the coarcted segment and primary end to end anastomosis. In neonates and infants up to 5 cm of aorta can be excised because of the elasticity of the remaining aorta. Progressive fibrosis decreases the elasticity in older children to the point that only about half as much aorta can be excised, and thus subclavian arterial flap, angioplasty, or Dacron patch repair may be required. For prolonged seg-

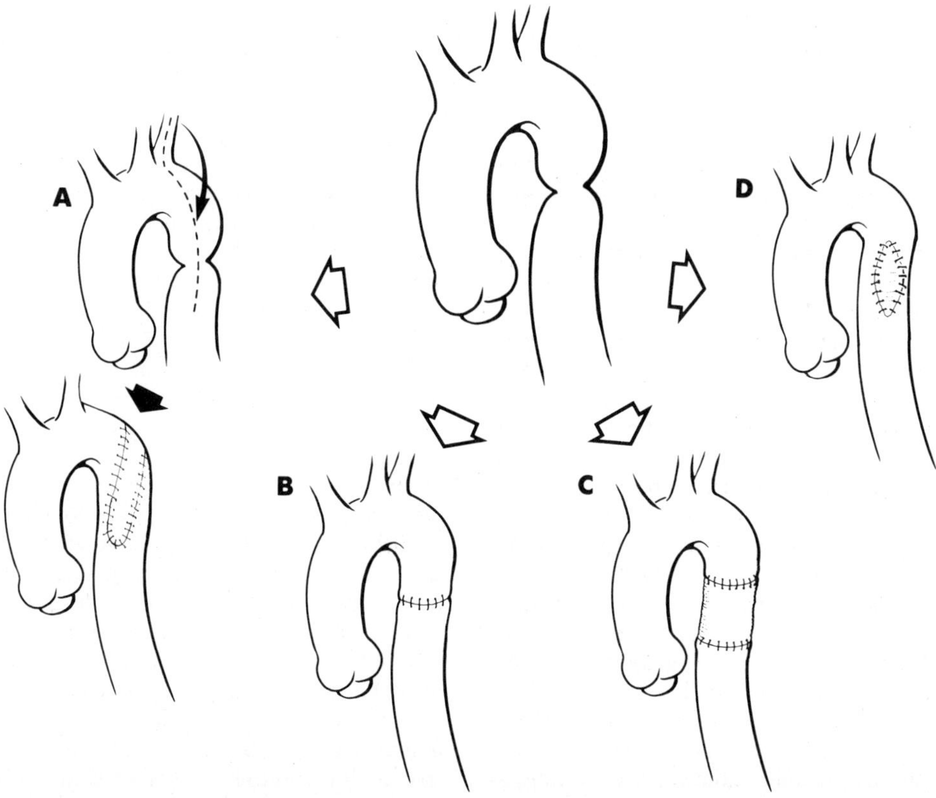


**Figure 24–6** Surgical techniques for correction of coarctation of the aorta. **A,** subclavian artery angioplasty. **B,** Resection and end to end anastomosis. **C,** Resection and repair with a Dacron graft. **D,** Repair with a Dacron patch.

ments of coarctation and for recurrent coarctation, use of Dacron interposition graft, or for a bypass, tube graft may be the only options. Adult coarctation often has sufficient degenerative fibrosis of the aorta that primary anastomosis is too hazardous, which mandates a prosthetic graft.

## ANESTHESIA MANAGEMENT

### Preoperative evaluation and preparation

Overall anesthetic management of the patient with coarctation of the aorta is guided, as for all cardiac lesions, by the patient's physical status and associated cardiologic and medical problems at the time of surgery. Especially heavy emphasis is placed upon an estimate of the patient's cardiopulmonary reserve and whether the current physical status has been optimally treated medically to put the patient in the best possible physical condition for the proposed anesthetic and surgical stresses. In this regard evaluation from the pediatric cardiologist, including the results of echocardiography and cardiac catheterization, as well as a thorough history as to the patient's exercise tolerance, are crucial. Obviously, it is important to know if the patient has had any prior surgery and the response to the stresses of anesthesia and surgery, particularly whether prior cardiac surgery has been performed. Thorough information about prior and current medical treatment is essential to plan perioperative continuation of essential cardiovascular pulmonary medications the patient may be taking, and to facilitate anticipation of drug interactions. Also essential is whether or not the patient has a functioning shunt between the right and left sides of the heart. Special care must always be taken in pediatric cardiac surgery patients to debubble scrupulously all intravenous fluid lines so as to avoid the possibility of right to left shunt of any air bubbles that might reach the coronary or cerebral circulation with devastating consequences.

Furthermore, factors that alter pulmonary blood flow must always be taken into account when planning the preanesthetic preparation, premedication, and intraoperative management of the patient who has coarctation of the aorta with associated VSD or other sources of potential for intracardiac shunting.

## Premedication

Physical status of patients presenting for repair of coarctation varies widely from the older asymptomatic individual who is an ASA PS-II patient to a sick neonate PS-IV in full congestive failure on vasopressor and diuretic support and likely digitalized for borderline cardiac function with minimal or no cardiac reserve. For the sick neonate, or in any child under approximately 6 to 9 months of age, premedication is as a rule inappropriate. Many patients up to 12 to 14 months of age do not require premedication; these decisions must of course be individualized regarding the patient's anticipated needs for sedation (i.e., predicted changes in emotional state) during the immediate preoperative period. For select calm older patients premedication may be unnecessary. Any sedation that is wanted can best be given in the operating room holding area immediately adjacent to the operating room because the patient can immediately be transferred from the holding area directly to the operating room should any unintended oversedation result. For patients with an intravenous line already in place, this also offers the advantage for the anesthesiologist to titrate the level of sedation under direct monitoring of oxygen saturation with supplemental oxygen as indicated by pulse oximetry and overall patient status.

In transfer of the patient from the hospital room or holding area to the operating room, particularly in the sicker patients and in infants and neonates, of crucial consideration is maintenance of a thermally neutral environment, so that there is no additional stress placed on the heart due to a change in systemic vascular resistance secondary to vasoconstriction or shivering induced by transit through cold hospital corridors and other areas. Passive warming measures such as clear plastic wrap and even somewhat active methods, for example, warming blankets, can be used to achieve this important goal. Anticholinergic premedication such as atropine often is best given in the operating room, as the primary benefit is that of blocking vagal response to direct laryngoscopy and endotracheal intubation. The onset of this benefit is prompt, but the dry mouth and warm, flushed skin that can result from anticholinergic premedication will last for quite some time and can be a distraction or discomfort to many patients.

Children approximately a year and a half and older, and occasionally some as young as a year, will often benefit from preoperative sedation. This is often best accomplished with the parents accompanying the child from their room or holding area to a location as near to the operating room as possible. The patient may receive oral midazolam 0.5 to 0.7 mg/kg if PS II, or 0.3 to 0.5 if PS III or IV, within 15 to 30 minutes of intended anesthetic induction if no intravenous line is in place. An alternative is atropine 10 to 20 μg/kg with morphine sulphate 0.1 to 0.15 mg/kg IM approximately 60 to 90 minutes prior to induction of anesthesia, again reduced by 30% to 50% for patients in PS-III or IV. All these doses, of course, may be reduced considerably, perhaps as much as 50% to 70%, according to the clinician's estimate of the severity of cardiac dysfunction. Patients with significantly reduced cardiopulmonary reserve who are given reduced dosages on the ward but judged to be insufficiently sedated at the time they arrive in the holding area may be given titrated supplemental sedation in the holding area under direct observation by the anesthesiologist. It is important to ensure provisions for continuous immediate availability of skilled patient assessment of airway and hemodynamic management once premedication is given, whether that be on the floor or in the holding room. Some transfer the unpremedicated patient to the holding area with the patient's family in attendance, resulting in an acceptably calm child who can there be premedicated with less risk from unintended overdosage or underdosage. Particularly with intramuscular premedication, if the dose is too low, the patient may receive only the stress of the painful injection, with little pharmacologic benefit but adverse consequences of increased muscle activity, vasoconstriction, and increased systemic vascular reserve. Any of these, although inconsequential to the patient with normal cardiac reserve, may threaten the patient with reduced cardiac reserve. Preoperative antibiotic chemoprophylaxis is targeted for common gram negative and especially gram positive organisms, particularly *Staphylococcus*, for all patients with associated bicuspid aortic valve or any other lesion predisposing to bacterial endocarditis.

## Monitoring

A left arm blood pressure cuff placement is not used, since the left subclavian artery may be clamped or used for surgical repair of coarctation. Right arm blood pressure cuff values can provide valuable information concerning cerebral circulation during periods of left subclavian artery occlusion. Invasive arterial blood pressure determination is essential if the aorta will be cross-clamped at any level. A preexistent umbilical artery catheterization placed by the neonatologist can be helpful. However, it will give very low or no readings at all during aortic cross-clamping. A right radial arterial line is used for the same reasons that a right arm blood pressure cuff is preferable. Pulse oximetry probe placement is limited by the same restrictions. Occasionally it may be useful to have a cuff on the patient's thigh or calf to measure the blood pressure gradient between upper and lower extremities both before and after the repair.

ECG lead placement must take into account the left lateral thoracotomy approach and right lateral decubitus position, which will be used intraoperatively.

### Induction of anesthesia and endotracheal intubation

Older asymptomatic patients often come to the operating room hemodynamically stable with a running IV in place, well premedicated, and in these patients, one may proceed with an IV induction of sodium thiopental 3 to 5 mg/kg when myocardial function is known to be essentially normal. Neuromuscular relaxation can proceed with succinylcholine 1.5 to 2 mg/kg after atropine 5 to 10 μg/kg and a defasciculating dose of nondepolarizing neuromuscular blocking drug have been given. This applies to patients who do not have ductal-dependent flow via a right to left shunt to the postcoarctation area of the circulation (see Chapter 14).

In patients with suspected or known decrease in myocardial function, rapid intravenous induction may be accomplished either with etomidate 0.15 to 0.3 mg/kg or ketamine 1 to 2 mg/kg, IV push. Alternatively, combined and gradually titrated benzodiazepine and narcotic induction may be used smoothly (e.g., midazolam 0.1 to 0.3 mg/kg and fentanyl 5 to 20 μg/kg or sufentanil 0.5 to 1.5 μg/kg). A major consideration concerning drug and dosage selection is whether or not to preserve the option for early postoperative extubation should the remainder of the patient's operative course be compatible with that objective. In patients with bicuspid aortic valve and significant aortic stenosis or aortic insufficiency, drugs such as ketamine that tend to increase systemic vascular resistance should be avoided. Likewise, if the patient has ductal-dependent physiology (see Chapter 14), high arterial oxygen pressure and probably succinylcholine should be avoided, as they tend to decrease flow through the PDA. Nondepolarizing neuromuscular blockers such as vecuronium 0.1 mg/kg can be used to facilitate endotracheal intubation.

When the patient has no IV line in place, often adequate sedation can be achieved with oral midazolam for placement of an intravenous cannula on arrival in the operating room. When IV access cannot be achieved prior to induction, either an inhalational induction with halothane in low to moderate concentrations or IM ketamine in the range of 5 to 10 mg/kg may be used. If ketamine was the initial agent, IV access is still not possible, and sedation is not yet as deep as required, induction can be completed with the inhalational agent, and IV placement then can be the next step. When necessary, the patient may be masked for lengthy periods, even if cutdown for intravenous access is required on patients with poor prospects of percutaneous venipuncture for such reasons as prematurity or prior operations with multiple past venipunctures. It is important to restrict inhaled concentrations of halothane to less than about 1.5 MAC (less than about 1% to 1.5% maximum inhaled concentration) because of the risk of bradycardia, severe myocardial depression, and even complete heart block.

### Effects of shunting

Left to right shunting may cause a slight reduction in the rate of IV induction, but probably only of theoretical interest. Left to right shunting does not appear to have any clinically significant effects on inhalational induction unless the shunt is very large, for example over 80% of left cardiac output, in which case this may slightly increase inhalational induction. Right to left shunting may slightly hasten inhalational induction, but it is not of major clinical significance.

Once the patient is sufficiently anesthetized, IV access has been established, and the trachea has been intubated, arterial and central lines are placed; this is generally much easier than while the patient is conscious except in the case of an older patient with an IV already in place.

### Maintenance of anesthesia

For sicker patients with physiologically significant associated cardiac lesions and/or depressed myocardial function for whom there are appropriately no plans for early postoperative extubation, a primarily narcotic-based anesthesia (e.g., fentanyl 10 to 25 μg/kg or sufentanil 1.0 to 2.5 μg/kg total doses) can be combined with low dose inhalational anesthetic for maintenance. Continued titration of short-acting benzodiazepine or use of longer-acting agents such as lorazepam is essential to avoid the possibility of the paralyzed, narcotized patient who is nonetheless aware with potential for recall postoperatively. For patients with normal physiology other than the coarctation, lower doses of narcotic with moderate doses of titrate inhalational agent facilitate the goal of early extubation, perhaps in the operating room, otherwise in the early postoperative period. Many cardiac anesthesiologists avoid the use of nitrous oxide because of the potential for myocardial depression in patients with abnormal cardiac function who are also receiving narcotics, and particularly because of the potential for enlargement of any air bubbles accidentally entrained in the IV fluid. Neuromuscular relaxation is achieved with a medium- to long-acting agent such as vecuronium, doxacurium, or pancuronium, the choice being based on the side effects of the drug if any such cardiovascular side effects are desired at all.

Ductal manipulation may cause abrupt bradycardia, so atropine always must be immediately available. Also, it is essential to alert the surgeon to suspend such manipulation momentarily until full onset of the atropine is achieved.

Neonatal patients with an associated VSD may have their pulmonary artery banded in association with coarctation repair. Considerations to prevent or minimize any increase in left to right shunting are in order: avoidance of respiratory alkalemia and hyperoxemia, excessive reductions in hematocrit or pulmonary vascular resistance, and increases in systemic vascular resistance (see Chapter 17).

### Fluid and blood product therapy

Hypervolemia must be scrupulously avoided to avoid any increase in left to right shunt in patients with VSD as well as to avoid a tendency toward increased pulmonary artery pressure and pulmonary vascular congestion with increased myocardial strain and further myocardial depression. Sicker neonates and infants with coarctation in particular are quite vulnerable to excessive preload.

Fluids should generally be dextrose-free except for neonates, insulin-requiring diabetics, and other patients known to be prone to hypoglycemia. Blood should be used judiciously to avoid significant reduction in oxygen delivery and administered at rates not likely to provoke myocardial ischemia or failure. Coagulation products generally are not required in noncardiopulmonary bypass cases.

## COMPLICATIONS

### Paraplegia

Complications include paraplegia (with a reported incidence of 0.14% to 1.25%) after aortic cross-clamping, postcoarctectomy syndrome (necrotizing mesenteric arteritis presenting with ileus, abdominal pain and distension), and persistent hypertension in all extremities, exacerbated by exercise.[11] In sicker neonates the incidence of recoarctation is higher, and postoperative renal failure is a common cause of death.

Preoperative identification of patients at a greater risk of paraplegia is problematic. The thoracic spinal cord of certain individuals appears to be at greater risk of ischemia from aortic cross-clamping because of anatomic interruptions of the anterior spinal artery that are poorly compensated for by intercostal arterial branches named radicular arteries. Spinal cord hypertension below the level of aortic cross-clamping may thus lead to cord infarction. Some have recommended that distal aortic pressure be continuously monitored during the period of aortic cross-clamping in the hope that interventions to maintain distal aortic pressure greater than 60 mm Hg would reduce the incidence of neurologic injury. Unfortunately, this practice has not been proven beneficial. With periods of aortic cross-clamping less than 20 minutes, spinal cord infarction rarely if ever occurs. When cross-clamp time will exceed 20 minutes, the surgeon may consider placement of a temporary shunt, although this decision is far from straightforward. Spinal angiography is considered to be riskier than aortic cross-clamping for patients with ischemia-prone anatomy and thus is not available for selection of shunt candidates. Some degree of hypothermia would logically be predicted to offer cord protection via reduced spinal cord oxygen requirements and consumption, but the proper degree of hypothermia is unknown.

### Hypertension

In the immediate postoperative period most patients develop hypertension.[12,13] Within the first 24 hours the hypertension—often exceeding the preoperative level—correlates with increased serum catecholamine levels, with especially dramatic increases in norepinephrine, that appear to result from aortic manipulation. Also, a significant increase in plasma renin activity after coarctation repair activates the angiotensin system. β-Adrenergic blocking drugs attenuate this first, catechol-induced, stage of hypertension and may delay or prevent the second, renin-induced increases in angiotensin-converting activity. Serum angiotensin–converting enzyme-inhibiting drugs may be effective therapy for the second phase of hypertension postcoarctation repair.

### Postcoarctectomy syndrome

Occurring in up to one fourth of patients undergoing coarctation repair, mesenteric arteritis is now less common than in earlier years because of increased success with control of postoperative hypertension.[14,15] Abdominal symptoms, including pain, tenderness, vomiting, melena, and fecal incontinence, correlate with plasma renin activity in both duration and severity. Untreated postoperative hypertension may eventuate in bowel necrosis and even be fatal. Current aggressive postoperative treatment of hypertension has greatly reduced the likelihood of this syndrome and improved the prognosis when it does occur.

## POSTOPERATIVE CARE AND VENTILATION

As with all other aspects of preoperative and intraoperative anesthesia management, the postoperative care of individuals with repair of coarctation, especially with regards to the decision whether or not to ventilate the patient mechanically postoperatively, must be individualized. A given individual patient's clinical status and cardiopulmonary reserve can be estimated from the preoperative evaluation and the intraoperative response to anesthetic management and surgical maneuvers. Generally, otherwise healthy older individuals who have coarctation repair can be extubated early in the postoperative period, even in the operating room at the end of the procedure, although often a period of several hours of careful observation for hemodynamic and coagulation stability of the patient is warranted before weaning a patient off mechanical ventilatory support in the early hours of the postoperative period. Obviously, the sicker patient with limited cardiopulmonary reserve and preoperative congestive heart failure is going to continue to require a greater level of cardiopulmonary support, and thus weaning may need to be delayed, perhaps for several days, according to the patient's overall clinical course. Usually the rapidity with which a patient is weaned from ventilator support is determined by cardiac status.

In addition to hemodynamic stability, the patient must be thoroughly rewarmed to a normal body temperature, and fluid, electrolyte, and coagulation status, hemoglobin levels, muscle strength, and neurologic status must all be acceptable prior to weaning, which often can be quite short in these patients, who as a rule have normal pulmonary function.

## INTERRUPTED AORTIC ARCH

Interrupted aortic arch, in which there is absence of a portion of aortic arch or atresia of an aortic segment, is invariably a ductal-dependent lesion in which the neonate is gravely ill with metabolic acidemia and circulatory failure. Approximately 12% of patients with coarctation have interrupted aortic arch.[17] Other than pulmonary atresia or tetralogy of Fallot, just about every known cardiac anomaly had been associated with interrupted aortic arch. The ECG shows right ventricular hypertrophy, chest x-ray film shows cardiac anomaly, and arterial blood gas analysis is essential to document and follow the serial response to treatment of the metabolic acidemia. Prostaglandin $E_1$ infusion and sodium bicarbonate therapy are the mainstay of temporizing medical treatment until stabilization can be achieved, allowing echocardiographic and perhaps cardiac catheterization data to be obtained prior to urgent surgery, without which fatality is 100%.

Recently reported discharge survival rates postoperatively for patients undergoing maximal or near maximal correction of interrupted aortic arch and associated cardiac anomalies has been reported to be as high as 90%.

Anesthetic management of repair of interrupted aortic arch is very similar to that of coarctation of the aorta.

## REFERENCES


1. Beekman RH, Rocchine AP, Behrendt DM et al: Long-term outcome after repair of coarctation in infancy: subclavian angioplasty does not reduce the need for reoperation, *J Am Coll Cardiol* 8:1406, 1986.
2. Bergdahl L, Bjork VO, Jonasson R: Surgical correction of coarctation of the aorta: influence of age on late results, *J Thorac Cardiovasc Surg* 85:532, 1983.
3. Campbell DB, Waldhausen JA, Pierce WS et al: Should elective repair of coarctation of the aorta be done in infancy? *J Thorac Cardiovasc Surg* 88:929, 1984.
4. Clarkson PM, Brandt PWT, Barratt-Boyes BG et al: Prosthetic repair of coarctation of the aorta with particular reference to Dacron onlay patch grafts and late aneurysm formation, *Am J Cardiol* 56:342, 1985.
5. Cobanoglu A, Teply TF, Grunkemeier GL et al: Coarctation of the aorta in patients younger than 3 months, *J Thorac Cardiovasc Surg* 89:128, 1985.
6. Crafoord C, Nylin G: Congenital coarctation of the aorta and its surgical treatment, *J Thorac Surg* 14:347, 1945.
7. Fyler DC, Buckley LP, Hellenbrand WE et al: Report of the New England Regional Infant Cardiac Program, *Pediatrics* 65:376, 1980.
8. Glancy DL, Morrow AG, Simon AL et al: Juxtaductal aortic coarctation: analysis of 84 patients studied hemodynamically, angiographically, and morphologically after age 1 year, *Am J Cardiol* 51:537, 1983.
9. Gross RE: Coarctation of the aorta: surgical treatment of 100 cases, *Circulation* 1:41, 1950.
10. Jacob T, Cobanoglu A, Starr A: Late results of ascending aorta–descending aorta bypass graft for recurrent coarctation of the aorta, *J Thorac Cardiovasc Surg* 95:782, 1988.
11. Maron BJ, Humphries JON, Rowe RD et al: Prognosis of surgically corrected coarctation of the aorta: a 20-year post-operative appraisal, *Circulation* 47:119, 1973.
12. Parker FB Jr, Streeten DHP, Phil D et al: Preoperative and postoperative renin levels in coarctation of the aorta, *Circulation* 66:513, 1982.
13. Rocchini AP, Rosenthal A, Barger AC et al: Pathogenesis of paradoxical hypertension after coarctation resection, *Circulation* 545:382, 1976.
14. Talner NS, Berman MA: Postnatal development of obstruction in coarctation of the aorta: role of the ductus arteriosus, *Pediatrics* 56:562, 1975.
15. Tawes RL, Berry CL, Aberdeen E: Congenital bicuspid aortic valves associated with coarctation of the aorta in children, *Br Heart J* 31:127, 1969.
16. Waldhausen JA, Nahrwold DL: Repair of coarctation of the aorta with subclavian flap, *J Thorac Cardiovasc Surg* 51:532, 1966.
17. Yee ES, Soifer SJ, Turley K et al: Infant coarctation: a spectrum in clinical presentation and treatment, *Ann Thorac Surg* 42:488, 1986.
18. Zeimer G, Jonas RA, Perry SB et al: Surgery for coarctation in the neonate, *Circulation 74*(suppl 1):I25, 1986.

# 25 Congenital Aortic Stenosis

*Jay Kambam*

Embryology
Pathologic anatomy
  Valvular aortic stenosis
    Deformed valves with primary aortic stenosis
    Bicuspid valves
  Subvalvular aortic stenosis
    Muscular type
    Fibrous type
  Supravalvular aortic stenosis
Pathophysiology
Clinical presentation
  Laboratory findings
    Chest x-ray film
    Electrocardiography
    Echocardiography
    Cardiac catheterization
Medical management
  Balloon valvuloplasty
Surgical management
  Valvular defects
  Subvalvular defects
  Supravalvular lesions
Anesthesia management
  Preoperative evaluation
  Preoperative sedation
  Monitoring
  Induction
  Maintenance
  Precautions
Management of children with idiopathic hypertrophic subaortic stenosis

## EMBRYOLOGY

The first major intraembryonic vessels appear as a pair of dorsal aortas, which form the continuation of the endocardial heart tubes. Between the fifth and sixth weeks of gestation the aortic arch system develops as six paired arches proliferating from the apex of the truncus arteriosus. These arches are never all present at the same time but develop successively. The first two aortic arches appear at the cranial portions of the dorsal aortas. The junction of the first aortic arches with the truncus arteriosus is somewhat dilated and is known as the aortic sac. It is from this aortic sac that the subsequent five pairs of aortic arches are formed as the heart and aortic sac undergo a caudal displacement. The ultimate fate of the aortic arch system is described in Chapter 1.

The various vascular systems are continually modified as they adapt to meet the demands of growth and development of the several organ systems. Although the final pattern of the vascular system is believed to be genetically determined, variations are inevitable in both the arterial and venous systems in cases of abnormally developed cardiovascular systems.

The semilunar valve of the aorta consists of three pouchlike cusps (the sinuses of Valsalva) of equal size (Figs. 25–1 and 25–2). These are the left coronary, the right coronary, and the noncoronary or posterior cusps. There is no well defined circular ring at the base of the aorta from which the aorta and its valve cusps arise. The embryologic explanation for congenital aortic valvular stenosis is not confirmed. Congenital aortic stenosis may be due to defective development of the endocardial cushions from which the aortic valve originates.[24] In the case of bicuspid aortic valve, stenosis arises from both developmental and acquired conditions.

## PATHOLOGIC ANATOMY

Aortic stenosis can be classified into three main types (see box on p. 282.). Any of the three valvular components (commissures, leaflet, and ring) may be involved in cases with congenital aortic valvular stenosis.

### Valvular aortic stenosis

The valvular type of aortic stenosis constitutes about 75% of cases of aortic stenosis. The incidence of valvular aortic stenosis among infants born with CHD is 2% to 5%.[9] Valvular aortic stenosis occurs far more frequently in boys than girls, with a ratio of about 4:1.[21] There is about a 20% incidence of associated cardiac anomalies in these

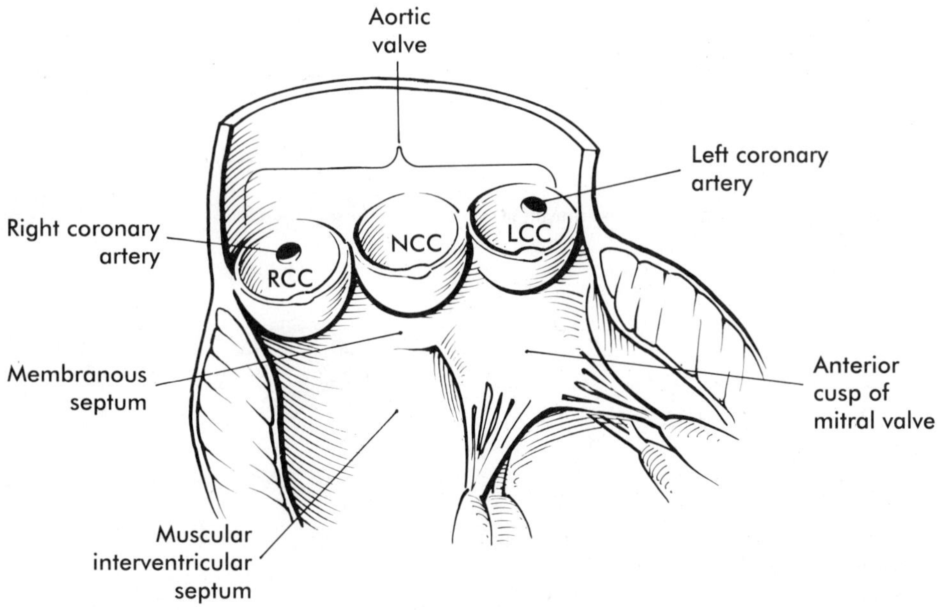


**Figure 25–1** Anatomy of the aortic valve. *RCC,* right coronary cusp; *LCC,* left coronary cusp; *NCC,* noncoronary cusp.

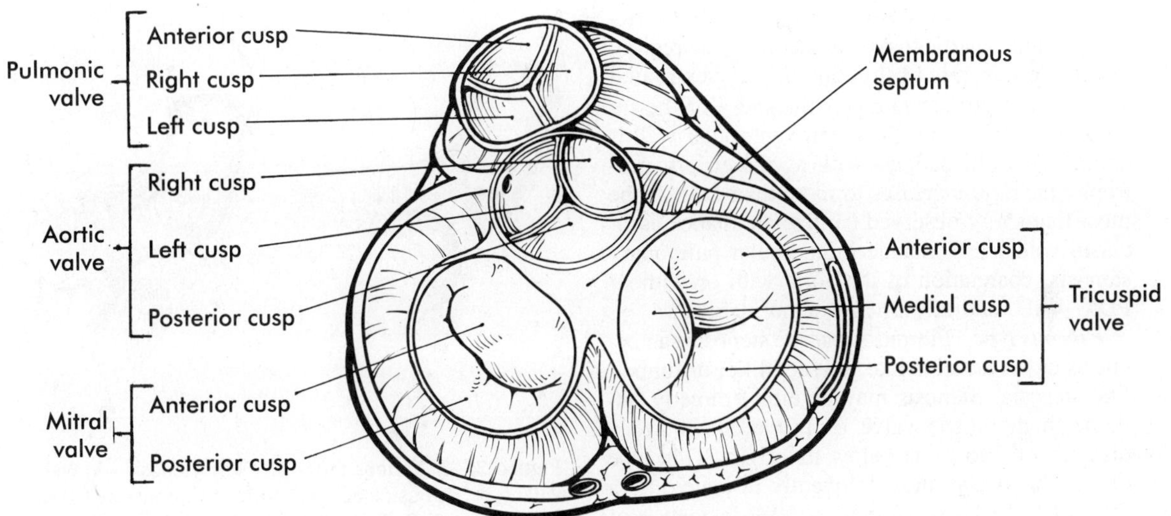


**Figure 25–2** Anatomy of the heart valves.

patients.[1,10] The frequent occurrence of endocardial fibroelastosis has been well described by many authors. Coarctation of the aorta with or without PDA occurs most frequently. VSD with or without pulmonary stenosis is present less frequently in patients with valvular aortic stenosis.

***Deformed valves with primary aortic stenosis.*** There may be an abnormal fusion of commisures, a single abnormally developed commisure, or abnormal development of leaflets in patients with a deformed aortic valve with primary stenosis, a deformed aortic valve with primary stenosis, (Fig. 25–3, *A*). In severe aortic stenosis the valve may be seen as a thick fibrous diaphragm pierced by a small orifice. A narrowed underdeveloped aortic ring is sometimes responsible for congenital aortic stenosis. The latter condition is sometimes associated with absence of the sinuses of Valsalva.

***Bicuspid valves.*** In persons born with bicuspid aortic valves (Fig. 25–3, *A*) stenosis of the valve usually does not occur until after the fourth decade. Valvular stenosis in these patients results from scle-

| CLASSIFICATION OF AORTIC STENOSIS |
|---|
| Valvular aortic stenosis (70% to 75%) |
| Primary stenosis (deformed valve) |
| Secondary stenosis (bicuspid valve) |
| Subvalvular aortic stenosis (20% to 25%) |
| Idiopathic hypertrophic subaortic stenosis (muscular type) |
| Discrete subaortic stenosis (fibrous type) |
| Supravalvular aortic stenosis (less than 5%) |

rosis and calcifications on both sides of the aortic valve.

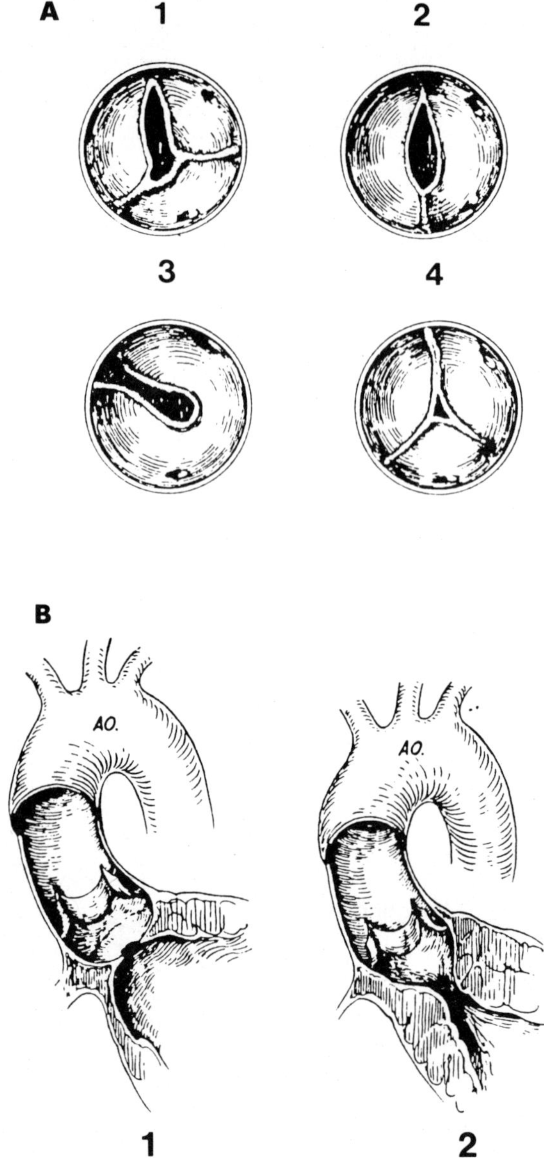


**Figure 25–3** Various types of aortic stenosis. **A,** Valvular type. **1,** Fusion of a well formed commissure (most frequent type). **2,** True bicuspid valve. **3,** Unicusp valve with an eccentric orifice. **4,** Commissural fusion of all commissures. **B,** Subvalvular type. **1,** Well localized (fibrous type), **2,** Diffuse (muscular type, also called IHSS). *AO,* aorta. (From Effler DB, editor: *Blades surgical disease of the chest,* ed 4, St. Louis, 1978, Mosby.)

### Subvalvular aortic stenosis

Subvalvular aortic stenosis can be divided into muscular and fibrous types (Fig. 25–3, *B*).

***Muscular type.*** This is also known as idiopathic hypertrophic subaortic stenosis (IHSS) or asymmetric septal hypertrophy. There is considerable hypertrophy of all the heart chambers, including the left ventricle. In addition there is extensive and disproportionate hypertrophy of the interventricular septum, particularly in the outflow region, leading to dynamic obstruction during ventricular systole. The normal ratio for thickness of the interventricular septum to the left ventricular wall is about 0.5:1. In patients with asymmetric hypertrophy the ratio increases to more than 1.3:1. The most frequently observed cardiac anomalies associated with IHSS include infundibular pulmonary stenosis, coarctation of the aorta with or without PDA, VSD, and mitral valve abnormalities.

***Fibrous type.*** Fibrous subaortic stenosis can occur as either annulus-like, crescentlike, or tunnel-like stenosis. Stenosis may be either directly underneath the aortic valve or further down, to a distance of 2 to 3 cm below its origin. This type of stenosis occurs most frequently in males, by a ratio of 2:1. There is about a 50% incidence of associated cardiac anomalies in patients with fibrous type subaortic stenosis. Coarctation of the aorta with or without PDA, VSD, aortic insufficiency, and mitral insufficiency occur most frequently.

### Supravalvular aortic stenosis

Supravalvular aortic stenosis is a rare form of CHD, equally distributed in both sexes. Stenosis can be seen as a localized or diffuse narrowing of the aorta, beginning at the superior margin of the sinuses of Valsalva and above the coronary arteries. Supravalvular stenosis can be the hourglass type, membranous type, hypoplastic type, or nonstenotic type with supravalvular membranes, bands, or cords. The bicuspid aortic valve, pulmonary stenosis, and a generalized arteriolar stenosis of cerebral, mesenteric, and other major vascular systems are sometimes associated with supravalvular aortic stenosis.

Supravalvular stenosis is manifested in patients with Williams-Beuren syndrome. This syndrome consists of infantile hypercalcemia, typical elfin facies, mental retardation, and osteosclerosis of the skull.[3-5,16,30]

## PATHOPHYSIOLOGY

The hemodynamic effects of all types of aortic stenosis on the left ventricle are fundamentally very similar, with some variations in cases with IHSS. The severity of the left ventricular outflow tract obstruction can be classified as mild, moderate, or severe. A peak systolic gradient between the left ventricle and poststenotic aorta of less than 50 mm Hg is considered mild, between 50 and 79 mm Hg is moderate, and greater than 80 mm Hg is severe or critical. When the aortic orifice in a child is less than 0.5 to 0.6 cm,[2] it is also considered a critical type. The obstruction of the left ventricular outflow tract, irrespective of the precise site, will impose a pressure overload on the left ventricle. The left ventricle in turn will respond with muscular hypertrophy. This may eventually result in myocardial ischemia and infarction. With time poststenotic dilatation of the ascending aorta is usually seen in patients with aortic stenosis.

In patients with valvular and subvalvular stenosis (obstruction proximal to the coronary ostia), myocardial ischemia can occur as a result of a mismatch between the myocardial blood flow and oxygen demand. In supravalvular aortic stenosis, the coronary arteries will be exposed to the same elevated pressures as the left ventricle. As a result the coronary arteries frequently become dilated and tortuous, and this may contribute to myocardial dysfunction.

In IHSS, or asymmetric septal hypertrophy, the hemodynamic changes vary greatly at different times. The degree of obstruction of the outflow tract, which is caused by septal hypertrophy and abnormal motion of the anterior leaflet of the mitral valve, is determined by the force of the left ventricular contraction, the size of the left ventricular cavity, and the transmural pressure transmitted to the outflow tract during systole. Decreased preload, reduced systemic vascular resistance, or increased contractile state intensify the obstruction. Increased left ventricular preload, elevated systemic vascular resistance, or decreased contractile state result in alleviation of obstruction.

## CLINICAL PRESENTATION

Children with mild to moderate aortic stenosis are usually asymptomatic.[25,29] In patients with critical

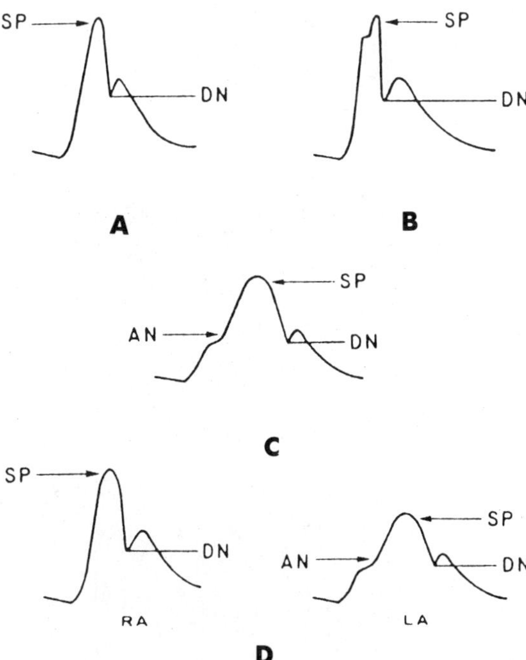


**Figure 25–4** Diagram of the various types of peripheral arterial pulse curves in the various forms of obstruction to left ventricular outflow. **A,** Normal. **B,** Idiopathic hypertrophic subaortic stenosis. **C,** Valvular aortic stenosis. **D,** Supravalvular aortic stenosis. *RA,* Right arm; *LA,* left arm; *AN,* anacrotic notch; *SP,* systolic peak; *DN,* Dicrotic notch.

stenosis exertional chest pain and syncope are commonly seen. Infants with critical stenosis usually develop CHF within the first few months of life. On physical examination one can palpate a systolic thrill, see a hyperactive precordium, and hear an ejection click and a harsh systolic ejection murmur. The peripheral pulses may be feeble, with a delayed upstroke, and these patients will typically have a narrow pulse pressure (Fig. 25–4). In patients with severe aortic stenosis, splitting of the second sound may be narrow or even reversed (paradoxical splitting). IHSS differs from other forms of aortic stenosis in that the obstruction in IHSS is dynamic and quite variable, so physical findings are equally variable. The diagnosis of IHSS is usually made in adolescent patients.

### Laboratory Findings

***Chest x-ray film.*** In mild to moderate cases of aortic stenosis one may see a normal chest roentgenogram. Left ventricular hypertrophy and signs of CHF may be seen in older infants with severe stenosis (Fig. 25–5). In neonates generalized car-

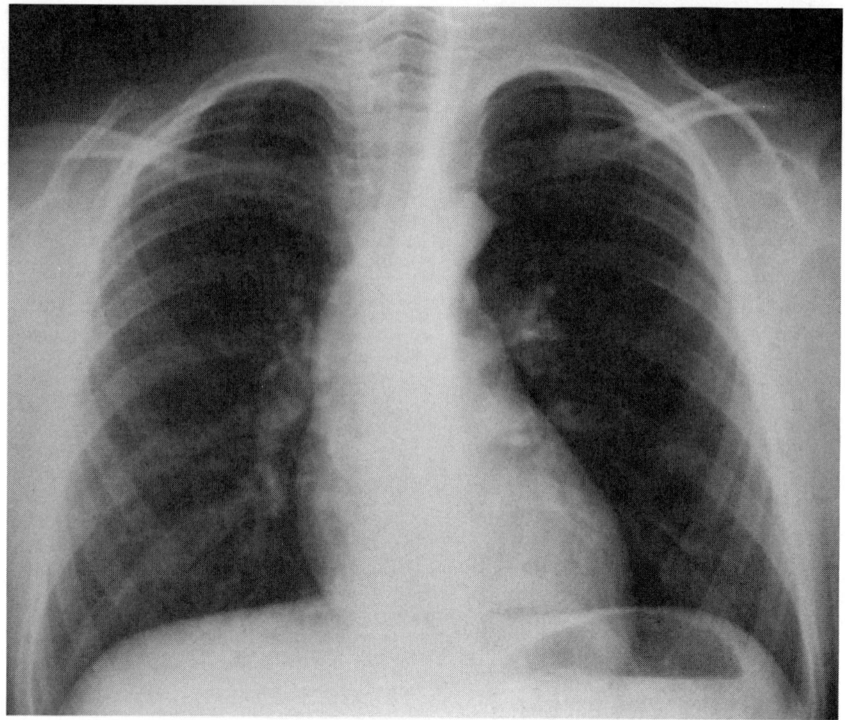

**Figure 25–5** Posterior chest radiograph of a 7-year-old boy with aortic stenosis due to a congenital bicuspid valve. The heart is not enlarged, but the shape is consistent with left ventricular hypertrophy. The ascending aorta is large. The pulmonary vascularity and main pulmonary artery segment are normal in appearance. (Courtesy of Sandra G. Kirchner, MD.)

diomegaly, left ventricular dilatation, and right ventricular hypertrophy are seen. Poststenotic dilatation may also be seen in older infants with severe form of aortic stenosis.

***Electrocardiography.*** Right ventricular hypertrophy is frequently seen in the first month of life. Left ventricular hypertrophy, with or without signs of myocardial ischemia, may be seen in children over 1 month of age with the severe form of aortic stenosis.

***Echocardiography.*** It is difficult to assess the severity of aortic obstruction based on history, physical signs, chest x-ray film, and ECG findings. However, the echocardiogram is quite useful in the diagnosis of aortic stenosis and may also be used to determine the type and extent of aortic stenosis and the presence of aortic insufficiency. The echocardiogram can also produce a noninvasive estimation of the pressure gradient across the stenotic area.

***Cardiac catheterization.*** The diagnosis can be confirmed with cardiac catheterization (Fig. 25–6). Cardiac catheterization is frequently performed in children with severe valvular stenosis and other types of aortic stenosis to confirm the diagnosis and to detect the other associated cardiovascular defects. Cardiac catheterization is less frequently used in mild to moderate valvular stenosis.

## MEDICAL MANAGEMENT

Infants with severe aortic valvular stenosis (critical stenosis with congestive heart failure and low perfusion) frequently receive preoperative inotropic support, supplemental oxygen with mechanical ventilation, and prostaglandin $E_1$ infusion to reopen the ductus arteriosus.[19,20,23,31] Once they are relatively stabilized, they are referred for surgical intervention.

Patients with IHSS may benefit from pharmacologic treatment with β-blockers and/or calcium channel blockers. Generally these patients should not receive inotropic agents, calcium, or digitalis preparations.

### Balloon valvuloplasty

Balloon valvuloplasty may be performed in selected cases to relieve the signs and symptoms of severe aortic stenosis and hopefully to delay the necessity of valve replacement.[2,7,8,15,28] This procedure may be tried at the time of cardiac cathe-

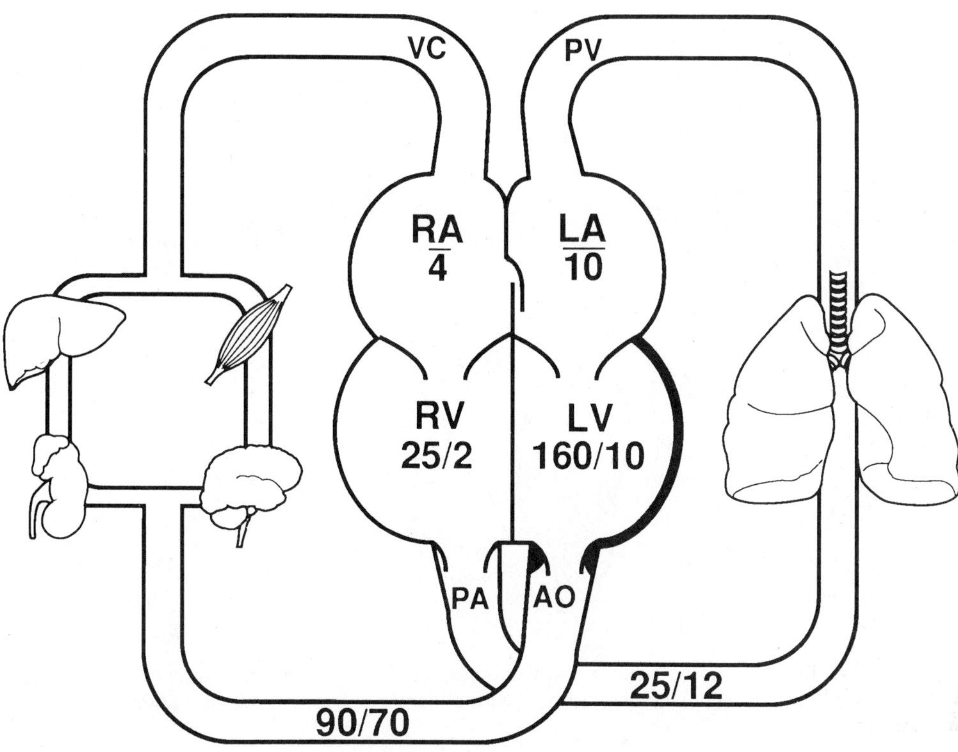


**Figure 25–6** Pressures in a patient with aortic stenosis. *VC*, Vena cava; *PV*, pulmonary vein; *RA*, right atrium; *LA*, left atrium; *RV*, right ventricle; *LV*, left ventricle; *PA*, pulmonary artery; *AO*, aorta.

terization in selected patients. Long-term results have not yet been compiled.

## SURGICAL MANAGEMENT

### Valvular defects

Children with a peak systolic pressure gradient of less than 80 mm Hg should be followed by a cardiologist, and surgery should be deferred until such time as a prosthetic valve of adult size can be used.[6,11,14,17,18,20,22,26,27] In general, children with pressure gradients of less than 50 mm Hg and with no symptoms do not need any kind of valvular surgery. However, surgery is indicated in these patients irrespective of their pressure gradient if angina or syncope is present along with signs of ischemic pattern on ECG. Also, a patient with CHF from critical aortic stenosis, irrespective of age, requires emergency medical management followed by surgical repair of the aortic valve. Closed aortic valvotomy without extracorporeal circulation may be performed in infants with critical aortic stenosis. Aortic valve commissurotomy with extracorporeal circulation is the procedure of choice in certain children (Fig. 25–7). Replacement of the aortic valve, preferably with an aortic homograft, may be necessary in certain valvular lesions (unicuspid or grossly deformed valve). Perioperative mortality rate depends in part on associated cardiac defects and is in the range of 25% to 50% for infants with critical aortic stenosis.

### Subvalvular defects

Since subaortic valvular stenosis is a progressive disease, surgery is usually recommended even when the pressure gradient is less than 50 mm Hg. Excision of fibromuscular tissue under direct vision is performed in patients with discrete membranous or endocardial cushion type subvalvular aortic stenosis. For patients with IHSS, surgical septectomy under cardiopulmonary bypass is the operation of choice. The mortality rate is low with these procedures and the chance of recurrence following surgery is small. A Konno procedure (valve replacement following aortic root enlargement) may be helpful for patients with tunnel type subvalvular aortic stenosis. Reoperation is often required for patients with tunnel defect.

### Supravalvular lesions

Surgery is usually indicated in these patients when angina or syncope is present or when the pressure gradient is above 50 mm Hg. Surgical correction

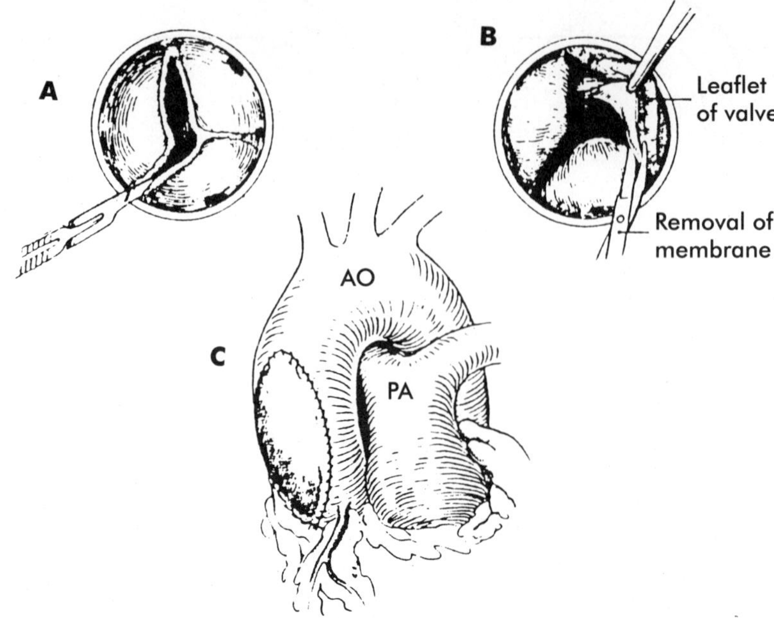


**Figure 25–7** Repair of aortic stenosis. **A,** Commissurotomy. **B,** Excision of discrete subvalvular stenosis. **C,** Repair of supravalvular stenosis with a diamond-shaped patch. *AO,* Aorta; *PA,* pulmonary artery.

of this lesion consists of a patch angioplasty of the ascending aorta (Fig. 25–7).

## ANESTHESIA MANAGEMENT

The principles of management of a child with aortic stenosis are essentially the same as those applied in an adult patient with aortic stenosis. One should keep in mind that in neonates with critical aortic stenosis, one is dealing with a compromised left ventricle with or without a strain pattern and with systemic hypoperfusion with or without a history of syncope. The primary goal of anesthetic management of a child with aortic stenosis is to preserve myocardial function and cardiac output. Children with IHSS are managed under somewhat different principles from those with valvular aortic stenosis and will be discussed separately.

### Preoperative evaluation

A thorough understanding of the pathologic anatomy and physiology of the type of aortic stenosis one is dealing with is absolutely necessary for optimal anesthetic management of these patients. Since the perioperative mortality rate is very high in children with critical aortic stenosis, one should pay utmost attention to all aspects of anesthetic management of these children.

Neonates with critical aortic stenosis quite often receive inotropic and mechanical ventilatory support preoperatively. In addition they are frequently treated with a prostaglandin infusion to maintain patency of the ductus arteriosus and a right to left shunt at the aortic level.

### Preoperative sedation

I frequently employ a narcotic infusion with muscle paralysis even before the child arrives in the operating room. A moderate to heavy preoperative medication may be necessary for older children, as anxiety can elevate blood catecholamine levels, leading to tachycardia and worsening of the signs and symptoms of aortic stenosis. Preoperative medications usually consist of either oral benzodiazepine (midazolam 0.5 to 0.6 mg/kg) or an IM dose of morphine sulphate (0.1 mg/kg) or both. Prophylactic antibiotic therapy to prevent bacterial endocarditis is recommended for these patients irrespective of the degree of aortic stenosis.

### Monitoring

Monitoring of children with critical aortic stenosis during surgery includes an ECG, invasive arterial pressure, noninvasive blood pressure, pulse oximeter, capnogram, body temperature (esophageal and nasopharyngeal), central venous pressure, and urinometer. Left atrial pressure monitoring may be useful. Arterial blood gases, serum potassium, and hematocrit should be checked frequently throughout the case. Monitoring of the prostaglandin infusion rate in these children needs special mention.

Both accidental stoppage and excessive prostaglandin infusion can result in an unacceptable condition. An abrupt discontinuation will result in a closure of the ductus arteriosus and sudden worsening of the patient's condition. On the other hand, an accidental increase in the rate of infusion will also result in a sudden worsening of the patient's clinical condition because of a decreased afterload.

### Induction

It is not difficult to start an IV line in a well sedated child before the induction of anesthesia. In these patients anesthesia can be induced with 1 to 2 mg/kg of intravenous ketamine. In children who are uncooperative and in small children who come to the operating suite without an IV line in place, anesthesia can be induced with 4 to 6 mg/kg of ketamine IM. Children with critical aortic stenosis always arrive in the operating room with an IV cannula. If the patient's trachea is not intubated, I induce anesthesia with 1 to 2 mg/kg of ketamine IV. A nondepolarizing muscle relaxant (mivacurium, vecuronium, doxacurium, or pipecuronium) can be used to facilitate the placement of the endotracheal tube. Even though succinylcholine is frequently used, I do not recommend for any patient in whom patency of the ductus arteriosus is critical. Since acetylcholine is known to constrict the ductus, it is possible that succinylcholine will do the same. I do not recommend atracurium or pancuronium in children with critical aortic stenosis because of their undesirable cardiovascular side effects. Inhalational induction is best avoided in these children, as excessive depression of left ventricular function with an unacceptable decrease in cardiac output may result.

### Maintenance

For a closed aortic valvotomy procedure without cardiopulmonary bypass pump, I use up to 50 μg/kg of fentanyl or 15 μg/kg of sufentanil IV. For procedures involving open commissurotomy, valvoplasty, or valve replacement, I use 100 μg/kg of fentanyl or 30 μg/kg of sufentanil as the main anesthetic agent. If deep hypothermia and circulatory arrest are planned (usually in children under 10 kg body weight), I administer 10 ml/kg of dextran 40 in a 5% dextrose solution before peripheral cooling is initiated (see Chapter 4 for complete details of deep hypothermia). Because peripheral cooling is associated with increased incidence of ventricular arrhythmias in patients with critical aortic stenosis, I do not employ it in children with this condition. In these patients deep hypothermia and circulatory arrest are achieved with a cardiopulmonary bypass pump without peripheral cooling. I administer 10 ml/kg of dextran 40 in a 5% dextrose solution before cooling is initiated using the cardiopulmonary bypass pump.

Normal ventilation with sufficient inspired oxygen concentrations is recommended in these children. One should avoid excessive positive pressure ventilation, as this may further decrease cardiac output. Frequent arterial blood gases, calcium, and glucose levels should be determined, and prompt correction of any abnormal values should be achieved.

Heparin is usually injected into the right atrium by the surgeon just before the placement of the vascular cannulas. Protamine is administered by the anesthesiologist at the conclusion of the extracorporeal circulation, following the removal of the cannulas. The majority of patients require inotropic support with either dopamine (3 to 6 μg/kg/min) or dobutamine (4 to 6 μg/kg/min) infusion after coming off bypass.

### Precautions

In all cases of a communication between the right and the left sides of the heart, it is absolutely necessary that all intravenous lines be free of air bubbles. In addition one should use extra caution not to introduce any air bubbles when injecting drugs through an IV line. Even though the use of nitrous oxide is not contraindicated in patients with an aortic stenosis, many anesthesiologists avoid the use of it, especially once the chest is opened, for fear of intravascular air bubble expansion.

Other precautions that should be observed in patients with aortic stenosis:

Avoid decrease in preload and afterload.
Maintain sinus rhythm and normal heart rate.
Avoid excessive tachycardia or bradycardia.
Avoid any kind of left ventricular depression.

I routinely leave the endotracheal tube in place in these patients at the end of the surgical procedure and mechanically ventilate these patients postoperatively for 1 or 2 days until they are stable.

## MANAGEMENT OF CHILDREN WITH IDIOPATHIC HYPERTROPHIC SUBAORTIC STENOSIS

IHSS may be seen at any age, including the neonatal period. In many ways the anesthetic management of a patient with IHSS is very similar to that of a patient with mitral valve prolapse syndrome (Chapter 32). The clinical picture usually mimics that of aortic valvular stenosis. Remember, children with IHSS have a dynamic outflow obstruction of the left or both ventricles. They frequently have mitral insufficiency, and their left ventricle may be compromised. The following circumstances are known to intensify outflow tract obstruction: (1) increased contractility, (2) de-

## ANESTHETIC MANAGEMENT OF A PATIENT WITH IDIOPATHIC HYPERTROPHIC SUBAORTIC STENOSIS

1. Maintain preload.
2. Avoid peripheral vasodilation.
3. Keep left ventricular contractility on the low side.
4. Use prophylactic antibiotic therapy.
5. Avoid inotropic drugs (ephedrine, calcium, epinephrine, and isoproterenol).
6. Use phenylephrine to treat hypotension.
7. Use atropine to treat bradycardia.
8. Treat hypertension and tachycardia with
   Esmolol
   Deepened anesthesia.
9. Use verapamil to treat supraventricular tachycardias.
10. Use a combination of a narcotic and minimal concentrations of inhalational anesthetics.

creased preload, and (3) decreased afterload. Anesthetic management of a patient with IHSS is summarized in the box.

## REFERENCES


1. Assey ME, Wisenbough T, Spann JF Jr et al: Unexpected persistence into adulthood of low wall stress in patients with congenital aortic stenosis: is there a fundamental difference in the hypertrophic response to a pressure overload present from birth? *Circulation* 75:973, 1987.
2. Beekman RH, Rocchini AP, Crowley DC et al: Comparison of single and double balloon valvuloplasty in children with aortic stenosis, *J Am Col Cardiol* 12:480, 1988.
3. Beuren AJ, Schulze C, Eberle P et al: The syndrome of supravalvular aortic stenosis peripheral pulmonary stenosis, mental retardation, and similar facial appearance, *Am J Cardiol* 13:471, 1964.
4. Beuren AJ, Apitz J, Harmjanz D: Supravalvular aortic stenosis in association with mental retardation and a certain facial appearance, *Circulation* 26:1235, 1962.
5. Black JA, Bonham-Carter RE: Association between aortic stenosis and facies of severe infantile hypercalcemia, *Lancet* 2:745, 1963.
6. Brown J, Stevens L, Lynch L et al: Surgery for discrete subvalvular aortic stenosis: actuarial survival, hemodynamic results, and acquired aortic regurgitation, *Ann Thorac Surg* 40:151, 1985.
7. Feldman T, Chiu YC, Carroll JD: Catheter balloon dilatation for discrete subaortic stenosis in the adult, *Am J Cardiol* 60:403, 1987.
8. Helgason H, Keane JF, Fellows KE et al: Balloon dilation of the aortic valve: studies in normal lambs and in children with aortic stenosis, *J Am Coll Cardiol* 9:816, 1987.
9. Hoffman JIE: The natural history of congenital isolated pulmonic and aortic stenosis, *Annu Rev Med* 20:15, 1969.
10. Johnson AM: Aortic stenosis, sudden death and the left ventricular baroreceptors, *Br Heart J* 33:I-35, 1971.
11. Jones M, Garhnart GR, Morrow AG: Late results after operations for left ventricular outflow tract obstruction, *Am J Cardiol* 50:569, 1982.
12. Keane JF, Driscoll D, Gersony W: Results of treatment of patients with aortic stenosis: the report of the Second Natural History Study of Congenital Heart Defects, *Circulation* 87:I16, 1993.
13. Keane JF, Fellows KE, LaFarge GC et al: The surgical management of discrete and diffuse supravalvular aortic stenosis, *Circulation* 54:112, 1976.
14. Konno S, Imai Y, Iida Y et al: New method for prosthetic valve replacement in congenital aortic stenosis associated with hypoplasia of the aortic valve ring, *J Thorac Cardiovasc Surg* 10:909, 1975.
15. Lababidi Z, Weinhaus L, Stoeckle H et al: Transluminal balloon dilation for discrete subaortic stenosis, *Am J Cardiol* 59:423, 1987.
16. Maisuls H, Alday LE, Thuer O: Cardiovascular findings in the Williams-Beuren syndrome, *Am Heart J* 114:897, 1987.
17. Messina LM, Turley K, Stanger P et al: Successful aortic valvotomy for severe congenital valvular aortic stenosis in the newborn infant, *J Thorac Cardiovasc Surg* 88:92, 1984.
18. Misbach GA, Turley K, Ullyot DJ et al: Left ventricular outflow enlargement by the Konno procedure, *J Thorac Cardiovasc Surg* 84:696, 1982.
19. Newfeld EA, Muster AJ, Paul MH et al: Discrete subvalvular aortic stenosis in childhood, *Am J Cardiol* 38:53, 1976.
20. Pelech AN, Dyck JD, Trusler GA et al: Critical aortic stenosis: survival and management, *J Thorac Cardiovasc Surg* 94:510, 1987.
21. Reynolds JL, Nadas AS, Rudolph AM et al: Critical congenital aortic stenosis with minimal electrocardiographic change, *N Engl J Med* 262:276, 1960.
22. Roberts WC, Morrow AG, McIntosh CC et al: Congenitally bicuspid aortic valve causing severe, rare aortic regurgitation without superimposed infective endocarditis: analysis of 13 patients requiring aortic valve replacement, *Am J Cardiol* 47:206, 1981.
23. Rosing DR, Kent KM: Verapamil therapy: a new approach to the pharmacologic treatment of hypertrophic cardiomyopathy I: hemodynamic effects, *Circulation* 60:1201, 1979.
24. Serck-Hanssen A: Congenital valvular aortic stenosis, *Acta Pathologica et Microbiologica Scandinavica* 72:465, 1968.
25. Shem-Tov A, Schneeweiss A, Motro M et al: Clinical presentation and natural history of mild discrete subaortic stenosis: follow-up of 1 to 17 years, *Circulation* 66:509, 1982.
26. Somerville J, Ross D: Homograft replacement of aortic root with reimplantation of coronary arteries: results after 1 to 5 years, *Br Heart J* 47:473, 1982.
27. Somerville J, Stone S, Ross D: Fate of patients with fixed subaortic stenosis after surgical removal. *Br Heart J* 43:629, 1980.
28. Vogel M, Benson LN, Burrows P et al: Balloon dilatation of congenital aortic valve stenosis in infants and children: short-term and intermediate results, *Br Heart J* 62:148, 1989.
29. Wagner HR, Ellison RC, Keane JF et al: Clinical course in aortic stenosis: report from the Joint Study of the Natural History of Congenital Heart Defects, *Circulation* 56:I47, 1977.
30. Williams JCP, Barrett-Boyes BG, Lowe JB: Supravalvular aortic stenosis, *Circulation* 24:1311, 1961.
31. Wright GB, Keane JF, Nadas AS et al: Fixed subaortic stenosis in the young: medical and surgical course in 83 patients, *Am J Cardiol* 52:830, 1983.

# 26 Congenital Mitral Stenosis

***Jay Kambam, Frank Fish,*** *and* ***Walter Merrill***



Congenital mitral stenosis (CMS) seldom occurs as an isolated anomaly.[4] More often it occurs as part of a generalized hypoplasia of the left heart. The incidence of CMS is about 0.2% of all congenital heart defects. Associated cardiac defects may include PDA, ASD, VSD, pulmonary stenosis, tricuspid stenosis, and endocardial fibroelastosis.

## EMBRYOLOGY

The cardiac valves are formed after the cardiac septa are completed, and all four valves are found at sites of endocardial cushion tissue (Fig. 26–1). The atrioventricular valves apparently develop from loose folds in the endocardial cushions, which then erode in a selective fashion, leaving the atrioventricular valves connected by chordae tendineae to papillary muscles in the ventricle. An alternative hypothesis is that portions of the atrioventricular valves develop from the ventricular muscle. The atrioventricular valves develop by undermining of ventricular muscle tissue (with tissue on the atrial side). The process of undermining extends until the atrioventricular junction is reached. Subsequent resorption of the muscle results in normal-appearing valve leaflets and chordae tendineae. If the developing leaflets fuse during development, then stenosis of the valve will result. If the obstruction is severe, then fetal flow patterns are altered. The opposite side of the heart, carrying more flow, becomes hypertrophic, and the ventricle of the obstructed side becomes hypoplastic. If the obstruction is mild, then no abnormality is evident until later in life. Valvular insufficiency is less common, but in utero it is more likely to be tricuspid than mitral, and it may be poorly tolerated by the fetus.

## PATHOLOGIC ANATOMY

Various components of the mitral valve complex are shown in the box on p. 290. The mitral valve has two leaflets, an anterior and a posterior leaflet. The base of the leaflets is attached to the annulus, or ring, and the free edges of the leaflets are tethered by delicate chordae tendineae to the papillary muscles. The papillary muscles are firmly attached to the endocardium of the ventricular cavity.

The anterior leaflet of the mitral valve is in close association with the outflow tract of the left ventricle. The open anterior leaflet forms the lateral aspect of the left ventricular outflow tract, and the closed leaflet forms the floor of the left atrium. The most important function of chordae tendineae is to prevent prolapse of leaflets into the left atrium when left ventricular pressure rises. During ventricular systole, as the ventricular radius rapidly decreases, contraction of the papillary muscle maintains the tension of the chordae tendineae on the valvular leaflets. An abnormal function of any component of the mitral valve complex can result in a dysfunction of the mitral valve itself.

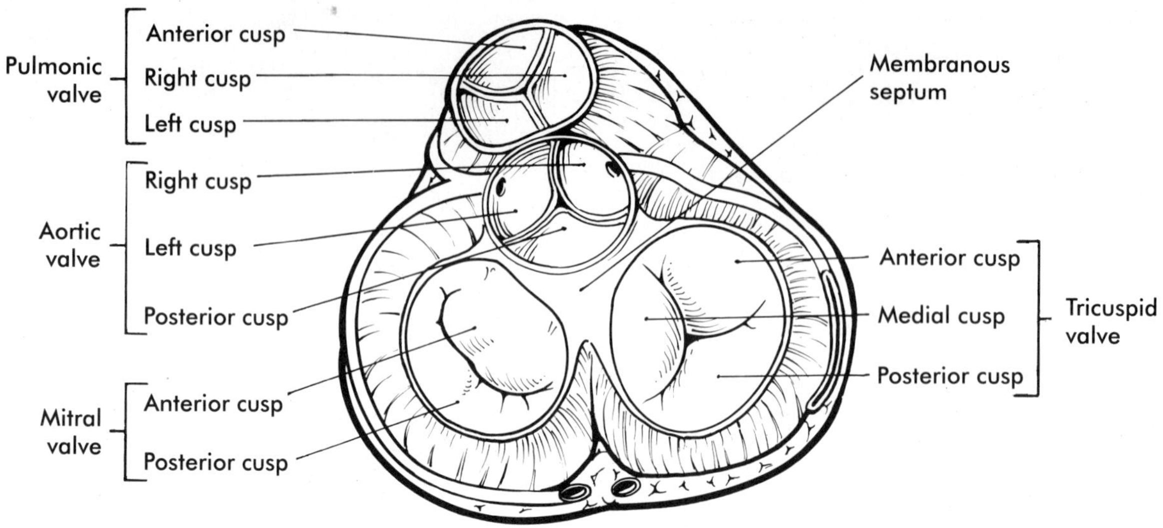


**Figure 26–1** Normal anatomy of the heart valves.

**MITRAL VALVE COMPLEX**

Anterior and posterior leaflets
Annulus, or ring
Chordae tendineae
Papillary muscles (anterolateral and posteromedial)

**VARIOUS TYPES OF CONGENITAL MITRAL STENOSIS**

1. Valvular stenosis
   - Diaphragmatic type
   - Funnel type
   - Accessory mitral valvular tissue
2. Parachute mitral valve
3. Anomalous mitral arcade
4. Supravalvular stenosis

The annulus of the mitral valve is composed of fibromuscular tissue and is part of the fibrous skeleton of the heart. Normal mitral valve orifice values in children are dependent on body surface area. In adults the normal mitral valve orifice area is 4 to 6 $cm^2$. An orifice of 2 $cm^2$ usually causes mild symptoms of mitral stenosis, and a 1-$cm^2$ orifice often causes severe symptoms.

Various types of CMS[12] are listed in the box at upper right.

### Obstruction at the valvular level

This lesion is subdivided into three main categories.

***Diaphragmatic type.*** In this deformity the mitral valve is short and suspended over the mitral aperture like a rigid diaphragm. Other defects of the mitral valve complex include absent or poorly formed commissures and short and fused papillary muscles and chordae tendineae. The mitral valve aperture usually measures less than 1 cm in diameter.

***Funnel type.*** As its name implies, this mitral valve has a conical or funnel-shaped appearance with its apex extending into the left ventricular cavity. Other deformities include fusion of the mitral valve commissures and short and fused chordae tendineae.

***Accessory mitral valvular tissue.*** With this defect mitral valve obstruction is due to a large, grayish white mass of accessory valvular tissue connected to the posterior mitral leaflet.

### Supravalvular stenosis

In this condition the mitral valve and its complex are entirely normal.[6,18] The obstruction is due to a circumferential ridge of connective tissue attached to the base of the mitral leaflets in the left atrium and protruding into the valvular aperture.

### Parachute mitral valve

The pathology in this anomaly is in the chordae tendineae and papillary muscles.[14] Chordae tendineae are short and fused, and they converge and insert into a single large papillary muscle. Although the valvular leaflets and commissures are normal, the abnormal papillary muscle will draw the leaflets into close opposition.

### Anomalous mitral arcade

In this defect the posterior, posteromedial, and anterolateral papillary muscles of the left ventricle and the anterior leaflet of the mitral valve together form an arcade.[2] The chordae tendineae are short and thickened. Fibrous tissue extends from the anterior leaflet and forms an arch between the two papillary muscles.

## PATHOPHYSIOLOGY

Obstruction at or just above the mitral valve results in elevated left atrial and pulmonary venous pressure, producing pulmonary arterial and right ventricular hypertension. Transmission of increased left atrial pressure into the pulmonary capillary circulation results in dyspnea and orthopnea. In severe mitral stenosis right ventricular dysfunction adds to the symptoms of low output and fluid overload. In patients with severe stenosis cardiac output is low even at rest.

## CLINICAL PRESENTATION

The age at presentation of children with CMS is usually dependent on the severity of mitral valve obstruction. The symptoms of mitral stenosis in children under 2 years of age are almost always due to a congenital condition. Children with mitral stenosis usually have dyspnea and tachypnea as their primary symptoms. Other signs and symptoms include recurrent respiratory infections, mild cyanosis, growth retardation, and signs of right-sided heart failure. Dysrhythmias and syncope can occur. On physical examination a middiastolic rumble secondary to the pressure gradient during diastole is best audible at the apex on auscultation. Mitral stenosis may occasionally produce an apical diastolic thrill in patients with congenital heart disease. Wheezing is a common consequence of pulmonary venous congestion. Findings indicative of aortic valvular or subvalvular stenosis or coarctation may also be evident.

### Laboratory findings

***Chest x-ray film.*** Chest x-ray may reveal pulmonary edema or pulmonary venous congestion, left atrial enlargement, and in some cases right ventricular hypertrophy.

***Electrocardiography.*** The ECG is normal in patients with minimal stenosis. However, in patients with moderate to severe mitral stenosis, one can see the signs of right ventricular hypertrophy as well as left atrial hypertrophy. Atrial fibrillation may also be detected in patients with severe mitral stenosis.

***Echocardiography.*** Echocardiography is the hallmark in the evaluation of mitral valve abnormalities. The contour, excursion, and aperture at the valve, the orientation of the papillary muscles, and the annulus size can be determined. Left atrial enlargement and right ventricular hypertension may also be evident. The severity of obstruction can be further assessed by Doppler estimates at the peak diastolic gradient and by a prolonged decline in diastolic flow velocity. The aortic valve, subaortic region, and aortic arch should also be carefully inspected for multiple left-sided obstructions (Shone's syndrome). A small mitral valve orifice, and abnormal tethering and restricted motion of the valve leaflets can be demonstrated by echocardiography (Fig. 26–2).

***Cardiac catheterization.*** Cardiac catheterization is often indicated preoperatively in patients with mitral stenosis, especially when associated with other congenital heart defects. One can measure left atrial and left ventricular pressures and estimate blood flow across the mitral valve. Typical oxygen saturations and chamber pressures are shown in Fig. 26–3.

## MEDICAL MANAGEMENT

Patients with mild to moderate mitral stenosis can be managed medically with a diuretic. The majority of children with atrial fibrillation can be converted to sinus rhythm with cardioversion. Digoxin and/or a class 1A antiarrhythmitic drug and anticoagulation therapy are necessary for patients with persistent atrial fibrillation.

## SURGICAL MANAGEMENT

Surgical management of CMS consists of either closed commissurotomy, open valvuloplasty, or replacement of the mitral valve.[1,3,5,7-11,13,15-17] Operation is indicated in patients with severe CMS if they have symptoms of persistent atrial fibrillation, CHF, thromboembolic phenomena, or severe pulmonary hypertension that are refractory to medical management. In many patients with CMS the results of surgery are less than ideal. Commissurotomy or valvuloplasty does not reliably relieve the symptoms for prolonged duration in many children, and these procedures frequently produce mitral regurgitation. The mortality rate for mitral repair procedures is at least 3%. Replacement of the mitral valve is not desirable in infants and small children. Porcine valves are no longer used in children because of decreased longevity from rapid valve degeneration. Mechanical prostheses may be inserted, but they require long-term maintenance of coumadin therapy. As a general rule one should delay mitral valve replacement as long as possible to give the child time to grow so that as large a

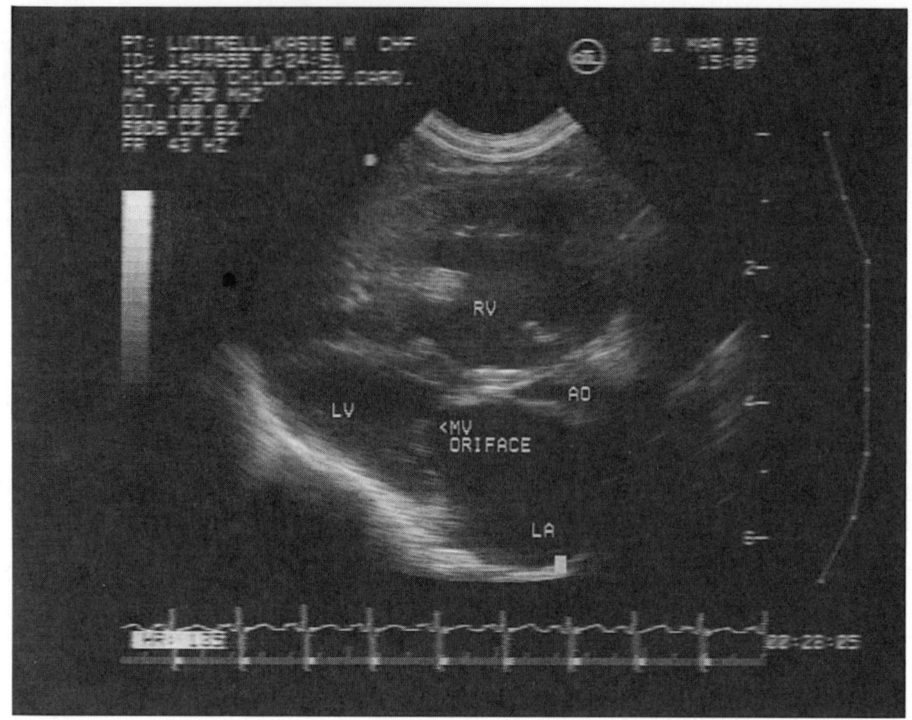


**Figure 26–2** Echocardiogram of a child with congenital mitral stenosis.

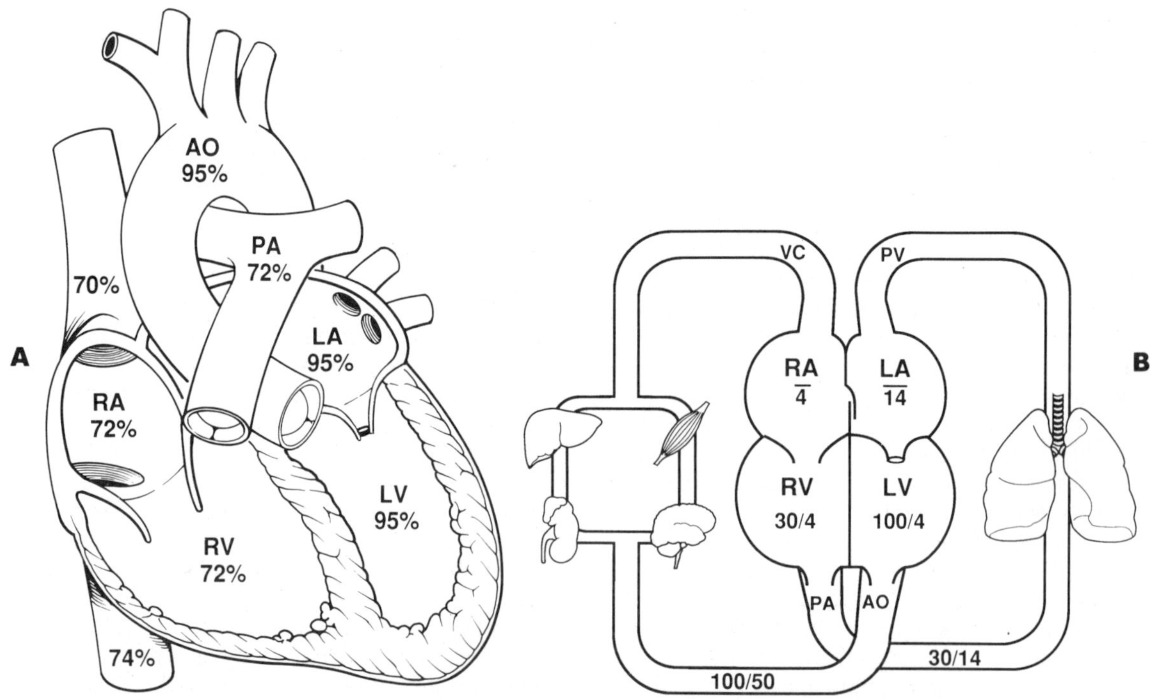


**Figure 26–3** Oxygen saturations, **A,** and chamber pressures, **B,** in a child with congenital mitral stenosis.

prosthesis as possible can be inserted. Small children commonly outgrow their prosthesis as their body surface area and cardiac output increase. Eventually a large prosthesis will have to be inserted, and this may be technically difficult. The mortality rate for mitral valve replacement is about 8%. Various other surgical modalities, including insertion of a left atrial to left ventricular conduit containing a prosthesis, have been tried with less than satisfactory results.[5-8,11]

## ANESTHESIA MANAGEMENT

An understanding of pathologic anatomy and physiology and of the pharmacology of various drugs that may alter the systemic and pulmonary blood flows is essential in managing patients with a congenital mitral valvular disease. Special problems one may encounter in a patient with congenital mitral valvular disease include pulmonary venous congestion, pulmonary edema, and decreased right ventricular function. A few of these patients may present with atrial fibrillation. One should watch for perioperative atrial arrhythmias in patients undergoing repair of CMS. In patients with severe mitral stenosis a decrease in resting cardiac output is an additional problem. Mitral regurgitation following commissurotomy is a frequent postsurgical problem in these patients. One should avoid tachycardia, as it causes shortening of the atrial emptying time and a decrease in cardiac output. Patients with CMS poorly tolerate any increase in pulmonary vascular resistance or decrease in ventricular contractility.

### Preoperative assessment

Preoperative evaluation of a patient with CMS should include a thorough history, including past and present medications and physical examination; laboratory tests including chest x-ray film, ECG, echocardiogram, catheterization data, hemoglobin, glucose, and electrolyte levels; any history of palliative or corrective surgery (PDA or coarctation of aorta) or noncardiac surgery; and a pediatric cardiologist's consult note.

Depending on the severity of the defect children with mitral stenosis may present with various degrees of CHF and decreased lung compliance. Signs and symptoms of CHF may be absent in a patient with a mild defect and in patients who are being treated medically with diuretic preparations.

### Premedication

Preoperative sedation in these patients depends upon the age of the child and severity of the defect. Advantages of preoperative sedation include a decrease or elimination of anxiety, reduction of oxygen demand, and avoidance of further hemodynamic deterioration. However, one should not oversedate these babies, as hypoventilation will have detrimental effects on oxygen saturation and pulmonary blood flow. Preoperative sedation should ideally be achieved in the holding room, where one can watch for any undesirable side effects. A narcotic and an anticholinergic drug combination (meperidine 2 mg/kg or morphine 0.1 mg/kg and atropine 10 μg/kg) can be given IM 90 to 120 minutes before the scheduled time of operation. Oral midazolam (0.6 mg/kg) may also be given 30 minutes before the scheduled time of operation, depending on the evaluation of the child in the holding room.

### Monitoring

Monitoring of the children with CMS during surgery includes an ECG, invasive arterial pressure, noninvasive blood pressure, pulse oximeter, capnogram, body temperature (esophageal and nasopharyngeal), central venous pressure, and urinometer. Left atrial pressure monitoring is helpful in the management of patients with severe CMS, especially after they come off cardiopulmonary bypass. Arterial blood gases, serum potassium, glucose and calcium, and hematocrit levels are monitored frequently throughout the operation.

### Induction of anesthesia

The majority of patients come to the operating room with no IV catheter. However, it is not difficult to start an IV line in a well sedated child before the induction of anesthesia. In patients who arrive with a functioning IV line, anesthesia can be induced with fentanyl 10 to 15 μg/kg and/or 1 mg/kg of ketamine. In children who are uncooperative and in small children who come to the operating suite without an IV line in place, anesthesia can be induced with either halothane by mask or ketamine by IM injection. We recommend low inspired concentrations of halothane under 1%, as severe myocardial depression and/or complete heart block may result with concentrations in excess of 1% to 1.5% in patients with CMS. Once the IV line is secured, tracheal intubation can be performed with either succinylcholine or a nondepolarizing muscle relaxant. Atropine 5 to 10 μg/kg should be given prior to the administration of succinylcholine (1 to 2 mg/kg IV). An arterial cannula and a central venous catheter are usually inserted after the airway is secured.

### Maintenance

Anesthesia is maintained with an IV narcotic (fentanyl 50 to 100 μg/kg or sufentanil 15 to 30 μg/kg). Patients with CMS may not tolerate inhaled anesthetic agents, as most of these patients have decreased ventricular function and cardiac output. We recommend avoiding pancuronium, as it can cause supraventricular tachycardia in these patients. Vecuronium or one of the newer nondepolarizing muscle relaxants (doxacurium or pipecuronium) can be used to maintain muscle paralysis throughout the operation. Excessive amounts of atropine should also be avoided, as tachycardia would further reduce cardiac output in these patients.

One should closely watch the administration of IV fluids in these patients. Both hypovolemia and hypervolemia are detrimental to these patients.

If deep hypothermia and circulatory arrest are planned (usually in children under 10 kg body weight), we administer 10 ml/kg of dextran 40 in 5% dextrose solution before peripheral cooling is initiated (see Chapter 4 for complete details of deep hypothermia).

Heparin is usually injected into the right atrium by the surgeon just before the placement of cannulas. Protamine is administered by the anesthesiologist at the conclusion of extracorporeal circulation following the removal of cardiac cannulas. The majority of patients require either isoproterenol (0.01 to 0.05 μg/kg/min) or dobutamine (3 to 6 μg/kg/min) infusion after coming off bypass.

One should avoid conditions that increase pulmonary vascular resistance in these patients, as an increase in PVR can cause worsening of right ventricular function (see the box). Since patients with CMS will have pulmonary venous congestion, they may benefit from hyperventilation, high inspired oxygen concentrations, and other measures that are known to cause a decrease in PVR (box).

**INCREASED PULMONARY VASCULAR RESISTANCE**

**Causes**

1. Hypoxemia
2. Hypercarbia
3. Acidosis
4. High mean airway pressure
5. Hypervolemia
6. Cough and laryngeal spasm
7. Crying and straining
8. Nitrous oxide (?) (in children with compromised myocardium)
9. Restriction of diaphragmatic movement from raised intraabdominal pressure
10. Surgical manipulation of the heart and great vessels
11. Noxious stimuli

**Treatment measures**

1. Oxygenation
2. Hyperventilation
3. Alkalosis
4. Prostaglandins (E type)
5. α-adrenergic antagonists
6. Vasodilators (nitroglycerin and nitroprusside)
7. $\beta_2$ Stimulants (isoproterenol)
8. High fractionated inspired oxygen concentration
9. Nitric oxide

## Precautions

In all cases where there is a communication between right and left sides of the heart, it is absolutely necessary that all intravenous lines be free of air bubbles. In addition, one should use extra caution not to push any air bubbles when injecting drugs through an IV line. Although the use of nitrous oxide is not contraindicated in patients with a CMS, many anesthesiologists avoid the use of it, especially once the chest is opened, for fear of intravascular air bubble expansion. Appropriate antibiotic prophylaxis is also required for patients with CMS.

## Postoperative ventilation

Patients with CMS are usually left intubated and mechanically ventilated postoperatively. Once the patient is awake, stable, and rewarmed to a normal body temperature, the trachea can be extubated safely in the cardiac recovery room.

## REFERENCES


1. Almeida RS, Elliott MJ, Robinson PJ et al: Surgery for congenital abnormalities of the mitral valve at the Hospital for Sick Children, London, from 1969 to 1983, *J Cardiovasc Surg* 29:95, 1988.
2. Castaneda AR, Anderson RG, Edwards JE: Congenital mitral stenosis resulting from anomalous arcade and obstructing papillary muscles: report of correction by use of a ball valve prosthesis, *Am J Cardiol* 24:237,1969.
3. Coles JG, Williams WG, Watanabe T et al: Surgical experience with reparative techniques in patients with congenital mitral valvular anomalies, *Circulation* 76(suppl 3):117, 1987.
4. Collins-Nakai RL, Rosenthal A, Castaneda AR et al: Congenital mitral stenosis: a review of 20 years experience, *Circulation* 56:1039, 1977.
5. Corno A, Giannico S, Leibovich S et al: The hypoplastic mitral valve: when should a left atrial–left ventricular extracardiac valved conduit be used? *J Thorac Cardiovasc Surg* 9:848, 1986.
6. Glaser J, Yakirevich V, Vidne BA: Preoperative echographic diagnosis of supravalvular stenosing ring of the left atrium, *Am Heart J* 108:169, 1984.
7. John S, Baghi VV, Jairaj PS: Closed mitral valvotomy: early results and long-term follow up of 3,724 consecutive patients, *Circulation* 68:891, 1983.
8. Laks H, Hellenbrand WE, Kleinman C et al: Left atrial–left ventricular conduit for relief of congenital mitral stenosis in infancy, *J Thorac Cardiovasc Surg* 80:782, 1980.

9. Lansing AM, Elbl F, Solinger RE et al: Left atrial–left ventricular bypass for congenital mitral stenosis, *Surgery* 35:667, 1983.
10. Mazzera E, Corno A, DiDonato R et al: Surgical bypass of the systemic atrioventricular valve in children by means of a valved conduit, *J Thorac Cardiovasc Surg* 96:321, 1988.
11. Midgley FM, Perry LW, Potter BM: Conduit bypass of mitral valve: a palliative approach to congenital mitral stenosis, *Am J Cardiol* 56:493, 1985.
12. Ruckmann RN, VanPraagh R: Anatomic types of congenital mitral stenosis: report of 49 autopsy cases with consideration of diagnostic and surgical implications, *Am J Cardiol* 42:592, 1978.
13. Scott WC, Miller DC, Haverich A et al: Operative risks of mitral valve replacement: discriminant analysis of 1,329 procedures, *Circulation* 72(suppl 2):108, 1985.
14. Shone JD, Sellers RD, Anderson RC et al: The developmental complex of parachute mitral valve: supravalvular ring of the left atrium, subaortic stenosis, and coarctation of the aorta, *Am J Cardiol* 11:714, 1987.
15. Spencer FC, Colvin SB, Culliford AT et al: Experiences with the Carpentier techniques of mitral valve reconstruction in 103 patients (1980-1985), *J Thorac Cardiovasc Surg* 90:341, 1985.
16. Spevak PJ, Freed MD, Castaneda AR et al: Valve replacement in children less than 5 years of age, *J Am Coll Cardiol* 8:901, 1986.
17. Stellin G, Bortolotti U, Mazzucco A et al: Repair of congenitally malformed mitral valve in children, *J Thorac Cardiovasc Surg* 95:480, 1988.
18. Sullivan ID, Robinson PJ, de Laval M et al: Membranous supravalvular mitral stenosis: a treatable form of congenital heart disease, *J Am Coll Cardiol* 8:159, 1986.

## Section D MISCELLANEOUS DEFORMITIES

# 27 Hypoplastic Left Heart Syndrome

*P. Syamasundar Rao, Volker Striepe and Walter H. Merrill*



The term hypoplastic left heart syndrome (HLHS) was proposed by Noonan and Nadas[34] to describe a clinical syndrome in neonates and infants with hypoplasia of the left ventricle, the same group of disorders characterized as hypoplasia of the aortic tract complex by Lev.[31] This syndrome is anatomically characterized by underdevelopment of the left side of the heart, with atresia or severe stenosis of the mitral and/or aortic valves and hypoplasia of the left ventricle and/or aorta with concomitant enlargement of the right side of the heart. To the best of our knowledge the earliest description of this syndrome (aortic atresia) is by Dilg[13] in 1883. While the clinical,[34] pathologic,[31,34,45] and pathophysiologic[45] features have been of interest to physicians who care for patients with congenital heart disease, the major recent increased interest in this entity was sparked after the description of innovative staged surgical therapy by Norwood and his associates[36,37] and allograft heart transplantation by Bailey and his colleagues.[1,3]

HLHS constitutes 1.2% to 1.5% of all CHD.[18,22] The reported prevalence varies between 0.16 and 0.27 per 1000 live births.[13,17,21] It represents 9% of serious CHD and 25% of deaths in the first week of life.[35] There is a slight male preponderance, with a male to female ratio of 3:2.[33] While reduction of blood flow into the left heart either by premature closure of the foramen ovale[24,32,38] or by malalignment of the atrial septum to the left[50] has been postulated as a causative factor of this syndrome, it is generally believed that it is a developmental anomaly similar to other CHD. Familial cases with autosomal recessive inheritance[42,44,48] have been reported, but HLHS is generally postulated to occur on a multifactorial inheritance basis.

This chapter discusses pathologic anatomy, pathophysiology, clinical features, invasive and noninvasive studies, management, and prognosis of HLHS.

## PATHOLOGIC ANATOMY

In general there is hypoplasia of the left-sided structures with enlargement and hypertrophy of the right heart structures. As do patients with other CHD, patients with HLHS show a spectrum of severity: in the most severe form there is aortic valve and mitral valve atresia, with a diminutive ascending aorta and severely hypoplastic left ventricle. The *left atrium* is usually smaller than normal, although it may be normal in size or enlarged, and it receives all the pulmonary veins. Pulmonary venous stenosis is an important but rare abnormality in HLHS. The *mitral valve* may be atretic, hypoplastic, or severely stenotic. With mitral atresia there is usually fibromuscular tissue in the plane of the mitral valve rather than a membranous atresia. With a stenotic mitral valve, the entire mitral valve apparatus, including the valve annulus, chordae tendineae, and papillary muscles, are small and hypoplastic. The *left ventricle* is often a thick-walled, slitlike cavity, especially when the mitral valve is atretic. Or it may be a small cavity when the mitral valve is perforate. Endocardial fibroelastosis is often present. The *aortic valve* is either atretic or severely stenotic. The *ascending aorta* is usually severely hypoplastic (2 to 3 mm in diameter), carrying blood toward the coronary arteries in a retrograde fashion. However, the ascending aorta may approach normal dimensions.[6,12,19] Aortic coarctation[6,15,28,36,37,49] may be present in a significant number of patients with HLHS, but interruption of the aortic arch is rare.

The right atrium, right ventricle, and pulmonary artery are markedly enlarged. ASD is uncommon, but a patent foramen ovale with herniation of the valve of the septum is frequently seen. Sometimes the patent foramen ovale is completely closed. A large PDA is usually seen. VSD is not considered an integral part of HLHS but may be present in the syndrome of mitral atresia with normal aortic root.

HLHS hearts usually have visceroatrial situs solitus with D-ventricular loop and concordant atrioventricular and ventriculoarterial connections, and the heart is in the left side of the chest (levocardia). Rarely, dextrocardia and visceroatrial heterotaxy can be present.

Severe hypoplasia of the left ventricle can also be present in patients with double-outlet right ventricle and common AV canal with malalignment. In some series these variants constitute up to 25% of HLHS.[35]

## PATHOPHYSIOLOGY

In utero the fetal circulatory pathways are such that there is no impairment of fetal growth or survival.[43] The oxygenated blood from the placenta is returned to the inferior vena cava, (see Chapter 2) and instead of being shunted preferentially into the left atrium, it mixes with the superior vena caval blood in the right atrium and enters the right ventricle and pulmonary artery. The pulmonary venous return to the left atrium flows across the patent foramen ovale. It, along with coronary sinus flow, also enters the right atrium, right ventricle, and pulmonary artery. Because of the widely patent ductus arteriosus and high pulmonary vascular resistance in the fetus, only a small portion of the blood from the right heart enters the lungs, and the majority of the blood flows into the aorta. Because there is essentially no forward flow in the ascending aorta and arch of the aorta, blood from the pulmonary artery, once it enters the aorta, gets distributed into the bracheocephalic vessels, the ascending aorta, and the descending aorta. The relative amounts of flow to these vascular beds is dependent upon their relative resistances. The blood in the ascending aorta flows in a reverse (when compared with normal) direction, and it supplies the coronary arteries.

These changes in circulation in the fetus with HLHS result in the following physiologic differences from the normal fetus:

1. A larger amount of flow across the PDA with a greater $Po_2$. It is not clear whether these factors influence the development of ductal musculature, which in turn may influence the ductal closure postnatally.
2. Lower $Po_2$ and questionably lower blood flow to the brain. Although there are no detailed studies of cellular development of the brain, its weight is generally normal. However, it is not known whether the recently reported association between brain anomalies and HLHS is related to these abnormalities in $Po_2$ and blood flow to the brain.[23]
3. Higher $Po_2$ in the pulmonary artery. It is generally believed that the normally low $Po_2$ in pulmonary arterial blood is responsible for progressive development of muscular pulmonary arteries in the fetus.[9,11,40] A higher than normal $Po_2$ may lead to a lack of normal medial muscular hypertrophy,[43] which may result in a rapid decline in PVR after birth.
4. Retrograde coronary flow through a long channel that carries blood with a lower than normal oxygen pressure. This is believed not to interfere with the supply of normal quantities of oxygen and nutrients to the myocardium. However, it is not clear whether myocardial reserve is adversely affected with relative asphyxia and other types of stress.

Postnatally, the circulation in HLHS depends upon three major factors: adequacy of interatrial communication, patency of the ductus arteriosus, and level of pulmonary vascular resistance. The pulmonary venous return to the left atrium must exit into the right atrium because of atresia or severe stenosis of the mitral valve (Fig. 27–1). In most infants with HLHS a patent foramen ovale is present and is small and partially obstructive.[45] Large interatrial communications such as true ASD, though they result in prompt egress of left atrial blood, cause a rapid and marked fall in pulmonary vascular resistance, which may be detrimental to the infant (see next section). A very small and markedly obstructive patent foramen ovale may produce pulmonary venous hypertension, marked elevation of pulmonary vascular resistance, and pulmonary edema.

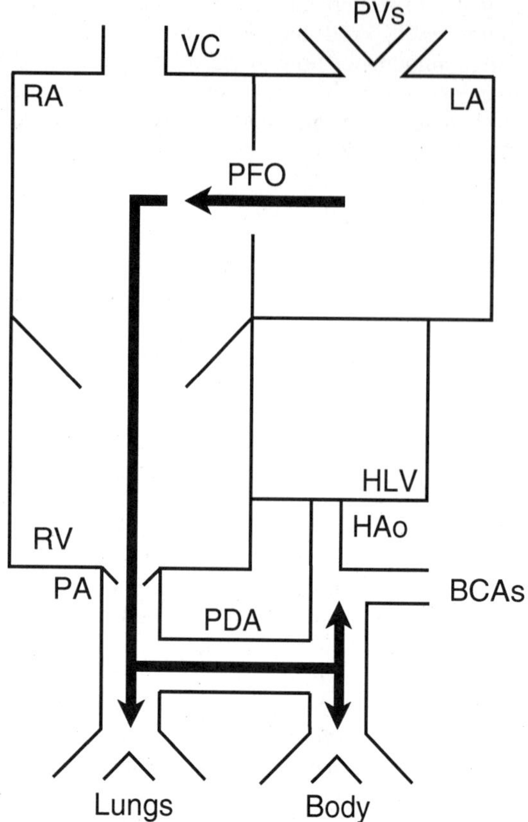


**Figure 27–1** Box diagram of circulation in hypoplastic left heart syndrome. In hypoplastic left heart syndrome (or mitral atresia) pulmonary venous *(PV)* return cannot exit into the hypoplastic left ventricle *(HLV)*, and its egress has to be into the right atrium *(RA)*. If the foramen ovale *(PFO)* is obstructive, the infant will develop signs of pulmonary venous obstruction. This blood mixes with systemic venous return and enters the right ventricle *(RV)* and pulmonary artery *(PA)*. Because there is no forward flow from the HLV into the hypoplastic aorta *(HAo)*, the systemic perfusion depends on the patency of the ductus arteriosus *(PDA)*. *BCA*s, Brachiocephalic arteries; *LA*, left atrium; *VC*, venae cavae. (From Rao PS: *Indian J Pediatr* 58:441, 1991.)

In HLHS the mitral valve, left ventricle, and/or aorta are markedly stenotic or atretic, and the entire systemic circulation depends upon the flow through the ductus arteriosus (Fig. 27–1). As the $Po_2$ increases, the ductus arteriosus tends to constrict, thus compromising the systemic perfusion. Infusion of prostaglandin $E_1$ will keep the ductus open, maintaining systemic perfusion.

Usually there is a drop in pulmonary vascular resistance following birth, mostly related to an increase in $Po_2$. This decrease in resistance increases pulmonary flow. Thus, a combination of ductal constriction and decrease in PVR results in a marked decrease in systemic perfusion with consequent acidemia. A rapid fall in PVR may be prevented by not administering ambient oxygen and even by providing lower fractional inspired oxygen concentration than room air. A slightly restrictive patent foramen ovale may also be helpful in preventing a rapid fall of pulmonary resistance.

Thus, maintenance of adequate systemic perfusion may be achieved by (1) administration of prostaglandin $E_1$ to keep open the ductus arteriosus and (2) maintaining a high pulmonary vascular resistance by administering fractional inspired oxygen concentration lower than room air or by adding carbon dioxide to the breathing gas mixture and by *not* opening the atrial septum widely.

## CLINICAL FEATURES

The clinical features will depend upon the status of the patent foramen ovale, PDA, and PVR. At birth the infant may be completely asymptomatic. As the ductus begins to close and PVR falls, tachypnea, tachycardia, and mild cyanosis are observed. Full-blown clinical features with signs of severe CHF (tachypnea, tachycardia, hepatomegaly), pale color, and poor pulses may develop within hours to days after birth. Flaring alae nasae, subcostal and/or intercostal retractions, fine rales in the lung bases, hyperdynamic precordium, and a nonspecific grade I-II/VI ejection systolic murmur (in about 60% of patients) may be found. Unless prompt administration of prostaglandin $E_1$ is begun (with other supportive measures), the infant may not survive.

### Noninvasive Evaluation

***Chest x-ray film.*** Moderate to severe cardiomegaly with increased pulmonary vascular markings is usually present (Fig. 27–2). There is evidence for both increased flow and pulmonary venous congestion (edema). Although no specific x-ray features are pathognomonic for HLHS, the presence of a large heart with increased pulmonary markings in a mildly cyanotic neonate should always prompt inclusion of HLHS in the list of differential diagnoses.[39]

***Electrocardiogram.*** The ECG findings are not sufficiently specific to diagnose HLHS. Most of these neonates have right axis deviation and right ventricular hypertrophy. In about half of the infants a QR pattern is present in the right chest leads, indicative of severe right ventricular hypertrophy. Right atrial enlargement, manifested by tall and peaked P waves in lead II and right chest leads, is not uncommon. The usual Q wave may be absent in lead $V_6$. While less than normal left ventricular voltages (S wave in $V_1$ and $V_2$ and R wave in $V_5$ and $V_6$) are present in most babies with HLHS, this feature is not specific because some normal newborns may have a similar pattern secondary to

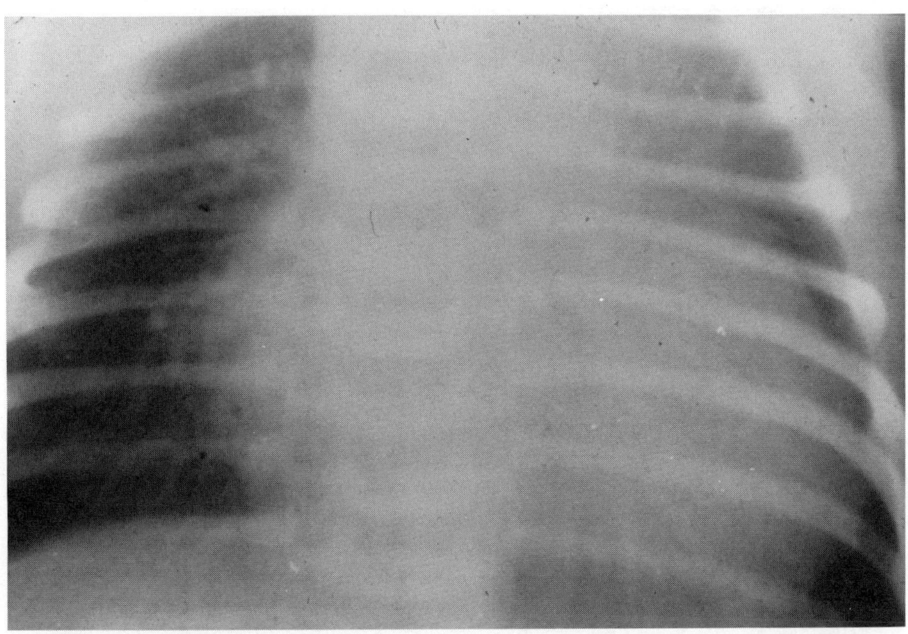

**Figure 27–2** Posteroanterior chest radiograph of a neonate with HLHS (confirmed by catheterization and angiographic studies) showing a markedly enlarged heart and increased pulmonary vascular markings.

their right ventricular preponderance. ST-T wave changes suggestive of myocardial ischemia may be present in some infants with HLHS.

***Echo-Doppler studies.*** Two-dimensional and Doppler echocardiographic features are sufficiently characteristic of HLHS that cardiac catheterization and angiography are no longer necessary for diagnosing this anomaly. The right ventricle is usually large, and its function should be evaluated. The tricuspid valve is also enlarged, and the degree of tricuspid insufficiency should be documented. The pulmonary valve, though large, is usually normal. The left atrium is usually small, and the atrial septum should be imaged in the subcostal view to assess the size of the ASD. High-velocity Doppler jets indicate restrictive defects. The ASD, usually a patent foramen ovale, becomes small with increasing age, and septal aneurysms may be seen more commonly in older infants. The mitral valve may be atretic or severely hypoplastic, with reduced excursion of the mitral valve leaflets. Less than 5-mm excursions are considered abnormal. The left ventricular cavity may exhibit varying degrees of hypoplasia. Multiple views must be examined to reach conclusions on its size. While the short-axis view may show only a minimal decrease in the left ventricular size, other views (long axis and four chamber) may show true hypoplasia of the ventricle. The ascending aorta should be evaluated in multiple views, and an ascending aorta less than 5 mm is reasonably characteristic of HLHS. However, a normal-size aortic root may be present with HLHS.[12] Retrograde flow in the ascending aorta can usually be documented by Doppler. Suprasternal notch views should be recorded to evaluate isthmic hypoplasia and aortic coarctation, especially if surgical options are under consideration. The ductus arteriosus with right to left shunt can usually be documented, although special echographic views may be necessary to do so. Several of these echo-Doppler features are demonstrated in Figs. 27–3 through 27–6.

### Invasive studies

Although cardiac catheterization and selective cineangiography are not necessary to diagnose HLHS, a focused catheterization may be necessary to resolve any peculiar echocardiographic features, especially if surgical options are considered.[4] It should also be noted that interventional catheterization may be indicated as an adjunct to palliative surgery or while awaiting cardiac transplantation.[7]

When catheterization is performed, the features reflect the pathophysiology described earlier and will be mentioned only briefly.

Oxygen saturation data document moderate to severe systemic venous desaturation with a step up at the right atrial level (secondary to entry of left atrial blood into the right atrium via an ASD). The oxygen saturations in the right ventricle, pulmonary artery, and aorta are similar, reflecting common mixing at the right atrial level. There is usually

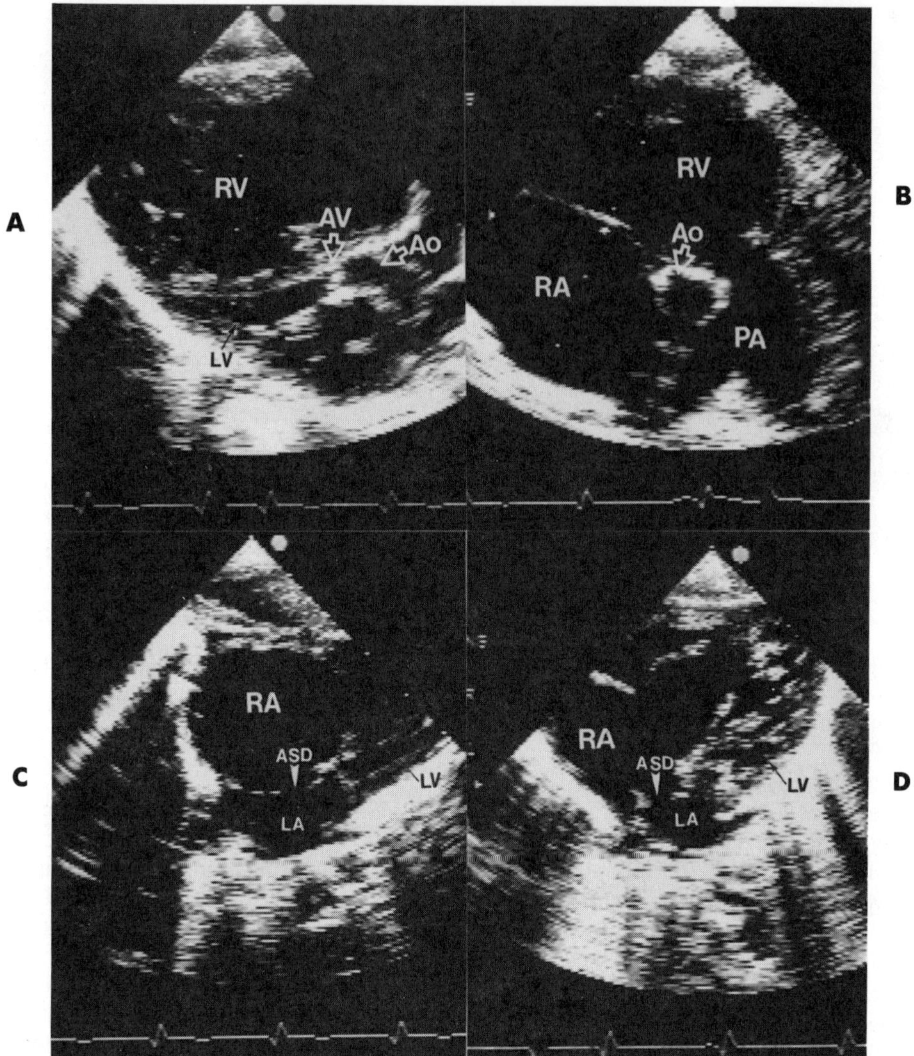


**Figure 27–3** Selected video frames from a two-dimensional echocardiographic study of a neonate wtih hypoplastic left heart syndrome. **A,** Precordial long-axis view showing a very small left ventricle *(LV),* aorta *(Ao),* severely stenotic aortic valve *(AV)* and a large right ventricle *(RV),* **B,** Precordial short axis view showing a small aorta and large RA, RV, and pulmonary artery *(PA).* **C,** Subcostal view showing a small LA, tiny, slitlike LV and a large RA. An ASD is also shown. **D,** A four-chamber view showing LV muscle mass with a slitlike cavity. Small LA and large RA and RV are also shown.

only mild systemic arterial hypoxemia unless severe pulmonary edema is present.

The right atrial pressure is mildly elevated, and the left atrial pressure is moderately to markedly elevated, unless there is a large ASD. The right ventricular and pulmonary arterial peak systolic pressures are at systemic level. If the ductus is constricted, these pressures may be higher than those in the aorta.

Angiography, though not necessary in all cases, demonstrates hypoplasia of the mitral valve, left ventricle, and aorta (Fig. 27–7 and Fig. 27–8). The ascending aorta is perfused in a retrograde fashion and serves as a common coronary artery supplying the right and left coronary arteries (Fig. 27–9).

## MANAGEMENT

There is no unanimity in the approach to treatment of neonates with HLHS. Supportive care, multistage surgical intervention, and cardiac transplantation are available options. A thorough explanation of each of these options, including their advantages and disadvantages, should be provided to the parents. Occasionally some anatomic features may favor one choice over the others. In the pres-

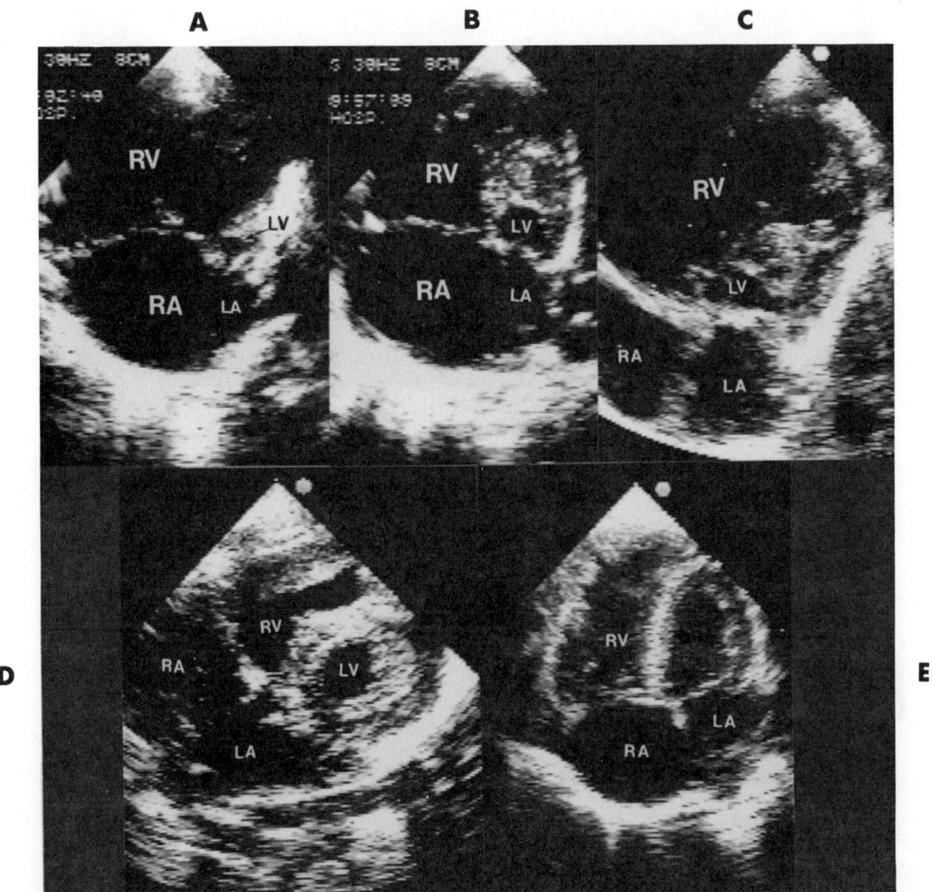


**Figure 27–4** Four-chamber views of the heart in five different neonates with varying degree of HLV.

ence of severe tricuspid or pulmonary valve anomalies, the multistage surgical intervention is not likely to be beneficial, and cardiac transplantation is the only surgical choice. If severe pulmonary venous anomalies are present, neither surgical option is feasible. However, in the majority of cases the choice of treatment is based on the parents' preference. While such a decision is being made, the infant should be stabilized.

Fundamental pathophysiologic principles outlined earlier should be taken into consideration in stabilizing the infant. IV infusion of prostaglandin $E_1$ (0.05 μg/kg/min) to keep the ductus widely patent is the mainstay of treatment. With a wide-open ductus the relative flows into the systemic and pulmonary circuits depend to a great degree on PVR. Factors that tend to decrease PVR should be avoided. Modest elevation of this resistance may result in better systemic perfusion. This may be achieved with controlled hypoventilation.[30] The fractional inspired oxygen concentration should be reduced to room air (0.21) or lower to maintain an arterial oxygen pressure of 30 torr. Similarly, the carbon dioxide pressure should be maintained at 40 torr and pH at 7.35 to 7.4, if need be, by adding carbon dioxide to the breathing gas mixture. Total pulmonary resistance may be increased by increasing positive end expiratory pressure. Finally, if the interatrial septum is markedly obstructive, causing severe pulmonary edema, relief of this obstruction is beneficial. However, wide-open atrial defects are likely to cause a rapid fall in PVR and a fall in systemic perfusion. Limited opening by balloon angioplasty of the atrial septum may be useful,[41] especially while waiting for cardiac transplantation.[7] Inotropic support, intermittent bicarbonate, and sodium nitroprusside (to decrease systemic vascular resistance) may occasionally be required to stabilize the patient.

### Supportive care

If only supportive care is chosen, the parents will need strong emotional support, as the condition is universally fatal without active treatment.

### Multistage surgical intervention

Sinha,[45] Caylor,[10] Dotty,[14] and their colleagues have proposed a variety of palliative operations.

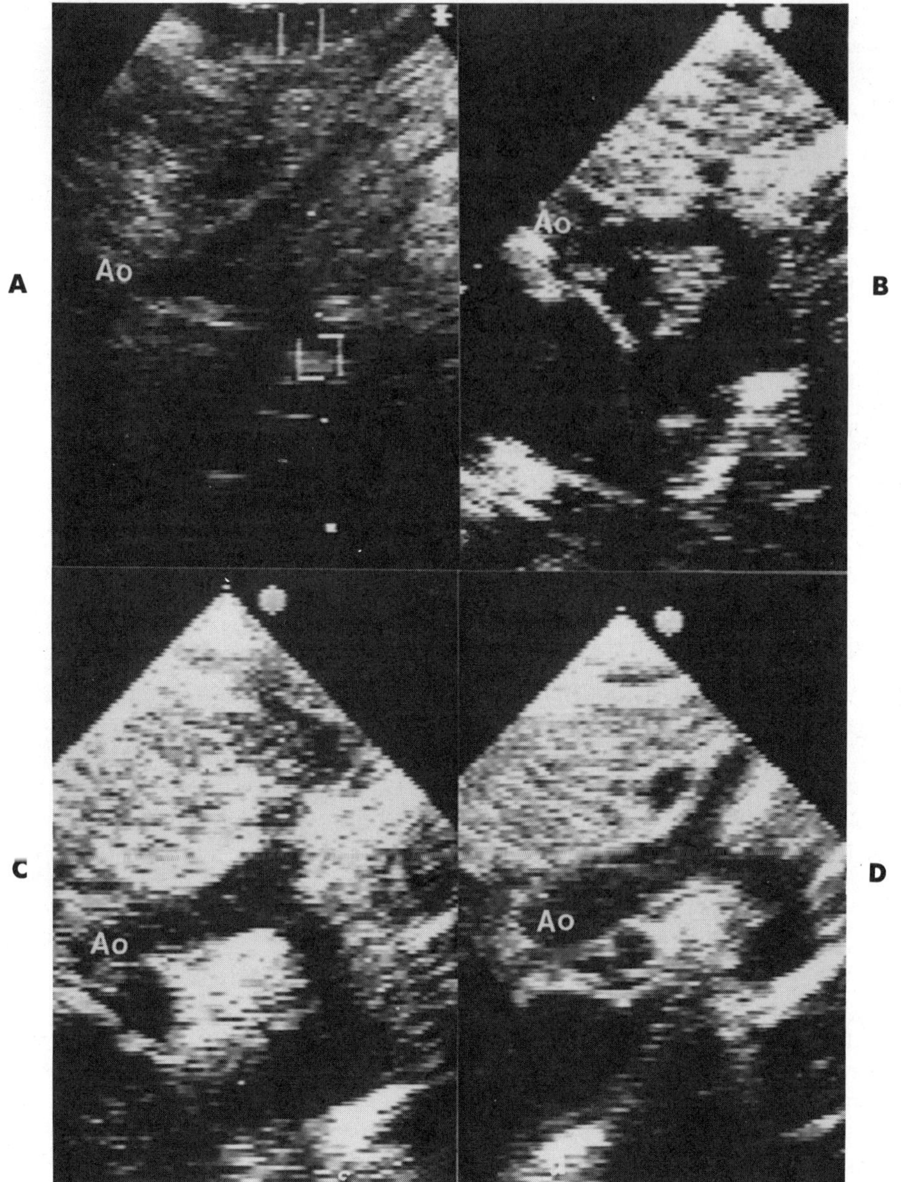


**Figure 27–5** Suprasternal notch views of the aortic arch, again showing different degrees of hypoplasia of the ascending aorta (Ao) and aortic arch in four different neonates with HLHS.

But it was not until Norwood and his colleagues[36,37] demonstrated that a multistage operative approach is feasible to palliate HLHS that this approach, now called the Norwood procedure, was adopted by other workers. This procedure has evolved and now consists of three stages.

***First-stage palliation.*** There are three basic principles to the first palliative procedure: (1) The aorta is to be connected to the right ventricle so as to permit unobstructed systemic blood flow. (2) Pulmonary blood flow is regulated for growth and development of the pulmonary vasculature. (3) A large interatrial communication is created to avoid pulmonary venous hypertension.[35]

This procedure is performed through a midline sternal incision. After pulmonary artery and right atrial appendage cannulation, cardiopulmonary bypass is initiated, and the infant is cooled to 20° C rectal temperature. During the cooling process the branch vessels of the aortic arch are dissected out and looped with suture tourniquets in preparation for circulatory arrest. Once cooling is complete, circulatory arrest is initiated, the venous and arterial cannulas are removed, and the following steps are carried out (Fig. 27–10)[35]:

1. Atrial septectomy

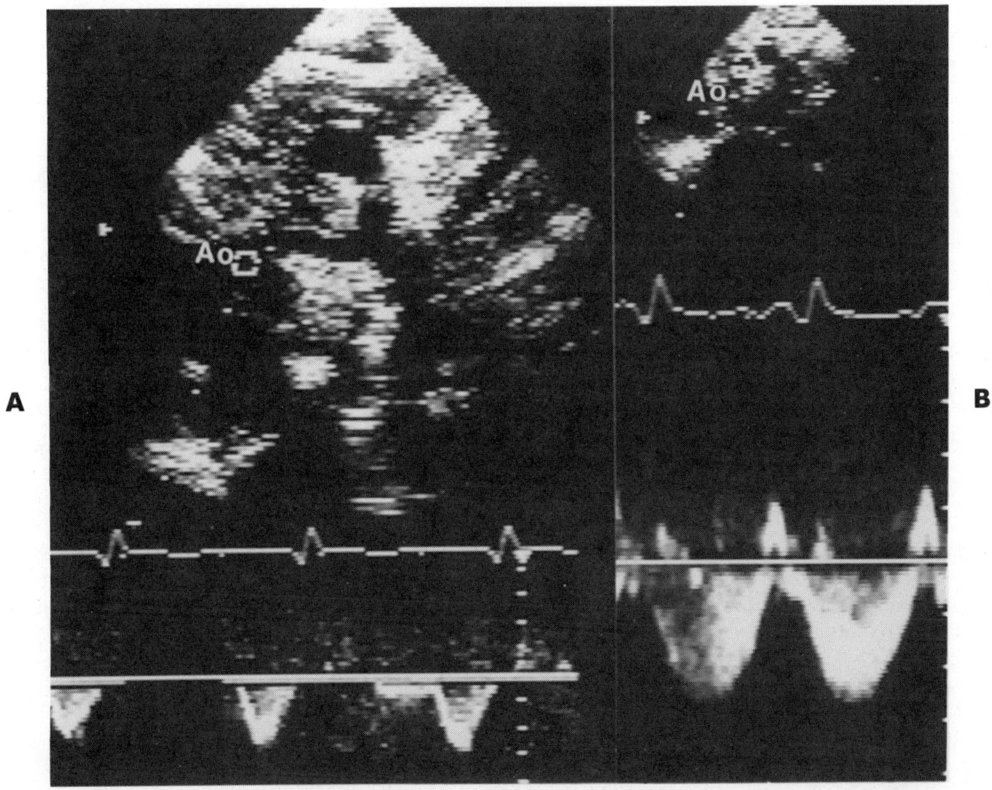


**Figure 27–6** Suprasternal notch two-dimensional echographic views of the aortic arch with a pulse-Doppler sample volume placed in the ascending aorta demonstrating reverse flow in the ascending aorta, supplying the coronary arteries. Examples in two neonates are shown.

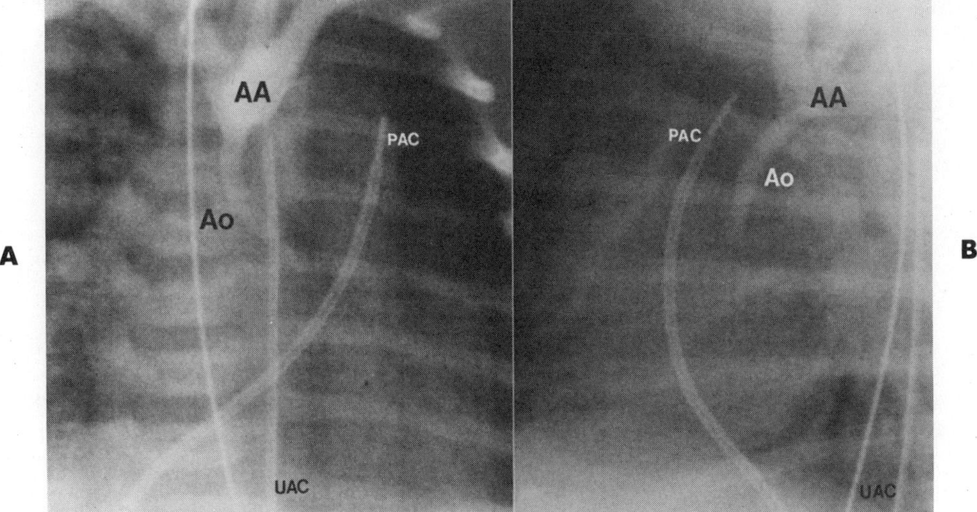


**Figure 27–7** Selected cine frames of aortic arch *(AA)* cineangiogram in posteroanterior *(A)* and lateral *(B)* views in a neonate with hypopolastic left heart syndrome. The angiogram was performed via the umbilical artery catheter *(UAC)*. Retrograde opacification of a very small hypoplastic ascending aorta is visualized. Pulmonary artery catheter *(PAC)* is also seen.

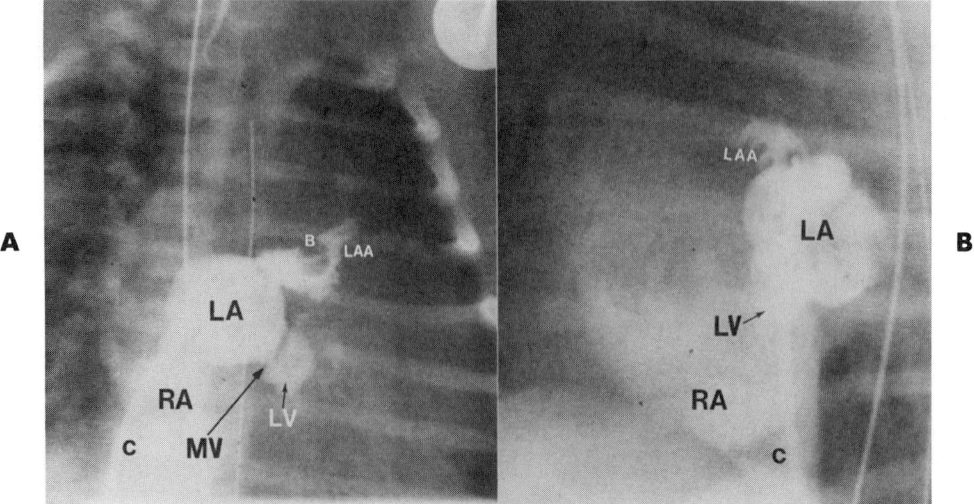


**Figure 27–8** Left atrial *(LA)* cineangiogram in posteroanterior *(A)* and lateral *(B)* views showing somewhat smallish LA, markedly hypoplastic LV opacified through a very stenotic mitral valve *(MV)*, and left-to-right shunting across an atrial defect opacifying the RA. Balloon *(B)* tipped catheter is in the left atrial appendage *(LAA)*. *C*, catheter.

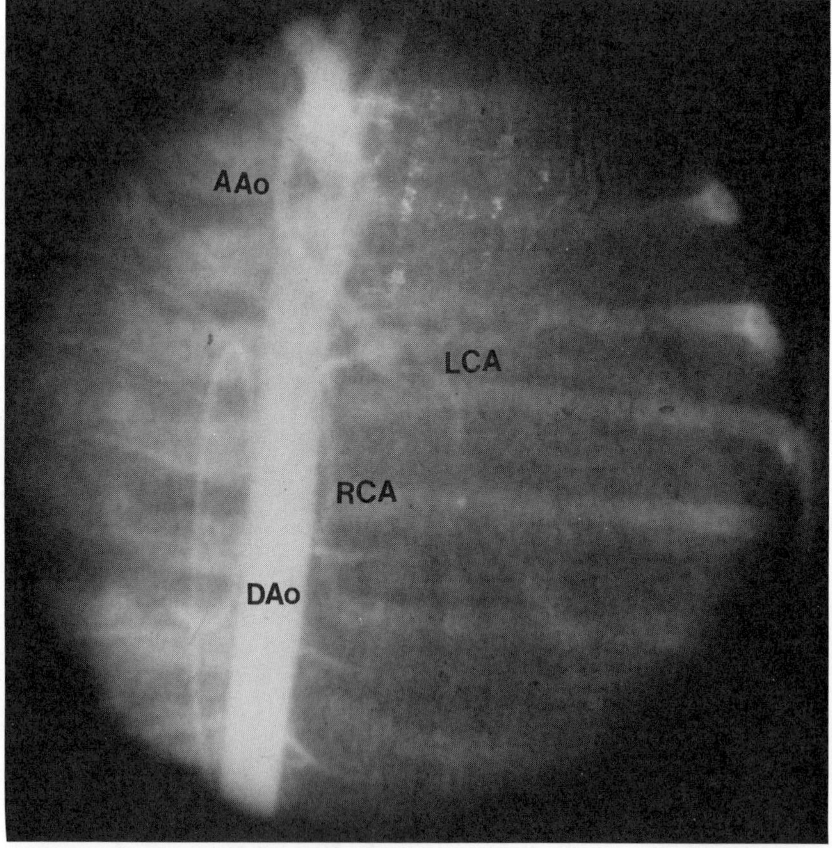


**Figure 27–9** Aortic arch cineangiogram in a posteroanterior view opacifying the descending aorta *(DAo)* and ascending aorta *(AAo)*, which is serving as a common coronary artery and supplying the right *(RCA)* and left *(LCA)* coronary arteries.

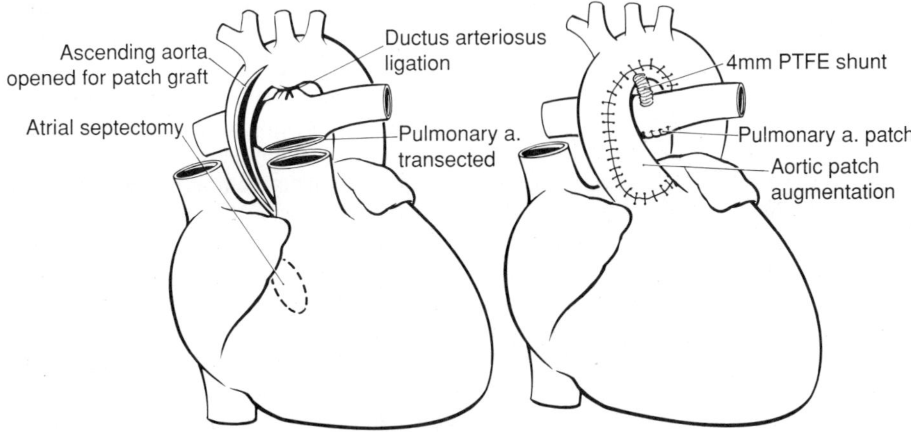


**Figure 27–10** First stage palliation of hypoplastic left heart syndrome by Norwood procedure. The initial steps include transsection of the PA, ductal ligation, incision of the undersurface of the aortic arch and ascending aorta, and atrial septectomy. Patch closure of the distal pulmonary artery, anastomosis of the proximal pulmonary artery to the incised aorta, most often with a homograft augmentation, and insertion of a 4-mm Gore-Tex® graft between the neoaorta and pulmonary artery.

2. Pulmonary artery transection just proximal to the takeoff of the right pulmonary artery
3. Repair of the pulmonary artery confluence with a patch
4. Ligation of the ductus arteriosus
5. Opening and augmentation of the aortic arch with a patch before it is anastomosed to the proximal transected pulmonary artery
6. Connection of a 4-mm polytetrafluoroethylene tube graft to the aorta and the branch pulmonary arteries

Cardiopulmonary bypass is resumed; the patient is rewarmed. After separation from cardiopulmonary bypass, hemostatsis is obtained and closure of the chest begun.

Complications of first-stage palliative surgery include (1) restrictive ASD, particularly in early operations in which the atrial septectomies were incomplete,[27] (2) neoaortic arch obstruction, (3) pulmonary artery distortion, (4) ventricular dysfunction and tricuspid regurgitation, and (5) pulmonary vascular obstructive disease. The latter complications in particular have led to the development of intermediate procedures, such as the bidirectional Glenn shunt, the fenestrated Fontan procedure, and extensive patch pulmonary angioplasty.[27]

***Second-stage palliation.*** Norwood and colleagues initially proposed a Fontan procedure for the patient between 1 and 2 years of age. But because of significant morbidity and mortality associated with early Fontan, they modified their approach, with resultant reduction of complications. A bidirectional Glenn (cavopulmonary) anastomosis directing the superior vena caval flow into both lungs with concomitant ligation of the aortopulmonary shunt is performed as a second-stage procedure. If there is interatrial obstruction, it should also be relieved. This is generally performed 6 months to a year after the first-stage procedure. The rationale behind this staged approach follows the observation that one cannot predict in which patients a rapid fall in end diastolic volume will develop after the Fontan procedure. This rapid fall in diastolic volume leads to an apparent increase in ventricular wall thickness, which results in diastolic dysfunction. The consequence may be a rise in end diastolic pressure, increased CVP, and decreased cardiac output. The ensuing low cardiac output state is very difficult to treat, since the muscle mass of the ventricle only gradually decreases. Staging the Fontan allows time for a gradual geometric adjustment, since only one third of the systemic venous return is obligated to flow passively through the pulmonary vasculature.

***Third-stage palliation.*** Six months to 1 year following the bidirectional Glenn procedure, the Fontan is completed by channeling of the flow from the inferior vena cava to the pulmonary artery. Interatrial obstruction, if present, should also be tackled at this time.

### Cardiac transplantation

The team at the Loma Linda University Medical Center has performed more than 100 pediatric cardiac transplants and has achieved actuarial survival in excess of 80% after 3 years.[2,16] These encouraging results have favored orthotopic transplantation as an important treatment option for HLHS.[46] Many centers have been unable to duplicate the good results Norwood has achieved with his palliative procedures, which has further encouraged transplantation programs.[46,47] The shortage of pediatric heart donors, however, has led to the development of treatment protocols which allow cross-over from the group of patients whose parents chose transplantation to the staged surgical palliation group when the patient deteriorated while awaiting a suitable donor.[2,8,46] As the success with cardiac transplantation became apparent, transplantation became an option for patients who had undergone the first-stage palliation but were unsuitable for a complete repair.[8] The transplantation is performed using hypothermic circulatory arrest. Surgical exposure is gained through a midsternal incision and opening of the pericardium. A thymectomy is followed by isolation of the aorta and its branches. The venous cannula is inserted into the right atrium. The aortic cannula is inserted through the main pulmonary artery into the ductus arteriosus, and the patient is placed on cardiopulmonary bypass. After core cooling to 18° C, circulatory arrest is established, and the heart is excised, leaving the posterior atrial walls and septum in place. Usually the hypoplastic aortic arch is opened from distal to the insertion of the patent ductus to proximal to the level of the innominate artery, and the ascending aorta is ligated. In rare cases, when the ascending aorta is 80% or more of the diameter of the descending aorta right below the inflow of the ductus, it may be feasible to leave the aorta, perform a classic end-to-end anastomosis with the donor aorta, and thereby decrease circulatory arrest duration.[8] More commonly the donor heart is sewn into place starting with the left atrial, then the right atrial and pulmonary artery anastomosis, and completed by an aortic reconstruction. This consists of an aortic onlay graft from the donor heart, which is especially prepared to retain more donor aorta, to augment the hypoplastic aorta. The presence of aortic coarctation (up to 80% of cases) must be carefully considered and corrected if present. Recannulation is performed and cardiopulmonary bypass resumed. Atrial pacing leads are placed and are frequently used when spontaneous ventricular rhythms are deemed too slow at the time of weaning. The patient is rewarmed to 37° C and weaned off bypass. Inotropic support is normally administered with dopamine 5 to 7 μg/kg/min and isoproterenol at an initial dose of 0.03 μg/kg/min, the most commonly used drugs. Prostaglandin $E_1$ is continued at 25 to 50 μg/kg/min.[16] Methylprednisolone 10 mg/kg is administered when flow to the donor heart is restored. The anesthesiologist may be asked to deliver other immunosuppressant drugs, including cyclosporine and azathioprine. The development of immunosuppressant protocols and drugs has been the single most important contributor to making cardiac transplantation feasible, and the low immune system activity of young infants has made them attractive candidates for this type of surgery. Neonatal survival in the Loma Linda experience was 87% after 5 years compared with 67% in older children.[16]

***Complications.*** Hypertension is a common complication after transplantation: 50% in one series,[46] 96% at Stanford,[46] but apparently lower in others.[8] Other cardiovascular problems include recurrent aortic coarctation and bradydysrhythmias. The majority of early and late deaths are due to either graft rejection or host infections.[16] Renal dysfunction occurs as an adverse effect of chronic cyclosporine therapy.[29] Other complications include pulmonary complications (pneumonia, atelectasis, pleural effusions, pulmonary hypertension), gastrointestinal (gastroesophageal reflux and peptic ulceration), and neurologic disorders (seizures and cerebrovascular accidents).

## ANESTHESIA MANAGEMENT

### Preoperative phase

Preoperative medical management must be continued. Patients are always on prostaglandin infusion and occasionally on inotropic support, which should not be interrupted for any reason. The prostaglandin infusion may be administered through a central or peripheral line (see dose under Management). Factors influencing ductus arteriosus patency are reviewed in Table 14–2. Remember that a potential complication of prostaglandin infusion is apnea, and ventilation must be monitored carefully. These infants are always stabilized prior to surgery, and this may include mechanical ventilation to achieve the best balance in vascular resistance between the systemic and pulmonary circulation. The goal is to maintain the ratio of pulmonary blood flow (Qp) to systemic blood flow (Qs) near unity. Carbon dioxide has an important direct effect on pulmonary vascular resistance. Hypocapnia and hyperoxia are avoided, since they will lower pulmonary vascular resistance and increase pulmonary blood flow. Carbon dioxide has been used in some circumstances to manipulate the pulmonary vascular resistance.[25,26] Insufficient pulmonary blood flow (Qp/Qs less than 1) may result in hypoxemia. Maneuvers to lower PVR and increase Qp should then be used. If the patient is no longer intubated and is stable on room air, the oxygen saturation is usually 80% to 85%. The hemoglobin is maintained at 10 g/dl or above. Minimal or no premedication is given if the patient is under 6 months of age. In older children oral premedication is preferred over the IM route. Midazolam 0.5 to 0.6 mg/kg is administered orally about 30 minutes prior to transfer into the operating room. The child must be under observation by a member of the anesthesia team skilled in airway management. Premedication and anesthetic considerations for patients undergoing the Fontan procedure are discussed in Chapter 23.

### Intraoperative phase

For management of anesthesia for pediatric cardiac transplantation see Chapter 30.

***First-stage palliation procedure.*** Preparation of the operating room should include the preparation of all emergency resuscitation drugs and equipment. It may be advisable to calculate doses of resuscitation drugs based on the infant's weight before the procedure to avoid any delay should an emergency arise. IV and arterial line systems must be carefully purged of all air. The operating room should be warm during the anesthesia induction phase and again after the patient is being rewarmed on cardiopulmonary bypass. For infants of 2 to 3 kg an operating room temperature of 80° to 84° F is recommended.[5] Once the patient's trachea is intubated and appropriate monitors are established, all warming devices are turned off, and the operating room is cooled in preparation for cardiopulmonary bypass. Monitoring for the anesthesia induction includes all routine monitors: ECG, pulse oximetry, capnography, temperature, and noninvasive blood pressure monitoring. In the stable patient, arterial and central venous pressure monitoring lines may be inserted after induction of anesthesia. The anesthesia induction is commonly by IV, since an umbilical catheter has usually been placed while the infant was in the neonatal intensive care unit. An opioid-based induction (fentanyl 50 to 75 μg/kg) or ketamine 1 to 2 mg/kg and atropine 10 to 15 μg/kg are good choices. Fentanyl is administered in small increments of 5 to 10 μg to minimize hemodynamic compromise. Muscle relaxation for tracheal intubation is achieved using a nondepolarizing muscle relaxant (pancuronium 0.1 to 0.15 mg/kg or vecuronium 0.1 to 0.2 mg/kg), since succinylcholine, by virtue of it acetylcholine-related structure, may constrict the ductus arteriosus. The prostaglandin infusion should not be interrupted, and the line used for its administration is not disturbed. Once a satisfactory plane of anesthesia is achieved, further IV access is sought. The oxygen saturation on pulse oximetry is often 80% to 85%, and excessive exogenous oxygen administration will vasodilate the pulmonary vasculature and lead to systemic hypoperfusion and acidosis (Qp/Qs above 1). This should be scrupulously avoided. High airway and therefore intrathoracic pressures during assisted or mechanical ventilation may decrease pulmonary perfusion and lead to hypoxemia. It is imperative to continually monitor the patient's response to changes in ventilation and fluid status. This is often best achieved by manual ventilation, unless sophisticated ventilators, such as the Siemens Servo 900, are available. Maintenance of anesthesia is preferably with an opioid-based agent for optimum hemodynamic stability. Fentanyl or sufentanil infusions or titrations are two alternatives. An important principle in anesthesia for neonates is that all anesthetic drugs must be titrated, since individual response varies considerably. Although isoflurane, halothane, ketamine, and fentanyl all induce hypotension with induction, this is almost completely reversed with surgical stimulation in patients maintained on fentanyl and ketamine, but not in those on the inhalational agents.[20] MAC varies with age: the MAC of halothane is 0.87% in the newborn, 1.2% in the infant, and 0.94% in the adult.

The operation is performed through a midline sternotomy. Low molecular weight dextran is administered at 10 ml/kg for its rheologic effects in preparation for cooling and circulatory arrest. The infant may be cooled exogenously, with continuation on cardiopulmonary bypass, or cooled actively on cardiopulmonary bypass only. The surgical procedure, performed during cardiopulmonary bypass and circulatory arrest, is described earlier. Inotropic support in the form of dopamine or isoproterenol is frequently needed to wean the patient off bypass. The most frequent problem in the postbypass phase is hypoxemia due to decreased pulmonary blood flow (Qp/Qs less than 1).[20] Hyperventilation to an arterial carbon dioxide pressure of 20 to 25 mm Hg and isoproterenol may help lower the pulmonary vascular resistance (Fig. 27–11). If the arterial partial pressure of oxygen is above 50 mm Hg, this may indicate too high a pulmonary blood flow, with systemic hypoperfusion and impending acidosis (Qp/Qs above 1). In this situation hypoventilation with intentional hypercapnia may be helpful in raising PVR. The patient is transferred to the cardiac recovery unit, mechanically ventilated and under residual anesthesia. The reactivity of the infant's pulmonary vasculature makes the continued vigilance of the entire team mandatory. Rapid fluctuations in the Qp/Qs ratio may require frequent adjustments in ventilation or drug therapy.

***Second-stage and third-stage palliation (Fontan procedure).*** This follows the principles outlined in Chapter 23 for the Fontan procedure.

## PROGNOSIS

Untreated, most babies with HLHS die in the neonatal period, although several reports document

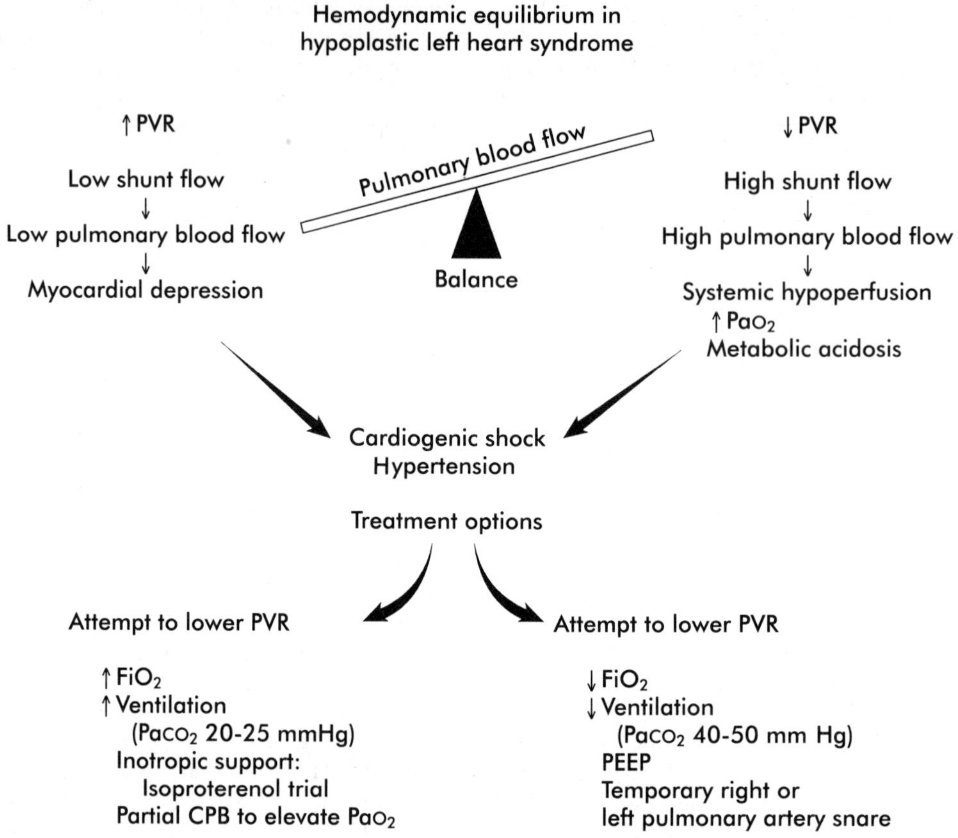

Hemodynamic equilibrium in hypoplastic left heart syndrome

↑ PVR

Low shunt flow
↓
Low pulmonary blood flow
↓
Myocardial depression

Pulmonary blood flow

Balance

↓ PVR

High shunt flow
↓
High pulmonary blood flow
↓
Systemic hypoperfusion
↑ $Pao_2$
Metabolic acidosis

Cardiogenic shock
Hypertension

Treatment options

Attempt to lower PVR

↑ $FiO_2$
↑ Ventilation
($Paco_2$ 20-25 mmHg)
Inotropic support:
Isoproterenol trial
Partial CPB to elevate $Pao_2$

Attempt to lower PVR

↓ $FiO_2$
↓ Ventilation
($Paco_2$ 40-50 mm Hg)
PEEP
Temporary right or
left pulmonary artery snare

**Figure 27–11** Hemodynamic equilibrium in hypoplastic left heart syndrome.

survival for several years in a very few patients. The latter appears to be related to an appropriate-sized interatrial communication, wide-open ductus arteriosus, and modest elevation of PVR. The prognosis is much improved with both multistage palliative operations and allograft transplantation. Because these are relatively new modalities of treatment, long-term prognosis remains unknown.

## REFERENCES


1. Bailey L, Concepcion W, Shattuk H et al: Method of heart transplantation for treatment of hypoplastic left heart syndrome, *J Thorac Cardiovasc Surg* 92:1, 1986.
2. Bailey LL, Gundry SR: Hypoplastic left heart syndrome, *Pediatr Clin North Am* 37:137, 1990.
3. Bailey LL, Nehlsen-Cannarella SL, Doroshow RW et al: Cardiac allotransplantation in newborns as therapy for hypoplastic left heart syndrome, *N Engl J Med* 315:949, 1986.
4. Bash SE, Huhta JC, Vick GW III et al: Hypoplastic left heart syndrome: is echocardiography accurate enough to guide surgical palliation? *J Am Coll Cardiol* 7:610, 1986.
5. Berry F: *Anesthetic management of difficult and routine pediatric patients,* ed 2, New York 1990, Churchill Livingstone.
6. Bharati S, Lev M: The surgical anatomy of hypoplasia of aortic tract complex, *J Thorac Cardiovasc Surg* 88:97, 1984.
7. Boucek MM, Mathis CM, Kanaknijeh MS et al: Management of the critically restrictive ASD awaiting infant cardiac transplantation, *Am J Cardiol* 70:559, 1992 (abstract).
8. Bove EL: Transplantation after first-stage reconstruction for hypoplastic left heart syndrome, *Ann Thorac Surg* 52:701, 1991.
9. Cassin S, Dawes GS, Mott JC et al: The vascular resistance of the fetal and newly ventilated lung of the lamb, *J Physiol (Lond)* 171:61, 1964.
10. Caylor GC, Smeloff EA, Miller GE: Surgical palliation of hypoplastic left side of the heart, *N Engl J Med* 282:780, 1970.
11. Cook CD, Drinker PA, Jacobsen HN et al: Control of pulmonary blood flow in the fetal and newly born lamb, *J Physiol (Lond)* 169:10, 1963.
12. Covitz W, Rao PS, Strong WB et al: Echocardiographic assessment of the aortic root in syndromes with left ventricular hypoplasia, *Pediatr Cardiol* 2:19, 1982.
13. Dilg J: Ein Beitrag zur Kenntniss seltener: Herzanomalien im Anschluss an einen Fall von angeborner linksseitiger Conusstenose, *Arch Pathol Anat* 91:193, 1883.
14. Dotty DB, Knott HW: Hypoplastic left heart syndrome: experience with an operation to establish functionally normal circulation, *J Thorac Cardiovasc Surg* 74:624, 1977.
15. Elzenga NJ, Gittenberger-de Groot AC: Coarctation and related aortic arch anomalies in hypoplastic left heart syndrome, *Int J Cardiol* 8:379, 1985.
16. Fabian JA: *Anesthesia for organ transplantation: a Society of Cardiovascular Anesthesiologists monograph,* Philadelphia, 1992, Lippincott.

17. Ferencz C, Rubin JD, McCarter RJ et al: Congenital heart disease: prevalence at live birth: the Baltimore-Washington infant study, *Am J Epidemiol* 121:31, 1985.
18. Freedom RM: Aortic atresia. In Keith JD, Rowe RD, Vlad P, editors: *Heart disease in infancy and childhood,* ed 3, New York, 1978, McMillian.
19. Freedom RM, Williams WG, Dishe MR et al: Anatomical variants in aortic atresia: potential candidates for ventriculoaortic reconstitution, *Br Heart J* 38:821, 1976.
20. Friesen RH, Henry DB: Cardiovascular changes in preterm neonates receiving isoflurane, halothane, fentanyl, and ketamine, *Anesthesiology* 64:238, 1986.
21. Fyler DC: Report of the New England Regional Infant Cardiac Program, *Pediatrics* 65(suppl):376, 1980.
22. Fyler DC: Prevalence/trends. In Fyler DC, editor: *Nadas' pediatric cardiology,* Philadelphia, 1992, Hanley & Belfus.
23. Glauser TA, Royke T, Weinberg PM et al: Congenital brain anomalies associated with hypoplastic left heart syndrome, *Pediatrics* 85:984, 1990.
24. Harh JY, Paul MH, Gallen WJ et al: Experimental production of hypoplastic left heart syndrome in the chick embryo, *Am J Cardiol* 31:51, 1973.
25. Jacobs ML, Murphy JD, Nicolson SC: Manipulation of inspired $Co_2$ in neonates with one ventricle and systemic-to-pulmonary artery shunt, *Circulation* 84(suppl 2):238, 1991 (abstract).
26. Jobes DR, Nicolson SC, Steven JM et al: Carbon dioxide prevents pulmonary overcirculation in hypoplastic left heart syndrome, *Ann Thorac Surg* 54:150, 1992.
27. Jonas RA: Intermediate procedures after first-stage Norwood operation facilitates subsequent repair, *Ann Thorac Surg* 52:696, 1991.
28. Jonas RA, Lang P, Hansen D: First stage palliation of hypoplastic left heart syndrome: the importance of coarctation and shunt size, *J Thorac Cardiovasc Surg* 92:6, 1986.
29. Kahan BD: Immunosuppressive therapy with cyclosporin for cardiac transplantation, *Circulation* 75:40, 1987.
30. Lang P, Fyler DC: Hypoplastic left heart syndrome, mitral atresia, and aortic atresia. In Fyler DC, editor: *Nadas' pediatric cardiology,* Philadelphia, 1992, Hanley & Belfus.
31. Lev M: Pathologic anatomy and interrelationship of hypoplasia of the aortic tract complexes, *Lab Invest* 1:61, 1952.
32. Lev M, Arcilla RA, Rimoldi HJA et al: Premature narrowing or closure of the foramen ovale, *Ann Heart J* 65:638, 1963.
33. Noonan JA: Hypoplastic left ventricle. In Moss AJ, Adams FH, editors: *Heart disease in infants, children and adolescents,* Baltimore, 1968, Williams & Wilkins.
34. Noonan JA, Nadas AS: The hypoplastic left heart syndrome, *Pediatr Clin North Am* 5:1029, 1958.
35. Norwood WI: Hypoplastic left heart syndrome, *Ann Thorac Surg* 52:688, 1991.
36. Norwood WI, Kirklin JK, Sanders SP: Hypoplastic left heart syndrome: experience with palliative surgery, *Am J Cardiol* 45:87, 1980.
37. Norwood WI, Lang P, Castaneda AR et al: Experience with operation for hypoplastic left heart syndrome, *J Thorac Cardiovasc Surg* 82:511, 1981.
38. Patten PM: Developmental defects of the foramen ovale, *Am J Dis Child* 33:585, 1928.
39. Rao PS: Management of the neonate with suspected serious heart disease, *King Faisal Specialist Hospital Medical Journal* 4:209, 1984.
40. Rao PS: Perinatal circulatory physiology, *Indian J Pediatr* 58:441, 1991.
41. Rao PS: Static balloon dilatation of the atrial septum, *Am Heart J* 125:1826, 1993 (editorial).
42. Rao SS, Gootman N, Platt N: Familial aortic atresia: report of a case of aortic atria in siblings, *Am J Dis Child* 118:919, 1969.
43. Rudolph AM: *Congenital diseases of the heart,* Chicago, 1974, Year Book Medical.
44. Shokeor MKH: Hypoplastic left heart syndrome: an autosomal recessive disorder, *Clin Genet* 2:7, 1971.
45. Sinha SN, Rusnak SL, Sommers HM et al: Hypoplastic left ventricle syndrome: analysis of 30 autopsy cases in infants with surgical considerations, *Am J Cardiol* 21:166, 1968.
46. Starnes VA, Griffin ML, Pitlick P et al: Current approach to hypoplastic left heart syndrome: palliation, transplantation, or both? *J Thorac Cardiovasc Surg* 104:189, 1992.
47. Starnes VA, Stinson EB, Oyer PE et al: Cardiac transplantation in children and adolescents, *Circulation* 76(suppl 5):43, 1987.
48. Van Egmond H, Orge E, Praet E et al: Hypoplastic left heart syndrome and 45X karyotype, *Br Heart J* 60:69, 1980.
49. Von Rueden TJ, Knight L, Moller JH et al: Coarctation of the aorta associated with aortic valve atresia, *Circulation* 52:951, 1975.
50. Weinberg PM, Chin AJ, Murphy JD et al: Postmortem echocardiography and tomographic anatomy of hypoplastic left heart syndrome after palliative surgery, *Am J Cardiol* 58:1228, 1986.

# 28 Double-Outlet Right Ventricle

*Scott H. Buck, P. Syamasundar Rao, Walter Merrill, and Jay Kambam*



Double-outlet right ventricle (DORV) is a congenital cardiac malformation characterized by both great vessels arising from the morphologic right ventricle. Defined by this ventriculoarterial connection, double-outlet right ventricle encompasses a heterogenous group of hearts further described in terms of atrial situs, atrioventricular connection, morphology and type of VSD, morphology of outflow tracts, and relationship of arterial trunks. The first description in English of a double-outlet right ventricle appeared in 1793.[38] Witham[39] is credited with the introduction of the term *double-outlet right ventricle* in 1957. Neufeld and associates[23] and Lev and colleagues[15] refined the understanding of double-outlet right ventricle by correlating pathophysiologic manifestations with the relationship of the VSD to the great vessels. Double-outlet right ventricle is rare, comprising less than 1% of congenital heart defects in pediatric patients.[21,24,38] Both sexes are equally affected.[10]

In this chapter the pathologic anatomy, pathophysiology, clinical features, invasive and noninvasive evaluation, management, and prognosis of children with double-outlet right ventricle will be discussed.

## PATHOLOGIC ANATOMY

The characteristic feature of double-outlet right ventricle is the ventriculoarterial connection relating both great vessels to the morphologic right ventricle. In spite of this seemingly unifying concept, there is considerable disagreement as to what constitutes double-outlet right ventricle. Various authors have defined it as both great vessels arising exclusively from the right ventricle with neither great vessel in continuity with the atrioventricular valve, as one complete arterial trunk and at least half of the other trunk arising from the right ventricle, and as more than half of each great vessel arising above the right ventricle.[7,8] A VSD is nearly universally present as the only egress of blood from the left ventricle. The location of the VSD is the major determinant of the pathophysiology and will be detailed below. An ASD is present in approximately 25% of patients. Double-outlet right ventri cle is normally associated with atrial situs solitus and concordant atrioventricular connections; when heterotaxy is present, abnormalities of systemic and pulmonary venous return are almost invariably present. In addition approximately 4% of patients have mitral valve abnormalities (straddling mitral valve, mitral stenosis, parachute mitral valve), frequently associated with left ventricular hypoplasia.[7,31]

## PATHOPHYSIOLOGY

The pathophysiology of double-outlet right ventricle is dependent on the location of the VSD relative to the great vessels, the relationship of the great vessels, and the presence or absence of outflow obstruction. The majority of VSD in patients with double-outlet right ventricle are perimembranous and are related to one or both great vessels (Fig. 28–1). Rarely, the septal defect is remote or noncommitted to either great vessel. Subaortic infracristal defects, which allow streaming of blood from the left ventricle to the aorta, are most com-

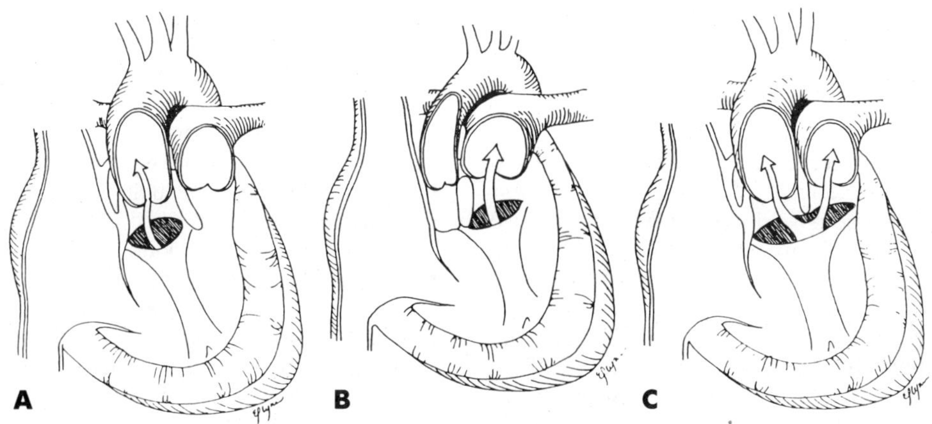


**Figure 28–1** Classification of DORV based on ventricular septal defect relationship to great vessels. **A,** Subaortic ventricular defect. **B,** Subpulmonic ventricular defect. **C,** Doubly committed ventricular defect. Not shown is noncommitted, remote defect. (From Fyler DC, editor: *Nadas' pediatric cardiology,* Philadelphia, 1992, Hanley & Belfus.)

| Relation of great arteries | Location of VSD (%) | | | | Total |
|---|---|---|---|---|---|
| | Subaortic | Subpulmonary | Subaortic & Subpulmonary | Remote | |
| Normal | 3% | 0 | 0 | 0 | 3% |
| Side-by-side | 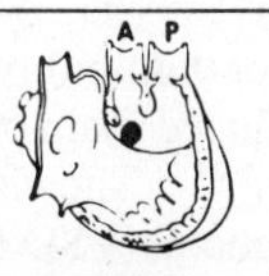 A P<br>46% | 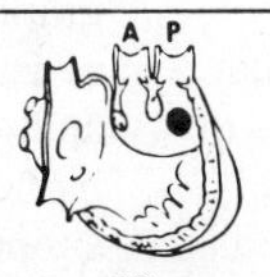 A P<br>8% | 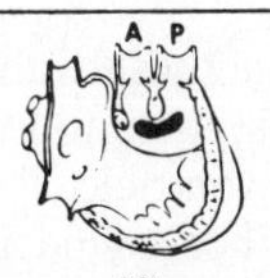 A P<br>3% | 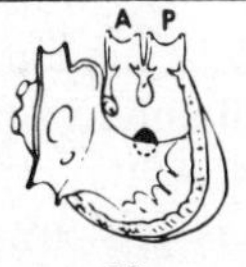 A P<br>7% | 64% |
| d - MGA | 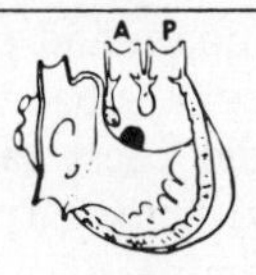 A P<br>16% | 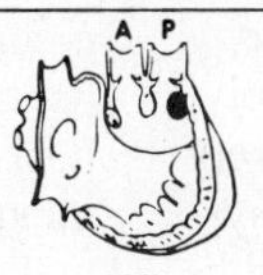 A P<br>10% | 0 | 0 | 26% |
| l - MGA | 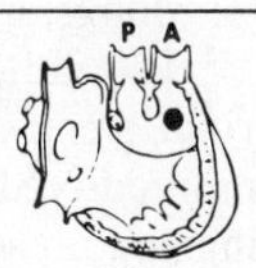 P A<br>3% | 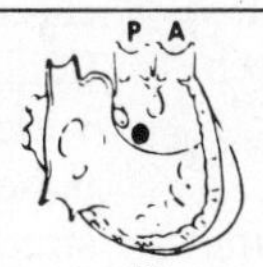 P A<br>4% | 0 | 0 | 7% |
| Total | 68% | 22% | 3% | 7% | |

**Figure 28–2** Relationship of great vessels and location of VSD in 70 patients with DORV. d-MGA and l-MGA, dextromalposition and levomalposition of great arteries, respectively. *A,* Aorta; *P,* pulmonary artery. (From Adams FH, Emmanouilides GC, Riemenschneider TA, editors: *Moss' heart disease in infants, children, and adolescents,* ed 4, Baltimore, 1989, Williams & Wilkins.)

mon, found in more than 50% of patients with double-outlet right ventricle (Fig. 28–2). Patients with such defects will present clinical features simulating isolated VSD. Subpulmonic VSD, present in nearly one quarter of patients, results in streaming of blood from the left ventricle to the pulmonary artery; the patients thus clinically resemble transposition patients. The Taussig-Bing malformation is double-outlet right ventricle with subpulmonic VSD and side by side great vessels.[36] In the remaining patients, the VSD is doubly committed (related to both great vessels) or noncommitted, remote from either semilunar valve. The VSD is usually large and nonrestrictive and is necessary for egress of left ventricular blood, so is essential for the patient's survival. Because of this, the septal defect is termed *physiologically advantageous.*[26-28] While most double-outlet right ventricular hearts have an open VSD, it can occasionally be congenitally absent,[1,2,17,34] causing left ventricular hypoplasia. Even in those in whom the VSD is initially open, the defect can become smaller and even completely close,[6,13,14,17-20,28,29] causing severe left ventricular outlet obstruction. Such spontaneous closure of physiologically advantageous VSD should be clinically recognized and appropriately dealt with.

The great vessel relationship is rarely normal (Fig. 28–2). Among the few patients with normally related great vessels, the VSD is usually subaortic and less commonly doubly committed or noncommitted. Approximately two thirds of patients have side by side great vessels; the majority of these patients have a subaortic VSD. Approximately one fourth of patients have d-malposed great vessels, and a small minority have l-malposed great vessels.

Pulmonary stenosis, predominantly subvalvular, is common and is found in almost three fourths of patients with double-outlet right ventricle. Rarely, pulmonary atresia is present. When found in association with subaortic VSD (50% to 60%), pulmonary stenosis results in Fallot-type physiology with right to left intracardiac shunting. Conversely, among patients with subpulmonic VSD (and rarely with doubly committed or subaortic defect), systemic arterial obstruction is frequent, with subaortic stenosis associated with the development of coarctation of the aorta or interrupted aortic arch.

## CLINICAL FEATURES

The clinical features of patients with double-outlet right ventricle are primarily defined by the relation of the VSD to the great vessels and the presence of pulmonary arterial outflow obstruction. Patients can be mildly symptomatic or have severe symptoms of CHF or cyanosis.[9,32,38] Nearly all children with double-outlet right ventricle present in early infancy.[8]

Patients with subaortic VSD and pulmonary stenosis (Fallot-type physiology) manifest cyanosis including hyperpneic and hypercyanotic spells, clubbing, and polycythemia due to right to left shunt. The parasternal precordial activity is increased, and auscultation reveals a single second heart sound and a systolic ejection murmur at the left sternal border attributable to pulmonary stenosis.[8,24] In the absence of pulmonary stenosis patients with double-outlet right ventricle and subaortic VSD manifest features of a large VSD with CHF, tachypnea, failure to thrive, and increased susceptibility to respiratory infections.[8] Physical examination demonstrates a loud second heart sound, a prominent left lower sternal border systolic murmur attributable to the VSD, and an apical diastolic rumble of increased mitral flow.[24]

Patients with subpulmonic VSD resemble patients with transposition of the great vessels with VSD.[24] Patients manifest symptoms of CHF and cyanosis in infancy with physical examination demonstrating left upper sternal border systolic murmur and apical diastolic rumble. Patients with doubly committed VSD or remote noncommitted VSD may mimic patients with a simple large VSD with manifestations of CHF or because of streaming or outflow obstruction may manifest cyanosis.

### Noninvasive evaluation

***Chest x-ray film.*** The chest radiograph of patients with double-outlet right ventricle varies according to the VSD's location relative to the great vessels and the presence of pulmonary outflow obstruction. In patients with Fallot physiology (subaortic VSD and pulmonary stenosis), the radiograph is similar to that of a patient with tetralogy of Fallot with pulmonary oligemia, upturned apex, and reduced main pulmonary artery segment prominence.[8,24,32] The chest radiograph of a patient with subpulmonic VSD (transposition physiology) demonstrates a globular heart with a narrow superior mediastinum and pulmonary plethora.[8,24,32] In the presence of subaortic VSD without pulmonary stenosis the chest radiograph demonstrates cardiomegaly, increased pulmonary blood flow, and eventual pruning of peripheral pulmonary vessels in cases of longstanding pulmonary overcirculation.[8,24,32] The radiographic appearance of double-outlet right ventricle with doubly committed or noncommitted VSD is dependent on intracardiac streaming and presence of arterial outflow obstruction.

***Electrocardiogram.*** There is no pathognomonic ECG appearance of double-outlet right ventricle. Right axis deviation and right ventricular hypertrophy are universally present, reflecting the connection of the aorta to the right ventricle. However, left axis deviation with counterclockwise loop in the frontal plane may be seen in some patients without and even in those with pulmonic stenosis.[3,23] Combined ventricular hypertrophy may be present in patients with markedly increased pulmonary flow, as is seen in patients without pulmonic stenosis. Severe left ventricular hypertrophy may be seen in the patient with left ventricular outlet obstruction (i.e., spontaneous closure of VSD).

***Echocardiogram.*** The goals of the echocardiographic examination are to localize the VSD and establish its function as the only egress of blood from the left ventricle, to determine the great vessel relationship, to determine the presence of arterial outflow obstruction, and to determine if additional complicating features may limit surgical intervention.[8,31] Because of the pathologic heterogeneity a thorough segmental evaluation is essential. Parasternal long-axis views do not readily demonstrate the origin of either great vessel directly from the left ventricle. However, modified parasternal long-axis view can typically demonstrate both great vessels arising from the right ventricle. In classic cases the lack of continuity between the atrioventricular and semilunar valves can also be shown.[10,31] The parasternal long-axis view also demonstrates the VSD as the only egress of blood from the left ventricle. The parasternal short-axis view frequently demonstrates the double-barrel end on appearance of malposed great vessels in the same plane (Fig. 28–3). In cases of normally related great vessels the short-axis view may be indistinguishable from that of tetralogy of Fallot.[31] Subarterial tissue separating the pulmonary and aortic outflow tracts may be seen in the parasternal views. The subcostal view is most advantageous in establishing the VSD's relationship to the great vessels[31] (Fig. 28–4) and in assessing outflow obstruction with Doppler echocardiography. Echocardiography is vital in determining the presence and severity of atrioventricular valve abnormalities that may dictate surgical options.[7,31,38]

### Invasive studies

Cardiac catheterization and selective cineangiography are indicated to confirm anatomic relations of the VSD to the great vessels, to determine if left ventricular or arterial outflow obstruction is present, and to determine whether complicating features may limit options for palliative or definitive surgical intervention. The catheter course and oxygen saturation data reflect the location of the VSD. Patients with subpulmonic VSD have higher pulmonary artery oxygen saturation than aortic saturation regardless of the presence of pulmonary stenosis or pulmonary vascular obstructive changes.[10,34] In the presence of other types of VSD no consistent relationship between systemic and pulmonary oxygen saturation is present. Ventricular and great vessel pressure measurement is essential to determine if the VSD is restrictive or if arterial outflow obstruction is present.[8,38] The angiographic diagnosis of double-outlet right ventricle is based upon demonstration of both great vessel arising from the right ventricle. Selective ventricular angiography is frequently best achieved with biplane images in anteroposterior and lateral projections.[9,33] Typically the lateral projection of the left ventriculogram profiles the VSD well; occa-

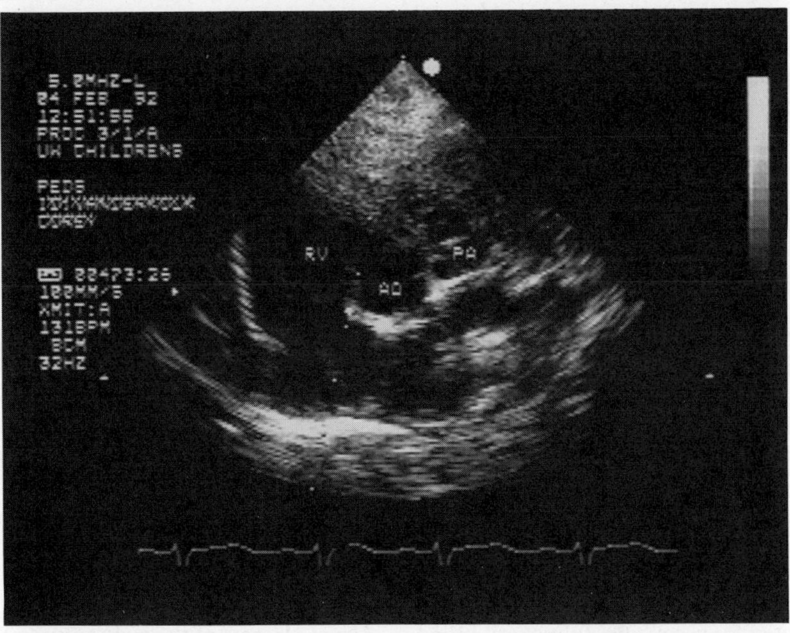


**Figure 28–3** Parasternal short-axis view of double-outlet right ventricle with side by side great vessels demonstrating down the barrel, or end on, appearance of great vessels. *Ao,* Aorta; *PA,* pulmonary artery; *RV,* right ventricle.

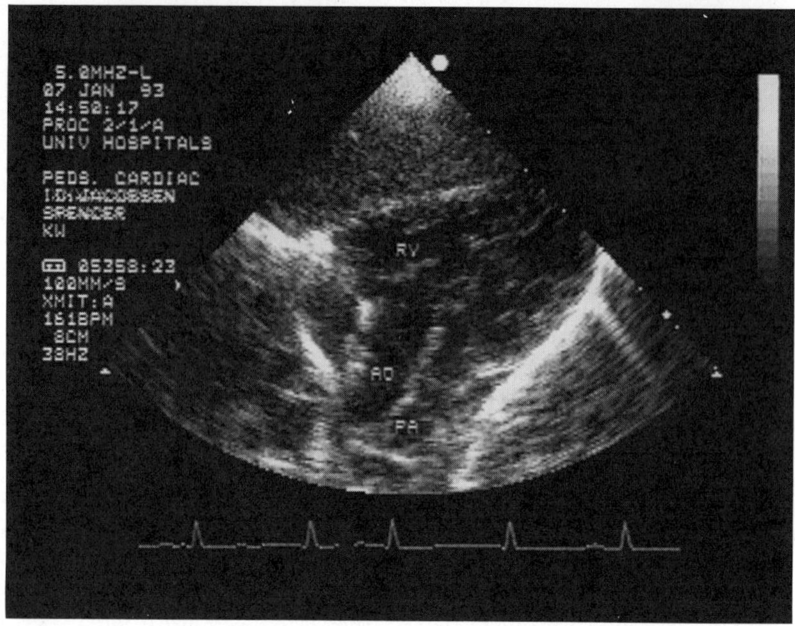


**Figure 28–4** Subcostal view of DORV with side by side great vessels demonstrating both great vessels arising from the right ventricle. *AO,* aorta; *PA,* pulmonary artery; *RV,* right ventricle.

sionally the long-axis oblique or hepatoclavicular projection is advantageous, particularly if the defect is remote from the semilunar valves.[7] The right ventriculogram demonstrates both great vessels' origins from the right ventricle, the relationship of the great vessels, and the great vessel outflow tract anatomy (Fig. 28–5).[11] In classic cases the right ventriculogram depicts both great vessels supported by and separated from each other by infundibular tissue and the semilunar valves at about the same level; however, these findings are not invariable. Although coronary artery anatomy is usually normal,[34] in one autopsy series 25% of specimens had a left anterior descending coronary artery, which arose anteriorly and coursed along the left ventricular free wall inferior to the origin of the pulmonary trunk.[37] Angiographic assessment of origin and course of the coronary arteries is required prior to definitive repair, including outflow tract reconstruction or use of an external conduit.

## MANAGEMENT

### Neonates and infants

The heterogeneity of pathophysiology dictates an individualized management approach to patients with double-outlet right ventricle. Management in infancy is directed to optimizing pulmonary blood flow and maintaining adequate systemic oxygen delivery. Systemic to pulmonary shunting may be required in cases of severe pulmonary stenosis.[8] At the opposite extreme, in cases of pulmonary plethora, as frequently seen with doubly committed VSD or subaortic VSD without pulmonary stenosis, pulmonary artery banding may be required to minimize CHF and reduce risk of pulmonary vascular obstructive disease.[8] Patients with subpulmonic VSD frequently require balloon or surgical atrial septostomy to improve atrial mixing and to relieve left atrial hypertension, if present.[8,24] Following palliation, hemodynamic reassessment is essential, particularly in patients following an unexpected course. Development of significant subaortic stenosis, presumably due to hypertrophy of the infundibulum, has been reported following pulmonary artery banding of double-outlet right ventricle with subpulmonic VSD.[7] In our personal experience subpulmonic stenosis can also develop rapidly following pulmonary artery banding.

### Children and adults

Approaches to surgical correction of double-outlet right ventricle are as varied as the pathophysiologic categories (Figs. 28–6 and 28–7). Patients with subaortic VSD can be treated with a patch-tunnel closure connecting the septal defect to the aorta. Usually repair of the right ventricular outflow tract by patch enlargement is necessary, analogous to that for patients with tetralogy of Fallot. Among 19 patients reported by Piccoli with classic

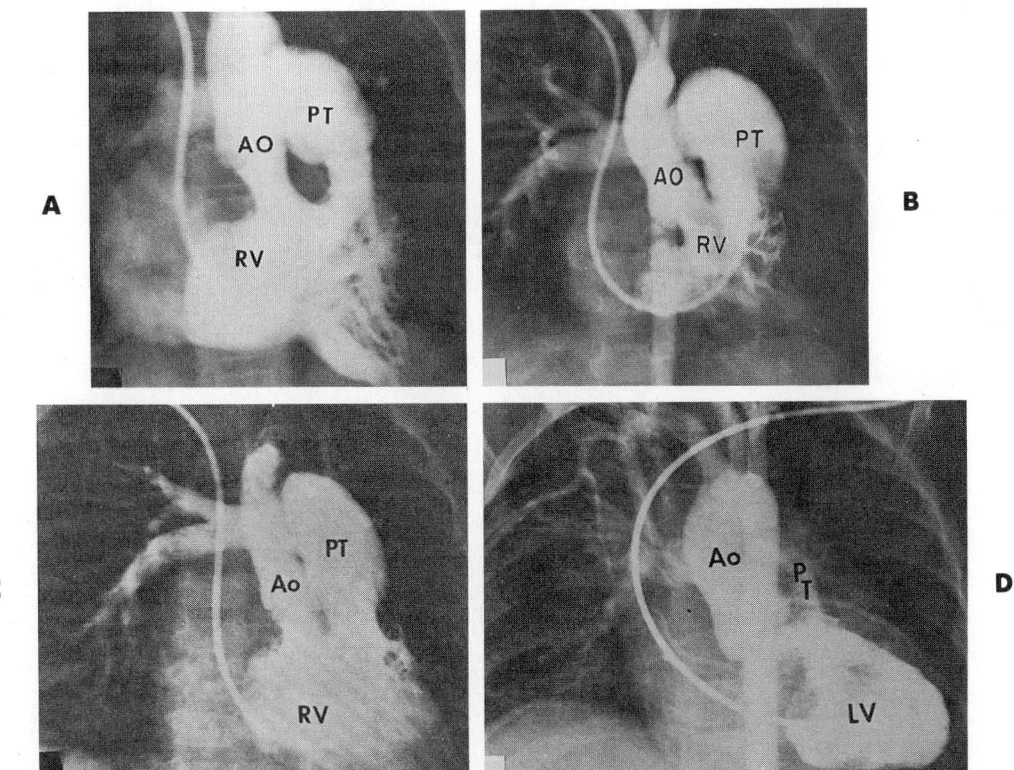


**Figure 28–5** DORV with side by side great vessels. **A,** Frontal view of right ventriculogram with subaortic VSD demonstrating aortic conus (right of aorta), conus septum (between aorta and pulmonary artery), and pulmonary conus (left of pulmonary trunk). **B,** Frontal view of right ventriculogram with subpulmonic VSD (Taussig-Bing anomaly). **C,** Frontal view of right ventriculogram with doubly committed VSD demonstrating aortic and pulmonary conus. **D,** frontal view of left ventriculogram demonstrating deformity of left ventricular outflow tract caused by abnormal insertion of left atrioventricular valve and deficiency of ventricular septum. *Ao,* aorta; *LV,* left ventricle; *PT,* pulmonary trunk; *RV,* right ventricle. (*A* from Hallerman FJ, Kincaid OW, Ritter DG et al: Angiographic and anatomic findings in origin of both great arteries from the right ventricle, *AJR Am J Roentgenol* 109:51, 1970. *B* and *C* from Sridaromont S, Ritter DG, Feldt RH et al: Double-outlet right ventricle: anatomic and angiocardiographic correlations, *Mayo Clin Proc* 53:555, 1978. *D* from Sridaromont S, Feldt RH, Ritter DG et al: Double-outlet right ventricle associated with persistent common atrioventricular canal, *Circulation* 52:933, 1975.).

double-outlet right ventricle (i.e., with subaortic VSD) repaired between 1978 and 1983, perioperative mortality was approximately 5% compared with 24% of patients with operation before 1978.[25]

Repair of double-outlet right ventricle with subpulmonic VSD by an intracardiac tunnel from the left ventricle to the aorta is ideal but has been associated with development of left and right ventricular outflow obstruction. Therefore, patch-tunnel closure of the VSD to the pulmonary artery in conjunction with atrial or arterial switch has been advocated.[8] The reported perioperative mortality of the former was high, approximately 60%.[35] Subsequently the application of the arterial switch procedure in conjunction with VSD closure to the pulmonary trunk (neoaorta) was associated with a reduction of perioperative mortality to approximately 15% to 20%.[12,22] When coronary artery abnormality or fixed subaortic stenosis precludes atrial or arterial switch procedures, the Damus-Kaye-Stansel operation has been advocated. In it, patch-tunnel closure of the VSD to the pulmonary artery is performed in conjunction with end to side anastomosis of the proximal pulmonary artery trunk to the aorta and placement of an external conduit from the right ventricle to the distal pulmonary artery to supply pulmonary flow.[4,5,8,37] In a recent small series of patients treated in this manner perioperative mortality was 16%. Of five survivors followed for an average of 62 months, two subsequently required balloon dilation of the conduit valve and three required reoperation.[5]

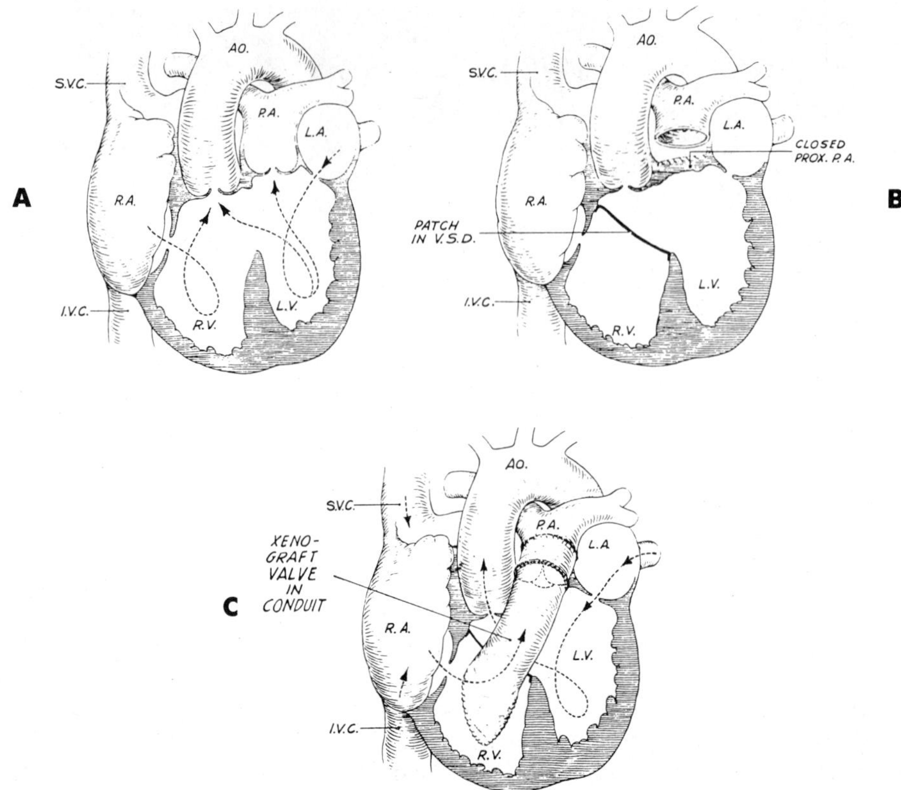


**Figure 28–6** DORV—valved conduit repair. **A,** This VSD is different from other types in that the aortic and pulmonary valves are on the same plane and immediately adjacent to each other. **B,** Patch commits the left ventricle to the aorta and leaves the right ventricle with no outlet. **C,** Right ventricular outlet is reconstructed with a valve-bearing Dacron conduit. (From Park MK, editor: *Pediatric cardiology for practitioners,* St Louis, 1988, Mosby.)

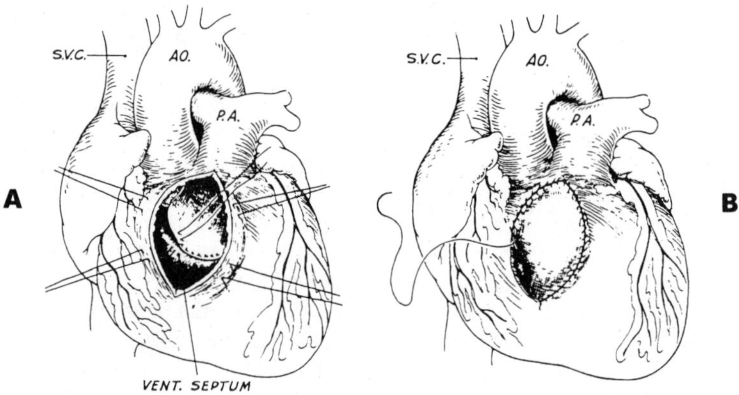


**Figure 28–7** DORV—alternative repair. **A,** Patch is sutured so as to produce a tunnel, allowing the left ventricle to empty through the VSD and into the aorta. The pulmonary artery maintains its continuity with the right ventricle with this method. **B,** Outflow tract patch is used to prevent obstruction. (From Park MK, editor: *Pediatric cardiology for practitioners,* St Louis, 1988, Mosby.)

Surgical management of double-outlet right ventricle with doubly committed or remote VSD involves patch-tunnel closure of the VSD to the aorta with or without an external right ventricle to pulmonary artery conduit.[8] In a recent series from the Brompton Hospital 16% surgical mortality for treatment of double-outlet right ventricle with doubly committed VSD was reported.[22] In the presence of complicating features such as left ventricle hypoplasia in which a biventricular repair is not deemed feasible, a staged modified Fontan procedure offers long-term palliation.

## PROGNOSIS

The heterogeneity of patients with double-outlet right ventricle precludes generalized predictions of long-term prognosis. As stated previously, double-outlet right ventricle constitutes less than 1% of congenital heart disease in children but represents 3% of infants dying with congenital heart disease in the first month of life. The long-term prognosis appears best for patients with subaortic VSD with or without pulmonary stenosis and less favorable for patients with subpulmonic VSD or complex anatomy requiring a univentricular repair.[16,25] In addition, late sudden death, presumably attributable to arrhythmia, has recently been reported in 16 of 89 patients following successful surgical repair of double-outlet right ventricle. The most important risk factors identified were older age at the time of operation, perioperative or postoperative ventricular arrhythmias, and third-degree atrioventricular block.[30]

## ANESTHESIA MANAGEMENT

An understanding of pathologic anatomy and physiology and of the pharmacology of various drugs that may alter the systemic and pulmonary blood flows is essential in managing patients with a functioning communication between the two sides of the heart. The anesthesia management of patients with double-outlet right ventricle may vary according to the type of VSD and the presence of associated defects such as pulmonary stenosis or aortic outflow obstruction. For example, the anesthesia management of patients with subaortic VSD and pulmonary stenosis is very similar to that of patients with tetralogy of Fallot (see Chapter 19); the management of patients with subaortic VSD without pulmonic stenosis is similar to that of a patient with large VSD (see Chapter 16); and the management of patients with subpulmonic VSD is similar to that of the patients with transposition of the great arteries (see Chapter 20).

### Preoperative assessment

Preoperative evaluation of a patient with double-outlet right ventricle should include a thorough history, including past and present medications and physical examination; laboratory tests including chest x-ray, ECG, echocardiogram, catheterization data, hemoglobin, glucose, and electrolyte levels; any history of palliative surgery (for example, shunt operation, PDA or coarctation of the aorta) or noncardiac surgery; and a pediatric cardiologist's consult note. In addition one should evaluate the status of both cardiac and pulmonary reserves.

Depending on the severity of the defect, children with double-outlet right ventricle may have various degrees of CHF and decreased lung compliance. These patients are frequently treated medically with digitalis and diuretic preparations.

### Premedication

Since anxiety and apprehension can worsen CHF, these children will benefit from preoperative medication. Premedication usually consists of an IM narcotic and anticholinergic drug combination (morphine 0.1 to 0.15 mg/kg and atropine 10 μg/kg) in the ward and/or oral midazolam (0.5 to 0.6 mg/kg) in the holding room.

### Monitoring

Monitoring of the children with double-outlet right ventricle during surgery should include an ECG, invasive arterial pressure, noninvasive blood pressure, pulse oximeter, capnogram, body temperature (esophageal and nasopharyngeal), central venous pressure, and urinometer. In patients who have undergone repair of coarctation of the aorta with a subclavian artery patch or a systemic to pulmonary artery shunt (children born with pulmonary stenosis), proper selection of an upper extremity for the placement of a blood pressure cuff, oxygen saturation probe, and arterial cannula should be made. Pulmonary arterial or left atrial pressure monitoring is not necessary in the majority of cases. Arterial blood gases, serum potassium, and hematocrit are monitored at frequent intervals throughout the perioperative period.

### Induction

The majority of patients come to the operating room with no IV catheter. In patients who arrive with a functioning IV line, anesthesia can be induced with IV narcotic and/or 1 to 2 mg/kg of ketamine. In children who are uncooperative and in small children who come to the operating suite without an IV line in place, anesthesia can be induced with either halothane by mask or ketamine by IM injection, depending on the underlying ventricular function. We recommend inspired concentrations of halothane under 2%, as severe myocardial depression and/or complete heart block may result with concentrations in excess of 2%.

The effects of a left to right or right to left shunt

on the speed of inhalational and IV inductions are discussed in Chapter 10, and these differences are of theoretic interest only. Once the IV line is secured, tracheal intubation can be performed with either succinylcholine or a nondepolarizing muscle relaxant. Atropine 5 to 10 μg/kg should be given prior to the administration of succinylcholine (1 to 2 mg/kg IV). An arterial cannula and a central venous catheter are usually inserted after the airway is secured.

### Maintenance

Anesthesia is usually maintained with an IV narcotic (fentanyl 50 to 100 μg/kg or sufentanil 15 to 30 μg/kg). If halothane or one of the inhalational agents is used as a sole anesthetic, one should administer a narcotic drug (fentanyl 15 μg/kg or sufentanil 5 μg/kg) and an amnestic agent such as lorazepam (30 μg/kg) at the time of rewarming during the extracorporeal circulation. For procedures that do not involve extracorporeal circulation (systemic to pulmonary shunt; pulmonary artery banding; atrial septectomy; repair of coarctation of the aorta), one should reduce these recommended narcotic drug doses by 50% to 75%. Vecuronium or one of the newer nondepolarizing muscle relaxants (doxacurium or pipecuronium) can be used to maintain muscle paralysis throughout the operation.

One should closely watch the administration of IV fluids in these patients, and only minimal amounts of fluids should be used in patients with increased pulmonary blood flow and CHF.

If deep hypothermia and circulatory arrest are planned (usually in children under 10 kg body weight), we administer 10 ml/kg of dextran 40 in 5% dextrose solution before peripheral cooling is initiated (see Chapter 4 for complete details of deep hypothermia).

Heparin is usually injected into the right atrium by the surgeon just before the placement of cannulas. Protamine is administered by the anesthesiologist at the conclusion of extracorporeal circulation following the removal of cardiac cannulas. The majority of patients, especially the ones with pulmonary hypertension, require either isoproterenol (0.01 to 0.05 μg/kg/min) or dobutamine (3 to 6 μg/kg/min) infusion after coming off bypass.

Patients with double-outlet right ventricle with increased pulmonary blood flow (isolated VSD type and transposition type) may benefit from the addition of slight PEEP. Hyperventilation and low hematocrit are known to increase left to right shunt and pulmonary blood flow; one should therefore maintain normal ventilation and normal hematocrit to reduce the chances of increased pulmonary blood flow and CHF (see Table 10–5). On the other hand, in patients with double-outlet right ventricle in whom there is decreased pulmonary blood flow (Fallot's type), one should avoid excessive airway pressures and all the factors that facilitate a decrease in pulmonary blood flow.

### Precautions

In all cases of communication between right and left sides of the heart, it is absolutely necessary that all intravenous lines be free of air bubbles. In addition, one should use extra caution not to push any air bubbles when injecting drugs through an IV line. Although the use of nitrous oxide is not contraindicated in patients with a double-outlet right ventricle, many anesthesiologists avoid the use of it, especially once the chest is opened, for fear of intravascular air bubble expansion. Appropriate antibiotic prophylaxis therapy is also required for patients with double-outlet right ventricle (see Chapter 9).

### Postoperative ventilation

Patients with double-outlet right ventricle are usually left intubated and mechanically ventilated postoperatively. Once the patient is awake, stable, and rewarmed to a normal body temperature, the trachea can be extubated in the cardiac recovery room.

## REFERENCES

1. Ainger LE: Double-outlet right ventricle: intact ventricular septum, mitral stenosis and blind left ventricle, *Am Heart J* 70:521, 1965.
2. Davachi F, Moller JH, Edwards JE: Origin of both great vessels from the right ventricle with intact ventricular septum, *Am Heart J* 75:790, 1968.
3. Dayem MKA, Preger L, Goodwin JF et al: Double-outlet right ventricle with pulmonary stenosis. *Br Heart J* 29:64, 1967.
4. DeLeon SY, Ilbawi MN, Tubeszewski K et al: The Damus-Stansel-Kaye procedure: anatomical determinants and modifications, *Ann Thorac Surg* 52:680, 1991.
5. Di Carlo DC, Di Donato RM, Carotti A et al: Evaluation of the Damus-Kaye-Stansel operation in infancy, *Ann Thorac Surg* 52:1148, 1991.
6. Edwards JE, James JW, DuShane JW: Congenital malformation of the heart: origin of transposed great vessels from right ventricle associated with atresia of the left ventricular outlet, double orifice of the mitral valve, and single coronary artery, *Lab Invest* 1:197, 1952.
7. Freedom RM, Culham JAG, Moes CAF: Double-outlet right ventricle. In *Angiography of congenital heart disease*, New York, 1984, Macmillan.
8. Freedom RM, Smallhorn JF: Double-outlet ventricle. In Moller JH, Neal W, editors: *Fetal, neonatal, and infant cardiac disease*, Norwalk, CT, 1990, Appleton and Lange.
9. Fyler DC: Double-outlet right ventricle. In Fyler DC, editor: *Nadas' pediatric cardiology*, Philadelphia, 1992, Hanley & Belfus.
10. Hagler DJ, Ritter DG, Puga FJ: Double-outlet right ventricle. In Adams FH, Emmanouildes GC, Riemenschneider TA, editors: *Moss' heart disease in infants, children, and adolescents*, Baltimore, 1989, Williams & Wilkins.

11. Hallerman FJ, Kincaid OW, Ritter DG et al: Angiocardiographic and anatomic findings in origin of both great arteries from the right ventricle, *AJR Am J Roentgenol* 109:51, 1970.
12. Kanter K, Anderson R, Lincoln C et al: Anatomic correction of double outlet right ventricle with subpulmonary ventricular septal defect (the Taussig-Bing anomaly), *Ann Thorac Surg* 41:287, 1986.
13. Lauer RM, DuShane JW, Edwards JE: Obstruction of the left ventricular outlet in association with ventricular septal defects. *Circulation* 22:110, 1960.
14. Lavoie R, Sestier F, Gilbert G et al: Double outlet right ventricle with left ventricular outflow tract obstruction due to small ventricular septal defect, *Am Heart J* 82:290, 1971.
15. Lev M, Bharati S, Meng CCL et al: A concept of double-outlet right ventricle, *J Thorac Cardiovasc Surg* 64:271, 1972.
16. Luber JM, Castaneda AR, Lang P et al: Repair of double-outlet right ventricle: early and late results, *Circulation* 68 (suppl 2):II144, 1983.
17. MacMahon HE, Lipa M: Double-outlet right ventricle with intact interventricular septum. *Circulation* 30:745, 1964.
18. Marino B, Loperfido F, Savin Sardi C: Spontaneous closure of ventricular septal defect in a case of double outlet right ventricle, *Br Heart J* 49:608, 1983.
19. Mason DT, Morrow AG, Elkins RC et al: Origin of both great vessels from right ventricle associated with severe obstruction to left ventricular outflow, *Am J Cardiol* 24:118, 1969.
20. Megarity AL, Chambers RG, Calder AL et al: Double outlet right ventricle with left ventricular–right atrial communication: fibrous obstruction of the left ventricular outlet by membranous septum and tricuspid valve tissue, *Am Heart J* 84:242, 1972.
21. Mitchell SC, Korones SB, Berendes HW: Congenital heart disease in 56,109 births: incidence and natural history, *Circulation* 43:323, 1971.
22. Musumeci F, Shumway S, Lincoln C et al: Surgical treatment for double-outlet right ventricle at the Brompton hospital, 1973 to 1986, *J Thorac Cardiovasc Surg* 96:278, 1988.
23. Neufeld HN, Lucas RV Jr, Lester RG et al: Origin of both great vessels from the right ventricle without pulmonary stenosis, *Br Heart J* 24:393, 1962.
24. Park M: Cyanotic congenital heart disease. In *Pediatric cardiology for practitioners,* Chicago, 1988, Mosby.
25. Piccoli G, Pacifico AD, Kirklin JW et al: Changing results and concepts in the surgical treatment of double-outlet right ventricle: analysis of 137 operations in 126 patients, *Am J Cardiol* 52:549, 1983.
26. Rao PS: Left ventricular obstruction in double outlet right ventricle (letter), *Am Heart J* 83:289, 1972.
27. Rao PS: Physiologically advantageous ventricular septal defects (letter), *Pediatr Cardiol* 4:59, 1983.
28. Rao PS, Sissman NJ: Spontaneous closure of physiologically advantageous ventricular septal defects, *Circulation* 43:83, 1971.
29. Serratto M, Arevalo F, Goldman EJ et al: Obstructive ventricular septal defect in double outlet right ventricle, *Am J Cardiol* 19:457, 1973.
30. Shen WK, Holmes DR, Porter CJ et al: Sudden death after repair of double-outlet right ventricle, *Circulation* 81:128, 1990.
31. Snider AR, Serwer GA: Abnormalities of ventriculoarterial connection. In *Echocardiography in pediatric heart disease,* Chicago, 1990, Mosby.
32. Sondheimer HM, Freedom RM, Olley PM: Double-outlet right ventricle: clinical spectrum and prognosis, *Am J Cardiol* 39:709, 1977.
33. Sridaromont S, Ritter DG, Feldt RH et al: Double-outlet right ventricle associated with persistent common atrioventricular canal, *Circulation* 52:933, 1975.
34. Sridarmont S, Ritter DG, Feldt RH et al: Double-outlet right ventricle: anatomic and angiographic correlations, *Mayo Clic Proc* 53:555, 1978.
35. Stewart RW, Kirklin JW, Pacifico AD et al: Repair of double-outlet right ventricle: an analysis of 62 cases, *J Thorac Cardiovasc Surg* 78:502, 1979.
36. Taussig HB, Bing RJ: Complete transposition of the aorta and a levoposition of the pulmonary artery, *Am Heart J* 37:551, 1949.
37. Wilcox BR, Ho SY, Macartney FJ et al: Surgical anatomy of double-outlet right ventricle with situs solitus and atrioventricular concordance, *J Thorac Cardiovasc Surg* 82:405, 1981.
38. Wilkinson JL: Double outlet ventricle. In Anderson RH, Macartney FJ, Shinebourne EA et al, editors: *Pediatric cardiology,* New York, 1987, Churchill Livingstone.
39. Witham AC: Double outlet right ventricle, *Am Heart J* 53:929, 1957.

# 29 Ebstein's Malformation of the Tricuspid Valve

*P. Syamasundar Rao and Jay Kambam*

- Pathologic anatomy
- Pathophysiology
- Clinical features
  - Noninvasive evaluation
    - Chest roentgenogram
    - Electrocardiogram
    - Echocardiography
  - Invasive studies
    - Catheter course
    - Oxygen saturation
    - Pressures
    - Electrode catheter studies
    - Angiography
- Management
  - Neonates and young infants
  - Children and adults
- Prognosis
- Anesthesia management
  - Premedication
  - Monitoring
  - Induction
  - Maintenance
  - Precautions
  - Postoperative ventilation

Ebstein's anomaly is a congenital cardiac malformation in which the septal and posterior leaflets of the tricuspid valve are displaced downward into and are adherent to the inflow portion of the right ventricle. In addition there is a redundancy or dysplasia of the tricuspid valve apparatus. In 1866 Wilhelm Ebstein[9] described the autopsy findings of the tricuspid valve and right ventricle in a 19-year-old laborer who had a history of cyanosis and dyspnea since early childhood. This tricuspid valve abnormality is now known by its eponym, Ebstein's anomaly. Although several reports of autopsy cases of this anomaly appeared in the literature in the later part of the nineteenth century and the early part of the twentieth century, it was not until 1949 that the first report of diagnosis during life appeared in the literature.[60] Ebstein's anomaly is rare, comprising 0.3% to 0.6% of congenital heart defects in pediatric patients.[31,52] Both sexes are equally affected.[31,52] Although familial cases have been reported, the majority are sporadic in nature. Exposure to lithium in utero has been implicated in the causation of this anomaly.[43,44,65]

In this chapter we will discuss pathologic anatomy, pathophysiology, clinical features, noninvasive and invasive evaluation, management, prognosis, and anesthetic management of Ebstein's anomaly of the tricuspid valve.

## PATHOLOGIC ANATOMY

The two characteristic features of Ebstein's anomaly are downward displacement of the tricuspid valve leaflets with adherence to the right ventricular muscle and redundancy or dysplasia of the tricuspid valve leaflets (Fig. 29–1). There is a marked variability in the pathology. The septal and posterior leaflets are displaced downward, away from the true tricuspid valve annulus, and adhere to the right ventricular wall. The extent of the displacement varies from patient to patient. In slight displacement the true annuli and the apparent, or false, tricuspid valve annuli are close together. In extensive displacement the false annulus is displaced down to the level of the parietal band and crista supraventricularis. The inflow portion of the right ventricle between the true and false annuli of the tricuspid valve forms a common chamber with the right atrium and is described as an atrialized portion of the right ventricle. The nonatrialized portion of the right ventricle is usually normal. The degree of adherence of the displaced tricuspid leaflets is also variable; it ranges from superficial attachment to the trabeculae carneae with minimal loss of right ventricular muscle to extensive adherence such that the right ventricular wall becomes a paper-thin fibrous sac simulating Uhl's anomaly.[61] The anterior leaflet of the tricuspid valve is usually spared in

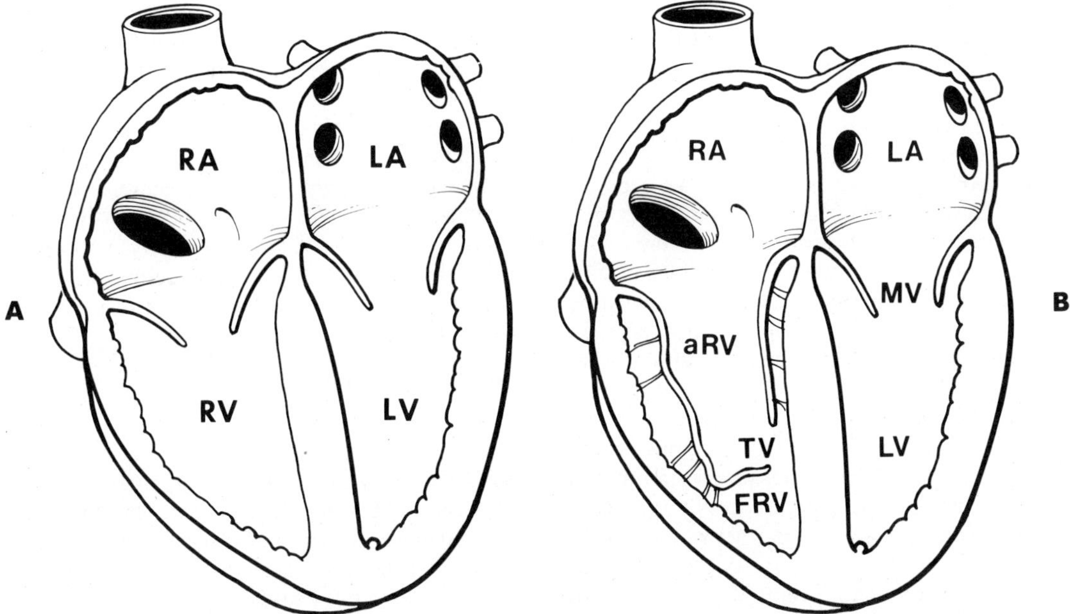


**Figure 29–1** Anatomy of the heart. **A,** Normal. **B,** With Ebstein's anomaly.

this pathologic process. The redundancy and dysplasia are seen in the free portions of the valve leaflets, and again the anterior leaflet is less affected. The free portions of the tricuspid valve leaflets are abnormally formed, with nodular appearance. The effective or false orifice of the tricuspid valve may be unobstructed and is usually incompetent. It may be stenotic,[58] is rarely atretic,[49] and may have more than one opening. Sometimes the redundant tricuspid valve causes right ventricular outflow obstruction mimicking pulmonary valve stenosis or atresia.[12,42]

Right atrial enlargement is usual and massive. Interatrial communication, usually a patent foramen ovale or a secundum ASD, is present in most cases. Other associated defects, especially in the neonatal period, include pulmonary stenosis, pulmonary atresia, and VSD. Occasionally PDA, tetralogy of Fallot, right aortic arch, coarctation of the aorta, transposition of the the great arteries, and mitral prolapse may be associated with Ebstein's malformation.

This type of malformation, "Ebsteinization", occurs only with the morphologic tricuspid valve. Therefore, in corrected transposition of the great arteries (ventricular inversion), the Ebstein type of malformation occurs only with this left atrioventricular valve, which is the atrioventricular valve of the left-sided, morphologic right ventricle. The occurrence of an anomaly of Ebstein's type in the left-sided, morphologic right atrioventricular valve is well described with corrected transposition.[3,34,45,51,53,62]

## PATHOPHYSIOLOGY

The pathophysiology of Ebstein's malformation is as variable as the pathologic anatomy. In patients with only a minor degree of abnormality the tricuspid valve function may be normal, and the malformation may not be detected until adulthood. In moderate to severe cases elements of stenosis or even atresia and insufficiency of the tricuspid valve raise the right atrial pressure above that in the left atrium, causing right to left atrial shunt across the patent foramen ovale or ASD, causing systemic arterial desaturation. With each right atrial contraction the blood is propelled into the atrialized right ventricle. With ventricular contraction a major portion of the blood in the right ventricle is forced back into the right atrium, only to be propelled back into the atrialized ventricle. This Ping-Pong effect further increases right atrial pressure and consequent right to left shunting. As a result of the right to left shunting, the pulmonary blood flow is decreased.

In the neonate with high pulmonary artery pressure and resistance the magnitude of tricuspid insufficiency and the right atrial pressure are high, causing a greater right to left shunting and systemic arterial desaturation. Thus neonates with Ebstein's anomaly have severe cyanosis, which is relieved as the pulmonary vascular resistance and pressure fall. However, the abnormality recurs during late childhood and early adolescence because of decreased efficiency of the tricuspid valve apparatus.

## CLINICAL FEATURES

Approximately half of the patients with Ebstein's malformation have cyanosis during the neonatal period.[31,54] Cyanosis is the initial complaint in most, if not all, infants who become symptomatic during the neonatal period.[39,52] Cardiac murmurs and signs of congestive heart failure are seen less often as presenting complaints. Cyanosis, dyspnea on exertion, and fatigue are usual in children. Dysrhythmias may also be presenting findings in some children. Paroxysmal supraventricular tachycardia, atrial flutter, and fibrillation are the most common rhythm disturbances. They may occur in nearly half the children.

Physical examination in an average case shows no distress or cyanosis and shows normal pulses and blood pressure and a quiet precordial impulse without thrills. Despite increased right atrial pressure, distended neck veins and hepatomegaly are not prominent features because of the compliant right atrium and systemic veins. If there is severe tricuspid insufficiency, hyperdynamic precordium and a thrill at the lower sternal border may be felt, and neck vein distention and hepatomegaly may be observed.

The first heart sound may be normal, diminished, or loud, but it is found to be delayed when referenced to the onset of QRS complex in the ECG. In neonates the second heart sound is usually single but may be split. Loud third and fourth heart sounds are usual, giving the so-called triple or quadruple rhythm, which is a characteristic feature of this anomaly. Faint or no cardiac murmurs are the usual findings, but in the presence of severe tricuspid insufficiency a loud holosystolic murmur may be heard at the left lower sternal border. A scratchy, superficial-sounding middiastolic murmur may be heard; this is presumed to be related to absolute or relative tricuspid stenosis. These murmurs tend to change in intensity with respiration, although this is difficult to demonstrate in the newborn because of typically rapid respirations in that group.

### Noninvasive evaluation

***Chest roentgenogram.*** Chest x-ray film usually shows severe cardiomegaly (Fig. 29–2, *A*), and a substantial portion of this enlargement is due to massive right atrial enlargement. The lung fields are oligemic. Some infants have normal to minimally enlarged heart size (Fig. 29–2, *B*); presumably these are mild cases.

***Electrocardiogram.*** Classic ECG features of Ebstein's anomaly are right atrial enlargement, low QRS precordial voltages, and right bundle branch block pattern (Fig. 29–3). Right bundle branch block is not as common in the neonate as in older children.

The rhythm is usually sinus, although occasionally supraventricular tachycardia or atrial flutter may be present. Right atrial enlargement with tall peaked P waves in lead II and right chest leads is

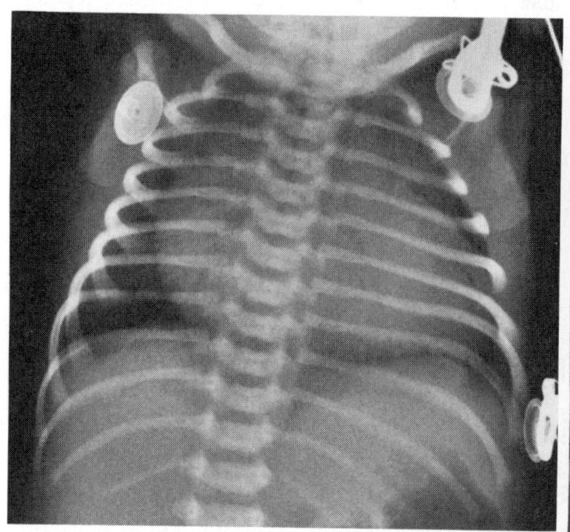


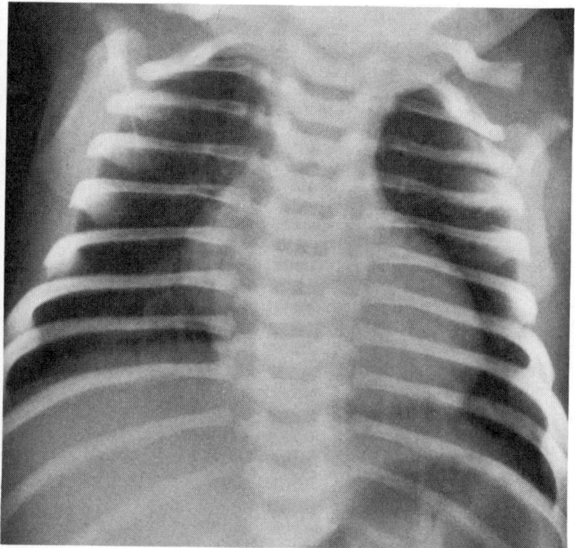


**Figure 29–2 A,** Chest roentgenogram of a day-old infant with severe cyanosis diagnosed as having Ebstein's anomaly by cardiac catheterization, and later at autopsy. Note markedly enlarged heart, dilated right atrium, and decreased pulmonary vascular markings. **B.** Chest radiograph of a 2-day-old infant with catheterization-proved Ebstein's anomaly. Note mildly enlarged heart with decreased pulmonary vascular markings. This infant improved on supportive measures.

present in most of the patients. Prolonged PR interval is present in more than two thirds of neonates.[52] Wolff-Parkinson-White syndrome (short PR interval with δ-wave) pattern may be present in some newborns. There is usually a right axis deviation of the QRS complex, but sometimes left axis deviation is seen.[4,32,52,54] Right bundle branch block is usually present. When it is present, the QRS voltages in right precordial leads are low. When it is associated with other lesions such as pulmonary stenosis or atresia and VSD, right ventricular hypertrophy pattern may be present, especially in the absence of right bundle branch block.

***Echocardiography.*** Features from both M-mode and two-dimensional echocardiography are

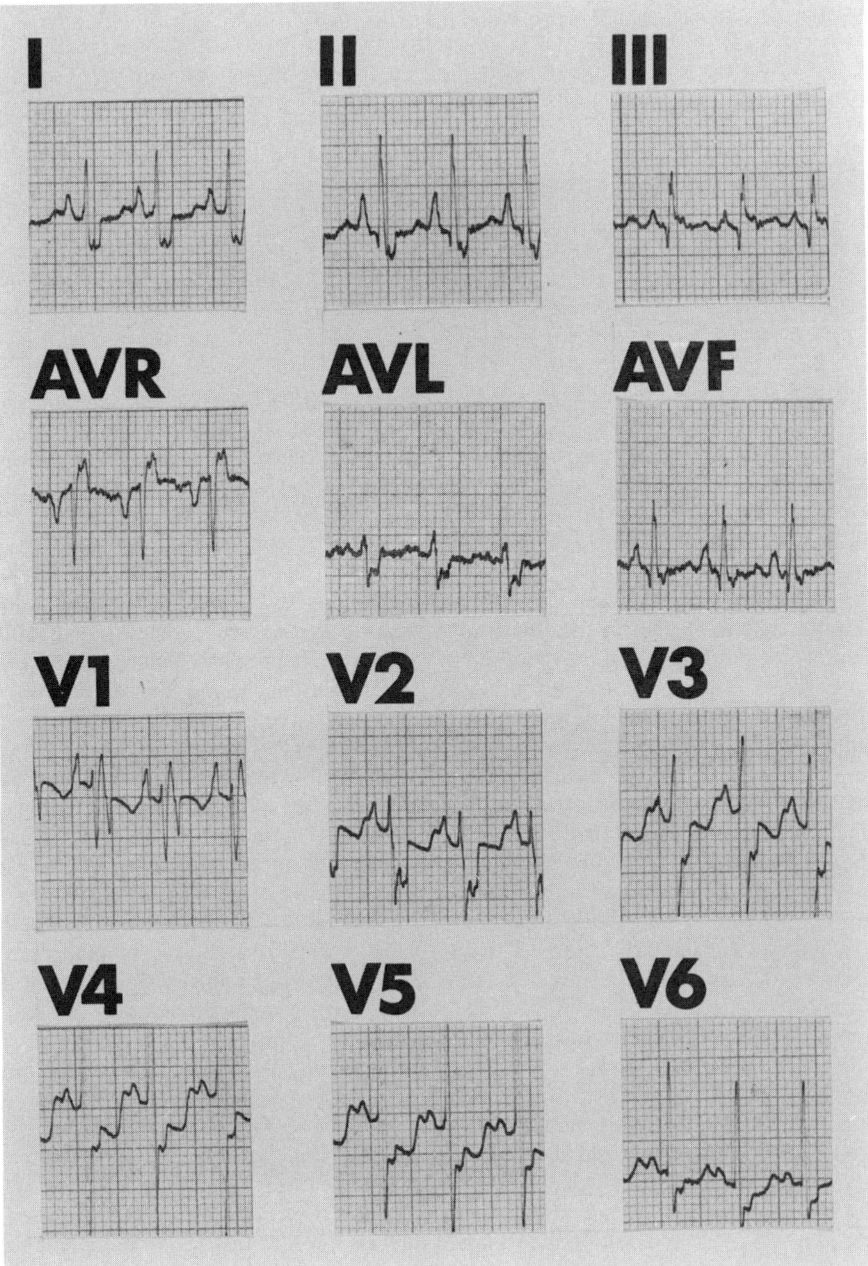


**Figure 29–3** Twelve-lead ECG of a 7-day-old infant with Ebstein's anomaly. Note right atrial enlargement, right bundle branch block pattern, and low QRS voltages in the right chest leads. (From Rao PS: Other tricuspid valve anomalies. In Long WA, editor: *Fetal and neonatal cardiology*, Philadelphia, 1990, Saunders.)

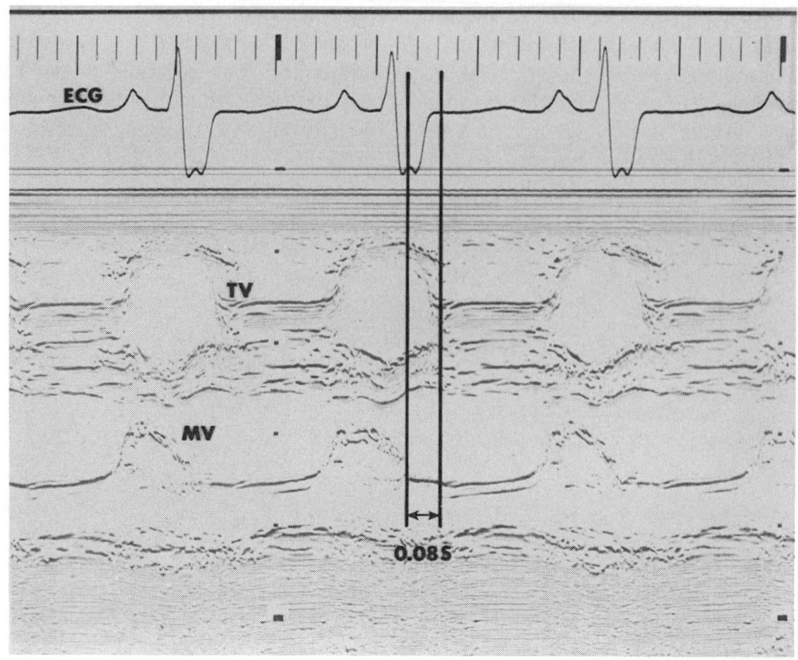


**Figure 29–4** M-mode echocardiogram of an infant with Ebstein's anomaly showing delayed closure of the tricuspid valve *(TV)*. The closure occurred 0.08 second after mitral valve *(MV)* closure. (From Rao PS: Other tricuspid valve anomalies. In Long WA, editor: *Fetal and neonatal cardiology*, Philadelphia, 1990, Saunders.)

helpful in the diagnosis of Ebstein's anomaly. On M-mode study the anterior leaflet of the tricuspid valve can be recorded further to the left of the sternum than normal,[11] tricuspid valve closure is delayed (0.06 second or later than mitral valve closure) (Fig. 29–4),[37] and the interventricular septal motion is abnormal.[68] The late closure of the tricuspid valve was initially thought to be due to the right bundle branch block, but in view of its presence in patients without the right bundle branch block and even in patients with preexcitation syndrome,[57] this is thought to be related to some other factor, possibly a mechanical factor.[37] These M-mode features, though helpful, may not be diagnostic because they can be seen in patients with other types of right ventricular volume overload.[16]

Two-dimensional echocardiographic findings, which are more reliable than M-mode features, include enlarged right atrium, thick and dysplastic tricuspid valve leaflets, and displacement of the attachment of the tricuspid valve leaflets into the right ventricle (Fig. 29–5).[47] In addition the status of the pulmonic valve and the presence and extent of right to left shunting across the patent foramen ovale by contrast study can also be evaluated by two-dimensional echocardiography.

Doppler evaluation may be of value in determining the degree of tricuspid insufficiency and right to left interatrial shunting and in the assessment of tricuspid and pulmonic flows.

### Invasive studies

Because of the incidence of dysrhythmias and deaths associated with cardiac catheterization in Ebstein's anomaly patients,[6,39,64] it has been recommended in the past that catheterization not be performed in these patients. However, because of the availability of more flexible catheters and balloon catheters, greater experience in catheterization, and better monitoring and treatment modalities, cardiac catheterization in Ebstein's anomaly does not at this time carry any higher risk than in other anomalies. However, with the availability of noninvasive techniques, particularly two-dimensional echocardiography, the diagnosis of this entity can be made with ease, and catheterization may not be necessary for diagnosis.

***Catheter course.*** Entrance into the right ventricle may be difficult, and the catheter may coil up in a large right atrium. These features, though suggestive, are not diagnostic of Ebstein's anomaly. It is easy to advance the catheter into the left atrium (from the femoral approach) across the pa-

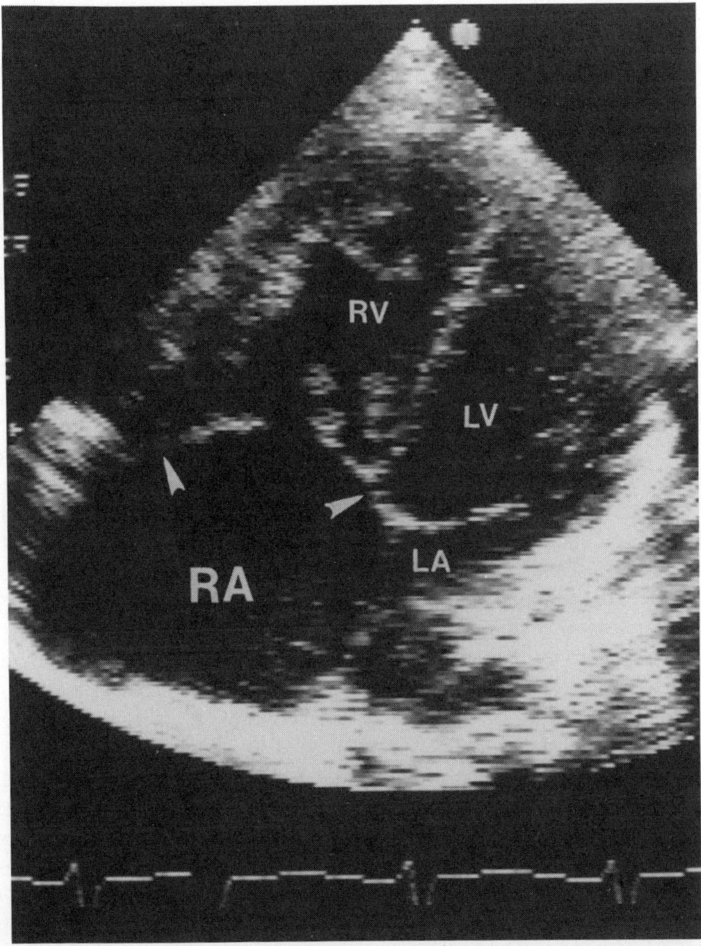


**Figure 29–5** Four-chamber, two-dimensional echocardiographic views of an infant with Ebstein's anomaly. Note downward displacement of the septal and posterior leaflets of the tricuspid valve *(arrows)*. The right atrium *(RA)* is enlarged. *LA*, left atrium; *LV*, left ventricle; *RV*, right ventricle.

tent foramen ovale, and from there into the left ventricle.

***Oxygen saturation.*** Systemic venous oxygen saturations are usually decreased, and the extent of decrease is related to the systemic arterial desaturation. There is usually no evidence for left to right shunt in the right side of the heart unless there is associated VSD or PDA. There is usually evidence for right to left shunting at the atrial level with resultant systemic arterial desaturation. The degree of right to left shunting and arterial unsaturation is inversely proportional to the pulmonary flow, which is in turn related to the degree of dysplasia and obstruction caused by the malformed tricuspid valve.

***Pressures.*** The mean right atrial pressure may be normal or slightly increased. The right atrial a waves are prominent but may be extremely tall if there is associated tricuspid obstruction (stenosis) and restrictive patent foramen ovale. The v waves may be prominent in the presence of tricuspid insufficiency, but more often than not they are not that well seen because of dissipation of the pressure wave in the large, compliant right atrium. The right ventricular systolic pressures are usually normal, although they may be elevated because of pulmonic stenosis, large VSD, or elevated pulmonary artery pressure, especially in the neonate. The right ventricular end diastolic pressure may be elevated. The pulmonary artery pressures are usually normal but may be increased if there is an associated large VSD or high pulmonary resistance of the newborn. The left atrial pressures are normal to low. The left ventricular and aortic pressures are normal.

***Electrode catheter studies.*** The use of intracavitary ECG studies to confirm the diagnosis of Ebstein's anomaly was first suggested by Sodi-Pallares and Marsico.[55] The simultaneous recording of the intracavitary ECG and pressure at cardiac catheterization to confirm the diagnosis of Ebstein's anomaly was first reported by Hernandez and associates.[22] In three patients with this malformation these investigators showed that recording of typical right ventricular intracavitary ECG pattern with simultaneously obtained atrial-type pressure curves was diagnostic of this condition. This was confirmed by subsequent reports by other investigators.[13,18,67] As a platinum-tipped end-hole catheter (with which the intracavitary ECG and pressure could be simultaneously recorded) is withdrawn from the right ventricle, ventricular ECG and ventricular pressure, ventricular ECG and atrial pressure (atrialized ventricle), and atrial ECG and atrial pressure (Fig. 29–6) are successively recorded. Such recordings are characteristic of Ebstein's anomaly. However, a false-negative recording may be obtained if the catheter slides along the normally attached anterior leaflet of the tricuspid valve, especially when the femoral approach is used during the catheterization.

***Angiography.*** Selective right ventricular angiography is optimal for diagnosing this anomaly. It will show displaced tricuspid valve leaflets (Fig. 29–7), size and function of the right ventricle, and the pulmonary valvular and arterial anatomy. Tricuspid insufficiency may also be observed. Opacification of the entire right side of the heart, either during right ventricular angiography or after right atrial angiography, reveals a trilobed heart, right atrium, atrialized right ventricle, and the distal right ventricle. The notch separating the first two structures is formed by a true tricuspid annulus, and the notch separating the last two is formed by the origin of the displaced tricuspid valve leaflets.

## MANAGEMENT

### Neonates and young infants

Cyanotic neonates with Ebstein's anomaly who are otherwise asymptomatic do not need any treatment unless they are markedly hypoxemic. They will improve as the pulmonary vascular resistance and pressure fall. If severe hypoxemia is present, especially in association with right ventricular outflow obstruction, infusion of prostaglandin $E_1$, 0.05 to 0.1 μg/kg/min, may open the ductus arteriosus, increase the pulmonary flow, and improve systemic arterial saturation. As the neonatal pulmonary vascular resistance regresses, the need for prostaglandin may be obviated. Some of these infants may become candidates for systemic artery to pulmonary artery anastomosis if they do not tolerate discontinuation of prostaglandins.

Neonates with signs of CHF secondary to tricuspid insufficiency will benefit by anticongestive measures (digitalis and diuretics).

Although replacement of the tricuspid valve with a prosthetic valve with the exclusion of the abnormally contracting atrialized ventricle[35,48] may be beneficial in older children and adults, such procedures in the neonatal period have not been successful and are not recommended.[40]

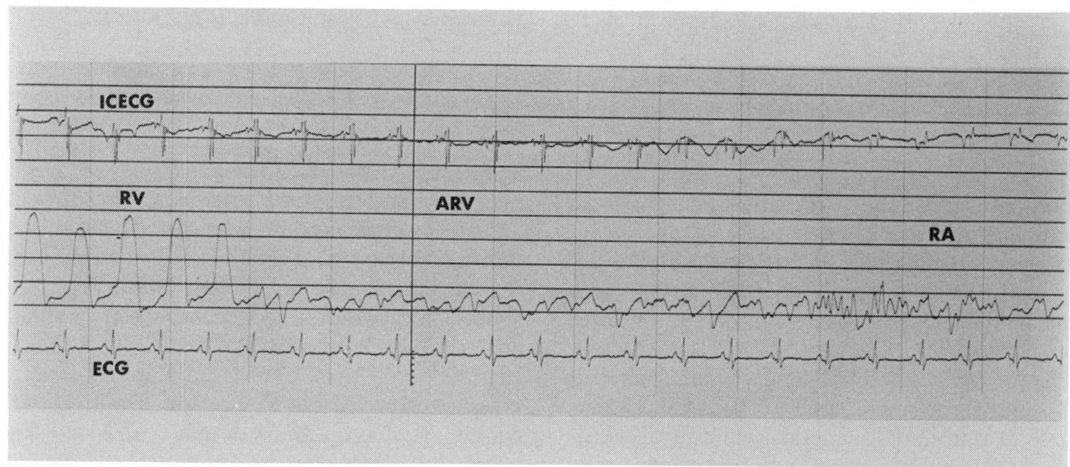


**Figure 29–6** Simultaneous intracavity ECG *(ICECG)* and pressures as the catheter is withdrawn from the right ventricular *(RV)* body to the right atrium *(RA)*. Surface ECG is shown at the bottom. Note the ventricular pressure and ventricular ECG in the body of the right ventricle, ventricular ECG and atrial pressure in the atrialized right ventricle *(ARV)* and atrial ECG and atrial pressure in the right atrium. This is characteristic for Ebstein's anomaly. (From Rao PS: Other tricuspid valve anomalies. In Long WA, editor: *Fetal and neonatal cardiology,* Philadelphia, 1990, Saunders.)

### Children and adults

Total surgical correction of Ebstein's anomaly is feasible (Fig. 29–8).[1,2,8,35,36,46] The procedure of choice appears to be prosthetic valve replacement after excision of the tricuspid valve leaflets.[1,2,8,35,36,46] Lilehei and associates[35,36] recommend leaving the interatrial communication open to allow a right to left shunt in case the right ventricle fails to maintain adequate output. They suggest that the ASD be closed at a subsequent operation.[35,36] Alternatively, closure by transcatheter occlusion[7,50] or creation of fenestrated atrial defect,[5] which could be closed in the postoperative period, may be considered.

Repositioning of the deformed leaflets of the tricuspid valve to their normal plane and thus excluding the abnormally contracting atrialized ventricle from circulation may be the logical physiologic approach.[19,20,28] With similar reasoning surgical reconstruction of the tricuspid valve to produce a competent monocuspid valve along with plication of the atrialized portion of the right ventricle has been performed with success.[38]

Aneurysmorrhaphy of the right ventricle to exclude atrialized right ventricle and replacement of the tricuspid valve with a prosthetic valve (heterograft) in selected children may also be beneficial.[30,38,48,49]

## PROGNOSIS

Ebstein's anomaly diagnosed during infancy appears to have higher mortality than when diagnosed during childhood or adulthood.[14] Approximately 50% of patients diagnosed during the neonatal period do not survive through the first birthday.[52] Signs of CHF, tricuspid insufficiency, very tall P waves on the ECG, complete right bundle branch block, and arrhythmia in the newborn period are considered to be poor prognostic signs.[52]

Patients surviving infancy do well for many years. There is a small but uniform distribution of mortality throughout childhood and adolescence. The mean age at death is about 20 years; however, some patients survive into the sixth decade of life.[63] Some of these deaths are related to surgical intervention and others are sudden. The latter is more common in adolescence and adulthood. Thus the prognosis is guarded for patients with Ebstein's anomaly of the tricuspid valve despite surgical and other advances in the management of these patients.

## ANESTHESIA MANAGEMENT

In determining the appropriate anesthesia strategy it is important to understand the pathologic anatomy and physiology of the heart lesion. Other associated cardiac and extracardiac deformities also influence anesthesia management. Establishing systemic and pulmonary pressures is also helpful for choosing the appropriate drugs.

When anesthetizing children with Ebstein's anomaly, one should remember that most of these patients are prone to cardiac dysrhythmias, especially atrial type. These patients' tricuspid valve is

A

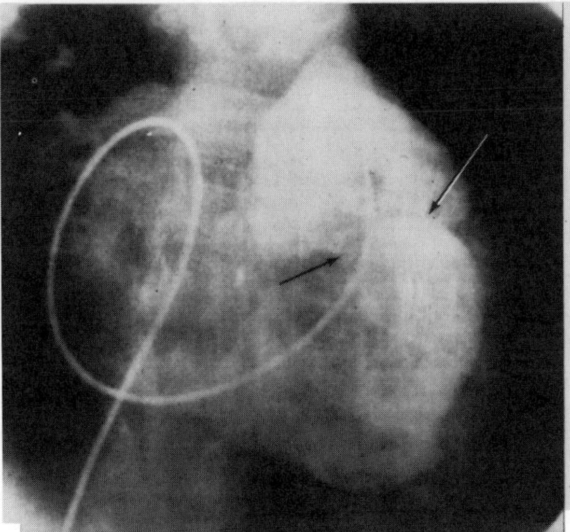

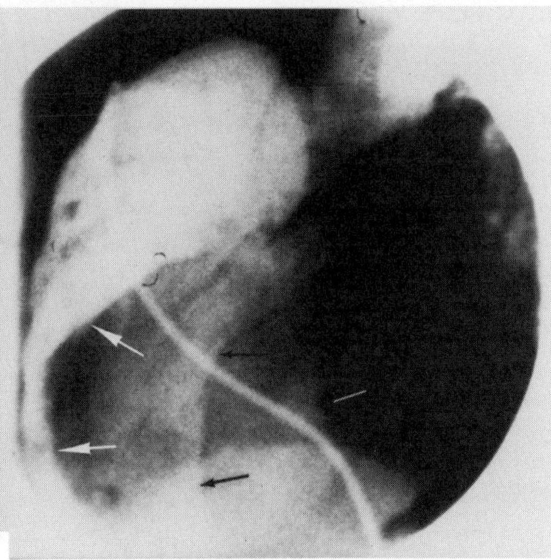

B

**Figure 29–7** Right ventricular cineangiogram in a patient with Ebstein's anomaly of the tricuspid. **A,** Posteroanterior view with displaced tricuspid valve leaflets. **B,** Lateral view. The small black arrows and black arrowhead point to the true tricuspid valve annulus, and the large white arrows show the false annulus with displaced tricuspid valve leaflets. (From Rao PS: Other tricuspid valve anomalies. In Long WA, editor: *Fetal and neonatal cardiology,* Philadelphia, 1990, Saunders.)

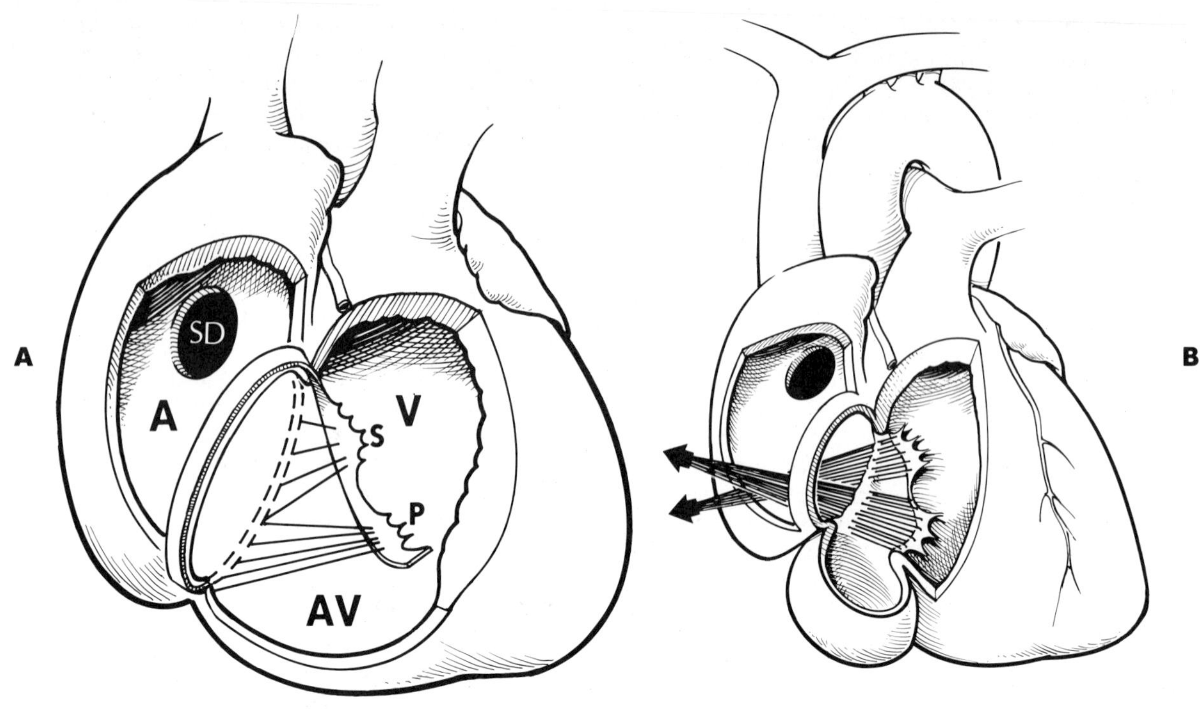


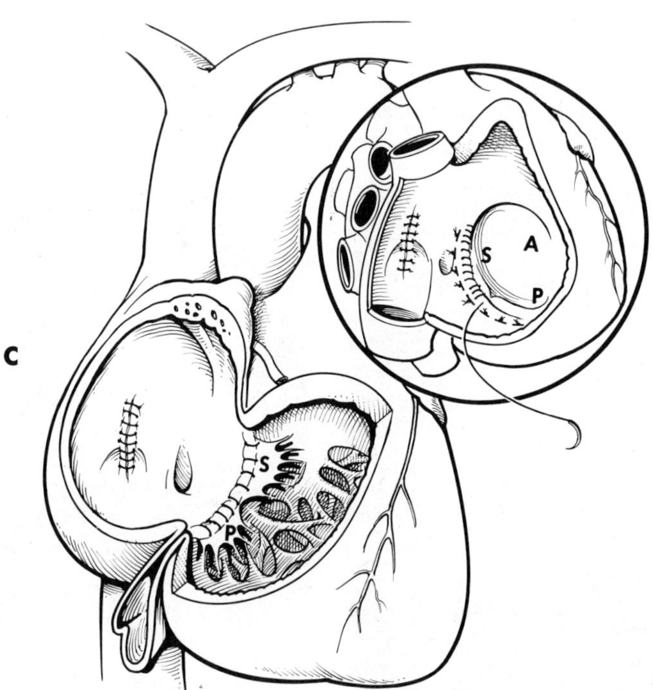


**Figure 29–8** Repair of Ebstein's anomaly. Operative technique consists of **A,** restoring the spiral line of valve attachment to an oval annulus to produce an orifice. **B** and **C,** Abnormal leaflets transposed to normal functional position, annulus reduced in size and atrialized ventricle excluded. (*Inset,* superior view of competent eccentric valve closure is shown). (From KL Hardy et al: Ebstein's anomaly, further experience with definitive repair, *J Thorac Cardiovasc Surg* 58:556, 1969.)

deformed, and as a result any increase in pulmonary vascular resistance will cause worsening of right to left shunt via right ventricle and right atrium to left atrium. In addition right ventricular failure is very common in these patients after they come off cardiopulmonary bypass and in the immediate postoperative period.

### Premedication

Preoperative sedation in these patients depends upon the age of the child and severity of the defect. One should not oversedate these patients, as hypoventilation will have detrimental effects on oxygen saturation and pulmonary blood flow. Preoperative sedation should ideally be achieved in the holding room, where someone can watch for any undesirable side effects. A narcotic and an anticholinergic drug combination (meperidine 2 mg/kg or morphine 0.1 mg/kg and atropine 10 μg/kg) can be given intramuscularly (IM) 90 to 120 minutes before the scheduled time of operation. In addition oral midazolam (0.5 to 0.7 mg/kg) may also be given 30 minutes before the scheduled time of operation, depending on the evaluation of the child in the holding room.

### Monitoring

Monitoring during surgery should include an ECG, invasive arterial pressure, noninvasive blood pressure, pulse oximeter, capnogram, body temperature (esophageal and nasopharyngeal), central venous pressure, and urinometer. Arterial blood gases, serum potassium, and hematocrit are monitored frequently throughout the surgery.

### Induction of anesthesia

Recent data from several investigators suggest in general that a number of induction techniques such as IM and IV ketamine, IV narcotics, and halothane with or without nitrous oxide can be used safely in the management of a child with cyanotic CHD.* Unlike in adult patients, both nitrous oxide and ketamine have been shown to have no worsening effects on the pulmonary vasculature of young children with CHD.[23,24] However, one should choose an optimal technique for a particular cardiac defect based on the preoperative evaluation. In general for sicker children with poor ventricular function induction with IV ketamine and/or IV narcotics has been shown to be safe and effective. In these children all inhalational agents, including nitrous oxide, have been shown to depress myocardium and reduce systemic blood pressure to a greater degree than ketamine or narcotics.[25,66]

*References 15, 17, 21, 23-27, 33, 41, 66.

A right to left shunt should theoretically prolong the uptake and induction time of insoluble anesthetics (nitrous oxide, desflurane, and sevoflurane) and shorten the onset of intravenous anesthetics. The least effect should be seen with the most soluble anesthetics (diethyl ether and cyclopropane) and intermediate results with the intermediate soluble anesthetics (isoflurane, halothane, and enflurane).[10,56] Clinical data to support this theory have not yet been presented, but the computerized models somewhat support it.[29,59] Theoretically a right to left shunt should slightly accelerate the onset of IV anesthetics. Again there are really no clinical data to support or contradict this theory.

Right to left intracardiac shunts are associated with an increase in dead space ventilation and a decrease in end tidal carbon dioxide pressure for a given arterial carbon dioxide pressure. As long as adequate ventilation is maintained, an increase in dead space ventilation has no effect on the uptake and induction time of the inhaled anesthetics.[10] However, if dead space ventilation is increased and alveolar ventilation is inadequate as a result of an increased right to left shunt (decreased pulmonary blood flow), the induction time of most soluble anesthetics will be delayed, and intermediate and least soluble anesthetics will be least effective.

The majority of patients come to the operating room with no IV catheter. It is not difficult, however, to start an IV line in a well sedated child before the induction of anesthesia. In these patients anesthesia can be induced with intravenous fentanyl or sufentanil and/or 1 to 2 mg/kg of ketamine. In children who are uncooperative and in small children who come to the operating suite without an IV line in place, anesthesia can be induced with either halothane by mask or ketamine by IM injection, depending on the underlying ventricular function. Once the IV line is secured, tracheal intubation can be performed with either succinylcholine or a nondepolarizing muscle relaxant. Atropine 5 to 10 μg/kg should be given prior to the administration of succinylcholine (1 to 2 mg/kg IV). An arterial cannula and a central venous catheter are usually inserted after the airway is secured.

### Maintenance

Children with Ebstein's anomaly and limited right ventricular function may not tolerate inhalational agents as a sole anesthetic and usually tolerate an IV narcotic (fentanyl 50 to 100 μg/kg or sufentanil 10 to 20 μg/kg). Vecuronium or one of the newer nondepolarizing muscle relaxants (doxacurium or pipecuronium) can be used to maintain muscle paralysis throughout the operation. We do not recommend pancuronium for children with Ebstein's anomaly, as it may cause supraventricular tachyarrhythmias, especially in patients prone to arrhythmias. Also we do not recommend the use of succinylcholine in neonates receiving prostaglandin $E_1$ infusion and in whom patency of the ductus arteriosus is critical for hemodynamic stability.

If deep hypothermia and circulatory arrest are planned (usually in children under 10 kg body weight), we administer 10 ml/kg of dextran 40 in 5% dextrose solution before peripheral cooling is initiated to prevent the aggregation of red cells and platelets in the microcirculation (see Chapter 4 for complete details of deep hypothermia).

Heparin is usually given into the right atrium by the surgeon just before the placement of cannulas. Protamine is administered by the anesthesiologist at the conclusion of extracorporeal circulation following the removal of cardiac cannulas. These patients commonly require either isoproterenol (0.01 to 0.05 μg/kg/min) or dobutamine (3 to 6 μg/kg/min) infusion after coming off bypass. Right ventricular dysfunction is one of the well recognized complications of repair of Ebstein's anomaly.

### Precautions

In all cases of communication between right and left sides of the heart, it is absolutely necessary that all IV lines be free of air bubbles. In addition one should use extra caution not to introduce any air bubbles when injecting drugs through an IV line. One should avoid factors that increase pulmonary vascular resistance (see the box) in patients with Ebstein's anomaly to minimize a right to left shunt. One should also pay utmost attention to ventilation and oxygenation along with the other measures (see the box) that may be necessary to reduce the pulmonary vascular resistance and right to left shunt. The correct placement of the endotracheal tube is very important in these patients. Since their oxygen status is marginal to start with, it is absolutely necessary to make sure that the tracheal tube is not advanced too far down into one of the bronchi. Care must be exercised during the insertion of wires and central catheters in these patients, as they are prone to cardiac arrhythmias.

### Postoperative ventilation

We routinely ventilate the patients mechanically for a day or two postoperatively, as the majority of our patients receive intravenous narcotic agents in high doses during surgery. In addition, patients usually become somewhat hypothermic at the end of the surgery. Once a patient is awake, stable, and rewarmed to a normal body temperature, the trachea can be extubated safely in the cardiac recovery room.

### INCREASED PULMONARY VASCULAR RESISTANCE

**Causes**

1. Hypoxemia
2. Hypercarbia
3. Acidosis
4. High mean airway pressure
5. Sympathetic stimulation (alpha)
6. Hypervolemia
7. Cough and laryngeal spasm
8. Crying and straining
9. Nitrous oxide (?) (in children with compromised myocardium)
10. Restriction of diaphragmatic movement from raised intraabdominal pressure
11. Surgical manipulation of the heart and great vessels
12. Noxious stimuli

**Treatment**

1. Oxygenation
2. Hyperventilation
3. Alkalosis
4. Prostaglandins (E type)
5. α-Adrenergic antagonists
6. Vasodilators (nitroglycerin and nitroprusside)
7. $\beta_2$ Stimulants (isoproterenol)
8. High $FIo_2$
9. Nitric oxide

## REFERENCES


1. Bahnson HJ, Bauersfled SR, Smith JW: Pathological anatomy and surgical correction of Ebstein's anomaly, *Circulation* 31(suppl 1):3, 1965.
2. Barnard CN, Schrire V: Surgical correction of Ebstein's malformation with prosthetic tricuspid valve, *Surg* 54:302, 1963.
3. Becu LM, Swan HJC, DuShane JM et al: Ebstein's malformation of the left atrioventricular valve in corrected transposition of the great vessels with ventricular septal defect, *Proc Staff Meet Mayo Clin* 30:483, 1955.
4. Bialostozky D, Medrano GA, Munoz L et al: Vectorcardiographic study and anatomic observations in 21 cases of Ebstein's malformation of the tricuspid valve, *Am J Cardiol* 30:354, 1972.
5. Billingsly AM, Laks H, Boyce SM et al: Definitive repair in patients with pulmonary atresia and intact ventricular septum, *J Thorac Cardiovasc Surg* 97:746, 1989.
6. Blacket RB, Sinclair-Smith BC, Palmer AJ et al: Ebstein's disease: a report of five cases, *Australas Ann Med* 1:26, 1952.
7. Bridges ND, Lock JE, Castaneda AR: Baffle fenestration with subsequent transcatheter closure: modification of the Fontan operation for patients at increased risk, *Circulation* 82:1681, 1990.
8. Cartwright RS, Smeloff EA, Cayler GC et al: Total correction of Ebstein's anomaly by means of tricuspid replacement, *J Thorac Cardiovasc Surg* 47:755, 1964.
9. Ebstein W: Uber einen sehr seltenen Fall von Insufficienz der Valvula tricuspidalis, bedingt dwich eine tangeborene hochgradige Missbildung derselben, *Arch Anat Physiol*

*Wissensch Med* 238, (Translated, *Am J Cardiol* 22:867, 1968).
10. Eger EI: Uptake of inhaled anesthetics: the alveolar to inspired anesthetic difference: effect of ventilation/perfusion abnormalities. In *Anesthetic uptake and action,* Baltimore, 1974, Williams & Wilkins.
11. Farooki ZQ, Henry JG, Green EW: Echocardiographic spectrum of Ebstein's anomaly of the tricuspid valve, *Circulation* 53:63, 1976.
12. Freedom RM, Culham G, Moes F et al: Differentiation of functional and structural pulmonary atresia: role of aortography, *Am J Cardiol* 41:914, 1978.
13. Gandhi MJ, Datey KK: The value of electrophysiologic changes at the tricuspid valve in the diagnosis of Ebstein's anomaly, *Am J Cardiol* 12:169, 1963.
14. Giuliani ER, Fuster V, Brandenburg RO et al: Ebstein's anomaly: the clinical features and natural history of Ebstein's anomaly of the tricuspid valve, *Mayo Clin Proc* 54:163, 1979.
15. Greeley WJ, Bushman GA, Davis DP et al: Comparative effects of halothane and ketamine on systemic arterial oxygen saturation in children with cyanotic congenital heart disease, *Anesthesiology* 65:666, 1986.
16. Gussenhoven WJ, Spitaels SEC, Bom N et al: Echocardiographic criteria for Ebstein's anomaly of tricuspid valve, *Br Heart J* 43:31, 1980.
17. Hansen DD, Hickey PR: Anesthesia for hypoplastic left heart syndrome: use of high-dose fentanyl in 30 neonates, *Anesth Analg* 65:127, 1986.
18. Hansen JF, Wennevold A: The diagnosis of Ebstein's disease of the heart. *Acta Med Scand* 189:515, 1971.
19. Hardy KL, May IA, Webster CA et al: Ebstein's anomaly: a functional concept and successful definitive repair, *J Thorac Cardiovasc Surg* 48:927, 1964.
20. Hardy KL, Ross BB: Ebstein's anomaly: further experience with definitive repair, *J Thorac Cardiovasc Surg* 58:553, 1969.
21. Hensley FA, Larach DR, Martin DE et al: The effect of saturation in cyanotic heart disease, *J Cardiothoracic Anes* 1:289, 1987.
22. Hernandez FA, Rochkind R, Cooper HR: The intracavitary ECG in the diagnosis of Ebstein's anomaly, *Am J Cardiol* 1:181, 1958.
23. Hickey PR, Hansen DD, Cramolini GM et al: Pulmonary and systemic hemodynamic responses to ketamine in infants with normal and elevated pulmonary and vascular resistance, *Anesthesiology* 62:287, 1985.
24. Hickey PR, Hansen DD, Straford M et al: Pulmonary and systemic effects of nitrous oxide in infants with normal and elevated pulmonary vascular resistance, *Anesthesiology* 65:374, 1986.
25. Hickey PR, Hansen DD, Wessel DL et al: Blunting of stress responses in the pulmonary circulation of infants, *Anesth Analg* 64:1137, 1985.
26. Hickey PR, Hansen DD, Wessel DL et al: Pulmonary and systemic hemodynamic responses to fentanyl in infants, *Anesth Analg* 64:483, 1985.
27. Hislop A, Reid L: Pulmonary arterial development during childhood: branching pattern and structure, *Thorax* 28:129, 1973.
28. Hunter SW, Lilehei CW: Ebstein's malformation of the tricuspid valve: study of a case together with suggestions of a new form of surgical therapy, *Dis Chest* 33:297, 1958.
29. Kambam JR, King P: Effect of right to left cardiopulmonary shunt on the uptake and distribution of inhaled anesthetics. *Int J Clin Monit Comput* 8:169, 1991 (abstract).
30. Kay JH, Tsuji HK, Redington JV et al: The surgical treatment of Ebstein's malformation with right ventricular aneurysmorrhaphy and replacement of tricuspid valve with a disc valve, *Dis Chest* 51:537, 1967.
31. Keith JD, Rowe RD, Vlad P: *Heart disease in infancy and childhood,* ed 3, New York, 1978, Macmillan.
32. Kumar AE, Fyler DC, Miettinen OS et al: Ebstein's anomaly: clinical profile and natural history, *Am J Cardiol* 28:84, 1971.
33. Laishley RS, Burrows FA, Lerman J et al: Effect of anesthetic induction regimens on oxygen saturation in cyanotic congenital heart disease, *Anesthesiology* 65:673, 1986.
34. Lev M, Rowlatt UF: The pathologic anatomy of mixed levocardia: a review of 13 cases of atrial or ventricular inversion with or without corrected transposition, *Am J Cardiol* 8:216, 1961.
35. Lilehei CW, Gannon PG: Ebstein's malformation of the tricuspid valve: method of surgical correction utilizing a ball-valve prosthesis and delayed closure of atrial septal defect, *Circulation* 31(suppl 1):9, 1965.
36. Lillienchei CW, Kalke BR, Carlson RG: Evolution of corrective surgery for Ebstein's anomaly, *Circulation* 35(suppl 1):111, 1967.
37. Lundstrom NR: Echocardiography in the diagnosis of Ebstein's anomaly of the tricuspid valve, *Circulation* 47:597, 1973.
38. Mair DD, Seward JB, Driscoll DJ et al: Surgical repair of Ebstein's anomaly: selection of patients and early and late operation results, *Circulation* 72(suppl 2):70, 1985.
39. Mayer FE, Nadas AS, Ongley PA: Ebstein's anomaly: presentation of 10 cases, *Circulation* 16:1057, 1957.
40. McFaul RC, Davis Z, Giuliani ER et al: Ebstein's malformation: surgical experience at the Mayo Clinic, *J Thorac Cardiovasc Surg* 72:910, 1976.
41. Meretoja OA, Takkunen O, Heikkila H et al: Haemodynamic response to nitrous oxide during high-dose fentanyl pancuronium anaesthesia, *Acta Anaesthesiol Scand* 29:137, 1985.
42. Newfeld EA, Cole RB, Paul MH: Ebstein's malformation of the tricuspid valve in the neonate: functional and anatomic outflow obstruction, *Am J Cardiol* 19:927, 1967.
43. Nora JJ, Nora AH, Toews AH: Lithium, Ebstein's anomaly and other congenital heart defects, *Lancet* 2:594, 1975.
44. Park JM, Sridaromont S, Ledbetter EO et al: Ebstein's anomaly of the tricuspid valve associated with prenatal exposure to lithium carbonate, *Am J Dis Child* 134:703, 1980.
45. Paul MH, VanPraagh S, VanPraagh R: Corrected transposition of the great arteries. In Watson H, editor: *Paediatric Cardiology,* St Louis, 1968, Mosby.
46. Perez-Alvarez JJ, Perez-Trevino C, Gaxiola A et al: Ebstein's anomaly with pulmonic stenosis: implantation of a tricuspid valvular prosthesis, *Am J Cardiol* 20:411, 1967.
47. Ports TA, Silverman NH, Schillder NB: Two-dimensional echocardiographic assessment of Ebstein's anomaly, *Circulation* 58:336, 1978.
48. Rao PS: Tricuspid valve anomalies other than tricuspid atresia. In Long WA, editor: *Fetal and neonatal cardiology,* Philadelphia, 1988, Saunders.
49. Rao PS, Jue KL, Isabel-Jones J et al: Ebstein's malformation of the tricuspid valve with atresia, *Am J Cardiol* 32:1004, 1973.
50. Rao PS, Wilson AD, Chopra PS: Transcatheter closure of atrial septal defect by "buttoned" devices, *Am J Cardiol* 69:1056, 1992.
51. Rogers JH Jr, Rao PS: Ebstein's anomaly of the left atroventricular valve with congenital corrected transposition of the great arteries: diagnosis by intracavitary electrocardiography, *Chest* 72:253, 1977.

52. Rowe RD, Freedom RM, Mehrizi A et al: The neonate with congenital heart disease. In *Major problems in clinical pediatrics,* vol 5, ed 2, Philadelphia, 1981, Saunders.
53. Schiebler GL, Edwards JE, Burchell HB et al: Congenital corrected transposition of the great vessels: a study of 33 cases, *Pediatrics* 27(suppl):851, 1961.
54. Schiebler GL, Adams P Jr, Anderson RC et al: Clinical study of 23 cases of Ebstein's anomaly of the tricuspid valve, *Circulation* 19:165, 1959.
55. Sodi-Pallares D, Marsico F: The importance of ECG patterns in congenital heart disease, *Am Heart J* 49:202, 1955.
56. Stoelting R, Longnecker DE: Effect of right-to-left shunt on rate of increase in arterial anesthetic concentration, *Anesthesiology* 365:352, 1972.
57. Tajik AJ, Gau GT, Giulani ER et al: Echocardiogram in Ebstein's anomaly with Woolf-Parkinson-White preexcitation syndrome, type B, *Circulation* 47:813, 1973.
58. Takayasu S, Obunai Y, Konno S: Clinical classification of Ebstein's anomaly, *Am Heart J* 95:154, 1978.
59. Tanner GE, Angers DG, Barash PG et al: Effect of left-to-right, mixed right-to-left, and right-to-left shunts on inhalational anesthetic induction in children: a computer model, *Anesth Analg* 64:101, 1985.
60. Tourniaire A, Deyrieux F, Tartulier M: Maladie d'Ebstein: Essai de diagnostique clinique, *Arch Mal Coeur* 42:1211, 1949.
61. Uhl HSM: A previously undescribed congenital malformation of the heart: almost total absence of the myocardium of the right ventricle, *Bull Johns Hopkins Hosp* 91:197, 1952.
62. VanMierop LHS, Alley RD, Kausel HW et al: Ebstein's malformation of the left atrioventricular valve in corrected transpositions with subpulmonary stenosis and ventricular septal defect, *Am J Cardiol* 8:270, 1961.
63. VanMierop LHS, Kutsche LM, Victorica BE: Ebstein's anomaly. In Adams FH, Emmanouilides GC, Riemenschneider TA, editors: *Moss' heart disease in infants, children, and adolescents,* ed 4, Baltimore, 1983, Williams & Wilkins.
64. Watson H: Natural history of Ebstein's anomaly of the tricuspid valve in childhood and adolescence: an international cooperative study of 505 cases, *Br Heart J* 36:417, 1974.
65. Weinstein MR, Goldfield MD: Cardiovascular malformation with lithium use during pregnancy, *Am J Psychol* 132:529, 1975.
66. Wessel DL, Hickey PR, Hansen DD: Pulmonary and systemic hemodynamic effects of hyperventilation in infants after repair of congenital heart disease, *Anesthesiology* 67:A526, 1987.
67. Yim BJB, Yu PN: Value of an electrode catheter in diagnosis of Ebstein's disease, *Circulation* 17:543, 1958.
68. Yuste P, Minguez I, Aza V et al: Echocardiography in the diagnosis of Ebstein's anomaly, *Chest* 66:273, 1974.

# 30 Heart Transplantation in Infants and Children

***Steven J. Hoff, Jay Kambam,*** *and* ***William H. Frist***



Improved survival and quality of life in adults undergoing heart transplantation set the stage for the emergence of heart transplantation in neonates and children with end stage heart disease. Experience with patient selection, improvement in preoperative and postoperative care and surgical techniques, and refinements in immunosuppression have allowed heart transplantation in children to become an established mode of therapy. The Registry of the International Society for Heart and Lung Transplantation (ISHLT) reports that more than 1400 heart transplant procedures have been performed in patients less than 19 years of age since 1980. Current 1-year survival reported by individual centers is 75% to 86%,* with similar rates maintained at 5 years of follow-up. Expanding the recipient selection to include young children and neonates was a natural progression of the earlier success in adolescent children.

As experience in pediatric heart transplantation has grown, it has become evident that transplantation in general and cardiac transplantation in particular present unique challenges and opportunities. Evidence suggests that the neonatal immune system may present a window of opportunity for allograft tolerance. Concern exists regarding the long-term

*References 11, 29, 36, 38, 79, 80, 92, 103.

sequelae of prolonged immunosuppression in children with the potential for retardation in growth and development as well as the potential for the development of neoplasms and lymphoproliferative disorders. There is a significant impact of congenital cardiac malformations and their effects on pulmonary vascular pressure and resistance on surgical techniques and outcome. Recipient size affects donor availability as well as postoperative monitoring for rejection. Social and ethical concerns regarding xenotransplantation and anencephalic donors for neonatal transplantation are highlighted in scientific and lay publications alike.

Cardiac transplantation for infants and children with end stage heart disease has shown remarkable early success in providing long-term survival with excellent quality of life without the need for multiple palliative procedures.

## HISTORICAL PERSPECTIVE

In 1967 the first successful orthotopic heart transplant operations were performed by Barnard[17] in South Africa and Shumway[100] in the United States. That same year Kantrowitz and colleagues[68] at Maimonides/Downstate Medical Center in New York performed an orthotopic heart transplant in a 3-week-old patient with tricuspid atresia who had undergone a previous palliative procedure. The donor organ was procured from an anencephalic donor. The child survived only 6½ hours after the transplant. In 1968 Cooley and associates[39,40] performed the first heart-lung transplant in a 2-month-old child with an atrioventricular canal defect. The child required an exploratory thoracotomy for bleeding 6 hours after transplantation and died 14 hours postoperatively due to respiratory insufficiency. The first successful pediatric heart transplants were performed in adolescents at Stanford.[107] Poor results after cardiac transplantation in the 1970s tempered early enthusiasm. This period saw continued investigation into the fundamental problems of immunosuppression and rejection by Shumway and colleagues[100] at Stanford. The development of techniques for percutaneous endomyocardial biopsy to monitor allograft rejection and the discovery of the immunosuppressive properties of cyclosporine by Borel[27] in 1980 led to a 20% improvement in survival after heart transplantation in adults and paved the way for expansion of transplantation in the pediatric population as the addition of cyclosporine allowed reduction in corticosteroid dosages to recipients.

In the early 1980s, pediatric heart transplantation was limited primarily to adolescents. As results improved, the age limit for recipients continued to be pushed lower. In 1986 Bailey and co-workers[16] reported the first series of successful heart transplants for neonates with hypoplastic left heart syndrome. Since that time pediatric heart transplantation has been limited by donor availability. The first xenograft in a pediatric recipient was performed by Bailey[15] at Loma Linda University in 1985, using a baboon as a donor in the controversial Baby Fae case. Ethical issues surrounding xenotransplantation and the use of organs from anencephalic donors have yet to be resolved but may affect the limitation of donor availability on modern pediatric heart transplantation.

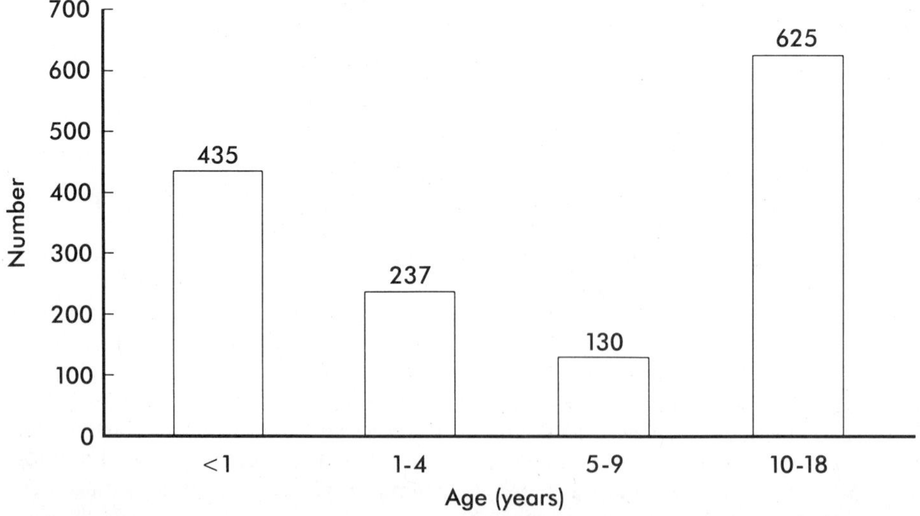


**Figure 30–1** Number of heart transplantations performed in children by age. (From ISHLT Registry, November 1992.)

## RESULTS

### The world experience with pediatric heart transplantation

Experience with pediatric heart transplantation continues to expand worldwide. Before 1980 only 14 pediatric heart transplant procedures had been performed. Since 1980 the IHSLT has maintained a voluntary registry of thoracic transplantation worldwide. As of December 1992 1427 heart transplants had been performed in children 18 years of age and younger at 137 centers worldwide (Fig. 30–1).

With growing experience and improved survival for heart transplantation in neonates, this age group has become the most common group undergoing transplantation; however, 44% of transplants performed were in children 10 to 18 years of age.

As the age distribution has evolved to younger recipients, indications for transplantation have changed as well (Fig. 30–2). Cardiomyopathy is the indication in 49% and congenital heart disease in 44%. The rate of retransplantation has remained stable at approximately 2% to 4% of all transplant procedures performed each year.[69]

Thirty-day perioperative mortality, which has shown a gradual decline over time (Fig. 30–3), is 16.7%. The increasing number of neonatal transplant recipients has a slightly higher mortality rate

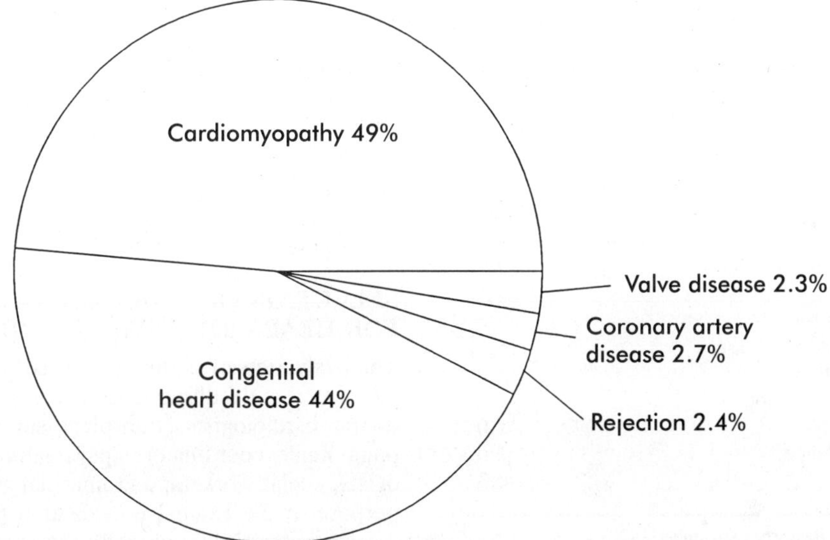


**Figure 30–2** Indications for heart transplantation in children. (From ISHLT Registry, November 1992.)

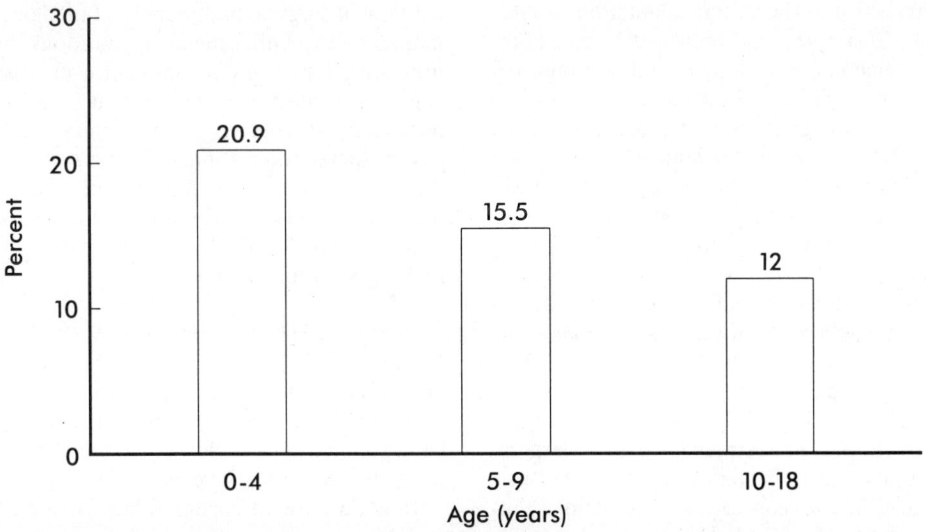


**Figure 30–3** Operative (30-day) mortality by age. (From ISHLT Registry, November 1992.)

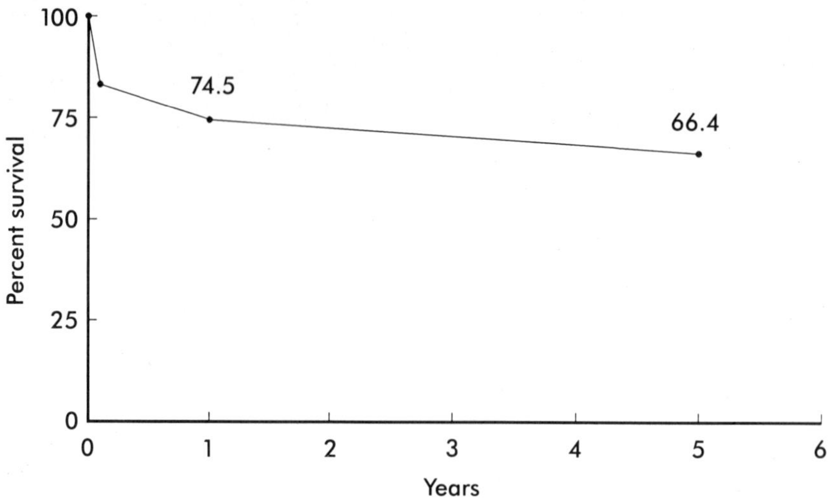


**Figure 30–4** Actuarial survival after heart transplantation in children. (From ISHLT Registry, November 1992.)

**Table 30–1** Cause of early postoperative death after heart transplantation in children (%)

| | |
|---|---|
| Nonspecific graft failure | 27.9 |
| Infection | 22.9 |
| Acute rejection | 22.6 |
| Coronary artery disease | 16.7 |
| Sudden death | 5.0 |
| Hyperacute rejection | 2.6 |
| Malignancy | 1.0 |
| Non-compliance | 1.0 |
| Suicide | 0.3 |

From ISHLT Registry, November 1992.

(20.9%) than older children, although experienced centers report mortality rates as low as 10%. Actuarial survival after heart transplantation in children is 74.5% at 1 year and 66.4% at 5 years (Fig. 30–4). Cardiac complications including donor organ preservation failure, right heart failure due to elevated pulmonary artery pressures, cardiac arrest, bleeding, and nonspecified technical problems are the leading cause of early postoperative death (Table 30–1). Rejection, infection, and graft coronary artery disease are the most common causes of late death.

Recipients under 1 year of age have an improving operative and long-term survival, although this remains higher than in older children ($p = .0024$, Fig. 30–5). Actuarial survival in recipients less than a year of age is 70.5% at 1 year and 65.8% at 5 years. Some 34 recipients have undergone retransplantation at 19 centers worldwide. The primary indication for reoperation is rejection. Operative mortality (27.5%) is higher, and 1- and 3-year actuarial survival is markedly poorer (53% and 35% respectively) than after initial transplantation (Figs. 30–6 and 30–7).

## SELECTION OF PEDIATRIC PATIENTS FOR HEART TRANSPLANTATION

The evaluation of children referred for transplantation is a multi-disciplinary matter including pediatric cardiologists, transplant surgeons, transplant nurse coordinators, psychiatrists, psychologists, social workers, and financial advisers. The purpose of the extensive evaluation process is to determine the child's suitability as a transplant candidate and the family's ability to withstand the lifelong demands involved with this therapy. Transplantation is considered only after conventional medical or surgical treatment has failed or is judged inappropriate. Other medical conditions that might limit long-term survival must also be absent. Because posttransplant management is complex and potentially disruptive to the family unit, certain psychosocial criteria must also be met by the candidate and family. The family (and child, depending on age) must clearly understand the risks, limitations, and benefits of the transplant before making an informed decision.

### Medical criteria and indications for operation

Children who are candidates for heart transplantation have end stage heart disease with severe functional limitations. The primary indications can be classified as complex congenital heart disease or cardiomyopathy (box on p. 339, top left).[22,79,103]

In children with cogenital heart disease the natural history of the specific cardiac lesion and the

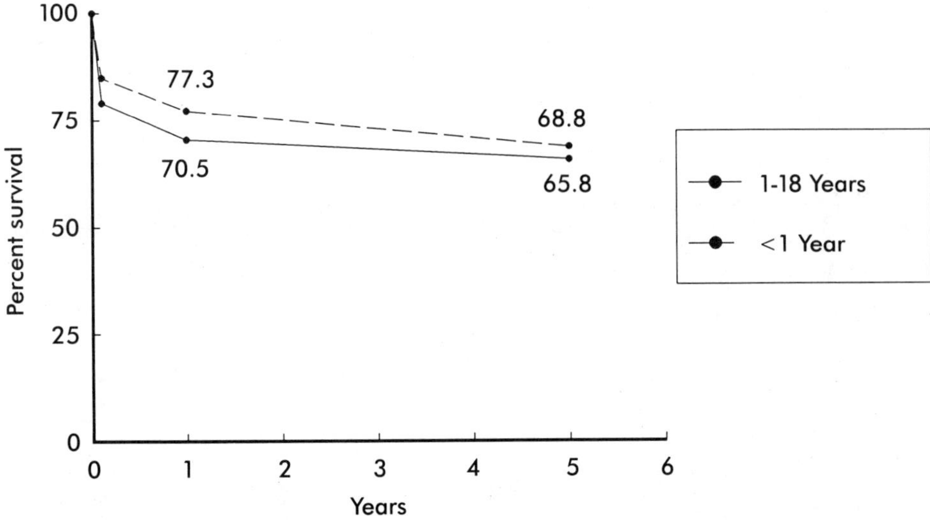


**Figure 30–5** Actuarial survival after heart transplantation in children by age. (From ISHLT Registry, November 1992.)

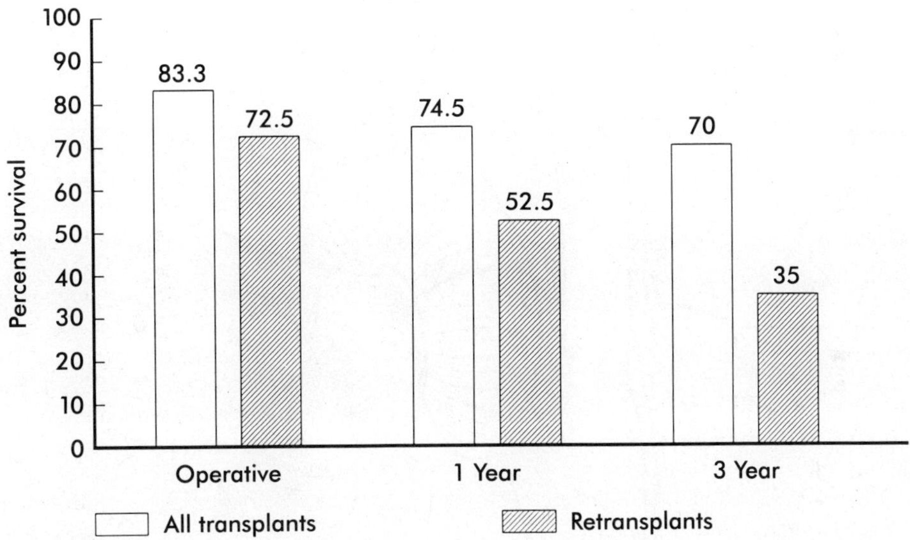


**Figure 30–6** Actuarial survival rate after heart retransplantation in children. (From ISHLT Registry, November 1992.)

risks and long-term benefits of conventional palliative treatment must be weighed against the risks and benefits of transplantation. Many clinicians advise surgical palliation as initial therapy because of the lack of suitable donors, particularly for infants. These children often present for transplantation once irreversible myocardial dysfunction has developed. Previous palliative procedures can create difficult technical challenges for the transplant surgeon. Proponents of early transplantation cite the improved survival of infants undergoing cardiac transplantations as well as the receptive nature of the immune system, with its potential for reduction of immunosuppressive therapy.[106]

The hypoplastic left heart syndrome (HLHS) is becoming the most common congenital lesion for which transplantation is a viable therapeutic option.[13] Although many neonates with HLHS undergo staged palliative reconstruction of this otherwise lethal defect with the Norwood and Fontan procedures,[29,52] long-term success with these procedures has been unsatisfactory at many centers.

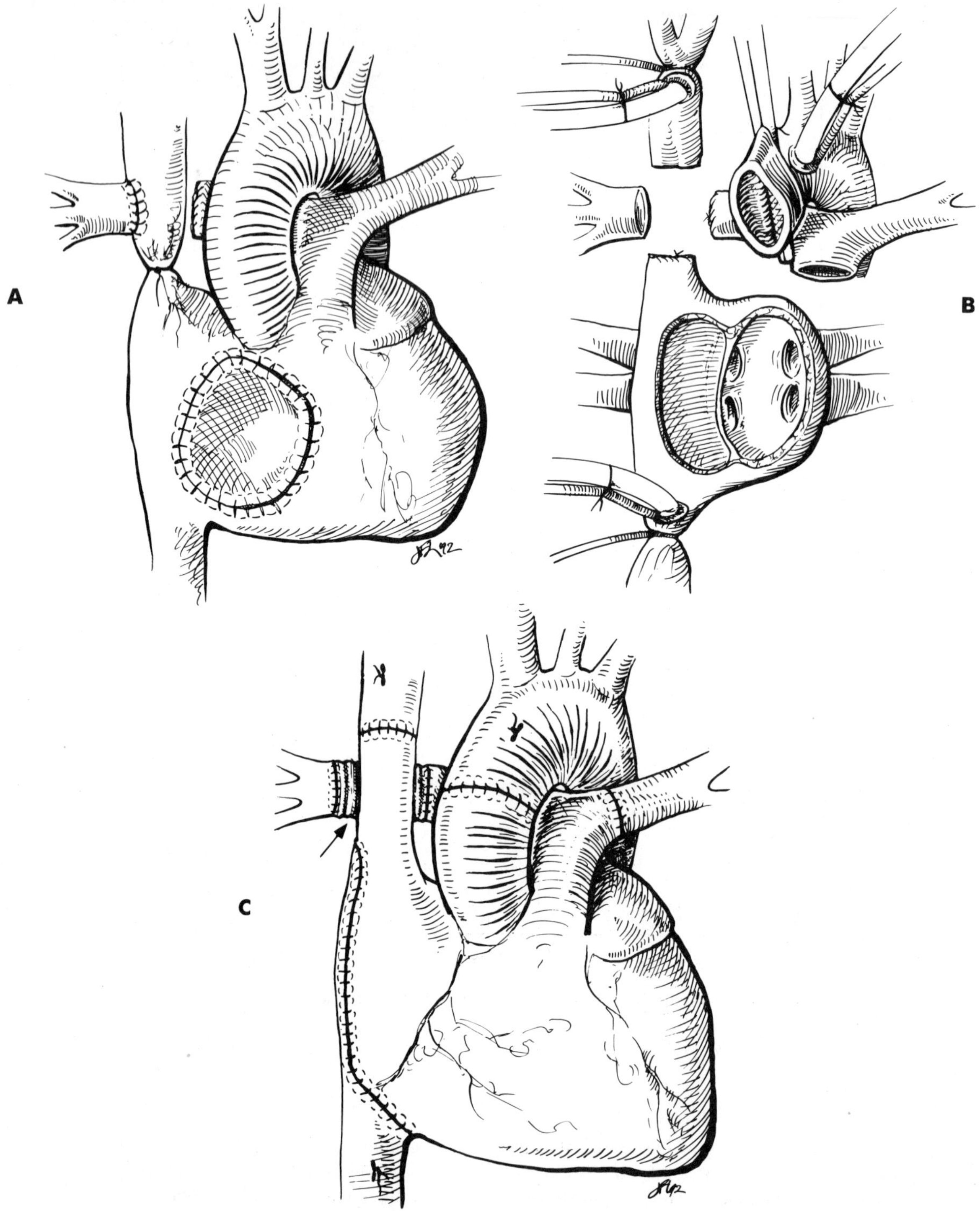


**Figure 30–7** Case study of transplantation for complex congenital heart disease. A child born with tricuspid atresia and ventricular septal defect underwent left Blalock-Taussig shunt at 18 months of age and Glenn shunt at 4 years of age prior to Bjork modification of the Fontan procedure at age 8. He developed progressive cyanosis and right heart failure requiring heart transplantation at 18 years of age. **A,** Native heart prior to transplantation demonstrating anatomy and previous operative procedures. **B,** Recipient's anatomy after excision of the native heart. **C,** Donor heart after completion of the transplant procedures. Modifications of implantation technique included direct superior vena cava to superior vena cava and left pulmonary artery to left pulmonary artery anastomoses, with interposition graft in the right pulmonary artery *(arrow)*.

### INDICATIONS FOR TRANSPLANTATION IN INFANTS AND CHILDREN

**Cardiomyopathy**
- Idiopathic
- Dilated
- Hypertrophic
- Restrictive

**Congenital malformations**
- Hypoplastic left heart syndrome
- D-Transposition of the great arteries with or without atrial baffle repair
- Pulmonary atresia with hypoplastic right ventricle and coronary fistulae
- Severe tricuspid insufficiency secondary to Ebstein's anomaly
- Single ventricle with atrioventricular (AV) valve incompetence and/or subaortic stenosis
- Atrioventricular canal with straddling AV valve
- Truncus arteriosus with interrupted aortic arch
- Congenital coronary artery anomalies

### CONTRAINDICATIONS TO HEART TRANSPLANTATION

**Absolute**
- Active infection
- Fixed pulmonary hypertension

**Relative**
- Anatomically inadequate pulmonary vessels
- Recent pulmonary infarction
- Severe renal or hepatic dysfunction
- Chronic pulmonary disease
- Insulin-dependent diabetes mellitus
- Malignancy
- Active peptic ulcer disease
- Extracardiac anomalies that would limit survival
- Drug addiction or alcoholism (parents or transplant candidate)
- Repeated noncompliance with medical regimens (parents or transplant candidate)

In addition anatomic considerations may obviate palliation. These include valvular pulmonic stenosis, tricuspid valvular abnormalities, and congenital stenosis of the pulmonary veins.[25,118]

There is no consensus regarding the natural history of cardiomyopathy in children. Dilated cardiomyopathy represents at least 90% of all cardiomyopathies in children. The cause is usually unknown. Intensive medical treatment with diuretics, vasodilators, inotropes, β-adrenergic blockers, and anticoagulation may improve function and influence survival. Little is known regarding the proper timing of cardiac transplantation,[3] but current practice is to palliate medically in the absence of elevated pulmonary artery pressures or end organ damage as long as possible. Results after transplantation are excellent.[105.]

## Limitations to transplantation unique to children

Absolute and relative medical contraindications to transplantation in children are similar to those in adults (box at top right). Active infection requires delay in transplantation until fully treated to prevent progression of the infectious process after induction of immunosuppression.

Markedly elevated pulmonary vascular resistance (PVR) can lead to acute failure of the normal donor right ventricle, which is not capable of adequate function in the face of markedly elevated pulmonary artery pressure and resistance. Some degree of pulmonary hypertension is common in children with end stage heart disease. Therefore right heart catheterization must be performed to determine pressures, PVR, and the degree to which increased pulmonary artery pressure and resistance will respond to vasodilator therapy. Infusion of vasodilator agents such as nitroprusside or prostaglandin $E_1$ and administration of 100% oxygen are useful to test the reactivity of the pulmonary vasculature. Generally, with appropriate acute intervention the pulmonary artery systolic pressure should fall to less than 50 mm Hg and the vascular resistance to less than 3 Wood units. In addition, the transpulmonary gradient (TPG is mean pulmonary artery pressure minus pulmonary capillary wedge pressure) should be less than 15 mm Hg. However, these criteria, developed from experience in adult transplantation, do not account for the varied body surface area in children. Therefore use of PVR index may be more appropriate for the pediatric population. It has been suggested that a PVR index of less than 4 to 6 Wood units and a TPG of less than 15 decreases perioperative morbidity.[2,47]

In many children with congenital heart disease, especially those with systemic to pulmonary artery shunts, accurate measurement of PVR may not be possible because of unevenly distributed regional pulmonary blood flows and pressures. Determination of the degree of reversibility of pulmonary hypertension by the use of vasodilator agents is less predictable in patients with systemic to pulmonary artery shunts. In children with elevated PVR, implantation of an oversized donor heart may help overcome elevated resistance and may provide better postoperative function.[47]

Distortion of the pulmonary artery anatomy, either by a previous systemic to pulmonary artery shunt or a pulmonary artery band, may create technical difficulties during implantation of the donor heart that lead to increased perioperative risk. Anomalous pulmonary venous return also poses technical challenges. The potential to reconstruct adequately abnormal pulmonary artery or venous anatomy must be considered when selecting patients for transplantation.[47,112]

Recent pulmonary embolism with infarction remains a relative contraindication to transplantation; however, successful transplantation in this setting is possible.[34] Anticoagulation prior to transplantation may limit embolic complications in children with poor ventricular function. Severe renal or hepatic dysfunction limits the use of cyclosporine, which is metabolized in the liver and can affect renal function, thereby limiting transplantation in these patients. Major systemic diseases such as chronic obstructive pulmonary diseases (bronchopulmonary dysplasia or cystic fibrosis), insulin-dependent diabetes mellitus, and malignancy are relative contraindications to transplantation.

### Psychosocial evaluation and financial considerations

A comprehensive psychosocial evaluation is necessary to assess the family's (and an older child's) compliance to previous medical regimens and overall commitment to health care demands. A stable and supportive family environment is crucial to success. This can be provided by single parents as well as by married parents if strong support is available from other relatives or friends who are equally committed to the child's welfare. Long-term survival depends on the patient's and the family's ability to learn the medical regimen and to follow instructions given by the medical staff. Parents must administer medications in a conscientious manner and promptly report signs and symptoms of complications to the medical team. In addition parents must be prepared to accept the social disruption caused by the development of complications, frequent visits to physicians' offices, and the likely need for repeated hospitalizations.

Heart transplantation is an expensive procedure. The candidate's family must have the means to cover expenses related to the pretransplant evaluation, waiting period, transplant procedure, hospitalization, and long-term care, including medications. Fortunately, most private insurers offer policies that cover heart transplantation. In addition many state Medicaid programs offer partial reimbursement.

## THE TRANSPLANT PROCESS

The transplant process begins with the identification of a suitable donor. Only increased awareness on the part of practitioners to counsel parents grieving for the loss of their child can affect the shortage of donor organs and death of children awaiting transplantation.[87] When a potential donor is identified, suitability of the heart is determined by the local transplant coordinator.[48] Echocardiography is invaluable in the assessment of cardiac function. Final determination of suitability is made at the time of explantation.

### Donor-recipient matching

The donor and recipient are matched according to three criteria: (1) ABO blood group, (2) body weight, and (3) cytotoxicity. Blood group compatibility is mandatory; otherwise immediate humoral rejection will develop with subsequent loss of the graft. The tolerable limit for weight discrepancy between donor and recipient varies according to age. A difference of as much as 300% may be appropriate in the neonatal population, but a difference of 50% may be more reasonable in older children. Case by case considerations must include the recipient's native heart size and PVR. For example, a small recipient with marked cardiomegaly can receive the heart from a much larger donor without compromise of the thoracic contents. In patients with pulmonary hypertension, a large donor heart may be preferred to overcome elevated PVR. A comparison of echocardiographic measurements between donor and recipient may facilitate the matching process. Panel for reactive antibodies (PRA) is routinely performed preoperatively to determine the lymphocytic cytotoxicity of a potential recipient. It measures the recipient's cytotoxic antibodies against different lymphocyte antigens in a sample population that may typify potential donors. Patients with a high PRA, usually greater than 5% to 10%, should if at all possible have a negative lymphocyte cross-match with a specific donor heart. For logistical reasons, if the PRA is 0% to 5%, cross-matches generally are performed retrospectively.

In addition donor and recipient cytomegalovirus (CMV) status is assessed. The risk of CMV infection is high when a seropositive organ is transplanted into a seronegative recipient. However, this does not preclude transplantation. Under these conditions prophylactic antiviral treatment with acyclovir or ganciclovir appears to be beneficial. Finally, proximity of donor procurement is important. Current recommendations are that donor procurement be limited to the distance a procurement team can safely travel in a graft ischemia time of no more than 4 hours. Some centers adhere to an upper limit of 6 hours, most notably those involved in neonatal transplantation. New methods of graft preservation will likely extend safe graft ischemia time. Human leukocyte antigen (HLA) matching has not been shown to affect survival or incidence of rejection significantly but is generally performed retrospectively.[6]

### Preoperative care of the recipient

Special medical concerns after the child has been listed as a suitable transplant candidate are to maintain hemodynamic stability and nutritional status and to prevent infection. Inotropic support such as dobutamine and amventirinone and the use of mechanical ventilation, extracorporeal membrane oxygenation, and the intraaortic balloon pump may be necessary to maintain cardiac function prior to transplantation.[51,116] In the neonate with HLHS continuous intravenous prostaglandin infusion is required to ensure ductal patency and adequate systemic perfusion. Oxygen saturation is maintained at 75% to 85% by use of a low-oxygen environment (fractional inspired oxygen concentration less than 0.21) to promote some degree of pulmonary vasoconstriction and create a balance between pulmonary and systemic blood flow.[42,79] Strict attention to nutritional intake is essential to meet metabolic requirements and maintain strength and growth prior to transplantation. Supplemental enteral feedings may be necessary to maintain positive nitrogen balance and prevent postoperative complications such as the inability to wean from mechanical ventilation, poor wound healing, and greater risk of pulmonary infection. Particularly in the neonate with HLHS, total parenteral nutrition is initiated if there is concern about mesenteric ischemic injury caused by poor systemic perfusion and acidosis. Infection (especially pneumonia or catheter-induced septicemia) is a risk in patients requiring endotracheal intubation or multiple invasive monitoring lines. Because active infection precludes transplantation, preventive measures are mandatory. IV lines are monitored closely. In addition frequent hand washing, adherence to strict sterile technique, and chest physiotherapy are practices that reduce the risk of infection.

While awaiting transplantation, growth and cardiac function are continually assessed. Additionally, repeated screening for infection and fixed pulmonary hypertension helps determine the child's continued candidacy for transplantation.

Once a child is listed for transplantation, the family must endure the emotional stress of waiting for a suitable donor. The parents may feel guilty because the attention required by the ill child may arouse jealousy and anger in siblings. Also, parents may feel inadequate in trying to comfort their sick child. Members of the transplant team and nursing staff help the child and family maintain hope and encourage them to deal constructively with their fear and anxiety. Meeting other waiting candidates, transplant recipients, and family members of both may provide additional hope, insight, and reassurance from those who understand the emotional experience.

## SURGICAL TECHNIQUES

### Donor procurement and preservation techniques

Procurement of the donor heart proceeds in a fashion similar to that in the adult. Heparin is given intravenously prior to skin incision if the heart is the only organ to be harvested; it is given prior to abdominal aortic cannulation in the setting of multiple organ harvesting. Through a median sternotomy the thymus is removed and innominate vein ligated unless a central venous catheter runs through it or it is needed for venous reconstruction in the recipient. After complete dissection, which includes the entire aortic arch, the superior vena cava is ligated and aortic cross-clamp applied. Cardioplegic arrest is accomplished using a single dose of 250 ml (amount adjusted to size) of cold crystalloid cardioplegia instilled in the ascending aorta. The group at Loma Linda prefer a calcium-free solution first advocated by Roe[5]; however, Kempsford and Hearse[70] suggested that solutions containing calcium such as St. Thomas solution may provide better myocardial protection of the immature myocardium. Free radical scavengers such as human recombinant superoxide dismutase may provide additional protection to the neonatal heart.[109] Topical cooling is accomplished with surface application of 4° C crystalloid solution. The inferior vena cava and a pulmonary vein are divided to decompress the heart.

After the cardioplegia the descending aorta, arch vessels, remaining pulmonary veins, pulmonary arteries, and superior vena cava are divided. Sufficient aortic, pulmonary artery, and caval tissue is removed with the specimen to accomplish anatomic repair of the recipient heart. The heart is removed, rinsed in iced saline solution, placed in saline, packed in ice, and transported in an insulated container.

### Implantation techniques

Graft implantation proceeds under moderate hypothermia and cardiopulmonary bypass in older children; in neonates deep hypothermia and circulatory arrest are used. The recipient then undergoes cardiectomy, leaving long segments of native pulmonary artery and aorta for implantation as well as cuffs of the right and left atrium. The left atrial anastomosis is performed first, followed by the right atrial, aortic, and pulmonary artery anastomoses in that order. The patient is then rewarmed, separated from cardiopulmonary bypass, and decannulated.

Infants with hypoplastic left heart syndrome requiring aortic arch reconstruction due to aortic atresia provide special technical challenges.[12,104] Modifications to standard implantation techniques have been summarized by Mavroudis.[5] These technical considerations allow for shorter circulatory arrest and donor heart ischemia times by modifications in the conduct of cardiopulmonary bypass, myocardial protection, intracavitary air removal, and precision suture techniques to ensure proper neoaortic reconstruction.

Children with complex congenital heart disease who may have undergone previous palliative procedures require modification of implantation techniques as well. In patients with transposition of the great vessels, complete mobilization and preservation of maximal length of the aorta and pulmonary trunks in the recipient allows end to end anastomosis without tension or kinking.[5,75] The pulmonary artery anastomosis must usually be performed prior to aortic anastomosis. Anomalies of pulmonary arteries and veins may require reconstruction at the time of implantation.[35,37,41] Children who have undergone Blalock-Taussig or Glenn shunts require ligation of the shunt and often require repair of the pulmonary artery. Patients with previous pulmonary artery banding may require pulmonary artery reconstruction using native or graft material.[61] Transplantation after Fontan or Senning repair require reconstruction of the atria.[75,77,78]

### Retransplantation

Indications for retransplantation in children are similar to those for adults. They include hyperacute graft rejection, graft failure because of inadequate preservation, and late graft failure. As survival improves, graft atherosclerosis is becoming a more common cause for retransplantation.[30]

As with all reoperative procedures, adhesions can make cannulation and cardiectomy difficult. Increased bleeding may require special attention to blood salvage or the need for transfusion. Previous reconstructive procedures during the first transplant (for example aortoplasty in recipients with hypoplastic left heart syndrome) may complicate retransplantation. Often the new graft can be implanted into the donor tissue left intact from the initial repair.[5]

## ANESTHESIA TECHNIQUES

Anesthesia management of a neonate or a child undergoing heart transplantation is similar to that of others with CHD for corrective surgery up to the time of institution of extracorporeal circulation.[59] If the body weight of a child is less than 10 kg, profound hypothermia and circulatory arrest for up to 75 minutes are usually used in many centers, including ours. A thorough understanding of the physiologic changes that occur in a transplanted heart after bypass is essential for optimal anesthetic management of a patient undergoing heart transplantation.

### Physiology of the transplanted heart

Cardiac transplantation interrupts the continuity of the sympathetic fibers and the parasympathetic fibers to the donor heart. Sympathetic innervation of the myocardium, the conduction system, and the coronary vascular system are all interrupted. On the parasympathetic side cardiac transplantation interrupts the vagal innervation to the sinus node and the atrioventricular node. As a result of this interruption in parasympathetic innervation the transplanted heart exhibits loss of vagal effects on the sinus node and the AV node. Available data also suggest that after transplantation both mechanoreflexes and chemoreflexes are impaired.[7,32,83,117] The remnants of the atria of the recipient heart are the only parts of the heart that retain autonomic innervation. For example, sinus arrhythmia related to respiration, which is seen in normal hearts, still occurs in the remnants and the sinus node of the native heart but not in the transplanted heart.[45,101]

The state of cardiac denervation in the post-transplant patient has important clinical, physiologic, and pharmacologic consequences. The heart transplant recipient is not able to sense cardiac pain, so these patients will experience silent myocardial ischemia. The physiologic responses to stress and pharmacologic responses to many drugs differ markedly in the donor heart from those of a normal heart with intact autonomic innervation. The resting heart rate of a transplanted heart is much higher than the usual heart rate.[55] In a normal heart the resting rate is mainly dependent on the input from the autonomic nervous system (ANS). The tone of the ANS is in turn under the influence of both internal and external factors. The ANS retains its influence on the sinus node and the remnants of the original atria, but the donor heart, lacking autonomic innervation, is not under the influence of the ANS. The rate of automaticity is thus not the same in the remnants of the native heart and the donor heart. Thus, two P waves are present in the ECG of a heart recipient. The resting coronary arterial blood flow of the donor heart is also higher because of the lack of α-sympathetic tone.[88] The coronary arteries, however, remain responsive to normal metabolic demands as well as to the α- and β-sympathetic agonists and antagonists. Although reinnervation has been demonstrated in animal models within 2 years after transplantation and there is increasing evidence that some elements of reinnervation occur in human beings, clinically significant innervation has not yet been demonstrated.[45,81,82,98,101,102,111] Nevertheless, the donor heart appropriately responds to many physiologic needs, mainly because of the Frank-Starling mechanism and direct catecholamine response and partly because of intact peripheral vascular reflexes. However, the responses of the donor and normal hearts to physiologic needs differ from one another. For example, the adaptive response to exercise in the transplanted heart is based on the Frank-Starling mechanism. The cardiac output in the transplanted heart is thus mainly increased by the stroke volume, and only in the later part of the exercise does the heart rate increase in response to elevated catecholamines.[108] In contrast, the increase in cardiac output in a nontransplanted normal heart is initially the result of an increased heart rate and only later of an increased stroke volume.[94]

Many cardiac drugs affect the heart directly or indirectly with or without involvement of the ANS. The comparative effects of various drugs on transplanted and normal hearts are listed in Table 30–2.[20,33,121] Following cardiac transplantation the denervated heart retains its automaticity and conductivity, and $\alpha$- and $\beta$-sympathetic receptors show no evidence of denervated postsynaptic hypersensitivity.[32,33,55,94] Because of the loss of uptake-1 system (presynaptic), adrenergic supersensitivity to catecholamines such as epinephrine and norepinephrine has been demonstrated, with high affinity for the neuronal uptake system.[53] As a result the direct-acting drug, epinephrine, will have a higher inotropic to vasoconstrictor ratio (beta to alpha ratio) in transplanted recipients than in normal patients.[53] The transplanted human heart has been shown to have a higher percentage of $\beta_2$-adrenergic receptors than $\beta_1$-adrenergic receptors.[96] Therefore one should use a nonselective $\beta$-agonist such as epinephrine, isoproterenol, or dobutamine to achieve optimal inotropy rather than norepinephrine, which is a $\beta_1$-selective drug. Also, because of the absence of neuronal norepinephrine stores in the transplanted heart, the indirect-acting drugs such as ephedrine and dopamine will be less effective inotropic agents.[95] Dopamine possesses predominantly dopaminergic and $\alpha$-adrenergic actions in cardiac transplant patients, unlike its action in normal patients. On the other hand, drugs such as atropine and other anticholinergic agents, anticholinesterases, pancuronium, and others that exert their effects on the heart indirectly via the ANS will have virtually no effect on the heart rate.[44,54,74,94]

### Preoperative evaluation

Understanding of the physiologic changes that occur with heart transplantation is essential for a safe anesthesia management, as is an appreciation of the pathologic anatomy and physiology of the basic CHD of the heart recipient. Children with severe hypoxemia are prone to metabolic acidosis, hypoglycemia, and hypocalcemia. Measurement of arterial blood gas and electrolyte concentrations and preoperative correction of metabolic derangements in children with severe hypoxemia are essential to avoid hypotensive and hypoglycemic episodes at the time of induction. Appropriate type of blood and blood products (washed red cells, fresh frozen plasma, and platelets) are ordered preoperatively to be given during the postbypass period. All blood products must be checked for CMV, and only CMV-negative units are given. Many centers irradiate all blood products after red cell antibody screening cross-matches are accomplished.[12]

### Preoperative medication

Preoperative sedation depends upon the age of the child and severity of the defect. Advantages of preoperative sedation include decrease or elimination of anxiety, reduction of oxygen demand, and avoidance of further hemodynamic deterioration. However, one should not oversedate these children, as hypoventilation will have detrimental effects on oxygen saturation and pulmonary blood flow. Preoperative sedation should ideally be achieved in the holding room, where someone can watch for any undesirable side effects. A small dose of narcotic and a paralyzing dose of a neuromuscular blocker may be given to certain patients, especially those on a ventilator and receiving prostaglandin $E_1$, for a smooth transport from the ICU. Bigger children can be given either oral benzodiazepine (midazolam 0.5 to 0.6 mg/kg) or an IM dose of morphine sulphate (0.1 mg/kg), or both as preoperative medications.

### Intraoperative monitoring

Intraoperative monitoring should include an ECG, invasive arterial pressure, noninvasive blood pressure, pulse oximeter, capnogram, temperature (esophageal and nasopharyngeal), central venous pressure, and urinometer. Whenever possible right internal jugular catheterization should be avoided to preserve the site for posttransplantation cardiac biopsies. Arterial blood gases, serum glucose, calcium, potassium, and hematocrit levels are monitored frequently throughout the operation. Appropriate bleeding and coagulation tests should be performed post bypass, as these patients frequently require blood and blood products.

### General precautions

Whenever there is a communication between the right and left sides of the heart, it is absolutely necessary that all IV lines, including the injection ports, be completely free of air bubbles. In addition one should use extra caution not to push any air bubbles when injecting drugs through an IV line. Even though there is sufficient evidence to show that nitrous oxide does not change PVR or worsen pulmonary hypertension in pediatric patients, many anesthesiologists avoid the use of nitrous oxide in patients undergoing heart transplantation because of the fear of intravascular expansion of air bubbles. One should also take extreme precautions for the prevention of infections, as these children will be immunosuppressed. Appropriate perioperative prophylactic antibiotic therapy is used, with initial dosages administered 1 hour before skin incision.

### Induction of anesthesia

Almost all anesthesia induction techniques, such as mask induction by an inhaled anesthetic, IM or IV administration of ketamine, and IV administration of a narcotic, are usually tolerated by children with CHD if these techniques are carefully conducted with appropriate monitoring.* However, one should choose a technique that is optimal for a given patient based on the preoperative evaluation. In general, for sicker children with poor ventricular function, induction with IV ketamine and/or IV narcotics has been shown to be safe and effective. In these children all inhalational agents, including nitrous oxide, have been shown to depress myocardium and reduce systemic blood pressure to a greater degree than ketamine or narcotics.[46,64]

Most critically ill children arrive in the operating room with an IV line in place. In these children anesthesia can be induced either with small incremental doses of a narcotic (fentanyl 15 to 25 μg/kg or sufentanil 5 to 10 μg/kg) or an IV dose of ketamine (1 to 2 mg/kg) followed by a narcotic. Either a depolarizing (succinylcholine 2mg/kg) or a nondepolarizing muscle relaxant can be used to facilitate endotracheal tube placement. In children who come to the operating room without IV access, there are at least two techniques by which one can induce anesthesia. One is by slow mask induction with low concentrations of halothane (0.75% to 1%) and the other way is by an IM injection of ketamine (4 to 5 mg/kg). Once an adequate level of anesthesia is achieved, an IV line is placed, and then the trachea is intubated with the administration of atropine and a muscle relaxant.

*References 46, 56, 60, 62-64, 71, 85, 86.

### Maintenance of anesthesia

Once the trachea is intubated and IV access is established, we recommend turning off the inhaled anesthetic. Desired levels of anesthesia can be achieved with additional doses of either fentanyl (maximum total dose of 100 μg/kg) or sufentanil (maximum total dose of 30 μg/kg). Vecuronium, pancuronium, atracurium, or one of the newer nondepolarizing muscle relaxants (doxacurium or pipecuronium) can be used to maintain muscle paralysis throughout the operation. In patients in whom deep hypothermia and circulatory arrest are used, we routinely give 10 ml/kg of dextran 40 in dextrose 5% solution IV before the initiation of peripheral cooling (see Chapter 4 for more details). Heparin is administered by the surgeon into the right atrium just before placement of cannulas. Once the transplantation procedure is completed, the patient is rewarmed (with recirculation in patients with circulatory arrest) to normal body temperature and weaned from the ECC. Protamine is administered by the anesthesiologist at the conclusion of ECC. The majority of children require either isoproterenol (0.01 to 0.05 μg/kg/min), and/or dobutamine (4 to 6 μg/kg/min) infusions for hemodynamic stability both before and after coming off bypass. Atrial, junctional, and ventricular dysrhythmias are frequently seen in patients with denervated hearts, especially during the first 6 months following transplantation; these arrhythmias must be treated appropriately. One should remember the alterations of physiologic and pharmacologic responses to various stresses and drugs in the transplanted patient (Table 30–2).

### Fluid and blood management

Minimal amounts of crystalloid solution should be used for maintenance in patients with CHF before they go on bypass. Once a patient is disconnected from the ECC, blood loss should be replaced with an appropriate type of banked blood in addition to the maintenance crystalloid solution (usually 5% dextrose in 25% normal saline) to maintain a hematocrit of about 30%. One should avoid bradycardia and hypovolemia in transplant patients after bypass, as those conditions are poorly tolerated by these patients. As mentioned earlier, these children frequently require blood and blood products for hemostasis, as the length of suture lines and number of anastomotic sites are more extensive than seen in a typical operation.

### Ventilation

In the prebypass period, patients with an increased pulmonary blood flow and CHF may benefit from low fractional inspired oxygen concentration, avoidance of hyperventilation, and addition of low

**Table 30–2** Effects of various physiologic stimuli and drugs on the transplanted and normal hearts

| | Transplanted heart | | Normal heart | |
|---|---|---|---|---|
| | HR | AV cond | HR | AV cond |
| Anticholinergics | | | | |
| Atropine | — | — | ↑ | ↑ |
| Glycopyrrolate | — | — | ↑ | ↑ |
| Sympathetic Drugs | | | | |
| Methoxamine | — | — | ↓ | — |
| Phenylephrine | — | — | ↓ | — |
| Isoproterenol | ↑ ↑ | ↑ ↑ | ↑ | ↑ |
| Epinephrine | ↑ ↑ | ↑ ↑ | ↑ ↑ | ↑ ↑ |
| Norepinephrine | ↑ | ↑ | ↑ | ↑ |
| Dobutamine | ↑ ↑ | ↑ ↑ | ↑ | ↑ |
| Dopamine | →/↑ | →/↑ | ↑ | ↑ |
| Propranolol | ↓ ↓ | ↓ ↓ | ↓ | ↓ |
| Ephedrine | →/↑ | →/↑ | ↑ | ↑ |
| Anticholinesterases | | | | |
| Neostigmine | — | — | ↓ | ↓ |
| Pyridostigmine | — | — | ↓ | ↓ |
| Other drugs | | | | |
| Digoxin (acute) | — | ↓ | ↓ | ↓ |
| Digoxin (chronic) | ↓ | ↓ | ↓ | ↓ |
| Quinidine | ↓ | ↓ | ↑ | ↓ |
| Verapamil | ↓ | ↓ | ↓ | ↓ |
| Pancuronium | ↓ | ↓ | ↑ | ↑ |
| Physiologic stimuli | | | | |
| Occulocardiac reflex | — | — | ↓ | ↓ |
| Carotid baroreflex | — | — | ↓ | ↓ |
| Other vagovagal reflex | — | — | ↓ | ↓ |
| Exercise (increased activity) | →/↑ | ↑ | ↑ | ↑ |

—, No effect; ↓, decreased effect; →/↑, slightly increased effect; ↑, increased effect; ↑ ↑, markedly increased effect. (HR, heart rate, AV cond, AV nodal conduction).

levels of PEEP. Patients with a decreased pulmonary blood flow require high fractional inspired oxygen concentration, slight hyperventilation and avoidance of excessive positive pressure ventilation.

In the immediate postbypass period pulmonary vascular resistance is typically elevated; these patients will benefit from slight hyperventilation during this period.

## Anesthesia management of a transplanted patient for reoperation

Heart transplant recipients may return to the operating room for various types of surgery, such as for complications related to the transplantation operation, or for various other types of routine surgery unrelated to the transplant operation. These patients may be safely anesthetized with any of a number of techniques provided one understands the physiologic and pharmacologic derangements associated with autonomic denervation of the transplanted heart.

Preoperative evaluation should include a review of cardiovascular and other systems, just as with other patients with CHD undergoing surgery and anesthesia. The type of surgery should dictate the selection of monitoring devices. One should also remember that whether one uses general or conduction anesthesia, acute hypovolemia is poorly tolerated by the autonomically denervated heart. One should avoid β-blockers and ganglionic blockers (for example, d-tubocurare), as they can cause marked hypotension and a decrease in cardiac output. The effects of various direct, indirect, and mixed-action drugs on a transplanted heart are listed in Table 30–2. For obvious reasons the direct-acting drugs (phenylephrine, isoproterenol, dobutamine, and epinephrine) are preferable in these patients. Since these patients are immunosuppressed and the most common cause of postoperative death in them is infection, one should take all precautions to prevent infection.[73] Invasive monitoring should be limited to that which is necessary because of the risk of infections. Heart transplant recipients are also prone to both atrial and ventricular dysrhythmias during the first 6 months after transplantation. Prophylactic perioperative steroid therapy should be given to patients on maintenance steroids.[31,84] Cyclosporine, azathioprine, and steroids are known to antagonize the nondepolarizing muscle relaxants.

## IMMUNOLOGY AND IMMUNOSUPPRESSION

The immune system of the child presents management challenges in the posttransplant care of patients. Growth and development as well as the processing of new antigens must proceed in the setting of immune suppression to allow graft tolerance for successful outcome.

Neonates seem to demonstrate some degree of immune tolerance to the transplanted graft that is unique to this age group. Although the phenomenon is not well understood, it is thought that this tolerance in the first few days or weeks of life is related to prenatal suppressor mechanisms that persist temporarily after birth.[14,120] Natural suppressor and T suppressor (CD4+) cells appear not to circulate but remain activated for a time postpartum. Immunologically naive infants who receive allografts during the first month of life, even despite poor matches of major histocompatibility antigens, demonstrate excellent graft survival rates with only single or double drug immunosuppression.[14]

Lifelong immunosuppression is necessary to prevent rejection of the transplanted heart. Immunosuppressive protocols vary among transplant centers in regard to the dosage and combination of immunosuppressive agents administered for maintenance and rejection therapy. Cyclosporine (5-10 mg/kg) with dosage depending on hepatic and renal function and azathioprine (2 mg/kg) are administered preoperatively. Methylprednisolone (7.5 mg/kg) is given just prior to cross-clamp release and every 8 hours (3.5 mg/kg) for three doses postoperatively.

Maintenance therapy consists of cyclosporine (10 mg/kg/day, in two doses) initially, with dose adjustment to maintain whole blood cyclosporine levels determined by high-pressure liquid chromatography at 200 to 300 ng/ml, and azathioprine (1 to 2 mg/kg/day) to maintain a white blood cell count of approximately 5000/mm$^3$. No prednisone is given to neonates.

The success of the Loma Linda Medical Center with neonatal transplantation has confirmed that prednisone usually can be avoided in this age group.[29] Older children receive 0.8 mg/kg/day tapered to 0.2 mg/kg/day by 6 weeks postoperatively and eventually discontinued in all patients under 6 years of age.[79] The goal is discontinuation of prednisone to avoid complications of long-term steroid use such as diabetes mellitus, osteoporosis, aseptic necrosis of the hip, cushingoid features (truncal obesity, buffalo hump, and moon facies), fragile skin with easy bruisability, and poor wound healing. Optional adjunctive therapy to the maintenance protocol includes a course of antithymocyte serum (ATS) or OKT3 for the first 7 to 14 days after transplantation.[49]

The choice of agents for treatment of acute graft rejection depends on the severity of the episode and point of time following transplantation. Inpatients receive methylprednisolone (15 mg/kg/day) for three days to treat the first two episodes of rejection. If a third episode of rejection occurs, ATS (0.2 ml/kg/day) is given intravenously for 7 days.[79] For recalcitrant rejection refractory to conventional therapy, methotrexate, vincristine, total lymphoid irradiation, and mechanical support have been used.[14,21,50,66,79] Outpatient treatment of mild to moderate rejection consists of augmentation of prednisone dose, which is tapered to the previous level over 3 weeks. Research into induction of immune tolerance and new specific immunosuppressive agents may allow for fewer complications of immunosuppressive therapy.[103]

### Early postoperative care

***Low cardiac output.*** Transient myocardial dysfunction and heart denervation contribute to low cardiac output in the immediate postoperative period. Myocardial dysfunction is related to global myocardial ischemia that develops during the donor heart transport and to increased right ventricular afterload from preexisting pulmonary hypertension. As discussed above, β-adrenergic receptors remain intact and functional; therefore, heart rate, conduction, and contractility of the denervated heart increase in response to circulating catecholamines released from the adrenal gland. Compensatory heart rate changes during periods of hypotension or exercise are gradual, not immediate.[24] Inotropic agents such as isoproterenol and dopamine, vasodilator agents such as prostaglandin $E_1$ and nitroprusside, and temporary AV sequential pacing are commonly used to maximize cardiac output.[119]

***Respiratory dysfunction.*** Existing preoperative pulmonary edema, use of cardiopulmonary bypass, and deep hypothermic circulatory arrest (infants) may cause alterations in respiratory function. Fluid restriction and aggressive diuresis allow progressive weaning from mechanical ventilatory support. Chest physiotherapy may be necessary to clear pulmonary secretions and prevent atelectasis.

***Rejection.*** Acute graft rejection is a major complication and one of the leading causes of death in both adults and children, primarily within the first 6 to 12 months. Most children experience at least one rejection episode within the first 6 months after transplantation, with a mean frequency of 1 to 2.5 per patient in the pediatric population.[21]

Clinical signs and symptoms of rejection include fever, tachycardia, a gallop rhythm, arrhythmias, hypotension, jugular venous distention (older children), dyspnea, edema, and malaise. In infants generalized irritability, poor feeding, sustained tachycardia, tachypnea, and hepatomegaly may herald acute rejection. Frequently, however, clinical signs and symptoms are nonspecific, and they may be absent during a rejection episode. Therefore ongoing surveillance is necessary to allow early diagnosis and successful treatment of rejection.

The transvenous endomyocardial biopsy of the right ventricle remains the gold standard for diagnosing rejection.[26] In children over 6 years of age routine surveillance biopsies are performed weekly for 4 to 6 weeks with progressive tapering in frequency as biopsies remain negative and the patient remains stable. Specific interpretive differences between the endomyocardial biopsies of children and adults include a larger potential for sampling error in children, an increase in the normal cellularity of the immature myocardium, and a higher frequency of dystrophic calcifications and quilty lesions, which do not require treatment.

In infants and small children the invasive technique of right ventricular endomyocardial biopsy poses specific risks and difficulties.[21,24] Possible problems include eventual loss of venous access secondary to venous thrombosis and scarring, myocardial perforation (especially in the newborn and infant), and need for anesthesia. The Vanderbilt program largely relies on noninvasive surveillance with serial echocardiography, a system developed jointly at Vanderbilt and Loma Linda, in children under age 6 years.[28,42] The echocardiographic manifestations of rejection include increased septal and posterior wall thickness, decreased left ventricular volume, measures of LV systolic function (LV shortening fraction and LV posterior wall thickening fraction), and LV diastolic function (LV wall thinning).[21,67] One study revealed that compared with endomyocardial biopsy findings, echocardiographic findings in infants were found to have a predictive accuracy for presence or absence of rejection of 93%.[21] Echocardiograms initially are performed twice weekly for the first three months post transplant, tapering to weekly, then bimonthly, and then monthly over the first year after transplantation.

Recent work at Vanderbilt has demonstrated that positron emission technology can noninvasively detect acute rejection post transplant in experimental animals.[65] Whether this technology will be of use in the noninvasive detection of acute transplant rejection in the pediatric population remains to be investigated.

***Infection.*** Infection is a major cause of morbidity and mortality in the pediatric transplant population.[24] Transplant recipients are susceptible to multiple nosocomial and opportunistic pathogens, including bacterial, viral, fungal, and protozoal organisms. The lungs are a common target.[57] The risk of infection is greatest in the early postoperative period and during treatment of rejection episodes, when the level of immunosuppression is higher. Measures to reduce the risk of exposure include frequent hand washing, strict adherence to sterile technique, and careful attention to all IV sites, wounds, and the patient's skin and mouth. Fever in the immunocompromised host is generally defined as 99.5° F or higher and requires immediate and aggressive investigation, including multiple cultures.

Prophylactic IV immunoglobulin is commonly administered to neonates in the early postoperative period and to infants and young children during treatment of rejection to provide passive immunity against opportunistic viral pathogens, particularly cytomegalovirus.[13] In addition acyclovir may be given for the first several months to protect against CMV. Sulfamethoxazole or trimethoprim is administered to protect against *Pneumocystis carinii*. Nystatin is used to prevent oral and esophageal *Candida*. The *Varicella zoster* immunoglobulin vaccine is administered for recent exposure (preferably within 48 hours) to chicken pox. *Varicella zoster* infections are treated with acyclovir and usually are well tolerated, although hospitalization may be required for treatment and closer observation.[15] Prophylactic immunoglobulin is administered for exposure to measles, mumps, and rubella.

***Neurologic complications.*** A recent report by Martin and associates[72] describes the frequency of early and late neurologic complications after heart transplantation in children. Seizure was the most common complication encountered. Long-term disability was rare.

## LONG-TERM CONCERNS

### Graft coronary artery disease

Accelerated coronary artery disease is a known chronic sequela in adult heart transplant recipients. There is increasing evidence that children also are at risk for this serious complication, limiting the probability of long-term survival.[93,97,113] The reported incidence ranges from 15% to 28% in children surviving 1 month to 6 years.[4,14,18,89,112] The pathogenesis is still unclear, although an immunologic injury to the coronary artery endothelium (a manifestation of chronic rejection) is thought to be the triggering mechanism.[89] An association with CMV infection has also been observed,[14] adding further credence to the theory that graft atherosclerosis is a manifestation of chronic graft rejection. Other theories suggest that it is a complication of immune suppression itself, possibly a side effect of a particular drug. The causes and interruption of graft atherosclerosis are under intensive investigation.

Graft coronary artery disease varies from the more typical coronary artery disease found in nontransplanted hearts in that the lesions tend to be concentric, with a diffuse distribution involving large epicardial arteries and small intramyocardial branches. The diffuse nature and small vessel distribution of the disease generally prohibit standard medical treatment such as balloon angioplasty or coronary artery bypass grafting. Because the transplanted heart is denervated, the clinical symptom angina pectoris is usually absent. Possible risk factors include hyperlipidemia, CMV infection, and frequent and recurrent rejection episodes.[4,24,47,89] Often the first indication of graft coronary artery disease is a myocardial infarction pattern on a routine ECG. Unfortunately, the first sign may be sudden death. Annual coronary arteriography is performed to screen for the development of graft coronary artery disease and to monitor progression of the disease. Positron emission tomography has recently shown utility in demonstrating alterations in myocardial blood flow consistent with this global atherosclerosis and may provide a method to diagnose graft atherosclerosis in its early stages and a means to assess therapy.

Currently retransplantation tends to be the only effective treatment. There is experimental evidence that calcium channel blockade may slow the progression of graft atherosclerosis.[99]

### Lymphoproliferative disease

There is an increased incidence of certain types of cancers in organ transplant recipients of all ages as compared with the general population. Lymphomas, the most common form of malignancy, account for 21% of all neoplasms in transplant recipients and seem to develop in response to severe immunosuppression.[91] It is suggested that some of the posttransplant lymphomas in children are associated with primary infection by Epstein-Barr virus.[24,115] Treatment includes reduction of immunosuppressive therapy and administration of acyclovir.

### Growth and development

Growth retardation is one of the major concerns in young children who receive heart transplants. Chronic administration of steroids is considered the offending agent. Although some children display a normal growth pattern while receiving steroid therapy, others do not.[47,103,115] Attempts to taper to alternate-day prednisone regimens and possibly to discontinue prednisone altogether may help prevent subnormal growth. Administration of recombinant growth hormone to children who continue to require prednisone therapy also may improve growth velocity.[110] Infants undergoing heart transplantation without prednisone therapy appear to grow and develop normally. In a study of linear growth at Loma Linda,[19] infants transplanted at less than 6 months of age were evaluated at 6-month intervals up to 2 years post transplantation. Some 86% exhibited normal linear growth measurements, defined as between the fifth and ninety-fifth percentile. Most of the children below the fifth percentile were receiving long-term steroid therapy. Of children undergoing bone age studies, 74% exhibitied normal bone maturation. Delayed bone maturation was thought to occur secondary to corticosteroid use.[23] Experimental evidence demonstrates that the heart does increase in size commensurate with the increased physiologic demands of growth,[23] but controversy exists as to whether this is true growth or simply adaptation to the increased metabolic needs of the body.[1]

Other studies have also documented favorable development in children after heart transplantation.[19] Of infants who survived transplantation, 89% were neurologically normal at an average follow-up of 14 months. In addition, 90% had normal audiologic evaluations.

### Patient and family education

Education of the pediatric recipient and family regarding the lifelong medical regimen is an ongoing process, starting preoperatively and continuing throughout the posttransplant period. Outpatient visits provide an excellent opportunity for discussion of educational and emotional concerns. Parents must cope with considerable stresses related to the uncertainty of the child's health and the increased demands on time and energy created by the child's chronic condition.[23] Once home, the healthy recipient will want to explore physical activities previously not possible due to the preoperative illness. Parents need to exercise reasonable caution without being overprotective. General educational needs of pediatric recipients of all ages and their families include the physiologic changes associated with transplantation; purpose, administration, and side effects of medications; dietary restrictions; and day to day monitoring of growth and well-being as well as surveillance for signs of infection or rejection. Specific educational needs related to certain pediatric age groups include administration of immunizations, activity guidelines, and unique problems of the adolescent population.

### Immunizations

Immunizations are administered according to the usual well-child schedule. However, only inactive vaccines are given. For polio the Salk inactivated vaccine is substituted for the Sabin active oral vaccine. Other family members who have not been immunized also should receive Salk vaccine, as the active virus is excreted in the stool for up to 2 months, with risk of transmission to the immunocompromised recipient. MMR (measles, mumps, rubella) is a live vaccine and is not recommended for the transplant recipient at this time, but siblings should receive MMR at the appropriate age. Immunizations are not given during an acute febrile illness, episodes of acute rejection, or immunoglobulin therapy. Antibody titers to inactivated vaccines have determined immunizations to be successful in 80% to 100% of children treated.[19] Consensus regarding immunization for hepatitis B has not been reached.

### Activity

For infants and preschool children, day care centers should be avoided during the early months after transplantation to minimize exposure to pathogens during this period of great immunosuppression. Returning to school usually can be considered 6 months postoperatively. Medical procedures should be scheduled to avoid excessive absenteeism from school. Participation in sports must be considered on an individual basis. Contact sports may be contraindicated in the patient requiring steroid therapy because of the predisposition to bone and joint injuries. Adolescents are encouraged to participate in a structured outpatient exercise rehabilitation program for approximately 6 weeks to improve physical conditioning and exercise tolerance for eventual return to school, work, or home-related responsibilities.

### Adolescence issues

Body image, identification with peer groups, and a sense of independence are important concerns during adolescence. Changes in physical appearance, for example, weight gain, obesity, cushingoid facies, acne related to steroid therapy, hirsutism, gingival hyperplasia, tremor (related to cyclosporine therapy), and the sternotomy scar can lead to feelings of "being different" from other teenagers and can create low self-esteem. Mood swings, exacerbated by steroid use, also contribute to the struggles. Posttransplant monitoring may require many invasive procedures. Preoperative counseling of children of appropriate age helps to create reasonable expectations. Interventions include tapering of steroid dosage, exercise and weight loss programs, aggressive treatment of acne, depilatory creams to remove excess hair, regular dental examinations, and psychologic counseling.[19] Meeting with other adolescent recipients may provide a supportive peer group that identifies with day to day adjustments. Adolescent recipients should assume primary responsibility for medications as soon as possible to provide them with a sense of control.

Noncompliance with the medication regimen can be a problem in this population and may lead to acute rejection.[18] Any noncompliant behavior must be explored carefully to determine and treat the cause. Administering medications before and after school hours diminishes the appearance of being different in the presence of peers and may help reduce the likelihood of noncompliance. Adolescent recipients who are sexually active need counseling on birth control methods and sexually transmitted diseases. Birth control pills should be used with caution by patients receiving cyclosporine because both medications can cause hypertension.

## SOCIAL AND ETHICAL ISSUES

### Diagnosis of brain death

Extraordinary emotions surround the death of a child. These affect both parents and caretakers and clearly influence initiation of discussions of organ donation by medical personnel and receptiveness to these ideas by parents. Concern over accurate diagnosis of brain death in infants and children with immature neurologic systems led to guidelines established by a multidisciplinary task force in 1987.[114] Ashwal and associates[8-10] found that these guidelines could reasonably be extended to preterm and term newborns and that accurate diagnosis of brain death required consideration of developmental influences and confounding factors such as phenobarbital administration, duration of asphyxia, developmental abnormalities, and hypotension as well as neurologic assessment, ECG and cerebral blood flow detection studies.

### Anencephalic donors

Despite current guidelines for determination of brain death, controversy exists regarding the ethical use of hearts from anencephalic donors for transplantation.[58,76] Current law does not allow determination of brain death in anencephalic children with signs of brain stem function. A study by Peabody and colleagues[90] describes the difficulty of treating anencephalic infants intensively from birth or waiting for signs of imminent cardiac death with subsequent resuscitation. The latter is often not associated with complete cessation of brain stem function and allows deterioration of organ function, often to the point of unsuitability for transplantation.

### Cost of transplantation

Rising health care costs and universal health insurance are matters of intense debate at state and national levels. New life-saving technologies such as heart transplantation in the pediatric population do not come without significant cost. Transplantation costs for the initial year range from $75,000 to $175,000. While the overall expense of pediatric heart transplant is clearly capped by the finite number of donors available, cost issues remain. Expanding limitations in pediatric heart transplantation may await changes in our health care delivery system.

## THE FUTURE

The future of heart transplantation in children will involve the development of new, more specific immunosuppressive agents to induce graft-immune tolerance without significant side effects, sensitive and specific noninvasive diagnosis of rejection, and prevention of accelerated coronary artery disease. In addition, quality of life issues in children require further study to establish the long-term benefits of transplantation in this population and to justify such aggressive and expensive therapy. The scarcity of donors will continue to limit the availability of the procedure to those in need. Changes in current organ donation practices and the use of xenografts remain possible alternatives. Continued efforts in education of lay persons and health professionals regarding organ donation and promotion of state and federal legislation that supports transplantation will be critical.

## REFERENCES


1. Addonizio LJ, Gersony WM: The transplanted heart in the pediatric patient: growth or adaptation *Circulation* 85(4):1624, 1992 (editorial).
2. Addonizio LJ, Gersony WM, Robbins RC et al: Elevated pulmonary vascular resistance and cardiac transplantation, *Circulation* 76(suppl 5):V52, 1987.
3. Addonizio LJ, Hsu DT, Fuzesi L et al: Optimal timing of pediatric heart transplantation, *Circulation* 80(suppl 3): 84, 189.
4. Addonizio LJ, Hsu DT, Smith CR et al: Late complications in pediatric cardiac transplant recipients, *Circulation* 82(suppl 5):295, 1990.
5. Allard M, Assaad A, Bailey L et al: Surgical techniques in pediatric heart transplantation, *J Heart Lung Transplant* 10(5 pt 2):808, 1991.
6. Alonso-de-Begona J, Gundry SR, Nehlsen-Cannarella SL et al: HLA matching and its effect on infant and pediatric cardiac graft survival, *Transplant Proc* 23(1 pt 2):1139, 1991.
7. Arrowood MA, Mohanty PK, Hodgson JMcB et al: Ventricular sensory endings mediate reflex bradycardia during coronary arteriography in humans, *Circulation* 80:1293, 1989.
8. Ashwal S: Brain death in the newborn, *Clin Perinatol* 16:501, 1989.
9. Ashwal S, Caplan AL, Cheatham WA et al: Social and ethical controversies in pediatric heart transplantation, *J Heart Lung Transplant* 10(5 pt 2):860, 1991.
10. Ashwal S, Schneider S: Brain death in the newborn, *Pediatr* 84:429, 1989.
11. Backer CL, Zales VR, Idriss FS et al: Heart transplantation in infants and children, *J Heart Lung Transplant* 11(2 pt 1):311, 1992.
12. Bailey LL, Concepcion W, Shattuck H et al: Method of heart transplantation for treatment of hypoplastic left heart syndrome, *J Thorac Cardiovasc Surg* 92:1, 1986.
13. Bailey LL, Assaad AN, Trimm RF et al: Orthotopic transplantation during early infancy as therapy for incurable congenital heart disease, *Ann Surg* 208:279, 1988.
14. Bailey LL, Kahan B, Nehlsen-Cannarella S et al: Session 5: the neonatal immune system: window of opportunity? *J Heart Lung Transplant* 10:828, 1991.
15. Bailey LL, Nehlsen-Cannarella SL, Concepcion W et al: Baboon to human cardiac xenotransplantation in a neonate, *JAMA* 254:3321, 1985.
16. Bailey LL, Nehlsen-Cannarella SL, Doroshow RW et al: Cardiac allotransplantation in newborns as therapy for hypoplastic left heart syndrome, *N Engl J Med* 315:949, 1986.
17. Barnard CN: A human cardiac transplant: an interim report of a successful operation performed at Groote Schur Hospital, Capetown, *S Afr Med J* 41:1271, 1967.
18. Baum D, Bernstein D, Starnes VA et al: Pediatric heart transplantation at Stanford: results of a 15-year experience, *Pediatr* 88:203, 1991.
19. Baum MF, Cutler DC, Fricker FJ et al: Session 7: physiologic and psychological growth and development in pediatric heart transplant recipients, *J Heart Lung Transplant* 10:848, 1991.
20. Baum V: Anesthesia for heart and heart-lung transplantation. In Kapoor AS, Laks H, Schroeder J et al, editors: *Cardiomyopathies and cardiopulmonary transplanation,* New York, 1990, McGraw-Hill.
21. Behrendt DM, Billingham ME, Boucek MM et al: Session 6: rejection/infection: the limits of heart transplantation success, *J Heart Lung Transplant* 10:841, 1991.
22. Benson L, Freedom RM, Gersony W et al: Cardiac replacement in infants and children: indications and limitations, *J Heart Lung Transplant* 10(5 pt 2):791, 1991.
23. Bernstein D, Kolla S, Miner M et al: Cardiac growth after pediatric heart transplantation, *Circulation* 85(4):1433, 1992.
24. Bernstein D, Starnes VA, Baum D: Pediatric heart transplantation, *Adv Pediatr* 37:413, 1990.
25. Bharati S, Nordenberg A, Brock RR et al: Hypoplastic left heart syndrome with dysplastic pulmonary valves with stenosis, *Pediatr Cardiol* 5:127, 1984.
26. Billingham ME: Diagnosis of cardiac rejection by endomyocardial biopsy, *J Heart Transplant* 1:25, 1982.
27. Borel JF: Immunosuppressive properties of cyclosporin A, *Transplant Proc* 12:233, 1980.

28. Boucek MM, Hodgkin DD, Mathis CM et al: Accuracy of echocardiographic rejection surveillance in infant cardiac transplantation, *J Heart Transplant* 9:63, 1990.
29. Boucek MM, Kanakriyeh MS, Mathis CM et al: Cardiac transplantation in infancy: donors and recipients, *J Pediatr* 116:171, 1990.
30. Braunlin EA, Hunter DW, Canter CE et al: Coronary artery disease in pediatric cardiac transplant recipients receiving triple-drug immunosuppression, *Circulation* 84(suppl 5):III303, 1991.
31. Bricker SRW, Sugden JC: Anesthesia for surgery in a patient with a transplanted heart, *Br J Anaesth* 57:634, 1985.
32. Cannom DS, Graham AF, Harrison DC: Electrophysiological studies in the denervated transplanted heart, *Circ Res* 32:268, 1973.
33. Cannom DS, Rider AK, Stinson EB et al: Electrophysiologic studies in denervated human heart II: response to norepinephrine, isoproterenol and propranolol, *Am J Cardiol* 36:859, 1975.
34. Cavarocchi N, Carp N, Mitra A et al: Successful heart transplantation in recipients with recent preoperative pulmonary emboli, *J Heart Transplant* 8:494, 1989.
35. Chartrand C: Pediatric cardiac transplantation despite atrial and venous return anomalies, *Ann Thorac Surg* 52(3):716, 1991.
36. Chartrand C, Dumont L, Stanley P: Pediatric cardiac transplantation, *Transplant Proc* 21(2):3349, 1989.
37. Chartrand C, Guerin R, Kangah M et al: Pediatric heart transplantation: surgical considerations for congenital heart disease, *J Heart Transplant* 9(6):608, 1990.
38. Chiavarelli M, Boucek MM, Nehlsen-Cannarella SL et al: Neonatal cardiac transplantation, *Arch Surg* 127:1072, 1992.
39. Cooley DA: Pediatric heart transplantation in historical perspective, *J Heart Lung Transplant* 10(5 pt 2):787, 1991.
40. Cooley DA, Bloodwell RD, Hallman GL et al: Organ transplantation for advanced cardiopulmonary disease, *Ann Thorac Surg* 8:30, 1969.
41. Cooper MM, Fuzesi L, Addonizio LJ et al: Pediatric heart transplantation after operations involving the pulmonary arteries, *J Thorac Cardiovasc Surg* 102(3):386, 1991.
42. Dodd DA, Frist WH, Merrill WH et al: Pretransplant and posttransplant management of the infant with hypoplastic left heart syndrome, *Transplant Science* 2:5, 1992.
43. Dodd DA, Merrill WH, Frist WH et al: Echo surveillance for rejection following infant heart transplantation, *J Heart Lung Transplant* 11:205, 1992, (abstract).
44. Dong E Jr, Hurley EJ, Lower RR et al: Performance of the heart 2 years after autotransplantation, *Surgery* 56:270, 1964.
45. Ellenbogen KA, Mohanty PK, Szentpetery S et al: Baroreflex abnormalities in heart failure: reversal after orthotopic cardiac transplantation, *Circulation* 79:51, 1989.
46. Friesen RH, Henry DB: Cardiovascular changes in preterm neonates receiving isoflurane, halothane, fentanyl, and ketamine, *Anesthesiology* 64:238, 1986.
47. Fricker FJ, Trento A, Griffith BP: Pediatric cardiac transplantation, *Cardiovasc Clin* 20:223, 1990.
48. Frist WH, Fanning WJ: Donor management and matching, *Cardiol Clin* 8:55, 1990.
49. Frist WH, Merrill WH, Eastburn TE et al: Nashville antithymocyte serum: a safe and efficacious agent for prophylaxis for heart transplantation, *Transplant Proc* 23:1160, 1991.
50. Frist WH, Winterland AW, Gerhardt EB et al: Total lymphoid radiation in heart transplantation: adjuvant treatment for recurrent rejection, *Ann Thorac Surg* 48:863, 1989.
51. Galantowicz ME, Stolar CJH: Extracorporeal membrane oxygenation for perioperative support in pediatric heart transplantation, *J Thorac Cardiovasc Surg* 102:148, 1991.
52. Gersony WM: Cardiac transplantation in infants and children, *Pediatrics* 116:266, 1990.
53. Gilbert EM, Eiswirth CC, Mealey PC et al: β-Adrenergic supersensitivity of the transplanted human heart is presynaptic in origin, *Circulation* 79:344, 1989.
54. Goodman DJ, Rossen RM, Cannom DS et al: Effect of digoxin on atrioventricular conduction: studies in patients with and without cardiac autonomic innervation, *Circulation* 51:251, 1975.
55. Goodman DJ, Rossen RM, Rider AK et al: The effect of cycle length on cardiac refractory periods in the denervated human heart, *Am Heart J* 91:332, 1976.
56. Greeley WJ, Bushman G, Davis DP et al: Comparative effects of halothane and ketamine on systemic arterial oxygen saturation in children with cyanotic heart disease, *Anesthesiology* 65:666, 1986.
57. Green M, Wald ER, Fricker FJ et al: Infections in pediatric orthotopic heart transplant recipients, *Pediatr Infect Dis J* 8:87, 1989.
58. Guidelines for the determination of brain death in children, *J Pediatr* 80:298, 1987.
59. Hansen DD, Hickey PR: Anesthetic technique for heart surgery in neonates. In Jacobs ML, Norwood WI, editors: *Pediatric cardiac surgery: current issues,* Boston, 1992, Butterworth-Heineman.
60. Hansen DD, Hickey PR: Anesthesia for hypoplastic left heart syndrome: use of high-dose fentanyl in 30 neonates, *Anesth Analg* 65:127, 1986.
61. Hehrlein FW, Netz H, Moosdorf R et al: Pediatric heart transplantation for congenital heart disease and cardiomyopathy, *Ann Thorac Surg* 52:112, 1991.
62. Hickey PR, Hansen DD: Fentanyl- and sufentanil-oxygen-pancuronium anesthesia for cardiac surgery in infants, *Anesth Analg* 63:117, 1984.
63. Hickey PR, Hansen DD, Cramolini GM et al: Pulmonary and systemic hemodynamic responses to ketamine in infants with normal and elevated pulmonary vascular resistance, *Anesthesiology* 62:287, 1985.
64. Hickey PR, Hansen DD, Strafford M et al: Pulmonary and systemic effects of nitrous oxide in infants with normal and elevated pulmonary vascular resistance, *Anesthesiology* 65:374, 1986.
65. Hoff SJ, Stewart JR, Frist WH et al: Noninvasive detection of heart transplant rejection with positron emission tomography, *Ann Thorac Surg* 53:572, 1991.
66. Hunt SA, Strober S, Hoppe RT et al: Total lymphoid irradiation for treatment of intractable cardiac allograft rejection, *J Heart Lung Transplant* 10:211, 1991.
67. Johnson J: A new beginning: current trends in pediatric heart transplantation, *Focus on Critical Care* 18:23, 1991.
68. Kantrowitz A, Haller JD, Joos H et al: Transplantation of the heart in an infant and an adult, *Am J Cardiol* 22:782, 1968.
69. Kaye MP, Kriett JM: Pediatric heart transplantation: the world experience, *J Heart Lung Transplant* 10(5 pt 2):856, 1991.
70. Kempsford RD, Hearse DJ: Protection of immature myocardium during global ischemia, *J Thorac Cardiovasc Surg* 97:856, 1989.
71. Laishley RS, Burrows FA, Lerman J et al: Effect of anesthetic induction regimens on oxygen saturation in cyanotic congenital heart disease, *Anesthesiology* 65:673, 1986.
72. Martin AB, Bricker JT, Fishman M et al: Neurologic complications of heart transplantation in children, *J Heart Lung Transplant* 11:933, 1992.

73. Mason JW, Stinson EB, Hunt SA: Infections after cardiac transplantation: relation to rejection therapy, *Ann Intern Med* 85:69, 1976.
74. Mason JW, Winkel RA, Rider AK et al: The electrophysiologic effects of quinidine in the transplanted human heart, *J Clin Invest* 59:481, 1977.
75. Mayer JE Jr, Perry S, O'Brien P et al: Orthotopic heart transplantation for complex congenital heart disease, *J Thorac Cardiovasc Surg* 99(3):484, 1990.
76. Medical Task Force on Anencephaly: The infant with anencephaly, *N Engl J Med* 322:669, 1990.
77. Menkis AH, McKenzie FN, Novick RJ et al: Expanding applicability of transplantation after multiple prior palliative procedures, *Ann Thorac Surg* 52(3):722, 1991.
78. Menkis AH, McKenzie FN, Novick RJ et al: Special consideration for heart transplantation in congenital heart diseases, *J Heart Transplant* 9:602, 1990.
79. Merrill WH, Frist WH, Stewart JR et al: Heart transplantation in children, *Ann Surg* 213:393, 1991.
80. Michler RE, Rose EA: Pediatric heart and heart-lung transplantation, *Ann Thorac Surg* 52(3):708, 1991.
81. Mohanty PK, Sowers JR, Thames MD et al: Myocardial norepinephrine, epinephrine and dopamine concentrations after cardiac autotransplantation in dogs, *Am J Coll Cardiol* 7:414, 1986.
82. Mohanty PK, Thames MD, Capehart J et al: Afferent reinnervation of the autotransplanted heart in dogs, *J Am Coll Cardiol* 7:419, 1986.
83. Mohanty PK, Thames MD, Sowers JR et al: Impairment of cardiopulmonary baroreflex following cardiac transplantation in humans, *Circulation* 75:914, 1987.
84. Moore FD: *Metabolic care of the surgical patient,* Philadelphia. Saunders.
85. Moore RA, Yang SS, McNicholas KW: Hemodynamic and anesthetic effects of sufentanil as the sole anesthetic for pediatric cardiac surgery, *Anesthesiology* 62:725, 1985.
86. Morray JP, Lynn AM, Stamm SJ: Hemodynamic effects of ketamine in children with congenital heart disease, *Anesth Analg* 63:895, 1984.
87. Morris JA Jr, Wilcox TR, Frist WH: Pediatric organ donation: the paradox of organ shortage despite the remarkable willingness of families to donate, *Pediatr* 89:411, 1992.
88. Orlick AE, Ricci DR, Alderman EL: Effects of $\alpha$-adrenergic blockade on coronary hemodynamics, *J Clin Invest* 62:459, 1978.
89. Pahl E, Fricker FJ, Armgwage J et al: Coronary arteriosclerosis in pediatric heart transplant survivors: limitation of long-term survival, *J Pediatr* 116:177, 1990.
90. Peabody JL, Emery JR, Ashwal S: Experience with anencephalic infants as prospective organ donors, *N Engl J Med* 321:344, 1989.
91. Penn I: Cancers complicating organ transplantation, *N Engl J Med* 323:1767, 1990.
92. Pennington DG, Noedel N, McBride LR et al: Heart transplantation in children: an international survey, *Ann Thorac Surg* 52(3):710, 1991.
93. Pennock JL, Oyer PE, Reitz BA et al: Cardiac transplantation in perspective for the future: survival, complications, rehabilitation and cost, *J Thorac Cardiovasc Surg* 83:168, 1982.
94. Pope SE, Stinson EB, Daughters JS et al: Exercise response of the denervated heart in long-term cardiac transplant recipients, *Am J Cardiol* 46:213, 1980.
95. Port JD, Gilbert EM, Larrabee P et al: Neurotransmitter depletion compromises the ability of indirect-acting amines to provide inotropic support in the failing human heart, *Circulation* 81:929, 1990.
96. Port JD, Skerl L, O'Connell JB et al: Increased expression of $\beta_2$-adrenergic receptors in surgically denervated, previously transplanted human ventricular myocardium, *J Am Coll Cardiol* 15:84A, 1990.
97. Radley-Smith R, Yacoub MF: Heart and heart-lung transplantation in children, *Circulation* 76(suppl 4):24, 1987.
98. Rowan RA, Billingham ME: Myocardial innervation in long-term heart transplant survivors: a quantitative ultrastructural survey, *J Heart Transplant* 7:448, 1988.
99. Schroeder JS, Gao S, Hunt SA et al: Accelerated graft coronary artery disease: diagnosis and prevention, *J Heart Lung Transplant* 11:S258, 1992.
100. Shumway NE, Dong E Jr, Stinson EB: Surgical aspects of cardiac transplantation in man, *Bull N Y Acad Med* 45:387, 1969.
101. Smith ML, Ellenbogen KA, Eckberg DL et al: Reversal of abnormal parasympathetic control of heart period following cardiac transplantation, *J Am Coll Cardiol* 14:106, 1989.
102. Smith ML, Ellenbogen KA, Eckberg DL et al: Subnormal parasympathetic activity after cardiac transplantation, *Am J Cardiol* 66:1243, 1990.
103. Starnes VA, Bernstein D, Oyer PE et al: Heart transplantation in children, *J Heart Transplant* 8:20, 1989.
104. Starnes VA, Griffen ML, Pitlick PT et al: Current approaches to hypoplastic left heart syndrome, *J Thorac Cardiovasc Surg* 104:189, 1992.
105. Starnes VA, Miller JA, Gamberg PL et al: Heart transplantation in children with cardiomyopathies. In Jacobs ML, Norwood WI, editors: *Pediatric cardiac surgery: current issues,* Butterworth-Heineman, 1992, Boston.
106. Starnes VA, Oyer PE, Bernstein D et al: Heart, heart-lung, and lung transplantation in the first year of life, *Ann Thor Surg* 53(2):306, 1992.
107. Starnes VA, Stinson EB, Oyer PE et al: Cardiac transplantation in children and adolescents, *Circulation* 76(suppl 5):V43, 1987.
108. Stinson EB, Griepp RB, Schroeder JS et al: Hemodynamic observations 1 and 2 years after cardiac transplantation in man, *Circulation* 45:1183, 1972.
109. Tatebe S, Nakayawa M, Mizamura H et al: Myocardial protection of neonatal heart by cardioplegic solution with recombinant superoxide dismutase, *Ann Thorac Surg* 54:124, 1992.
110. Tejani A, Ingulli E: Growth in children post transplantation and methods to optimize posttransplant growth, *Clinical Transpl* 5:214, 1991.
111. Thames MD, Zubair-ul-Hassan, Brackett NC Jr et al: Plasma renin responses to hemorrhage after cardiac autotransplantation, *Am J Physiol* 221:1115, 1971.
112. Trento A, Griffith BP, Fricker FJ, et al: Lessons learned in pediatric heart transplantation, *Ann Thorac Surg* 48:617, 1989.
113. Uretsky BF, Murali S, Reddy PS et al: Development of coronary artery disease in cardiac transplant patients receiving immunosuppressive therapy with cyclosporine and prednisone, *Circulation* 76:827, 1987.
114. Uzark K, Crowley D: Family stress after pediatric heart transplantation, *Progress in Cardiovascular Nursing* 4:23, 1989.
115. Uzark K, Crowley D, Callow L et al: Linear growth after pediatric heart transplantation, *Circulation* 78(suppl 2):492, 1988.
116. Veasy LG, Blalock RC, Orth JL et al: Intraaortic balloon pumping in infants and children, *Circulation* 68:1095, 1983.
117. Victor R, Scherrer U, Vissing S et al: Orthostatic stress activates sympathetic outflow in patients with heart transplants, *Circulation* 78:II365, 1988 (abstract).

118. Weinberg PM, Peiper K, Hackney JR: Fetal hydrops in a newborn with hypoplastic left heart syndrome: tricuspid valve "stopper," *J Am Coll Cardiol* 6:1365, 1985.
119. Whitehead B, James I, Helms P et al: Intensive care management of children following heart and heart-lung transplantation, *Intensive Care Med* 16(7):426, 1990.
120. Yacoub MH, Radley-Smith R: Heart transplantation in infants and children, *Sem Thorac Cardiovasc Surg* 2:206, 1990.
121. Yosuf S, Theodoropoulous S, Mathas CJ et al: Increased sensitivity of the denervated transplanted human heart to isoprenaline both before and after β-adrenergic blockage, *Circulation* 75:696, 1976.

# 31 Mitral Valve Prolapse Syndrome (Barlow's Syndrome)

***Jay Kambam** and **P. Syamasundar Rao***



Although mitral valve prolapse syndrome (MVPS) was described a century ago by Osler[17] and Griffith,[15] it was more widely recognized as a separate clinical entity only after Barlow in 1963 demonstrated angiographically the association of billowing of the mitral valve leaflets into the left atrium and late systolic mitral regurgitation with the clinical syndrome of midsystolic click and late systolic murmur.[1-3] The exact incidence of MVPS in pediatric population is not known, but it appears to be in the order of 1.4%, much lower than that reported in adult patients (6.3%).[8,16] It is commonly diagnosed in mid childhood or early adolescence.[16] Female patients are affected more than male patients by a ratio of 2:1.[5,12] Several names have been used to describe this syndrome, and some of them are listed in the box. The natural history of MVPS is benign in the great majority of cases. An occasional patient develops complications such as severe mitral valve regurgitation, cerebral complications, ventricular fibrillation, and sudden death.[8]

Since systolic prolapse of one or both mitral valve leaflets is the common denominator in these cases, the disorder is now generally called the mitral valve prolapse syndrome.

## CLASSIFICATION

MVPS can be classified into two principal types, cases associated with other conditions and sporadic cases without apparent secondary conditions.[6,8,9,13]

### Cases associated with other conditions

1. Familial or genetically predetermined conditions
   a. Homocystinuria
   b. Marfan's syndrome or similar syndromes
   c. Osteogenesis imperfecta
   d. Pseudoxanthoma elasticum
   e. Hurler's syndrome
   f. Von Willebrand's disease
   g. Pectus excavatum, scoliosis or other spinal bone abnormalities
   h. Polycystic disease
2. Nonfamilial or nongenetically predetermined conditions
   a. Kawasaki's syndrome
   b. Cardiomyopathy
   c. Hyperthyroidism (Graves' disease)
3. Other congenital heart defects

### Sporadic cases without apparent associated secondary conditions

Shortened platelet survival time
Thromboembolic phenomena

## PATHOLOGIC ANATOMY AND PHYSIOLOGY

These are the various components of the mitral valve complex:

Anterior and posterior leaflets
Annulus or ring
Chordae tendineae

Papillary muscles (anterolateral and posteromedial)

The mitral valve has two leaflets, an anterior and a posterior leaflet (Fig. 31–1). The base of the leaflets is attached to the annulus, or ring, and the free edges of the leaflets are tethered by delicate chordae tendineae to the papillary muscles. The papillary muscles are firmly attached to the endocardium. Main pathologic features are shown in the box.

The anterior leaflet of the mitral valve of the left atrium is in close association with the outflow tract of the left ventricle. The open anterior leaflet forms the lateral aspect of the left ventricular outflow tract, and the closed leaflet forms the floor of the left atrium. The most important function of chordae tendineae is to prevent herniation of leaflets into the left atrium when left ventricular pressure rises. During ventricular systole, as the ventricular radius rapidly decreases, the contraction of the papillary muscle maintains the tension of the chordae tendineae on the valvular leaflets. A malfunction of any component of the mitral valve complex can result in a dysfunction of the mitral valve itself.

In a normal heart anterior and posterior leaflets of the mitral valve are of equal size, and they open and close equally during ventricular diastole and systole respectively. In a child with mitral valve prolapse the posterior leaflet of the mitral valve is abnormally large and redundant, bulging into the left atrium (Fig. 31–2). In the majority of patients the posterior leaflet is severely involved and the

### TERMINOLOGY USED IN MITRAL VALVE PROLAPSE CASES

**Clinical**

Midsystolic click—late systolic murmur syndrome

**General**

Auscultatory—ECG syndrome
Barlow's syndrome
DaCosta's syndrome
Effort syndrome
Mitral prolapse
Neurocirculatory asthenia
Prolapsed leaflet

**Morphologic**

Mucinous degeneration of the mitral valve
Myxoid degeneration of the mitral valve
Myxomatous degeneration of the mitral valve

### PATHOLOGIC FEATURES OF MITRAL VALVE PROLAPSE

1. Leaflets increased in area
2. Folding convolution, and doming upward toward the atrium
3. Posterior leaflet more frequently and severely involved
4. Central, medial, and lateral scallops of posterior leaflet involved in that order
5. Medial scallop of anterior leaflet frequently involved

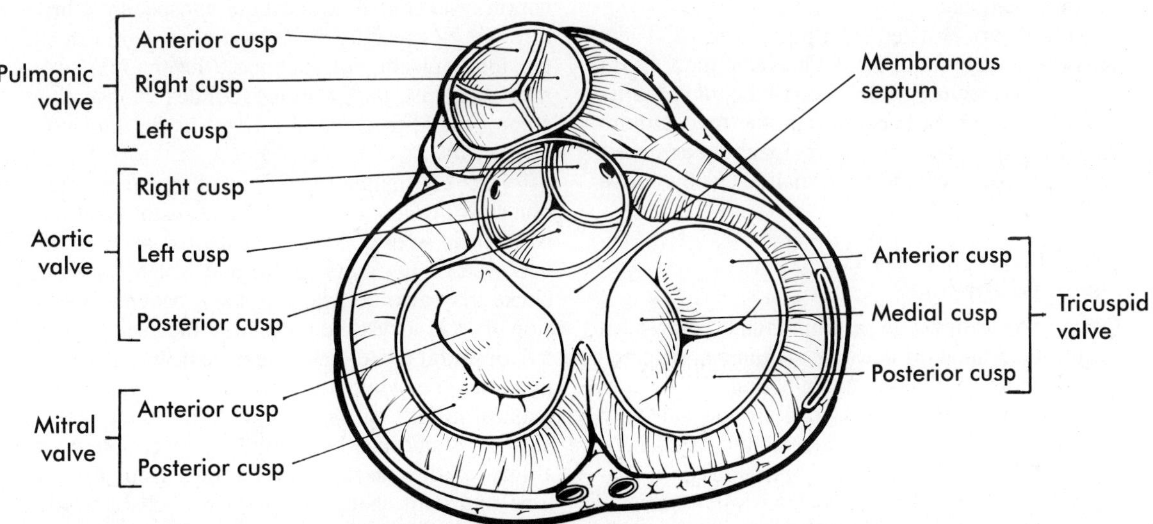


**Figure 31–1** Normal anatomy of the heart valves.

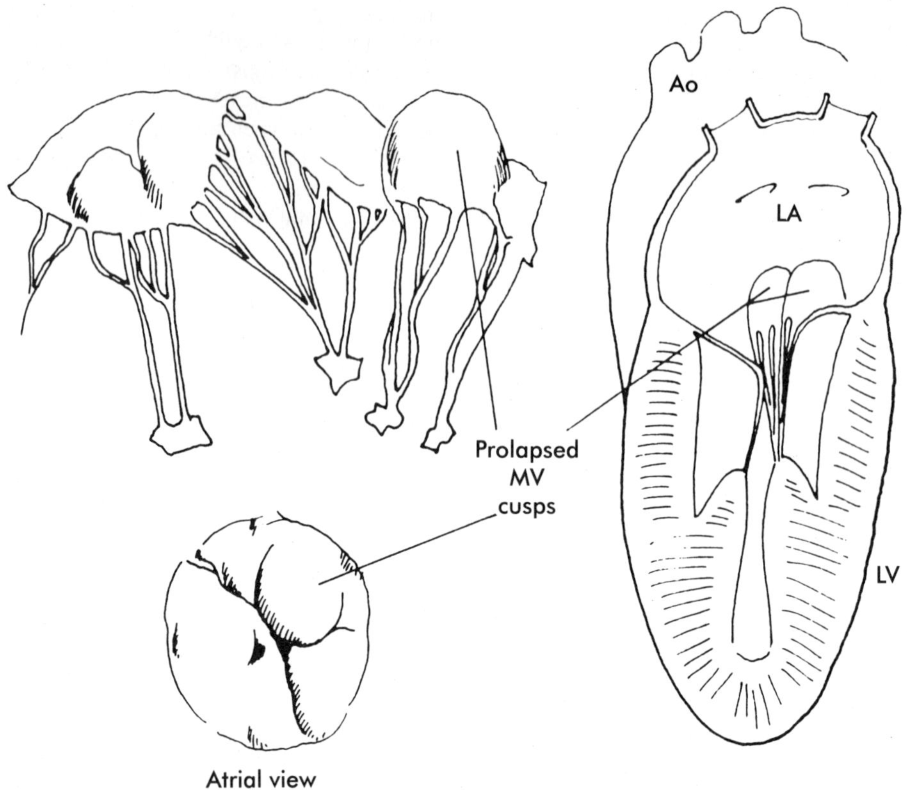


**Figure 31–2** Pathologic anatomy of a heart with mitral valve prolapse syndrome. *AO,* aorta; *LA,* left atrium; *LV,* left ventricle; *MV,* mitral valve. (In Gravanis MB, editor: *Cardiovascular pathophysiology,* New York, 1987, McGraw-Hill.)

anterior leaflet is only partially involved.[21] Both leaflets are involved in severe cases. Elongation, thickening, and tortuosity of the chordae tendineae are commonly present in patients with MVPS. The mitral valve ring is usually normal in circumference but may be dilated.

The cause of isolated MVPS is unknown. There are two major hypotheses.[12] The valve theory suggests myxomatous degeneration of the valve leaflet tissue as the principle cause, and the myocardium theory suggests that primary regional or segmental myocardiopathy causes abnormalities in the valve leaflets.

## CLINICAL PRESENTATION

### Signs and symptoms

Often these patients are asymptomatic and are referred for evaluation because of findings detected during a routine physical examination. This sometimes occurs as early as 3 years of age but more typically in adolescence. There is increased incidence of thromboembolic phenomena in certain patients with MVPS. The diagnosis is often made as a consequence of auscultatory findings of a midsystolic click with or without a late systolic murmur. These signs can be observed better with the patient standing, because of an acute postural decrease in left ventricular volume. In one study the MVPS was detected accidentally in two thirds of the patients, either on a routine physical examination or examination during a nonspecific febrile illness.[5] Nonspecific ill-defined chest pain (18%), previous episodes of rheumatic fever (7%), dysrhythmias (3%), and chronic fatigue (3%) were the complaints at the time of referral in the remainder of patients.[5]

Typical auscultatory finding of apical nonejection systolic click followed by late systolic murmur is heard in over 60% of the patients, and isolated late systolic murmurs (24%) and isolated systolic clicks may also be heard in some patients. Occasionally a holosystolic murmur at the apex suggestive of mitral insufficiency may be heard. The murmur may be whooping, honking, squeaking, or musical in 30% of the patients.[12] The click is usually single but may be multiple on occasion. Variability of the auscultatory findings from time to time and with change in posture is characteristic of MVPS. Patients may also experience a variety of symptoms such as palpitations, lassitude, anx-

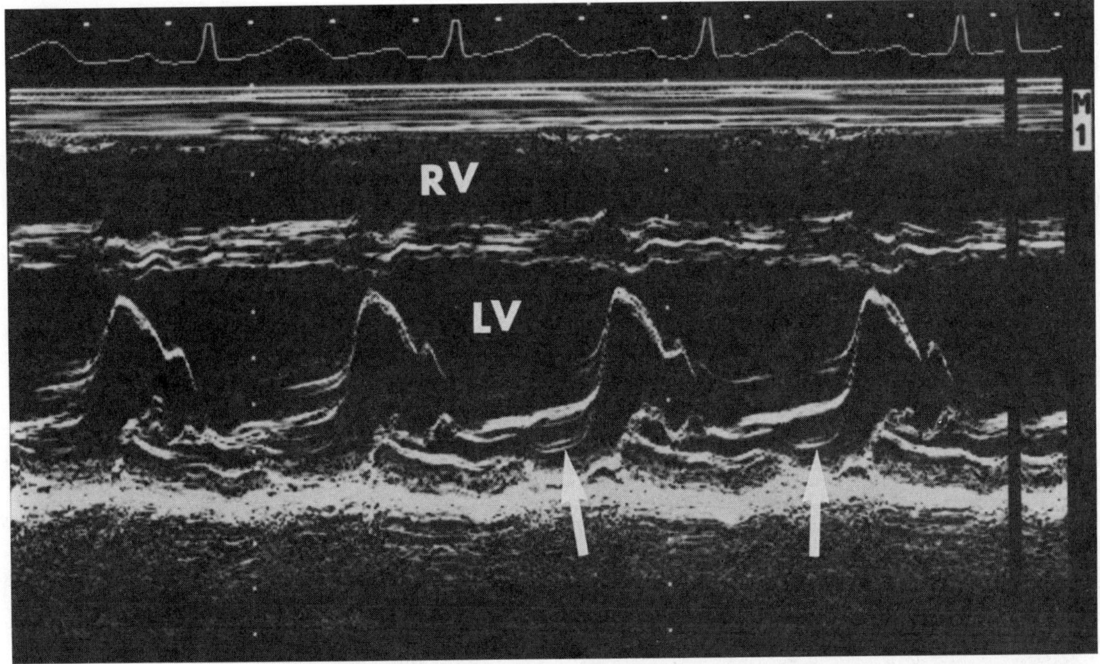


**Figure 31–3** M-mode echocardiogram showing mitral prolapse *(arrows)* in midsystole. *LV,* left ventricle; *RV,* right ventricle. (From Rao PS: Mitral valve prolapse syndrome, *Indian J Pediatr* 54:140, 1987.)

iety, dyspnea, hyperventilation, fatigue, syncope, orthostatic hypotension, neuropsychiatric symptoms, symptoms of left heart failure, transient cerebral ischemic episodes, and neurologic deficits.[10,11]

## Investigations

A thyroid profile and a coagulation profile may be necessary in certain patients, depending on the signs and symptoms.

***Electrocardiography.*** Abnormal resting ECG is present in about 60% of patients with MVPS.[5,16] The abnormalities may vary from time to time. The abnormal findings can be divided into four major categories: repolarization, conduction, rhythm, and chamber hypertrophy. Repolarization disturbances usually consist of flat to inverted T waves and ST segment depression in inferior leads and less frequently in left chest leads ($V_5$ and $V_6$). Conduction disturbances such as first degree or second degree (rarely complete) heart block, left anterior hemiblock, and RBBB may be present.[5,12] Arrhythmias in the form of atrial or ventircular premature contractions, junctional rhythm, and supraventricular tachycardia have been observed; most common among these is premature ventricular contractions.[5] Chamber hypertrophy consisting of left atrial, left ventricular, or right ventricular hypertrophy may be present in some cases.

***Chest x-ray film.*** The majority of patients will have normal chest x-ray findings. One can see signs of cardiac enlargement only in patients with significant mitral regurgitation. Thoracic cage abnormalities including pectus excavatum, straight back syndrome, and thoracic scoliosis may be present in some patients.

***Echocardiography.*** Echocardiography is the main method for making a definitive diagnosis of MVPS. However, false-positive results can be produced by positioning the transducer too high and angling it inferiorly. M-mode echocardiographic criteria include dorsal movement of the posterior and/or anterior leaflet of the mitral valve greater than 2 mm dorsal to an imaginary line drawn parallel to the chest wall from the closure point of the mitral valve echocardiogram (Fig. 31–3). Pansystolic posterior hammocking or late systolic dorsal movement may be present. The latter by itself or in association with pansystolic abnormality is considered to be a more reliable criterion than isolated pansystolic hammocking.[4] Demonstration of superior displacement of posterior, anterior, or both leaflets of the mitral valve superior to atrioventricular junction by two-dimensional echocardiography in long-axis or four-chamber view (Fig. 31–4) may be considered more specific than M-mode

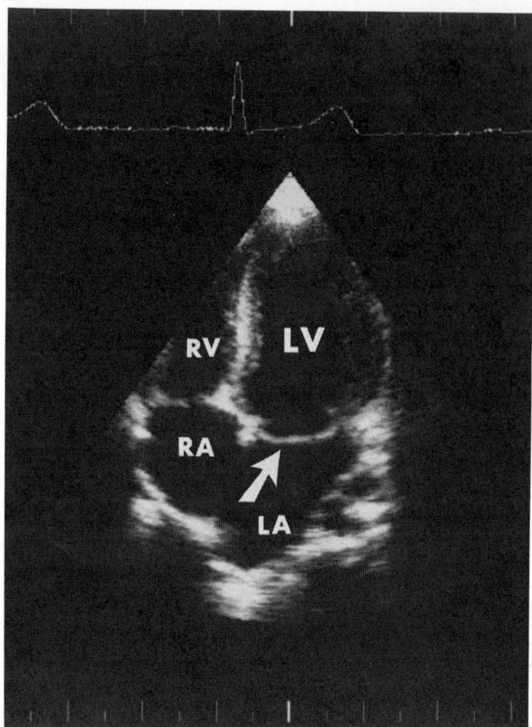


**Figure 31–4** Two-dimensional echocardiographic frame from an apical four-chamber view demonstrating prolapse of the mitral valve *(arrow)* into the left atrium. *LA,* left atrium; *LV,* left ventricle; *RA,* right atrium; *RV,* right ventricle. (From Rao PS: Mitral valve prolapse syndrome, *Indian J Pediatr* 54:140, 1987.)

findings.[14,18] Mitral valve regurgitation if present can also be demonstrated by color Doppler echocardiography.

***Cardiac catheterization.*** Unless there is an associated CHD, catheterization is not indicated for patients with MVPS.

### Complications

Major but infrequent complications of MVPS (box) include ventricular or supraventricular tachycardia, cerebrovascular accidents, disabling chest pain, bacterial endocarditis, and sudden unexpected death. Although there are no long-term follow-up studies of MVPS in children, it appears that this disease runs a relatively benign course in the pediatric population.

**COMPLICATIONS OF MVPS**

Cerebral or retinal ischemia
Noninfective endocarditis with subsequent thromboembolism
Infective endocarditis
Rupture of the chordae tendineae
Dysrhythmias and sudden death
Severe mitral valve regurgitation

## MEDICAL MANAGEMENT

Patients with isolated midsystolic click usually have a normal life expectancy and do not need any therapy. Antibiotic prophylaxis against infective endocarditis in patients with midsystolic click and late systolic murmur is recommended. Patients in the latter category should be followed carefully for progressive mitral regurgitation. The significance of associated chest pain should be explained to patients with that symptom. Patients presenting with cerebrovascular symptoms of transient ischemic attacks usually receive antiplatelet drugs or long-term anticoagulation therapy. β-Blockade is the preferred treatment for symptoms of chest pain, palpitations, and arrhythmias. Chest pain refractory to β-blockade may benefit from nitrates or quinidine.

## SURGICAL MANAGEMENT

Rupture of chordae tendineae with acute mitral regurgitation and CHF usually requires reconstructive surgery or replacement of the mitral valve. Moderate to severe mitral regurgitation from the valvular deformity also requires mitral valve replacement surgery. In general, left ventricular enlargement in patients with chronic signs and symptoms indicates the need for mitral valve repair or replacement. Although severe CHF requiring valvular surgery in infancy has been reported, the exact incidence of this condition is not known.[6,8,19,20]

## ANESTHESIA MANAGEMENT

The majority of patients with MVPS present to anesthesiologists for noncardiac surgery. Management of patients with benign MVPS and no symptoms should be straightforward (box). Only an occasional patient with moderate to severe mitral regurgitation undergoes mitral valve replacement surgery.

Preoperative evaluation should include a thorough evaluation of other systems besides the cardiac system (for example thyroid status), and the volume and electrolyte status of the patient. One should not make these patients fast for long periods, as hypovolemia causes excessive billowing of the leaflets.

A moderate to heavy preoperative medication may be necessary for these patients, as anxiety can result in excessive catecholamines leading to tachy-

**ANESTHESIA MANAGEMENT OF A PATIENT WITH MITRAL VALVE PROLAPSE**

1. Maintain preload.
2. Avoid peripheral vasodilation.
3. Keep left ventricular contractility on the low side.
4. Use prophylactic antibiotic therapy.
5. Monitor ECG lead II.
6. Avoid inotropic drugs (ephedrine, calcium, epinephrine, and isoproterenol).
7. Use phenylephrine to treat hypotension.
8. Use atropine to treat bradycardia.
9. Treat hypertension and tachycardia with esmolol and deepened anesthesia.
10. Use verapamil to treat supraventricular tachycardias.
11. Avoid epinephrine infiltrations during surgery.
12. Spinal and epidural anesthesia may exaggerate the signs (sudden decrease in preload and systemic vascular resistance) of mitral valve prolapse.

cardia and worsening of prolapse and regurgitation. Although there is some controversy, prophylactic antibiotic therapy is generally recommended for these patients, especially when they are symptomatic.

Monitoring of children with MVPS during surgery should include an ECG, noninvasive blood pressure, pulse oximeter, capnogram, and body temperature. The ECG changes are usually best seen in the inferior leads (leads II, III, and a $V_F$). The severity of disease and the type of surgery should dictate the necessity of invasive arterial pressure monitoring, central venous or pulmonary arterial pressure monitoring, and a urinometer. Since some patients with MVPS are known to have platelet abnormalities, their coagulation function should be monitored closely during the perioperative period.

By the time they are diagnosed, the majority of patients with MVPS are in adolescence and will agree to have an IV induction. One should avoid excessive decreases in preload and systemic vascular resistance and increases in inotropy and positive airway pressure, since all these situations are associated with excessive prolapse and may also provoke an arrhythmic incident.

Induction of anesthesia can be achieved with sodium thiopental, and the trachea can then be intubated using either succinylcholine or vecuronium. A β-blocker (esmolol) may be useful for the prevention or treatment of tachycardia and hypertension, which are sometimes seen with endotracheal stimulatior. Pancuronium, atracurium, and ketamine are not drugs of choice for a patient with MVPS. Because of the arrhythmogenic properties of halothane, its safety has not been established in patients with MVPS. Isoflurane may cause excessive reduction in systemic vascular resistance and exacerbate symptoms and signs of MVPS. Depending on the type of surgery an inhalational anesthetic with nitrous oxide and enflurane, a total IV with propofol, a narcotic with fentanyl or sufentanil, or a combination of narcotic and a low concentration of an inhalational anesthetic can be used. Unless the patient undergoes mitral valve surgery, the type of surgery and the general condition of the patient should dictate whether or not postoperative mechanical ventilation is required. Spinal or epidural anesthesia should be used with caution in these patients, as these may exaggerate the signs and symptoms of MVPS resulting from a sudden decrease in preload and systemic vascular resistance. One should maintain an optimal preload before the execution of spinal or epidural anesthesia. If the patient develops hypotension, administration of phenylephrine and IV fluids is recommended.

## REFERENCES


1. Barlow JB, Bosman CK, Peacock WA et al: Late systolic murmur and nonejection (mid-late) systolic clicks: an analysis of 90 patients, *Br Heart J* 30:203, 1968.
2. Barlow JB, Peacock WA: The problems of nonejection systolic clicks and associated mitral systolic murmurs: emphasis on the billowing mitral leaflet syndrome, *Am Heart J* 90:636, 1975.
3. Barlow JB, Peacock WA, Marchand P et al: The significance of late systolic murmurs, *Am Heart J* 66:443, 1963.
4. Baylen BG, Griley JM: Diseases of mitral valve. In Adams FH, Emmanouilides GC, editors: *Moss' heart disease in infants, children, and adolescents,* ed 3, Baltimore, 1983, Williams & Wilkins.
5. Bisset GS III, Schwartz DC, Meyer RA et al: Clinical spectrum and long-term follow-up of isolated mitral valve prolapse in 119 children, *Circulation* 62:423, 1980.
6. Boudoulas H, Kolibash AJ, Baker P et al: Mitral valve prolapse and the mitral valve prolapse syndrome: a diagnostic classification and pathogenesis of symptoms, *Am Heart J* 118:796, 1989.
7. Boudoulas H, Wooley CF: Mitral regurgitation: chronic versus acute: implications for timing of survery. In Bowen JM, Mazzaferri EL, editors: *Contemporary internal medicine,* vol 3, New York, London, 1991, Plenum Medical Book.
8. Boudoulas H, Wooley CF, editors: *Mitral valve prolapse and the mitral valve prolapse syndrome,* Mount Kisco, NY, 1988, Futura.
9. Bowen J, Boudoulas H, Wooley CF: Cardiovascular disease of connective tissue origin, *Am J Med* 82:481, 1987.
10. Coghlan CH, Phares P, Cowley M et al: Dysautonomia in mitral valve prolapse, *Am J Med* 67:236, 1979.
11. Gaffney AF, Bastain BC, Lane LB et al: Abnormal cardiovascular regulation in the mitral valve prolapse syndrome, *Am J Cardiol* 52:316, 1983.
12. Gingell RL, Vlad P: Mitral valve prolapse. In Keith JD, Rowe RD, Vlad P, editors: *Heart disease in infancy and childhood,* ed 3, New York, 1978, Macmillan.

13. Glesby MJ, Pyeritz RE: Association of mitral valve prolapse and systemic abnormalities of connective tissue, *JAMA* 262:523, 1989.
14. Goldberg SJ, Allen HD, Sahn DJ: *Pediatric and adolescent echocardiography,* New York, 1980, Mosby.
15. Griffith JPC: Mid-systolic and late-systolic murmurs, *Am J Med Sci* 104:285, 1892.
16. Lachman PD, Francheschi AD, Zamalloa O: Late systolic murmurs and clicks associated with abnormal mitral valve ring, *Am J Cardiol* 23:679, 1969.
17. Osler W: On a remarkable heart murmur, heard at a distance from the chest wall, *Can Med Surg J* 8:518, 1879-80.
18. Rao PS: Mitral valve prolapse syndrome, *Indian J Pediatr* 54:140, 1987.
19. Simpson JW, Nora JJ, McNamara DG: Marfan's syndrome and mitral valve disease: acute surgical emergencies, *Am Heart J* 77:96, 1969.
20. Wilcken DEL, Hickey AJ: Lifetime risk for patients with mitral valve prolapse of developing severe valve regurgitation requiring surgery, *Circulation* 78:10, 1988.
21. Wooley CF, Baker PB, Kolibash AJ et al: The floppy myxomatous mitral valve, mitral valve prolapse and mitral regurgitation, *Prog Cardiovasc Dis* 33:397, 1991.

# 32 Anomalous Origin of the Left Coronary Artery (Bland-White-Garland Syndrome)

*Jay Kambam* and *P. Syamasundar Rao*



Anomalous origin of the left or right coronary artery or of both arteries from the pulmonary trunk rarely occurs.[2,3,9,12,14] Unless the anomalous origin of the left coronary artery (ALCA) is diagnosed and treated early, death is often the outcome of this congenital disease. If the right coronary artery arises from the pulmonary trunk, the patient is usually asymptomatic. Blood flow usually occurs from the aorta via anastomoses between the left and right coronary arteries to the pulmonary artery. Myocardial ischemia is not seen in patients with anomalous origin of the right coronary artery, and the lesion is discovered as an incidental finding at autopsy.[13] Thus, the exact incidence of anomalous origin of the right coronary artery is not known. The incidence of ALCA is about 0.5% of patients with CHD. Little was known about ALCA until Bland and associates in 1933 described its clinical features (Bland-White-Garland syndrome).[12,14]

## EMBRYOLOGY

Early in the embryonic developmental stage the growing myocardium consists of muscle trabaculae (a loose meshwork of cardiac fibers) with large spaces between them containing blood that flows freely back and forth from the cavities.[7] As the myocardium gets thicker with growth, most of these spaces become flattened sinusoids, and the remaining few become clefts that are continuous with cardiac cavities. The coronary arteries arise as small buds from the posterior aspect of the truncus arteriosus (the future aorta) during the seventh week of fetal life. Each coronary artery proliferates swiftly over the epicardium and gives rise to branches that traverse the entire heart. The smaller branches of the coronary arteries form into a rich bed of fine capillaries in the growing myocardium. A few of these vessels make connections with ventricular cavities via the sinusoids.

In patients with coronary artery anomalies the formation of one or both of the coronary buds begins from the pulmonary trunk. It is postulated that one or both of the coronary buds originating from the truncus arteriosus become displaced anteriorly during its partition, resulting in the origin of left or both coronary arteries from the pulmonary trunk. In other patients an enlargement of connecting vessels between the coronary arteries and endothelial sinusoids form as coronary artery fistulas.

## ANATOMY

The coronary circulation arises from the ascending aorta as the right and left coronary arteries (Fig. 32–1). After its origin the left coronary artery

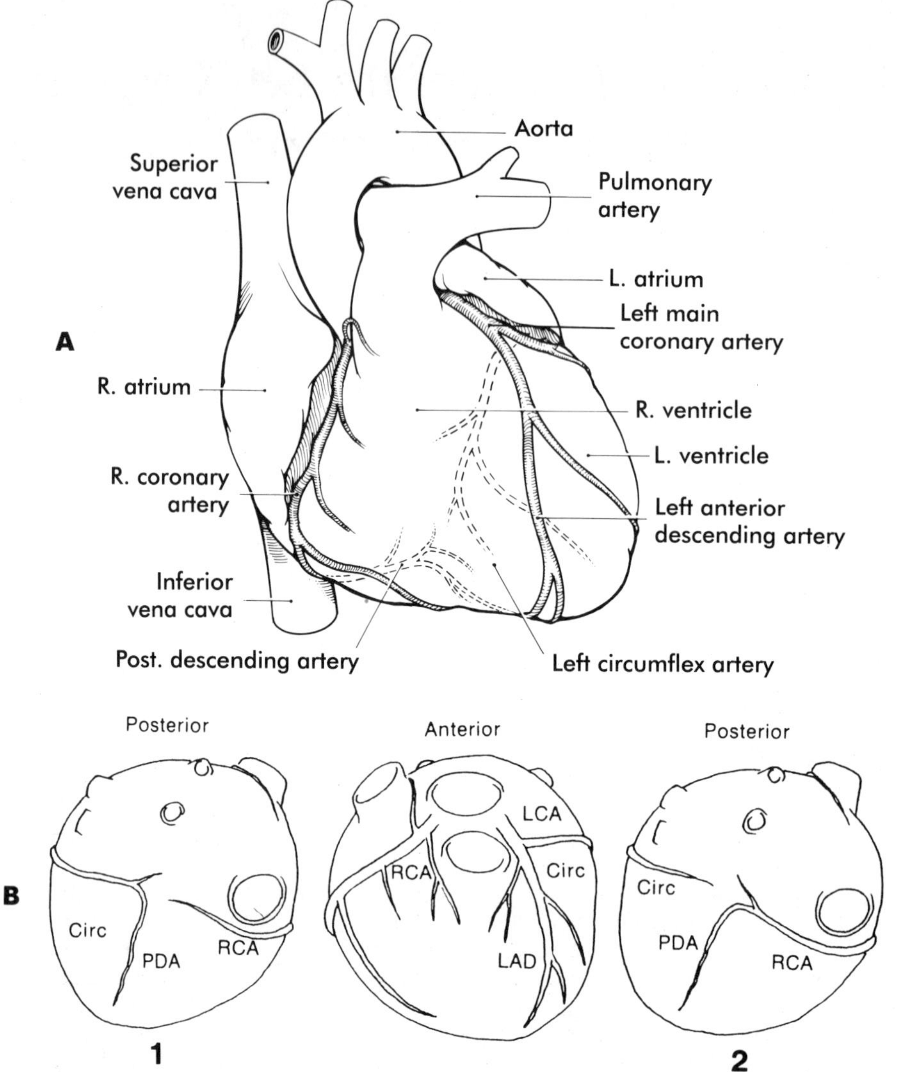


**Figure 32–1** **A,** anatomy of the normal coronary circulation; **B,** Patterns of distribution of coronary circulation. Note that posterior descending artery arises from **1,** the left circumflex artery (left coronary dominance), and **2,** the right coronary artery (right coronary dominance).

promptly divides into a left anterior descending artery and a circumflex artery. The left anterior descending artery is a larger branch that supplies blood to the right bundle branch, anterior fascicle of left bundle branch, anterolateral aspects of the left ventricle, and through septal perforator branches to the anterior two thirds of the interventricular septum. This artery extends to the apex of the heart and loops over the apex to supply a variable area of the inferior surface. The circumflex artery turns laterally to the left and extends for a variable distance between the left ventricle and left atrium in the atrioventricular (AV) groove. The circumflex artery gives off the obtuse marginal artery, which supplies the lateral aspect of the left ventricle. The circumflex artery usually supplies the posterior fascicle of the left bundle branch.

The right coronary artery runs between the right atrium and right ventricle in the AV groove to reach the posterior surface of the heart. There it usually gives off an important nutrient artery to the AV node and then divides into a posterior descending artery and a posterior left ventricular branch. Septal branches arising from the posterior descending artery supply blood to the posterior third of the interventricular septum. In 95% of female patients and in 85% of male patients the right coronary

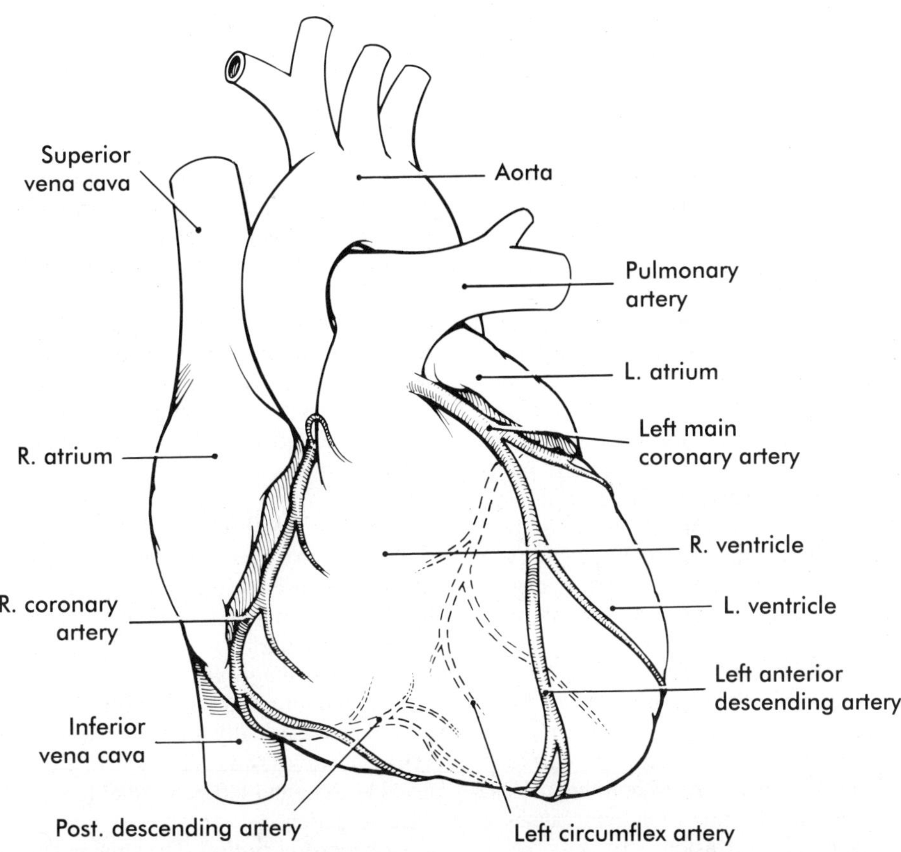


**Figure 32–2** Anomalous origin of the left coronary artery from the pulmonary trunk.

artery gives off the AV nodal artery and supplies the posterior descending artery. These persons are said to have a dominant right coronary artery. The remainder have a left dominant system, in which the circumflex artery extends to give rise to the AV nodal artery as well as the posterior descending artery. The S-A node is supplied by the right coronary artery in about 55% of human beings and by the left circumflex artery in the remaining 45%.

The coronary arteries penetrate the myocardium perpendicularly from the epicardium toward the endocardium, and many of these finer branches of coronary vessels in normal physiologic conditions are basically end-arteries. Collateral vessels up to several hundred microns in diameter can be demonstrated in the coronary circulation.

The principal drainage system of the heart is via the coronary sinus into the right atrium. There is also a deep drainage system directly into the heart chambers (thebesian venous drainage).

## PATHOLOGIC ANATOMY

As its name implies, the left coronary artery arises from the low-pressure pulmonary trunk (Fig. 32–2). Except for its abnormal origin the course of the left coronary artery is normal. One can demonstrate the collateral connections between the right and left coronary arteries in patients with anomalous origin of left coronary artery. The high-pressure right coronary artery is usually bigger than the left coronary artery, as it supplies blood flow to most of the myocardium through the collateral connections. One can also demonstrate a retrograde blood flow from the ALCA into the pulmonary artery in these patients.[10]

## PHYSIOLOGY

### Coronary blood flow

The heart receives about 5% of the cardiac output per minute. The blood flow of 60 to 90 ml/min/100 g of myocardium is usually required in the basal state. Oxygen extraction, even at resting state, is very high compared with that of any other vital organ in the body. The arteriovenous content difference ($C(a\text{-}v)o_2$) in the coronary circulation is about 12 vol%. Flow is ordinarily low, but in the case of normal coronaries there is a large reserve capacity. It can increase to five times the resting value. The normal coronary circulation is autoregulatory over a wide range of physiologic stresses. While the primary cause of myocardial ischemia is a defect in coronary blood supply, ischemia does not occur until the oxygen demand of myocardial tissue exceeds the oxygen supply. The normal myocardium is dependent solely on aerobic metabolism for continued contractile function.

### Coronary flow pattern

The coronary flow pattern to the right ventricle differs significantly from that to the left ventricle. Coronary flow to the right ventricle is normally pancyclic because of the low intramyocardial tension and lower intracavity pressure relative to the high systemic coronary perfusion pressure. Coronary flow to the left ventricle, however, is interrupted during systole because intramyocardial tension increases significantly from the epicardium to the endocardium and compresses the vessels. Furthermore, intracavity pressure of the left ventricle exceeds coronary perfusion pressure during ventricular systole.

***Coronary perfusion pressure.*** This is the difference between aortic diastolic pressure and left ventricular diastolic pressure or pulmonary capillary wedge pressure. Any reduction in diastolic pressure reduces flow in vessels to both ventricles. Tachycardia shortens diastole and thus causes a decrease in myocardial perfusion.

***Preload and afterload.*** In vivo the preload is the degree to which the myocardium is stretched before it contracts, and afterload is the resistance against which blood is expelled.

## PATHOPHYSIOLOGY

During fetal life pulmonary artery pressure and systemic pressure are about equal, and thus the myocardium enjoys satisfactory perfusion from the pulmonary artery via the aberrant left coronary artery. After birth, with the gradual decline of pulmonary vascular resistance and pressure, the antegrade perfusion of the left coronary artery decreases and will gradually be replaced by a retrograde perfusion into the pulmonary artery, resulting in a coronary artery steal. The high-pressure right coronary artery supplies most of the myocardium via collateral vessels. The pulmonary artery pressure pretty much dictates the pattern of blood flow via the aberrant left coronary artery. If the pulmonary artery pressure is high, the aberrant left coronary artery adequately oxygenates the myocardium. On the other hand, if the pulmonary artery pressure is low, the blood from the normal coronary artery (right coronary artery) flows through the collateral vessels and the aberrant left coronary artery into the pulmonary artery. This produces a left to right shunt into the pulmonary artery, resulting in a steal of blood from the normal right coronary artery.

## CLINICAL PRESENTATION

Typically children of 1 to 2 months of age will have the signs and symptoms of myocardial ischemia. Signs include episodes of irritability and distress from angina, excessive screaming attacks on exertion, pallor, sweating, tachypnea, and occasional brief episodes of loss of consciousness. Typically these episodes may occur with feedings, between which the infant is quite normal. These patients may show signs of CHF (most common) or signs of mitral regurgitation (systolic heart murmur) due to left ventricular dilatation and papillary muscle dysfunction.

### Laboratory findings

***Chest x-ray film.*** The heart size varies according to the severity of the disease, but in general the heart is enlarged without an increase in pulmonary vascularity.

***Electrocardiography.*** The ECG shows signs of anterolateral myocardial ischemia or infarction pattern. This classically shows as deep Q waves, inverted T waves, and ST segment abnormalities in leads I, aVL, and left precordial leads in the symptomatic patient.

***Echocardiography.*** The diagnosis is usually confirmed by demonstration of the origin of the left coronary artery from the pulmonary trunk. Other findings such as an enlarged and poorly functioning left ventricle, evidence of mitral regurgitation, and aneurysm of the left ventricular wall may also be present, depending on the severity of the disease.

***Cardiac catheterization.*** Definitive diagnosis can be made with cardiac catheterization and demonstration of an abnormal origin of left coronary artery from the pulmonary trunk. An angiogram may also show a retrograde filling of the anomalous vessel with some drainage into the pulmonary artery via collaterals from an enlarged right coronary artery.[10] Elevated left atrial pressure and left ventricular end diastolic pressure can also be seen during catheterization.

## MEDICAL MANAGEMENT

Once the diagnosis is made, the infant is usually treated medically with digitalis and diuretic drugs. Anemia, if present, also requires correction before the surgery. Nitroglycerin has no role in the treatment of these patients during the preoperative period, as the origin of ischemia is entirely different from that in adults. Nitroglycerin may make the condition worse in these patients by further reducing the pulmonary artery pressure.

## SURGICAL MANAGEMENT

Once the infant is stabilized, surgery is usually undertaken without any further delay, as these infants are at risk for sudden death from myocardial infarction. A variety of surgical procedures such as ligation of the left coronary artery near its origin, saphenous vein graft, subclavian artery anastomosis to the left coronary artery, and reattachment of the left coronary artery to the aorta by various methods have been tried with varied success in patients with ALCA from the pulmonary trunk (Fig. 32–3A, Fig. 32–3B).[1,4,5,6,8,11] Because of the

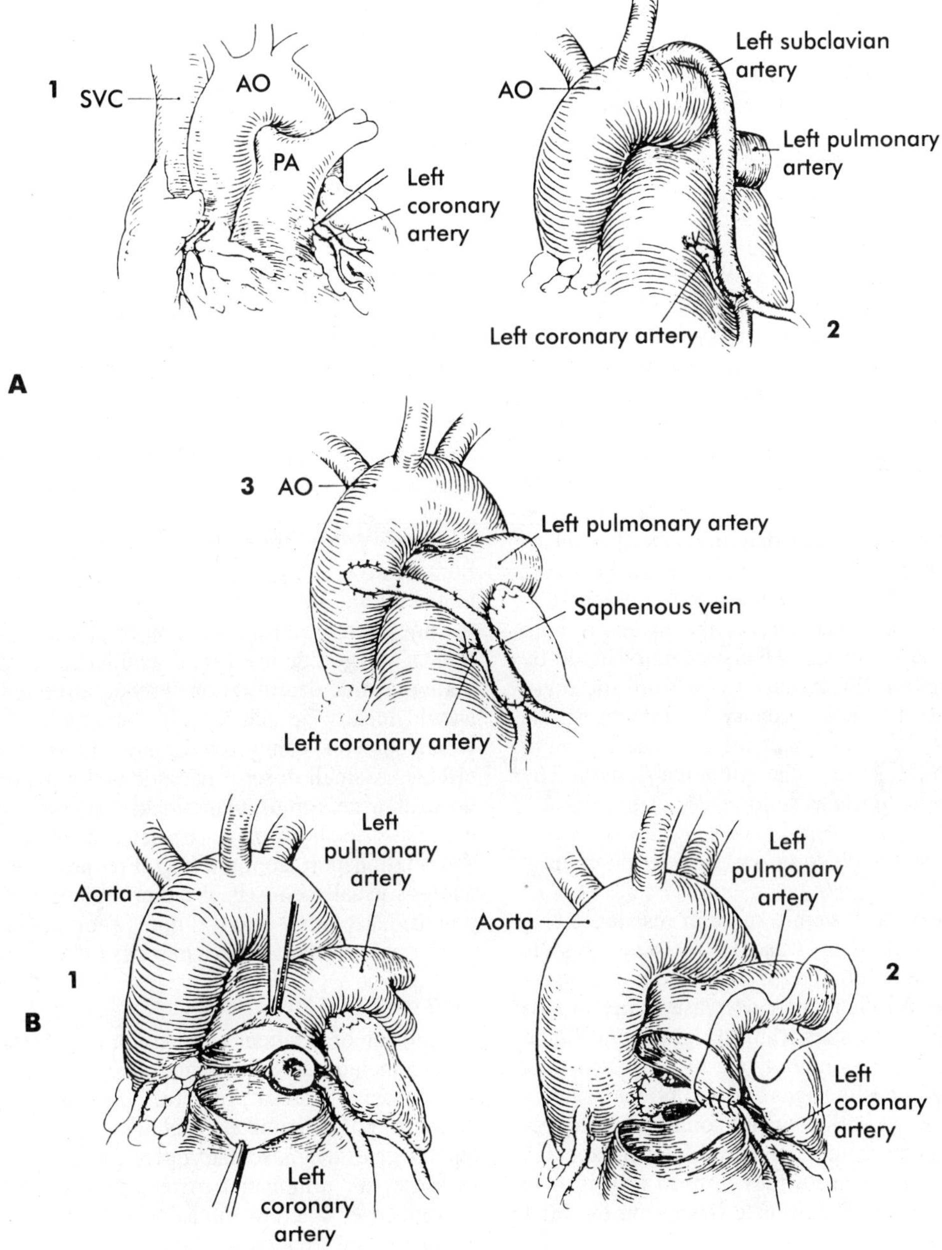


**Figure 32–3** Repair of anomalous left coronary artery. **A,** Arising from pulmonary artery. **1,** Simple ligation. **2,** Subclavian artery is turned down and anastomosed end to side to a proximally ligated left coronary artery. **3,** saphenous vein graft is used to reconstruct the coronary artery. **B,** Technique for direct anastomosis of anomalous left coronary artery to aorta. (From Effler DB, editor: *Blades' surgical diseases of the chest,* ed 4, St Louis, 1978, Mosby.)

poor long-term survival rates associated with ligation of the left coronary artery, this procedure is not considered one of the decisive operations for a patient with ALCA. Detachment of the left coronary artery from the pulmonary trunk and reconnection to the aorta is the preferred operation today. The signs and symptoms usually disappear after a successful operation.[5,6,8]

## ANESTHESIA MANAGEMENT

Follow these general precautions and principles:

1. Maintain higher than normal pulmonary vascular resistance.
2. Maintain slightly lower than normal systemic vascular resistance.
3. Prevent anemia.
4. Avoid hyperventilation.
5. Maintain high inspired oxygen fraction.
6. Avoid hypovolemia.
7. Maintain slightly decreased contractile state.
8. Maintain slightly decreased heart rate.
9. Remember that narcotic anesthesia is better than inhalation anesthesia.

It is essential to maintain higher than normal pulmonary vascular resistance and pressure and mixed venous oxygen content when anesthetizing these infants. The major determinants of myocardial oxygen supply and demand are shown in the box. One of the primary reasons for myocardial ischemia in these patients, unlike in adults with ischemic heart disease, is the stealing of blood by the low-pressure pulmonary trunk from the myocardium via the left coronary artery (retrograde flow of blood). As a result there is a left to right shunt from the aorta to the pulmonary artery. The direction of shunt is as follows:

Ascending aorta → right coronary artery → collateral vessels → left coronary artery → pulmonary trunk.

An increase in systemic vascular resistance or a decrease in pulmonary vascular resistance results in an increase in left to right shunt and a worsening of myocardial ischemia. A decrease in hematocrit (anemia) also promotes a left to right shunt. Since these infants are symptom free at birth and normally do not develop signs and symptoms of myocardial ischemia until their pulmonary vascular resistance is significantly decreased (usually about 1 or 2 months after birth), they also do well if their pulmonary vascular resistance is kept on the high side.

Since the left coronary artery arises from the pulmonary trunk and the blood it carries is relatively low in oxygen content, any decrease in cardiac output or systemic oxygenation or in hemoglobin may adversely affect the myocardium that is supplied by the left coronary artery.

**MAJOR DETERMINANTS OF MYOCARDIAL OXYGEN BALANCE**

**Oxygen supply**

Coronary blood flow
Oxygen content
P50 (oxyhemoglobin dissociation)

**Oxygen demand**

Heart rate
Contractility
Preload
Afterload

### Preoperative evaluation

An understanding of the pathologic anatomy and physiology of ALCA is important for a safe anesthesia management of these patients. Since these patients are usually treated with digoxin and a diuretic, checking electrolytes preoperatively is recommended. Patients with a hematocrit of less than 40% are likely to develop CHF and acidosis.

### Preoperative medication

Preoperative sedation depends upon the condition of the child. Advantages of preoperative sedation include decrease or elimination of anxiety, reduction of oxygen demand, and avoidance of further hemodynamic deterioration. Preoperative sedation should ideally be achieved in the holding room, where someone can watch for any undesirable side effects. A small dose of narcotic and a paralyzing dose of a neuromuscular blocker may be given, especially to those on a ventilator, to facilitate a smooth transport from the ICU. Preoperative medications usually consist of either oral benzodiazepine (midazolam 0.5 to 0.6 mg/kg) or an IM dose of morphine sulphate (0.1 mg/kg) or both.

### Intraoperative monitoring

Monitoring of a patient with ALCA during surgery should include an ECG (anterolateral leads I and $V_5$), invasive arterial pressure, noninvasive blood pressure, pulse oximeter, capnogram, temperature (esophageal and nasopharyngeal), central venous pressure, and urinometer. Arterial blood gases, serum glucose, calcium, potassium, and hematocrit are monitored frequently throughout the operation. One should be aware of an increased incidence of perioperative myocardial ischemia, ventricular dysfunction, and even frank myocardial infarction in these infants. It is therefore important to monitor for and treat these perioperative complications appropriately.

### Induction

Critically ill children usually arrive in the operating room with an IV line already in place. In these children anesthesia can be induced either with small incremental doses of a narcotic (fentanyl 15 to 25 μg/kg or sufentanil 5 to 10 μg/kg), or an IV dose of ketamine (1 to 2 mg/kg) followed by a narcotic. Either a depolarizing (succinylcholine 2 mg/kg) or a nondepolarizing muscle relaxant can be used to facilitate the endotracheal tube placement. If the child comes to the operating room without an IV, there are at least two ways to induce anesthesia. Our choice is by an IM injection of ketamine (4 to 5 mg/kg); the other way is by a slow mask induction with halothane (less than 2%). Once an adequate level of anesthesia is achieved, an IV line is placed and the trachea is intubated with the administration of atropine and a muscle relaxant.

### Maintenance

After the trachea is intubated and an IV line is established, we recommend turning off the inhaled anesthetic. The desired levels of anesthesia can be achieved by using additional doses of either fentanyl (up to a total dose of 100 μg/kg) or sufentanil (up to a total dose of 30 μg/kg) and a nondepolarizing type muscle relaxant. Vecuronium, pancuronium, or one of the newer nondepolarizing muscle relaxants (doxacurium or pipecuronium) can be used to maintain muscle paralysis throughout the operation. Infants who are not optimally stabilized preoperatively with digoxin usually benefit from dopamine infusion (5 to 7 μg/kg/min) during prebypass period. Heparin is usually given into the right atrium by the surgeon just before the placement of cannulas. Protamine is administered by the anesthesiologist at the conclusion of extracorporeal circulation following the removal of cannulas. The majority of patients require dopamine (3 to 6 μg/kg/min) infusion after coming off bypass. An occasional patient may develop spasms of the relocated left coronary artery after coming off bypass. If there are signs of myocardial ischemia and ventricular dysfunction, use of nitroglycerin in the postbypass period may be helpful.

### Fluid and blood management

One should avoid hypovolemia during the prebypass period in these patients, as this can increase a left to right shunt and worsen myocardial function. Once the patient is disconnected from the extracorporeal circulation, along with maintenance crystalloid solution (usually 5% dextrose in half normal saline) blood loss should be replaced with banked blood to maintain a hematocrit of 30% to 40%.

### Intraoperative ventilation

Patients are mechanically ventilated to maintain a near normal arterial $Pco_2$ (40 to 45 mm Hg). Addition of low levels of PEEP may be beneficial in these patients, as it may minimize the pulmonary steal of blood from the myocardium.

### Postoperative ventilation

We routinely ventilate these patients postoperatively for 1 to 2 days and administer adequate narcotic for pain relief.

## REFERENCES


1. Bunton R, Jonas RA, Lang P et al: Anomalous origin of left coronary artery from pulmonary artery: ligation versus establishment of a two coronary artery system, *J Thorac Cardiovasc Surg* 93:103, 1987.
2. Heifetz SA, Robinowitz M, Mueller KH et al: Total anomalous origin of the coronary arteries from the pulmonary artery, *Pediatr Cardiol* 7:11, 1986.
3. Menahem S, Venables AW: Anomalous left coronary artery from the pulmonary artery: a 15 year sample, *Br Heart J* 58:378, 1987.
4. Midgley FM, Watson DC, Scott LP et al: Repair of anomalous origin of the left coronary artery in the infant and small child, *J Am Coll Cardiol* 4:1231, 1984.
5. Moodie DS, Fyfe D, Gill CC et al: Anomalous origin of the left coronary artery from the pulmonary artery (Bland-White-Garland syndrome) in adult patients: long-term follow-up after surgery, *Am Heart J* 106:81, 1983.
6. Patten BM: The development of the heart. In Gould SE, editor: *Pathology of the heart,* Springfield, Ill, 1968, Charles C. Thomas.
7. Peerenboom PJHA, van Telligen C, Plokker HWM: Echocardiographic features after surgical treatment for Bland-White-Garland syndrome, *Int J Cardiol* 7:69, 1985.
8. Rein AJJT, Colan SD, Parness IA et al: Regional and global left ventricular function in infants with anomalous origin of the left coronary artery from the pulmonary trunk: preoperative and postoperative assessment, *Circulation* 75:115, 1987.
9. Roberts WC: Anomalous origin of both coronary arteries from the pulmonary artery, *Am J Cardiol* 10:595, 1962.
10. Shem-Tov AA, Hegesh J, Schneeweiss A et al: Visualization of left coronary artery in anomalous origin of left coronary artery from pulmonary artery, *Am Heart J* 108:621, 1984.
11. Takeuchi S, Imamura H, Katsumoto K et al: New surgical method for repair of anomalous left coronary artery from pulmonary artery, *J Thorac Cardiovasc Surg* 78:1, 1979.
12. Wesselhoeft HJS, Johnson AL: Anomalous origin of the left coronary artery from the pulmonary trunk, *Circulation* 38:403, 1968.
13. Worsham C, Sanders SP, Burger BM: Origin of the right coronary artery from the pulmonary trunk: diagnosis by two-dimensional echocardiography, *Am J Cardiol* 55:232, 1985.
14. Zmugg P: Variation des Blande-White-Garlands, *Virchows Arch Pathol Anat Histol* 363:89, 1974.

# 33 Eisenmenger's Syndrome

*Michael F. Sweeney and Kumar G. Belani*



In 1897 Victor Eisenmenger described a 32-year-old man with cyanosis and exercise intolerance. He died of heart failure associated with hemoptysis.[17] Postmortem examination revealed a VSD. Subsequently patients with VSD and similar clinical courses were found to have pulmonary arterial medial hypertrophy and intimal fibrosis. This constellation of findings was termed Eisenmenger's complex. Eventually other congenital cardiovascular malformations that, early in life caused large left to right shunts or elevated pulmonary venous pressures were related to similar later changes in the pulmonary vasculature. A common late feature is pulmonary hypertension with pressures approaching systemic level because of an extreme fixed elevation of resistance to pulmonary blood flow. Bidirectional or predominant right to left shunting through defects then occur. This broadened spectrum of involvement is termed Eisenmenger's syndrome. It represents the end-stage of pulmonary vascular disease (PVD) secondary to a CHD. Eisenmenger's syndrome has been recognized as a cause of significant morbidity and mortality, sometimes sudden, in children.[16]

Eisenmenger's syndrome can set in as early as 2 years of age in patients with very large left to right shunts and pulmonary hypertension, as seen in large VSD, truncus arteriosus, large aortopulmonary communications, or complete atrioventricular canal (box). Rapid onset may also occur in d-transposition of the great arteries, with or without a VSD.

This syndrome may also take decades to develop, as in ASD, moderate size ventricular or great vessel communications, or partial AV canal. It appears that the speed of progression is in large part related to the magnitude of the pulmonary artery pressure in early infancy and less affected by shunt size. An additional important factor is alveolar hypoxia. This may be due to pulmonary edema as seen in pulmonary venous obstruction syndromes or left-sided heart failure. Alveolar hypoxia may also happen in patients with superimposed chronic airway problems, especially during sleep.[45] Examples of the latter include Down's syndrome (hypotonic airway), severe tonsillar hypertrophy, and tracheobronchomalacia.

**CARDIAC LESIONS THAT CAN LEAD TO EISENMENGER'S SYNDROME**

1. VSD/truncus arteriosus
2. Aortopulmonary communications (e.g., PDA)
3. Complete atrioventricular canal
4. d-Transposition of the great arteries
5. ASD
6. Pulmonary venous or left heart obstruction

## NORMAL DEVELOPMENT AND PHYSIOLOGY

The pulmonary vasculature arises centrally from the left sixth aortic arch and the common or primitive pulmonary vein. These are of course connected to the embryonic heart. Distally, splanchnic mesoderm forms a vascular plexus invested into the developing tracheobronchial tree and primitive saccules, which eventually change into alveoli. By 16 weeks gestation, the vascular branching pattern is developed to the same degree as that of the adult, down to the airway level of the terminal bronchiole. Vessel size increases as airway size increases. Additional distal vessels develop as numbers of primitive saccules and alveoli increase, until age 8 years. Thereafter they increase in size as alveolar size increases with chest wall growth. Therefore, total vascular cross-sectional area at any level is increasing with growth. Obviously this growth, most prominent in the newborn, gradually slows until adult size is reached.

At birth pulmonary arterial medial muscle does not extend beyond the very small (below 0.02 mm) level. All arteries greater than 0.02 mm diameter are fully muscularized. Those greater than 2 mm diameter have prominent elastic layers. Between these sizes there is a transition. For a given lumen size, wall thickness is greater at all levels in the newborn than in the adult. At birth, with aeration of the lungs and termination of fetal circulation, vascular dilatation occurs, and wall thickness regresses over 3 days to several months of age.[53] The smaller the muscularized artery, the more rapid the regression. Pulmonary veins develop in a fashion similar to that of the pulmonary arteries but have less medial muscle and therefore wall thickness. Regression of venous wall thickness parallels that of arterial wall thickness. As a consequence of these normal changes pulmonary vascular resistance drops, and pulmonary arterial pressure falls to the adult level by the end of the first month of life (Figs. 33-1 and 33-2).[49]

In the systemic vasculature resistance is predominantly determined at the arteriolar level. This is not the case with pulmonary vessels, in which the resistance is more evenly distributed along the entire course, main pulmonary artery to large pulmonary vein. Normally the smooth muscle tone that modulates this resistance is very low. It can be increased by alveolar hypoxia, acidemia,[41] increased autonomic nervous system activity (α adrenergic agonism increases, but β adrenergic[36] and acetylcholine agonism decreases[12]), endogenous and exogenous humoral agents[58] and intrapulmonary reflexes triggered by stretching of large pulmonary arteries or air spaces.[33]

Mechanical factors also can increase pulmonary vascular resistance independent of smooth muscle tone elevations.[6] Lung volume is one, with a normal functional residual capacity (FRC) being the lung volume at which resistance is minimized.[62,65] Airway pressure that does not allow the lungs to ventilate about the FRC volume can elevate pulmonary vascular resistance independently of alveolar hypoxia.[14] Another important mechanical factor is pulmonary vascular blood volume. Hypovolemia can directly increase resistance via loss of distending pressure to the point of vascular closure.[24,29] Indirect effects may also be mediated via the sympathetic nervous system's response to inadequate cardiac preload. Severe elevations of hematocrit can also increase pulmonary vascular re-

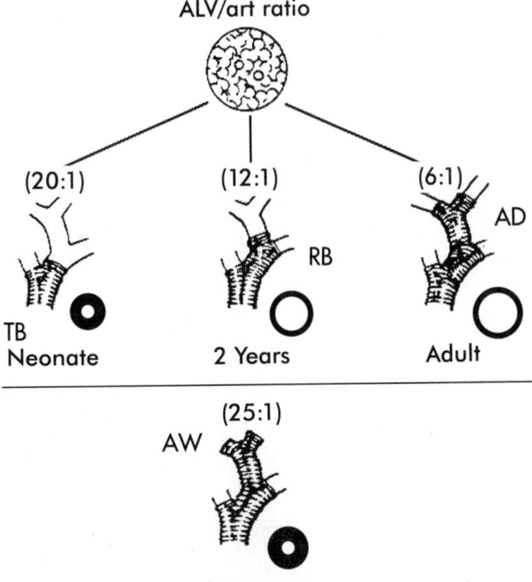


**Figure 33–1** A schematic representation of peripheral pulmonary artery development showing morphometric changes of extension of muscle into peripheral arteries, wall thickness and artery number as they relate to age. Top panel shows normal development *ALV/art,* alveolor arterial ratio. Lower panel demonstrates changes in all three features in a 2-year-old child with a hypertensive VSD. TB = artery accompanying a terminal bronchiolus, RB = artery accompanying a respiratory bronchiolus, AD = artery accompanying an alveolar duct, AW = artery accompanying an alveolar wall (From Rabinovitch M et al: Lung biopsy in congenital heart disease: a morphometric approach to pulmonary vascular disease, *Circulation* 58:1107, 1978.)

**FACTORS RESPONSIBLE FOR MODULATING PULMONARY VASCULAR RESISTANCE**

**Action on smooth muscle tone**
Alveolar hypoxia (↑)
Acidemia (↑)
Autonomic nervous system activity (↑ or ↓)
Humoral agents (↑ or ↓)
Active stretch (↑)

**Mechanical factors**
Lung volume
Pulmonary blood volume
Hematocrit

↑, Increase in tone; ↓, decrease in tone.

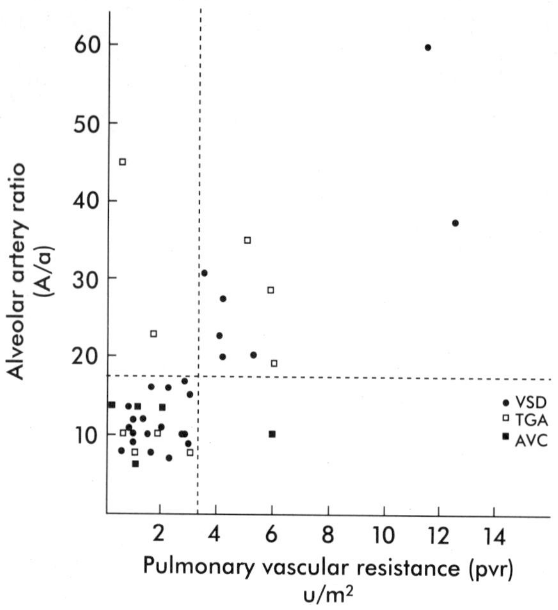


**Figure 33–2** Note relationship of pulmonary artery resistance and alveolar artery ratio. Normal or mildly abnormal patients are separated by the dotted lines from those that are clearly abnormal. Note the two extreme examples, one with transposition and pulmonary stenosis and the other with complete atrioventricular canal and severe mitral regurgitation. (From Rabinovitch M et al: Lung biopsy in congenital heart disease: a morphometric approach to pulmonary vascular disease, *Circulation* 58:1107, 1978.)

sistance via an increase in internal blood viscosity. These changes are most pronounced at a hematocrit of at least 55%.[28]

## PATHOPHYSIOLOGY

The person with congenital cardiac disease may not undergo the aforementioned changes in the pulmonary vasculature after birth. Three basic types of hemodynamic derangement can change this normally smooth course (Table 33-1). The first and most common is elevated pulmonary blood flow and pressure. This is due to a large communication between ventricles or great arteries or both. In this instance predominant arterial pulmonary vascular changes that deviate from normal can be seen in the first year of life. Some of the lesions are more likely to do this than others. High-risk lesions are complete AV canal, d-transposition of the great arteries with a large VSD, and truncus arteriosus.[5,19,30,34] Somewhat less accelerated development can be expected with a large VSD and/or PDA.[25,65]

The second hemodynamic group is elevated pulmonary flow with normal initial pressures. ASD predominates here.[18] Again, the histologic deviation is mainly arterial but tends to progress very slowly or even not at all. Adulthood is the usual time of occurrence. Another type of defect in this class is d-transposition of the great arteries with intact septum. The development here can be much quicker. This probably relates to the severe systemic hypoxemia and resultant polycythemia, which can cause pulmonary microthromboemboli. Another factor is the development of bronchial collaterals, which further increase pulmonary flow.[5] The third hemodynamic situation is normal or low pulmonary flow with increased pulmonary venous pressure. Congenital mitral stenosis, cor triatriatum, and pulmonary venous obstruction—almost always with total anomalous venous return—cause significant venous as well as arterial aberrations. These early-onset changes are very responsive to surgery that alleviates the obstruction. Therefore many patients in this group come to the operating room as neonates or young infants.

These deviations from normal development are all said to represent PVD. Heath and Edwards[25] described the histopathology of PVD secondary to congenital heart disease in 1958. A brief summary of their severity classification follows:

- Grade 1 Medial hypertrophy and medial extension into normally nonmuscular vessels
- Grade 2 Same as grade 1 with intimal proliferation
- Grade 3 Same as grade 2 with intimal fibrosis
- Grade 4 Same as grade 3 with significantly larger pulmonary arterial dilatation and thinning associated with occlusal fibrosis

**Table 33–1** Summary of types of pulmonary vascular derangement leading to Eisenmenger's syndrome

| Classification | Characteristic pulmonary features | Examples of cardiac defects |
|---|---|---|
| Type 1 | Elevated pulmonary blood flow and pressure | Complete AV canal<br>d-Transposition of great vessels<br>Large VSD<br>Truncus arteriosus |
| Type 2 | Elevated pulmonary blood flow with normal initial pressures | ASD<br>d-Transposition of great vessels with intact septum |
| Type 3 | Normal or low pulmonary flow with increased pulmonary venous pressure | Congenital mitral stenosis<br>Cor triatriatum<br>Pulmonary venous obstruction lesions |

Grade 5 Same as grade 4 with medial fibrosis
Grade 6 Same as grade 5 with necrotizing arteritis

A second classification scheme developed by Reid[48] is morphometric. It quantitates medial thickening, medial extension, and density of small vessels relative to alveoli:

Grade A Medial extension with medial thickness up to 1.5 times normal
Grade B Medial extension plus medial thickness more than 1.5 times normal
Grade C Same as grade B with decreased small vessels relative to alveoli

In summary, the earlier histopathologic changes of PVD are medial hypertrophy, medial extension, and intimal proliferation. With time the other features emerge (Figs. 33-1 and 33-2).

The hemodynamic consequence of PVD is increased resistance to blood flow. Pulmonary arterial hypertension results, and blood flow tends to fall. Left to right shunt size decreases and eventually reverses direction through defects. In the increased pulmonary venous pressure situation, normal pulmonary flow diminishes and right to left shunting can occur via coexistent defects or a patent foramen ovale. If it is severe enough, persistent fetal circulation can be seen in the neonate. The relative resistance contributions of smooth muscle tone versus hypertrophy, fibrosis, and decreased small vessel density vary among patients. A method of sorting out these factors is to administer 100% oxygen or a vasodilator while ensuring that the patient is not experiencing any significant vasoconstrictive influences (agitation, hypoventilation, hypothermia, acute pulmonary dysfunction).[37,52] If a large fall in resistance is noted, the vascular bed is said to be reactive. If little or no response is seen, the resistance elevation is called fixed. There tends to be a correlation between fixed resistance and more severe histopathologic grade. Lung biopsy for severity grading by either method has been used to try to predict outcome from surgical repair of congenital defects.[46,47] Unfortunately, it has added little to the basic hemodynamic evaluation and oxygen-vasodilator challenge, usually performed in the catheterization laboratory. In addition, some evidence suggests that if surgical correction is carried out in infancy, outcome is excellent regardless of underlying lesion or severity of PVD.[9,22,57,67] On the other hand, if repair is delayed beyond age 2 years (ASD closure excluded), postoperative pulmonary hypertension may persist, and PVD may actually continue to progress. This course of events significantly worsens prognosis. In summary, the best pulmonary vascular outcome can be expected in the infant with a normal calculated pulmonary vascular resistance. The poorest may be expected in the patient above 2 years of age with fixed systemic level resistance. Such a patient would probably be declared inoperable for defect closure. In the marginal patient with a pulmonary vascular resistance greater than twice normal, repair is attempted but may have to be reversed if the patient subsequently deteriorates despite maximum medical support. If defect correction at a young age is not feasible, banding of the main pulmonary artery can be done to protect the pulmonary vasculature, lessen CHF and allow for normal growth.[15,64] Then, when the patient is larger, the band can be removed and defects corrected. For example, this approach is fairly common when VSD is in the muscular septum. In effect, the best management of Eisenmenger's syndrome is prevention.

## CLINICAL FEATURES

As a result of current management schemes, the incidence of Eisenmenger's syndrome has decreased substantially. Some patients fall through the cracks, usually via inadequate follow-up. As the patient's PVD progresses, left to right shunt

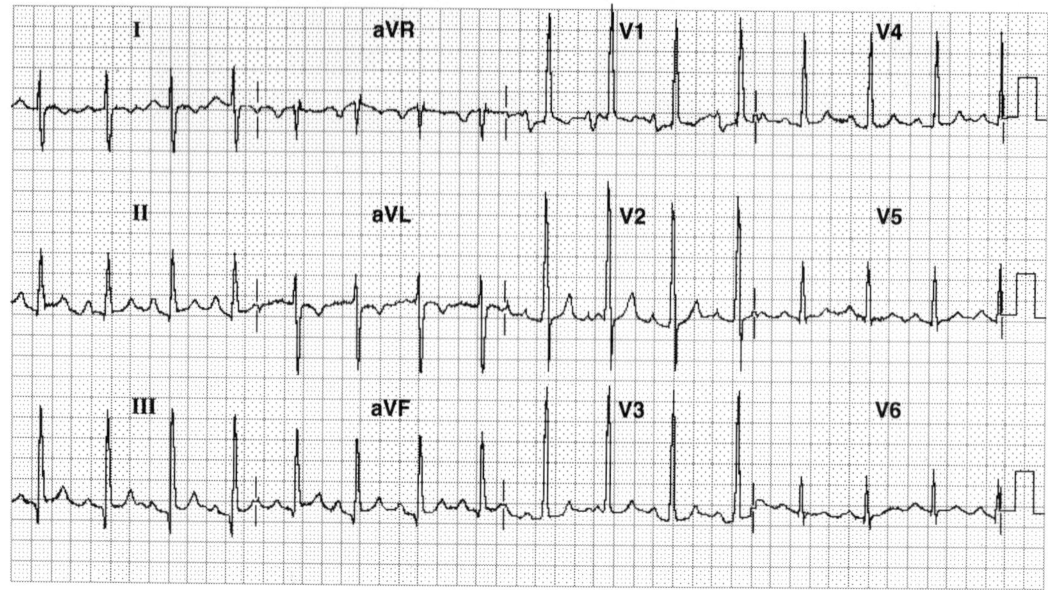


**Figure 33–3** A typical ECG in a patient with Eisenmenger's complex secondary to VSD. Note the biatrial enlargement, right ventricular hypertrophy, and ST-T wave abnormality in lead VI.

size diminishes, since resistance is increasing. CHF temporarily improves. Chest x-ray films demonstrate normalization of heart size and vascular markings. The ECG gradually shifts from baseline to a right ventricular pressure overload pattern, eventually with strain (Fig. 33–3). At this point shunt size is small and bidirectional, depending on circumstances. Echocardiography demonstrates this finding and displays the thickened and dilated right ventricle, along with features of pulmonary hypertension, which become evident radiologically (Fig. 33–4). Intermittent cyanosis, easy fatiguability, and exertion intolerance develop. Eventually continuous cyanosis, reactive polycythemia, dyspnea at rest, and biventricular heart failure ensue. Recurrent massive hemoptysis is not uncommon, and even pulmonary hemosiderosis has been seen. At this point 5-year survival is low.

Medical management of Eisenmenger's syndrome serves to provide better patient comfort. It may also stabilize the pathophysiology on a temporary basis, so that transplantation or other intercurrent procedures are more likely to be successful. Treatment commonly involves the following:

| | |
|---|---|
| Oxygen | Although resistance is usually nonreactive, it may help with intrapulmonary mismatch secondary to pulmonary edema or hemoptysis. Subjective dyspnea may be lessened. |
| Diuretics | These are administered for edema secondary to congestive heart failure. |
| Inotropes | Usually digoxin is given because of biventricular systolic cardiac dysfunction from chronic hypoxemia. |
| Polycythemia control | Hemoglobin levels above 20 to 22 g/dl secondarily worsen resistance and predispose the patient to thromboembolic problems and tracheobronchial hemorrhage. |
| Vasodilators | They have not been consistently helpful but are usually tried anyway. No known vasodilator is consistently a selective pulmonary vasodilator. Drugs reportedly used in humans include amrinone, captopril, phentolamine, nitroprusside, nitroglycerine, hydralazine, diazoxide, nifedipine, tolazoline and various prostaglandins.* Clinical experience regarding nitric oxide as a relatively selective inhaled pulmonary vasodilator has been favorable in newborns with persistent pulmonary hypertension (fetal circulation). It is much less likely to be of benefit where PVD is advanced and therefore reactivity is minimal or zero. |

## CONSIDERATIONS FOR ANESTHESIA

The anesthesiologist may encounter a patient with Eisenmenger's syndrome scheduled for lung transplantation with cardiac defect correction or heart-lung transplantation.[8,21] Such operations are potentially curative. The repair is performed with the help of cardiopulmonary bypass. As with any brain death organ donation lung transplant, short notice is given to both the patient and the anesthesiologist.

*References 1, 10, 32, 35, 39, 40, 42, 50, 53, 60, 61

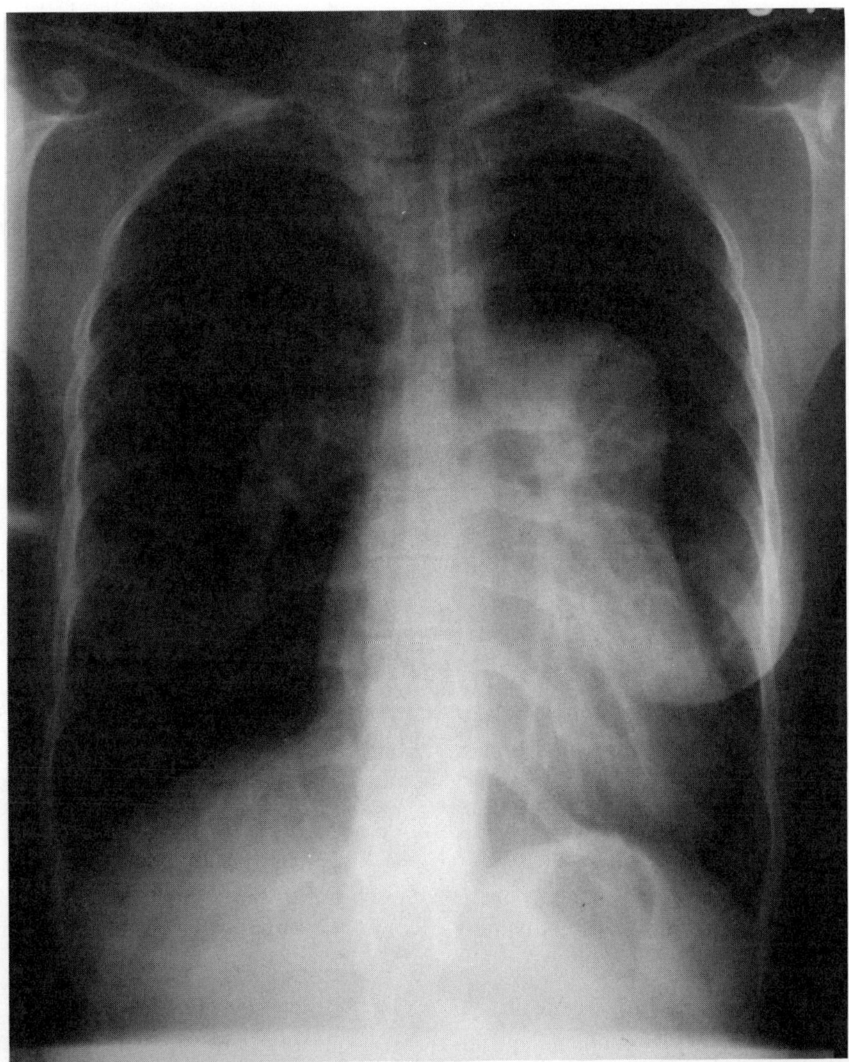

**Figure 33–4** Typical chest x-ray film of a patient with advanced Eisenmenger's complex because of VSD with coarctation of the aorta. Note the massive cardiomegaly with a huge main pulmonary artery and a large right pulmonary artery. This 25-year-old woman had a small left to right shunt and a moderate right to left shunt with a systemic oxygen saturation of 77 and a pulmonary artery saturation of 73. The pulmonary artery pressures were equal to systemic pressures. (Chest x-ray film provided by W. Castaneda, department of radiology, University of Minnesota.)

For this reason full stomach precautions must be taken during induction of general anesthesia. The patient is instructed to drink an antacid dose of sodium citrate. Preoperative anxiety is most easily treated with small to moderate doses of benzodiazepine by any route. In infants and young children the rectal administration of sedation has worked out well at the University of Minnesota.[7] Heavy sedation without an anesthetist in attendance is dangerous and potentially fatal, since even brief hypoventilation or hypotension is so poorly tolerated from an oxygenation standpoint. IV access for induction is recommended, since this will allow for rapid paralysis and control of the airway. Because of right to left shunting and a high possibility of paradoxical air embolism, special attention should be taken to avoid air in the IV lines.[31] Cricoid cartilage pressure is used to facilitate hyperventilation and protect against gastric content aspiration prior to endotracheal intubation. A typical basic sequence for induction is as follows:

1. Complete denitrogenation with oxygen ($Fio_2$ 1.0)
2. Atropine 0.02 mg/kg IV
3. Defasciculation or priming dose of nondepolarizing muscle relaxant

4. IV induction with ketamine (2 mg/kg) or etomidate (0.2 mg/kg)
5. Succinyl choline (2 mg/kg IV) or a large dose of nondepolarizer

The endotracheal tube inserted is as large a bore as possible, since postoperative bronchoscopy to assess bronchial anastomosis is always done, usually in the operating room at the termination of surgery. For added stability during induction and subsequent positive pressure ventilation, a moderate bolus (10 ml/kg) of isotonic crystalloid or colloid fluid is administered. Prebypass it is especially important to maintain euvolemia because of an increased right ventricular filling pressure requirement and the tendency for pulmonary vascular resistance to increase with hypovolemia. Also, oxygenation will be best at a higher systemic arterial pressure from increased bronchial collateral flow. Excessive crystalloid infusion (above 40 ml/kg) should be avoided. Diuretics are routinely given because the transplanted lung will initially have some degree of lymphatic insufficiency and capillary leak. Therefore, at some point colloid should be used for volume expansion prebypass. An oximetric thermodilution pulmonary artery catheter is inserted so that the tip is in the main pulmonary artery. Because of severe pulmonary hypertension, this procedure should not be taken lightly.[44] In some cases it may not be possible to position the pulmonary artery catheter without fluoroscopy.[55] The use of dual pulse oximetry (right upper extremity and a lower extremity) to monitor right to left shunting has been reported to be useful in some situations.[44] An arterial line is placed before or immediately post induction. If a heart-lung transplant is to be done, right internal jugular catheterization is avoided because there is a need postoperatively for repeated right ventricular endomyocardial biopsies, which are easiest performed via this site. General anesthesia is maintained with standard high-dose narcotic technique, loading taking place over the 30-minute period following induction and as tolerated. High concentrations of any potent inhalation agent are generally avoided, since some degree of heart failure is almost always present. In fact, a catecholamine (dobutamine) infusion can improve and provide for hemodynamic stability prebypass. Vasoconstricting inotropes are best avoided or kept at nonvasoconstricting doses. One should also avoid prebypass hypothermia (core temperature below 35° C), as this may result in endogenous catecholamine release. Occasionally an IV vasodilator is needed. Moderate hypocarbia (arterial carbon dioxide pressure about 30 mm Hg) with avoidance of excessive mean airway pressure is a major goal of ventilator management. Inspired oxygen concentration is adjusted to keep the arterial oxygen pressure above 100 mm Hg or oximetric saturation near 100%. If an orogastric tube is inserted, one should avoid suctioning for at least 4 hours because of orally administered immunosuppressives given shortly preinduction. Intraoperative transesophageal echocardiography is routinely performed for lung transplantation with intracardiac correction, since right ventricular outflow tract obstruction can occur after the repair. This is thought to happen because of significantly decreased pulmonary afterload in the presence of a severely hypertrophied right ventricle. Selected patients having heart-lung transplantation may also benefit from this monitor, as the transplanted heart's performance may be more of a problem. In addition to routine measures during weaning from bypass one should again provide moderate hyperventilation (arterial carbon dioxide pressure about 30 mm Hg), with tidal volume and rate adjusted to keep peak airway pressures no more than 30 cm $H_2O$ (almost always possible). The latter is helpful in lessening barotrauma to the fresh bronchial anastomosis. To minimize oxygen toxicity to the transplanted lung, the pulse oximeter is used to decrease expeditiously the inspired oxygen fraction to no more than 0.4, as tolerated, with a saturation of 90% generally being acceptable. A vasodilator such as prostaglandin $E_1$ is sometimes needed to help manage pulmonary resistance and therefore right ventricular afterload. Postbypass isoproterenol is always used to support heart rate when a heart-lung transplant is performed. If other inotropes are required, nonvasoconstricting ones (or nonvasoconstricting doses) should be selected.

Most patients with severe polycythemia have some degree of coagulopathy preoperatively. This is secondary to low plasma volume and small-vessel sludging with subsequent low-grade disseminated intravascular consumption of factors. For this reason and because of increased mediastinal vascularity from bronchial collaterals or any previous mediastinal procedures, bleeding post bypass is more of a problem. Desmopressin (0.3 μg/kg) is now routinely used. It is possible that prophylactic aprotinin may also be of use and be routine in the future. Nonetheless, administration of coagulation factors and platelets is commonplace in these patients. As in any patient undergoing an organ transplantation procedure, all blood products should be checked for CMV antigen. ϵ-aminocaproic acid is usually reserved for patients unresponsive to the above interventions. Overall short-term (up to 6 months) survival with these procedures is excellent (average 85%). Long-term survival (more than 5 years) is uncertain but probably approaches 50%. After transplantation the quality of life is much improved unless complications such as graft rejection, opportunistic infection, or bronchial anastomosis insufficiency ensue.

Patients with Eisenmenger's syndrome may also present to the anesthesiologist for nontransplant surgical procedures. Any nonessential surgical procedures are best avoided for obvious reasons. Maternal and neonatal death despite adequate anesthesia management have been reported.[27] Some of the common reasons for noncardiac surgery include dental extractions,[38] brain abscess drainage (more common with right-to-left shunting),[13] caesarean section,[3,23,43,44] hysterectomy, bilateral tubal ligation,[2,59] bronchoscopy, and thoracotomy with lung resection for massive hemoptysis,[4,66] Other uncommon but reported surgeries include inguinal herniorrhaphy,[56] resection of a carotid body tumor,[31] and excision of pheochromocytoma.[54]

During the administration of general anesthesia, all the previously discussed concerns apply to these patients. Regional anesthesia has been used successfully in adults,[3,11,23,43,44,56] though coagulation tests and platelet count should be checked prior to performing any block. Sympathetic blockade resulting from either spinal or epidural block can result in increased right to left shunt and further clinical deterioration[44] and should be used when the benefits outweigh the risks as judged on an individual basis.[3,56] Intrathecal morphine is well tolerated and therefore can be used to advantage in these patients.[44] Snabes and Poindexter[59] described the successful use of local anesthesia during laparoscopic tubal ligation in five patients with advanced Eisenmenger's syndrome. This may be the best choice in some situations. When polycythemia is severe, partial exchange transfusion (patient's blood for appropriate colloid) should be done so that the hemoglobin level is no more than 20 gm/dL. Lung resection for massive hemoptysis is usually done when all other management schemes have failed, since any loss of gas exchange surface area may be poorly tolerated from an oxygenation standpoint. A double-lumen endotracheal tube is used during thoracotomy in these patients to protect the down lung from massive blood aspiration. In addition, one should have sufficient vascular access and appropriate amounts of blood products available to maintain intraoperative hemodynamic stability.

There is no doubt that the patient with Eisenmenger's syndrome poses increased risk during anesthesia in any situation, but with careful attention to the pathophysiology, good outcomes should be routine. The continuation of medical management throughout the perioperative period can be expected to improve intraoperative management. Since the best treatment for Eisenmenger's syndrome is prevention, early detection and correction of cardiac lesions that lead to the syndrome play the most important role in the management of these patients.

## REFERENCES


1. Abbott TR, Rees CJ, Dickinson D et al: Sodium nitroprusside in idiopathic respiratory distress syndrome: case report, *Br Med J* 1:1113, 1978.
2. Asling JH, and Fung DL: Epidural anesthesia in Eisenmenger's syndrome: a case report, *Anesth Analg* 53(6):965, 1974.
3. Atanassoff PE, Alon ER, Schmid et al: Epidural anesthesia for cesarean section in a patient with severe pulmonary hypertension, *Acta Anaesthesiol Scand* 34(1):75, 1990.
4. Au J, Cusack SP, Walker WS: Successful pulmonary resection after spontaneous hemopneumothorax in the Eisenmenger syndrome, *Thorax* 46(7):540, 1991.
5. Aziz KU, Paul MH, Rowe RD: Bronchopulmonary circulation in d-transposition of the great arteries: possible role in genesis of accelerated pulmonary vascular disease, *Am J Cardiol* 39:432, 1977.
6. Baylen BG, Emmanouilides GC, Juratsch CE et al: Main pulmonary artery distension: a potential mechanism for acute pulmonary hypertension in the human newborn infant, *J Pediatr* 90:540, 1980.
7. Beebe DS, Belani KG, Chang PN et al: The effectiveness of preoperative sedation with rectal midazolam, ketamine or their combination in young children, *Anesth Analg* 75:880, 1992.
8. Bolman RM III, Shumway SJ, Estrin JA et al: Lung and heart-lung transplantation: evolution and new applications, *Ann Surg* 214(4):456, 1991.
9. Braunlin EA, Moller JH, Patton C et al: Predictive value of lung biopsy in ventricular septal defect: long-term follow-up, *Circulation* 68(suppl 3):III-A396, 1983.
10. Buch J, Wennevold A: Hazards of diazoxide in pulmonary hypertension, *Br Heart J* 46:401, 1981.
11. Camba, Rodriguez MA, Gonzalez AM et al: Epidural anesthesia for cesarean section in a patient with Eisenmenger's syndrome, *Rev Esp Anestesiol Reanim* 36(1):45, 1989.
12. Cassin S, Dawes GS, Ross BB: Pulmonary blood flow and vascular resistance in immature foetal lambs, *J Physiol (Lond)* 171:80, 1964.
13. Chaney MA: Craniotomy in a patient with Eisenmenger's syndrome, *Anesth Analg* 75(2):299, 1992.
14. Culver BH, Butler J: Mechanical influence on the pulmonary microcirculation, *Ann Rev Physiol* 42:187, 1980.
15. Dammann JF Jr, McEacchen JA, Thompson WM et al: The regression of pulmonary vascular disease after the creation of pulmonary stenosis, *J Thorac Cardiovasc Surg* 42:722, 1984.
16. Denfield SW, Garson A Jr: Sudden death in children and young adults, *Pediatr Clin North Am* 37(1):215, 1990.
17. Eisenmenger V: Die angeborenen Defekte Kammerscheidewand des Herzens, *Z Klin Med* 132(suppl):1, 1897.
18. Feldt RH, Edwards WD, Puga FJ et al: Heart disease in infants, children, and adolescents. In *Atrial septal defects and atrio-ventricular canal,* ed 3, Baltimore, 1983, Williams & Wilkins.
19. Ferencz C: Transposition of the great vessels: pathophysiologic considerations based upon a study of the lungs, *Circulation* 33:232, 1966.
20. Fishman AP: Respiratory gases in the regulation of the pulmonary circulation, *Physiol Rev* 41:214, 1961.
21. Fremes SE, Patterson GA, Williams WG et al: Single lung transplantation and closure of patent ductus arteriosus for Eisenmenger's syndrome, *J Thorac Cardiovasc Surg* 100(1):1, 1990.
22. Friedli B, Kidd BS, Mustard WT et al: Ventricular septal defect with increased pulmonary vascu ır resistance, *Am J Cardiol* 33:403, 1974.

23. Gilman DH: Caesarean section in undiagnosed Eisenmenger's syndrome: report of a patient with a fatal outcome, *Anaesthesia* 46(5):371, 1991.
24. Graham R, Skoog C, Oppenheimer L et al: Critical closure in the canine pulmonary vasculature, *Circ Res* 50:566, 1982.
25. Heath D, Edwards JE: The pathology of hypertensive pulmonary vascular disease: a description of six grades of structural changes in the pulmonary arteries with special reference to congenital cardiac septal defects. *Circulation* 18:533, 1958.
26. Heath D, Helmoholz HF, Burchell HB et al: Graded pulmonary vascular changes and hemodynamic findings in cases of atrial and ventricular septal defect and patent ductus arteriosus, *Circulation* 18:1155, 1958.
27. Heytens L, Alexander JP: Maternal and neonatal death associated with Eisenmenger's syndrome, *Acta Anaesthesiol Belg* 37(1):45, 1986.
28. Hoffmann JL, Rudolph AM, Heymann MA: Pulmonary vascular disease with congenital heart lesions: pathologic features and causes, *Circulation* 64:873, 1981.
29. Hyman AL: Pulmonary vasoconstriction due to nonocclusive distension of large pulmonary arteries in the dog, *Circ Res* 23:401, 1968.
30. Juaneda E, Haworth SG: Pulmonary vascular disease in children with truncus arteriosus, *Am J Cardiol* 54:1314, 1984.
31. Kraayenbrink MA, Steven CM: Anaesthesia for carotid body tumour resection in a patient with the Eisenmenger syndrome: a case report, *Anaesthesia* 40(12):1194, 1985.
32. Kulik TJ, Johnson DE, Green TP et al: Amrinone for pulmonary hypertension in infants and children, *Pediatr Res* 18:125A, 1984.
33. Kulik TJ, Reid LM: Neonatal pulmonary vasculature. In Moller JH, Neal WA, editors: *Fetal, neonatal, and infant cardiac disease,* Norwalk, CT, 1990, Appleton & Lange.
34. Lakier JB, Stanger P, Heymann MA et al: Early onset of pulmonary vascular obstruction in patients with aortopulmonary transposition and intact ventricular septum, *Circulation* 51(51):875, 1975.
35. Leier CV, Bambach D, Nelson S, et al: Captopril in primary pulmonary hypertension, *Circulation* 67:155, 1983.
36. Lloyd TC: Influence of blood pH on hypoxic pulmonary vasoconstriction, *J Appl Physiol* 21:358, 1966.
37. Lock JE, Einzig SE, Bass JL et al: The pulmonary vascular response to oxygen and its influence on operative results in children with ventricular septal defect, *Pediatr Cardiol* 3:41, 1982.
38. Lumley J, Whitwam JG, Morgan M: General anesthesia in the presence of Eisenmenger's syndrome, *Anesth Analg* 56(4):543, 1977.
39. Lupi-Herrera E, Sandoval J, Seoane M et al: The role of hydralazine therapy for pulmonary arterial hypertension of unknown cause, *Circulation* 65:645, 1982.
40. Niarchos AP, Whitman HH, Goldstein JE et al: Hemodynamic effects of captopril in pulmonary hypertension of collagen vascular disease, *Am Heart J* 104:834, 1982.
41. Packer M: Therapeutic application of calcium-channel antagonists, *Am J Cardiol* 55:196B, 1985.
42. Packer M, Greenberg B, Massie B et al: Deleterious effects of hydralizine in patients with pulmonary hypertension, *N Engl J Med* 306:1326, 1982.
43. Pitkin RM, Perloff JK, Koos BJ et al: Pregnancy and congenital heart disease, *Ann Intern Med* 112(6):445, 1990.
44. Pollack KL, Chestnut DH, Wenstrom KD: Anesthetic management of a parturient with Eisenmenger's syndrome, *Anesth Analg* 70(2):212, 1990.
45. Rabinovitch M: Heart disease in infants, children and adolescents. In Adams FH, Emmanouilides GL, editors: *Pulmonary Hypertension,* ed 3, Baltimore, 1983, Williams & Wilkins.
46. Rabinovitch M, Castaneda AR, Reid L: Lung biopsy with frozen section as a diagnostic aid in patients with congenital heart defects, *Am J Cardiol* 47:77, 1981.
47. Rabinovitch M, Haworth SG, Castaneda AR et al: Lung biopsy in congenital heart disease: a morphometric approach to pulmonary vascular disease, *Circulation* 58:1107, 1978.
48. Reid LM: The pulmonary circulation: remodeling in growth and disease, *Am Rev Respir Dis* 119:531, 1979.
49. Rowe RD, James LS: The normal pulmonary arterial pressure during the first year of life, *J Pediatr* 51:1, 1957.
50. Rubin LJ, Groves BM, Reeves JT et al: Prostacyclin-induced acute pulmonary vasodilation in primary pulmonary hypertension, *Circulation* 66:334, 1982.
51. Rudolph AM: Fetal and neonatal pulmonary circulation, *Annu Rev Physiol* 41:383, 1979.
52. Rudolph AM, Paul MH, Sommer LS et al: Effects of tolazoline hydrochloride (Priscoline) on circulatory dynamics of patients with pulmonary hypertension, *Am Heart J* 55:424, 1958.
53. Ruskin J, Hutter AM: Primary pulmonary hypertension treated with oral phentolamine, *Ann Intern Med* 90:772, 1979.
54. Rutter TW, Mullin V: Pheochromocytoma in a patient with Eisenmenger's complex, *Anesth Analg* 73(4):496, 1991.
55. Schwalbe SS, Deshmukh SM, Marx GF: Use of pulmonary artery catheterization in parturients with Eisenmenger's syndrome, *Anesth Analg* 71(4):442, 1990 (letter, comment).
56. Selsby DS, Sugden JC: Epidural anaesthesia for bilateral inguinal herniorrhaphy in Eisenmenger's syndrome, *Anaesthesia* 44(2):130, 1989.
57. Sigmann JM, Perry BL, Behrendt DM et al: Ventricular septal defect: results after repair in infancy, *Am J Cardiol* 39:66, 1977.
58. Smith RW, Morris JA, Assali NS: Effects of chemical mediators on the pulmonary and ductus arteriosus circulation in the fetal lamb, *Am J Obstet Gynecol* 89:252, 1964.
59. Snabes MC, Poindexter AN III: Laparoscopic tubal sterlization under local anesthesia in women with cyanotic heart disease, *Obstet Gynecol* 78(3):437, 1991.
60. Soifer SJ, Clyman RI, Heymann MA: Prostaglandin $D_2$ does not lower pulmonary arterial pressure or improve oxygenation in infants with persistent pulmonary hypertension syndrome, *Pediatr Res* 19:365A, 1985.
61. Szczeklik J, Dubiel JS, Mysik M et al: Effects of prostaglandin $E_1$ on pulmonary circulation in patients with pulmonary hypertension, *Br Heart J* 40:1397, 1978.
62. Thilenius OG: Effect of anesthesia on response of pulmonary circulation of dogs to acute hypoxia, *J Appl Physiol* 21:901, 1966.
63. Tibaldi G, Marchi L, Huscher M et al: Anesthesia for cesarean section in a pregnant woman with Eisenmenger's syndrome: description of a clinical case, *Minerva Ginecol* 40(2):145, 1988.
64. Wagenvoort CA, Wagenvoort N, Draulans-Noe Y: Reversibility of plexogenic pulmonary arteriopathy following banding of the pulmonary artery, *J Thorac Cardiovasc Surg* 87:876, 1984.
65. Whittenberger JL, McGregor M, Berglund E et al: Influence of state of inflation of the lung on pulmonary vascular resistance, *J Appl Physiol* 15:878, 1960.
66. Yamaki S, Haneda K, Yaginuma G et al: Surgical management of open lung biopsy in Eizenmenger's syndrome, *Kyobu Geka* 43(2):114, 1990.
67. Yeager SB, Freed MD, Keane JF et al: Primary surgical closure of ventricular septal defect in the first year of life: results in 128 infants, *J Am Coll Cardiol* 3:1269, 1984.

# Index

## W



## X